Brain Repair After Stroke

Brain Repair After Stroke

Edited by

Steven C. Cramer
University of California, Irvine

Randolph J. Nudo
Kansas University Medical Center

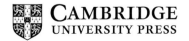

CAMBRIDGE UNIVERSITY PRESS
Cambridge, New York, Melbourne, Madrid, Cape Town, Singapore,
São Paulo, Delhi, Dubai, Tokyo, Mexico City

Cambridge University Press
The Edinburgh Building, Cambridge CB2 8RU, UK

Published in the United States of America by Cambridge University Press, New York

www.cambridge.org
Information on this title: www.cambridge.org/9780521515337

First published 2010

Printed in the United Kingdom at the University Press, Cambridge

A catalog record for this publication is available from the British Library

ISBN 978-0-521-51533-7 Hardback

Contents

Preface *page* vii
List of contributors viii

Section I. Basic Science and Animal Studies

1. **Motor map plasticity: a neural substrate for improving motor function after stroke** 1
   Jeffrey A. Kleim & Susan Schwerin

2. **Molecular mechanisms of neural repair after stroke** 11
   S. Thomas Carmichael

3. **Behavioral influences on neuronal events after stroke** 23
   Theresa A. Jones & DeAnna L. Adkins

4. **Post-stroke recovery therapies in animals** 35
   G. Campbell Teskey & Bryan Kolb

5. **Environmental effects on functional outcome after stroke** 47
   Barbro B. Johansson

6. **Functional and structural MR imaging of brain reorganization after stroke** 57
   Maurits P. A. van Meer & Rick M. Dijkhuizen

7. **Stroke recovery in non-human primates: a comparative perspective** 67
   Randolph J. Nudo

8. **Issues in translating stroke recovery research from animals to humans** 77
   J. Leigh Leasure, Andreas Luft & Timothy Schallert

Section II. Spontaneous Stroke Recovery in Humans

9. **Brain events in the acute period of stroke in relation to subsequent repair** 87
   Rüdiger J. Seitz

10. **Changes in cortical excitability and interhemispheric interactions after stroke** 103
    P. Talelli, O. Swayne & J. C. Rothwell

11. **Human brain mapping of the motor system after stroke** 113
    Nick S. Ward

12. **Recovery from aphasia: lessons from imaging studies** 125
    Cornelius Weiller & Dorothee Saur

13. **Brain mapping of attention and neglect after stroke** 133
    Alex R. Carter, Gordon L. Shulman & Maurizio Corbetta

14. **Depression and its effects after stroke** 145
    Thomas Platz

15. **Epidemiology of stroke recovery** 163
    Samir Belagaje & Brett Kissela

Section III. Treatment Strategies

16. **Issues in clinical trial methodology for brain repair after stroke** 173
    Steven C. Cramer

17. **Neuropharmacology in stroke recovery** 183
    Isabelle Loubinoux & François Chollet

18. **Robotic approaches to stroke recovery** 195
    David J. Reinkensmeyer

19. **Electromagnetic approaches to stroke recovery** 207
    Gottfried Schlaug & Leonardo G. Cohen

20. **Intensive physical therapeutic approaches to stroke recovery** 219
    Steven L. Wolf & Carolee J. Winstein

21. **Cognitive approaches to stroke recovery** 233
    Valerie M. Pomeroy, Stephen J. Page & Megan Farrell

22. **Electrical stimulation approaches to stroke recovery** 247
    John Chae & Leigh R. Hochberg

23. **Growth factors as treatments for stroke** 259
    Seth P. Finklestein & JingMei Ren

24. **Cellular approaches to stroke recovery** 267
    Yi Li & Michael Chopp

Index 275

The color plates will be found between pages 86 and 87.

Preface

For years, stroke was a disease with few treatment options. This changed in the mid 1990s with the approval of thrombolytic therapy. Despite this revolutionary change in acute stroke management, only a limited number of patients reach the hospital in time to benefit from such interventions; many who are so treated none the less have significant long-term disability. A need exists for therapies that are accessible and efficacious for a majority of patients beyond the current narrow treatment window.

Recent years have seen the dawning of a new field of clinical therapeutics based on the neuroscience of brain repair. With this approach, the aim is not to rescue threatened tissue, but to rewire, restore, repair, and rehabilitate. The current volume examines brain repair after stroke, from the latest basic science experiments performed in animal models of stroke recovery (Section I) to the process of spontaneous recovery in human stroke survivors, including results of modern neuroimaging studies (Section II) to treatment strategies in humans largely based on brain repair principles (Section III).

In the first section (Chapters 1–8), preclinical studies pave the way for evidence-based hypothesis testing in humans. Molecular data, derived from species ranging from rodents to primates, provide a mechanistic foundation. An important chapter focuses on MR imaging of stroke recovery in animals, with results relating directly to the human findings that are presented in the second section. Effects of environment, therapy, and behavior are also considered, topics particularly relevant to translational efforts.

In the second section (Chapters 9–15), the science of spontaneous stroke recovery in humans is reviewed.

The relationship to core aspects of the field of stroke, such as acute stroke therapy and epidemiology, is examined. Several brain systems are considered, including motor, language, attention, and affect, with many areas of overlap among the findings. These data provide a baseline against which interventional therapies will be compared, and also suggest key brain events whose measurement might help optimize prescription of repair-based therapies after stroke.

In the third section (Chapters 16–24), a range of emerging therapies is examined. Approaches include drugs, robotics, stimulation, physical therapies, cognitive approaches, growth factors, and cells. The progress and potential for each approach is considered. A separate chapter considers issues of clinical trial methodology that might be of particular importance to brain repair approaches.

The field of brain repair after stroke is young. However, already, animal and human sciences are converging on core principles. The literature is witnessing a blossoming of reports focused on this area of research. The current volume brings together international experts to review the current state of brain repair after stroke. We expect that the future will see increasingly successful efforts to reduce disability after stroke based on this approach.

This book will serve as a valuable reference for clinicians wanting to gain a better understanding of emerging brain repair therapies, for scientists and students wanting to gain increased knowledge of human stroke recovery and its underlying principles, and for basic scientists working with animal models to provide a comprehensive volume that covers the spectrum of stroke research from laboratory to clinic.

Contributors

DeAnna L. Adkins
Department of Psychology, University of Texas at Austin, Texas, USA

Samir Belagaje
University of Cincinnati College of Medicine, Cincinnati, Ohio, USA

S. Thomas Carmichael
Department of Neurology, University of California Los Angeles Geffen School of Medicine, Los Angeles, California, USA

Alex R. Carter
Department of Neurology, Washington University School of Medicine, St. Louis, Missouri, USA

John Chae
Department of Physical Medicine and Rehabilitation, Department of Biomedical Engineering, Cleveland Functional Electrical Stimulation Center, Case Western Reserve University, Stroke Rehabilitation MetroHealth Medical Center, Cleveland, Ohio, USA

François Chollet
INSERM, Institut des Sciences du Cerveau de Toulouse, and Department of Neurology, CHU Hospital, Toulouse, France

Michael Chopp
Department of Neurology, Henry Ford Health System, Detroit, Michigan and Department of Physics, Oakland University, Rochester, Michigan, USA

Leonardo G. Cohen
Human Cortical Physiology and Stroke Neurorehabilitation Section, National Institute of Neurological Disorders and Stroke, NIH, Bethesda, Maryland, USA

Maurizio Corbetta
Department of Neurology, Department of Radiology, and Department of Anatomy and Neurobiology, Washington University School of Medicine, St. Louis, Missouri, USA

Steven C. Cramer
Department of Neurology, and Department of Anatomy and Neurobiology, University of California, Irvine, California, USA

Rick M. Dijkhuizen
Department of Medical Imaging, Image Sciences Institute, University Medical Center Utrecht, Utrecht, The Netherlands

Megan Farrell
Department of Rehabilitation Sciences, University of Cincinnati, Academic Medical Center, Cincinnati, Ohio, USA

Seth P. Finklestein
Biotrofix Inc., Needham, Maryland, USA

Leigh R. Hochberg
Center for Restorative and Regenerative Medicine, Rehabilitation Research & Development Service, Department of Veterans Affairs, Providence Rhode Island; and Stroke and Neurocritical Care Services, Department of Neurology, Massachusetts General Hospital, Brigham & Women's Hospital, and Spaulding Rehabilitation Hospital; and Harvard Medical School, Boston, Massachusetts, USA

Barbro B. Johansson
Department of Clinical Neuroscience, Wallenberg Neuroscience Center, Lund, Sweden

Theresa A. Jones
Department of Psychology, University of Texas at Austin, Texas, USA

Brett Kissela
Department of Neurology, University of Cincinnati College of Medicine, Cincinnati, Ohio, USA

Jeffrey A. Kleim
McKnight Brain Institute, Department of Neuroscience, University of Florida, and Brain Research Rehabilitation Center, Malcom Randall VA Hospital, Gainesville, Florida, USA

Bryan Kolb
Canadian Centre for Behavioural Neuroscience, University of Lethbridge, Lethbridge, Alberta, Canada

J. Leigh Leasure
Department of Psychology, University of Houston, Houston, Texas, USA

Yi Li
Department of Neurology, Henry Ford Health System, Detroit, Michigan, USA

Isabelle Loubinoux
INSERM and Institut des Sciences du Cerveau de Toulouse, Toulouse, France

Andreas Luft
Department of Neurology, Johns Hopkins University, Baltimore, Mayland, USA

Randolph J. Nudo
Department of Molecular and Integrative Physiology and London Center on Aging, Kansas University Medical Center, Kansas City, Kansas, USA

Stephen J. Page
Department of Rehabilitation Sciences, University of Cincinnati Academic Medical Center, Cincinnati, Ohio, USA

Thomas Platz
Neurological Rehabilitation Centre, Ernst-Moritz-Arndt University, Greifswald, Germany

Valerie M. Pomeroy
Neurorehabilitation, University of East Anglia, UK

David J. Reinkensmeyer
Department of Mechanical and Aerospace Engineering and Department of Biomedical Engineering, University of California at Irvine, Irvine, California, USA

JingMei Ren
Biotrofix Inc., Needham, Maryland, USA

J. C. Rothwell
Sobell Department, University College London, Institute of Neurology, London, UK

Dorothee Saur
Neurologische Universitatsklinik Freiburg, Freiburg, Germany

Timothy Schallert
Department of Psychology, University of Texas at Austin, Austin, Texas, USA

Gottfried Schlaug
Department of Neurology, Neuroimaging and Stroke Recovery Laboratories, Beth Israel Deaconess Medical Center and Harvard Medical School, Boston, Massachusetts, USA

Susan Schwerin
McKnight Brain Institute, Department of Neuroscience, University of Florida, Gainesville, Florida, USA

Rüdiger J. Seitz
Department of Neurology, University Hospital Düsseldorf, Heinrich-Heine-University, Düsseldorf, Germany

Gordon L. Shulman
Department of Neurology, Washington University School of Medicine, St. Louis, Missouri, USA

O. Swayne
Sobell Department, University College London, Institute of Neurology, London, UK

P. Talelli
Sobell Department, University College London, Institute of Neurology, London, UK

G. Campbell Teskey
Department of Psychology, University of Calgary, Calgery, Alberta, Canada

Maurits P. A. van Meer
Department of Medical Imaging, Image Sciences Institute, and Department of Neurosurgery, Rudolf Magnus Institute of Neuroscience; University Medical Center Utrecht, Utrecht, The Netherlands

Nick S. Ward
Sobell Department of Motor Neuroscience, University College London Institute of Neurology, London, UK

Cornelius Weiller
Neurologische Universitatsklinik Freiburg, Freiburg, Germany

Carolee J. Winstein
Division of Biokinesiology and Physical Therapy, School of Dentistry, Department of Neurology, Keck School of Medicine, University of Southern California, Los Angeles, California, USA

Steven L. Wolf
Departments of Rehabilitation Medicine and Medicine, Department of Cell Biology, Emory University School of Medicine, Center for Rehabilitation Medicine; Health and Elder Care, Nell Hodgson Woodruff School of Nursing at Emory University; Atlanta VA Rehabilitation R&D Center, Atlanta, Georgia, USA

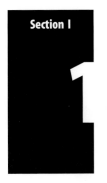

Motor map plasticity: a neural substrate for improving motor function after stroke

Jeffrey A. Kleim & Susan Schwerin

Motor map plasticity as a model for studying functional improvements after stroke

The loss of neural tissue associated with stroke induces profound neurophysiological changes throughout the brain that incite a wide range of behavioral impairments. Such impairments are not solely a manifestation of the damaged brain region, but are also an expression of the ability of the rest of the brain to maintain normal function. Indeed, the capacity to maintain function is often hindered by a cascade of neuronal events within residual neural tissue after stroke including inflammation, edema and deafferentation that can occur both proximal and distal to the infarction. In some instances, behavioral improvements can be attributed to the progressive resolution of these factors that allow for the compromised brain areas to regain control of lost function. However, functional gains can be brought about that are independent of simply resolving neural dysfunction resulting from edema or inflammation. These changes can be driven by rehabilitation and are supported by structural and functional adaptation of residual neural circuits. Identifying the specific neural mechanisms underlying rehabilitation-dependent neural plasticity for any given functional impairment after stroke is not trivial. It is difficult to obtain neurobiological measures that can be directly related to specific changes in behavior and thereby targeted for therapy. For example, even in healthy subjects we do not yet have a neural measure that directly reflects linguistic ability or capacity for memory, so it is difficult to identify specific adaptations in function related to recovery from aphasia or amnesia in brain-injured patients. Animal models provide a partial solution to the problem as they afford us the luxury of obtaining more specific neurobiological measures that may be more directly related to changes in behavior. The limitations of animal models of behavior, however, make studying the neural basis for improvements in complex behaviors such as language or memory after injury arduous.

Studies of motor behavior in animal models have several advantages for understanding the neural mechanisms of functional recovery after stroke for several reasons. First, it has long been known that the primary motor cortex is a critical brain area for the execution of skilled movement and most laboratory animals used to study stroke have highly evolved corticospinal systems (see Chapter 7). Second, primary motor cortex contains a well-characterized somatotopic map of movement representations that can be derived from surface or intracortical stimulation. Third, the topography of these representations is highly adaptable and reflects motor capacity both in the intact and injured nervous system. Fourth, changes in motor map organization can be related to adaptations in motor performance that occur both in response to injury and subsequent rehabilitation interventions. Finally, motor maps can be readily derived from most laboratory animals used to study stroke. The present chapter reviews the evidence for motor map plasticity after stroke and provides examples of how understanding the neural mechanisms underlying such plasticity can guide the development of adjuvant therapies. We propose that there is a fundamental set of neuroplastic mechanisms that operate throughout the nervous system and exist in order for new behaviors to be acquired in the intact CNS (learning) and for behavioral improvements in the damaged CNS (relearning or recovery). Thus, studies of motor map plasticity and improvements in motor performance may reveal potential treatment strategies that could be used for treating a wide range of both motor and non-motor impairments that occur after stroke.

Brain Repair After Stroke, ed. S. C. Cramer and R. J. Nudo. Published by Cambridge University Press.
© Cambridge University Press 2010.

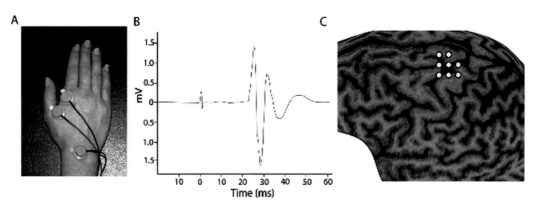

Figure 1.1 Transcranial magnetic stimulation (TMS) technique used to derive maps of movement representation in human motor cortex. **A**. Electrodes are placed over a target muscle to measure small changes in electrical potential associated with muscle contraction in response to magnetic stimulation of the motor cortex. In this example two electrodes are placed over the first dorsal interosseus (FDI) muscle and a ground electrode on the wrist. **B**. Electromyograph (EMG) showing a motor-evoked potential (MEP) within the FDI after TMS (at time 0). The amplitude and latency of the MEP can be measured and used to assess the strength of corticospinal output. **C**. The location of stimulation over the cortex can be integrated with a three-dimensional MRI of the subject's brain. This allows for the experimenter to determine the area and location in the cortex from which MEPs can be elicited by TMS.

Measuring corticospinal function: the motor map

John Hughlings Jackson was the first to suggest that movement control was organized somatotopically within the brain [1]. His inference was based in part on observations in epileptic patients that seizures often began in one area of the body and passed systematically to adjacent body parts and from the early studies by Fritsch and Hitzig who demonstrated that electrical current delivered through the surface of the precentral gyrus evoked movement in dogs [2]. His hypothesis was confirmed when more detailed cortical stimulation studies revealed that systematic stimulation across the precentral gyrus produced a somatotopically organized motor map. Modern motor mapping techniques involve either stimulation of the cortical surface such as with transcranial magnetic stimulation (TMS), or stimulation within layer V as with intracortical microstimulation (ICMS). In both cases, corticospinal neurons are trans-synaptically activated. With TMS, a single magnetic field is pulsed directly over the head, via a specialized coil, inducing a downward electrical current across the skull and into the cortex. Because neuronal axons have the highest density of ion channels, they become preferentially activated during a weak magnetic pulse and drive synaptic inputs onto large populations of neurons throughout the cortex, including layer V corticospinal neurons. TMS responses are measured ultimately as motor evoked potentials (MEPs) reflecting changes in electromyographic (EMG) activity within discrete muscles (Figure 1.1). ICMS techniques are typically used in animal studies, where a microelectrode is lowered into layer V of the exposed motor cortex stimulating more restricted patches of axons driving corticospinal neurons. In these studies the response is measured by visual confirmation of movement (Figure 1.2) and/or EMG activity.

Decades of cortical stimulation experiments have revealed four general principles of motor map organization.

1. *Fractured somatotopy*. Individual movements are represented multiple times and are highly interspersed with adjacent movement representations across discrete cortical regions. This functional redundancy can contribute to the capacity for the motor cortex to adapt to injury.
2. *Interconnectivity*. Corticospinal neurons from adjacent cortical areas are densely interconnected via reciprocal intracortical connections. This provides a platform for functional compensation after injury and facilitates the capacity for motor map reorganization.
3. *Area equals dexterity*. Movements requiring a greater degree of dexterity are more easily evoked in response to stimulation and occupy a larger proportion of the map. This provides a neural measure that can be compared to changes in motor behavior and used to relate changes in motor map

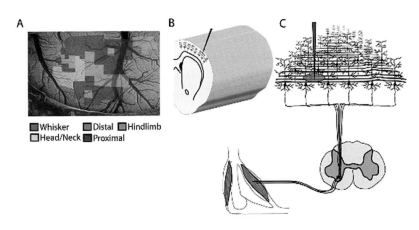

A

Whisker   Distal   Hindlimb
Head/Neck   Proximal

B

C

Figure 1.2 For the color version of this figure, see the Plate section. Intracortical microstimulation (ICMS) technique used to derive maps of movement representation in rat motor cortex. **A**. Motor map showing areas of the cortex in which stimulation evoked movement. **B**. Movements are produced by lowering a stimulating electrode into layer V of the motor cortex and activating corticospinal neurons. **C**. Corticospinal neurons are activated trans-synaptically. These neurons then project to motor neurons in the spinal cord that in turn cause muscle contractions in the periphery.

topography with changes in motor function after injury.

4. *Plasticity*. Motor map topography is highly dynamic and can rapidly change in response to a variety of internal and external pressures. Because motor maps can be considered as part of the motor engram, measures of motor map topography are a neurophysiological representation of motor capacity and can reflect adaptive responses that occur after stroke in order to support motor improvement [3].

Integrity of the corticospinal system is related to motor recovery after stroke

The corticospinal system is the final common path for motor output and the integrity of this system is directly related to the capacity for improvements in motor function after stroke. Acute stroke patients that exhibit TMS-elicited MEPs show better functional outcome than those without [4]. In chronic stroke patients, MEP amplitude is also positively correlated with hand function [5]. Improvements in upper extremity motor performance after constraint-induced movement therapy (CIMT) are associated with increases in the area of cortex from which MEPs can be elicited and increases in MEP amplitude [6]. Furthermore, level of recovery is positively correlated with the degree of change in corticospinal output [7]. Thus, understanding how corticospinal function can be adapted after stroke may provide some insight into how the brain adapts in order to support improvements in motor performance after stroke.

Neural strategies for motor improvement after stroke

Improvements in motor performance after stroke occur through either recovery and/or compensation, and these two processes can be described at either the neural or behavioral level (Table 1.1). At a behavioral level, motor recovery refers to the capacity to perform a previously lost or impaired motor task in exactly the same manner as before the injury. Motor compensation refers to the use of new movements or movement sequences to perform a task in a manner different from that used prior to injury. Studies of motor cortex plasticity after stroke have revealed that both recovery and compensation can be observed at a neurophysiological level. Recovery refers to the restoration of motor function within an area of motor cortex that was initially lost after injury. Compensation occurs when areas of motor cortex adapt to take on motor functions lost after the injury. Collectively, three neural strategies can be related to the processes of neural recovery and compensation within motor cortex after stroke.

Restoration

Restoration refers to the reactivation of brain areas that are dysfunctional after injury, and is therefore an example of neural recovery. Residual brain areas undergo profound neurobiological changes following brain injury or disease, resulting in dysfunction within structurally intact brain areas both proximal and distal to the infarction. This phenomenon was first described by Von Monakow and termed diaschisis [8], and is due to a number of pathological changes in metabolism, blood flow, inflammation, edema and neuronal

Table 1.1 Neural strategies for motor improvement after stroke

	Motor recovery	Motor compensation
Neural	Restoring motor function in neural tissue that was initially lost due to injury	Residual neural tissue takes over a motor function lost due to injury
Behavioral	Restoring the ability to perform movement in the same manner as it was performed prior to injury or disease	Performing a motor task in a manner different from how it was performed prior to injury
Strategy	Restoration	Recruitment, retraining

excitability. Diaschisis is particularly evident during the acute phase [9]. Functional improvement during this phase can occur in response to the progressive resolution of these secondary factors that allows the motor cortex to return to a more normal functional state and begin contributing to motor improvement. Indeed, the greatest gains in motor improvement after stroke are observed within the first 30–90 days, when restorative processes are most prominent [10]. However, restoration is also not limited to the acute phase after stroke, and one of the consequences of damage within the motor system is learned non-use. Many patients will avoid performing movements that engage compromised but intact regions of the motor cortex because it is simply too difficult or counterproductive. Patients may adopt compensatory behaviors that avoid the use of the compromised regions of motor cortex that continue well after the acute phase. This has distinct consequences for motor map topography, as the motor representations corresponding to the ignored movements may degrade despite maintaining some residual function. Rehabilitation training that forces or encourages the use of the avoided movements can re-engage the neglected neural circuits within the motor cortex and reinstate these movement representations, as has been demonstrated in both animal models and human patients. Randy Nudo's laboratory published a series of seminal papers demonstrating restoration, recruitment, and retraining in squirrel monkey motor cortex after focal cortical infarctions. The experiments involve first using ICMS to create very detailed maps of hand movement representations. A small cortical infarction stroke is then produced by devascularizing an area of cortex

containing wrist and digit representations. The monkeys exhibit difficulty in producing skilled wrist and digit movements when tested on a Kluver board where they are required to retrieve food pellets from a small well. The initial motor impairments are accompanied by a loss of hand representations that extends into undamaged areas of the map [11]. However, with several weeks of training on this task, the monkeys progressively improve, and the wrist and digit representations can be partially restored within the undamaged cortex [11].

The restoration of function is likely due to re-establishing neural connectivity within these areas. Within 24 h of a creating a small focal ischemic infarct within approximately 30% of forelimb movement representations in rat motor cortex, there is an additional loss of movement representations within the remaining 70% of the motor map that is in undamaged cortex (Figure 1.3). The loss of movement representations is accompanied by a loss of synapses, presumably from the neurons within the infarct. Thus, the neurons within these circuits have not been lost, but have become dysfunctional because of a lack of synaptic input. The loss of synapses and forelimb movement representations are accompanied by forelimb motor impairments, as rats have difficulty in reaching for food. With several days of motor rehabilitation (training on a forelimb reaching task), both the movement representations and the synapses can be restored.

In clinical studies, similar restoration of motor maps can be shown using TMS. Motor maps are smaller in patients with more severe impairments [12], and increases in motor map size and corticospinal output are correlated with motor improvement [7]. Some of these changes are also reminiscent of those evidenced in the healthy subjects during motor skill learning [13]. In other words, those neural circuits that normally contribute to the performance of arm movement were not being engaged after stroke. This may reflect diaschisis or learned non-use in these areas resulting from the injury. Motor rehabilitation may serve to re-engage these circuits and work to return them to a more normal state that is manifested as a restoration of movement representations and an overall expansion of motor map area.

Recruitment

Recruitment refers to enlisting motor areas that have the capacity to contribute to the lost motor function, but may not normally have been making significant

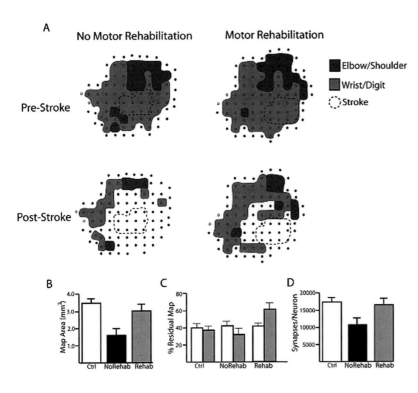

Figure 1.3 Example of resuscitation of function after injury with motor rehabilitation. **A.** Motor map of forelimb movement representations within rat motor cortex prior to and after stroke. Two weeks of motor rehabilitation restores movement representations within residual cortical areas. **B.** Residual motor map area is restored in animals receiving motor rehabilitation but not in animals without motor rehabilitation. **C.** Percentage of the residual motor map occupied by wrist and digit representations is increased with motor rehabilitation. **D.** The number of synapses per neuron is also restored with motor rehabilitation.

contributions to that behavior prior to the injury. These areas are asked to play a larger role in the performance of the impaired motor behavior compromised because of stroke, but are not necessarily acquiring new function (retraining). Within the motor cortex this can be demonstrated through the expansion of movement representations within areas outside of the original motor map. For example, recovery of dexterity after unilateral motor cortex lesions in macaque monkeys appears to be mediated by the premotor cortex in the damaged hemisphere, as inactivation of this region abolishes recovered movement but does not affect performance in non-damaged animals [14]. Large infarctions within the primary motor cortex of squirrel monkeys cause a profound expansion of movement representations within the premotor cortex [15]. In comparison to healthy controls, stroke patients can show significant increases in contralesional motor cortex activity during movement of the affected foot [16] or arm [17]. Although the contralesional hemisphere does have the capacity to contribute to movement on the ipsilateral side [18], it does not normally make any significant contribution. Some of the increased activity also occurs in the ipsilesional dorsal premotor cortex [19], and TMS-induced disruption of the function within this area impairs

recovered movement of the stroke-affected hand [20], suggesting that such activity is functionally relevant. The pattern of recruitment also appears to reflect the level of impairment and locus of the lesion. Lesions predominantly involving the primary motor cortex tend to result in increased contralesional activity, while lesions sparing the primary motor cortex increase the ipsilesional activity [21]. Increases in ipsilesional activity within cortical areas not normally engaged during movement have also been observed. Motor improvement is associated with enhanced activation of the dorsal premotor cortex in the affected hemisphere [20]. Further, TMS-induced disruption of this cortical area causes movement impairments in stroke patients but not healthy controls [22], demonstrating that the increased activity within the premotor cortex is indeed related to performance.

Retraining

In some cases areas of motor cortex may either adapt to an existing function or take on additional functions to support functional improvement. This strategy is integrally related to restoration and recruitment in that neural circuits do not simply use their existing functions to contribute to behavior, but begin to

5

perform novel or additional functions. As described above, focal lesions within the motor cortex cause a loss of movement representations within residual cortical areas that can be restored with motor rehabilitation. These same studies also provide clear examples of retraining. For example, when an area of motor cortex containing digit representations is removed, digit representations can be observed to re-emerge in areas of the remaining cortex that used to contain elbow or shoulder [23]. It is also important to point out that the emergence of a movement representation within an area previously occupied by a different representation does not mean that the original representation has been completely replaced. This is largely the result of the method used to derive motor maps. Movement representations are determined by lowering the amount of current delivered until only one movement can be observed. However, in many cases, if the stimulating current is increased, the previous movement appears. In other words, this particular cortical region has not lost the elbow representation, but has become biased towards wrist. In effect, the area has become capable of contributing to both movements. In support of this notion, there is an increase in the number of stimulation sites where such responses occur [11,24]. Operationally, dual responses are stimulation sites where two movements occur with the same stimulation current and the two movements cannot be clearly dissociated by reducing stimulation current. The number of these sites also positively correlates with the degree of functional improvement.

There is now evidence that motor map reorganization is not simply an epiphenomenon of rehabilitation but is indeed involved in supporting motor improvement. Conner et al. demonstrated that depleting cortical acetylcholinergic input by lesioning the nucleus basalis of Meynert reduced motor recovery and motor map reorganization [25]. They further showed that lesioning the reorganized areas of the motor map reinstated the motor deficits. Together these results provide strong evidence that motor map plasticity is a neural substrate for rehabilitation-dependent motor recovery.

Neural basis of motor cortex reorganization: synaptic plasticity

The above studies demonstrate that restoration, recruitment and retraining of motor maps within residual cortical tissue accompany motor recovery after stroke. Understanding the cellular basis and

key neural signaling pathways that drive such reorganization would aid in the development of adjuvant therapies that will enhance recovery. This first requires understanding the neurophysiological and anatomical properties of motor cortex that underlie motor maps.

The functional organization of primary motor cortex has long been defined by cortical stimulation experiments [26]. These studies have revealed two important characteristics of motor cortex organization. Neurons within the motor cortex are aggregated such that small groups of cells appear to encode elementary movement representations in that neighboring cells have similar output properties [27]. Further, these pools of neurons are interconnected by dense horizontal connections that can extend several millimeters [28]. ICMS evokes movement via direct [25] and indirect [30] activation of pyramidal tract neurons. In fact, the majority of pyramidal tract neurons that drive movement in response to stimulation are trans-synaptically activated [31], presumably through activation of horizontal afferents. Therefore, the spatial characteristics of motor maps, as defined by stimulation, are dependent upon the synaptic activation of localized groups of pyramidal tract neurons. Any alteration in motor map topography or loss of map area after damage must therefore involve changes in the pattern of intracortical connectivity through modifications in synaptic efficacy [26].

There are several lines of evidence that support the idea that motor map reorganization is dependent upon changes in synaptic efficacy within intracortical microcircuitry. First, manipulations that induce changes in synaptic strength also induce map reorganization. Long-term potentiation (LTP) causes map expansion and synaptogenesis [32], while long-term depression (LTD) induces map retraction and synaptic loss. Second, cortical kindling that drives increases in cortical excitatory postsynaptic potentials (EPSPs) also increases motor map area [33]. Third, synaptic potentiation that occurs in response to motor skill learning [32,34] is colocalized within regions of cortex that exhibit motor map reorganization [35]. Finally, learning-dependent motor map plasticity is also colocalized with synaptogenesis [36]. Thus, reorganization of motor maps after brain injury and in response to motor rehabilitation must be supported by changes in synaptic efficacy within motor cortex. Indeed, motor map reorganization is accompanied by synaptogenesis within residual motor cortex (Figure 1.2).

Adjuvant therapies that promote motor map plasticity enhance motor recovery after stroke

The reorganization of cortical movement representations is likely mediated by synaptic plasticity within intracortical microcircuitry. In normal motor learning, regions of motor cortex that undergo redistribution of movement representations during skill learning also show increases in synapse number [37]. Further, these same regions also demonstrate enhanced synaptic responses after skill learning [32]. In addition, manipulations that alter synaptic strength or number also change motor map topography. Finally, restoration of movement representations within residual cortical areas is accompanied by increases in synapse number (Figure 1.3). Given that such synaptic plasticity is a key neural mechanism mediating motor map plasticity and motor improvement after stroke, manipulations that enhance synaptic plasticity may serve to augment motor recovery. Molecular, genetic, pharmacological and electrophysiological studies in a variety of organisms have revealed several key neural signaling systems critical for orchestrating synaptic plasticity. These studies have inspired the development of several adjuvant, plasticity-promoting therapies for enhancing motor map plasticity and concomitant motor improvement after stroke.

Pharmacological stimulation

One approach to developing adjuvant therapies is to develop pharmacological manipulations that upregulate endogenous intracellular signaling pathways that drive synaptic plasticity. Although numerous signaling pathways have been identified, the most well characterized is the cAMP/CREB pathway. A variety of experimental models and systems have established the cAMP/CREB signaling pathway to be a key regulatory pathway in experience-dependent synaptic plasticity. Administration of the type IV-specific phosphodiesterase inhibitors (PDE 4) that enhance cAMP/CREB signaling facilitate memory in normal and aged rodents [3]. PDE treatment in combination with motor rehabilitation following a focal stroke significantly enhanced motor recovery [38]. Further, the drug increased motor map area in residual cortex (restoration), increased the proportion of the maps occupied by distal forelimb representations (retraining) and expanded movement representations into new cortical areas (recruitment).

In addition to drugs that enhance plasticity, several neurochemicals have been identified that may block plasticity inhibiting processes such as axonal sprouting. For example, myelin-associated inhibitory factors (such as Nogo-A or MAG) are present in neural tissue that block neurite outgrowth after damage. When antibodies for Nogo-A (IN-1) are applied to motor cortex following ischemic lesion, an increase in apical and basilar dendritic arborization and spine density is observed [39]. In addition, new projections to the de-afferented striatum [40] and red nucleus [41] have been observed. ICMS mapping of the intact hemisphere following treatment with monoclonal antibody IN-1 results in a substantial increase in ipsilateral movements [42]. Such manipulations could facilitate compensation through recruitment of distal brain areas.

Cortical stimulation

There is a growing body of evidence that electrically stimulating the motor cortex facilitates recovery of motor function after CNS injury. In humans, transcranial direct cortical stimulation (tDCS) improves motor function in patients with chronic motor impairments when anodal current is delivered over lesioned motor cortex or cathodal current was delivered over the contralesional motor cortex [43]. Clinical reports suggest that epidural motor cortex stimulation, used to reduce chronic pain after subcortical strokes, reduces hemiparetic impairments [44], motor weakness [45], motor spasticity [46], action tremor [47] and dystonia [14].

The efficacy of CS-RT (cortical stimulation rehabilitation therapy) at enhancing motor recovery after stroke has been demonstrated in rats [48,49] and in monkeys [50]. Furthermore, the enhanced motor recovery is associated with increased cortical dendritic hypertrophy [49] in comparison to animals in standard rehabilitation. The increased postsynaptic space is also accompanied by an enlargement of the polysynaptic component of motor cortical-evoked potentials [51]. Finally, CS-RT also induces a greater expansion of movement representations in rats [48] and monkeys [50]. All of these data demonstrate that CS-RT drives significantly greater motor recovery after stroke and that the functional gains are accompanied by an upregulation of the neuroplastic changes observed with standard rehabilitation. Although the means by which CS-RT enhances recovery and promotes cortical plasticity are unknown, upregulation of neurotrophins is one viable mechanism. Indeed, electrical stimulation of cortical tissue increases brain-derived neurotrophic factor (BDNF) levels [52].

Genetic factors

The neural signals that drive neural plasticity often involve altering the expression of specific genes that coordinate the synthesis of specific proteins required for synaptic plasticity and motor map reorganization. Naturally occurring genetic alterations in those plasticity-related genes may then influence the capacity for motor map plasticity. Indeed, such genetic polymorphisms have been identified in the human population that may influence both the capacity for motor map plasticity and functional improvement after stroke. For example, a polymorphism has been identified in the human *BDNF* gene (*BDNF* val^{66}met). *BDNF* polymorphic individuals show reduced training-dependent motor map expansion in comparison to non-polymorphic subjects [53]. Furthermore, val^{66}met subjects show reductions in motor cortex plasticity after paired association stimulation and intermittent theta burst stimulation [54]. This reduced capacity for cortical plasticity is proposed to be due to a reduction in the capacity for synaptic plasticity within motor cortical neurons. Because motor map plasticity supports motor improvement after stroke, it is possible that these individuals may not respond to motor rehabilitation the same way the non-polymorphic subjects do, limiting their capacity for recovery. Indeed, after subarachnoid hemorrhage patients with the polymorphism are three times more likely to have poor recovery than non-polymorphic individuals [55]. Thus, understanding the relationship between genotype and the capacity for motor cortex plasticity may be a critical step towards developing effective motor rehabilitation interventions. Such polymorphic individuals might require more or different forms of rehabilitation in order to drive motor cortex plasticity. Further, the efficacy of adjuvant therapies such as those described above may be affected by genotype.

Conclusions

There is now significant evidence that motor map plasticity is one of the key neural substrates supporting motor improvement after stroke. This plasticity appears to fall into one of three general strategies: restoration, retraining, and recruitment that are not mutually exclusive. All these three strategies also

appear to be mediated by synaptic plasticity within cortical circuits to allow for behavioral recovery and compensation. Understanding the neural signaling pathways that influence such synaptic plasticity may guide the development of novel, adjuvant therapies that can upregulate endogenous plasticity mechanisms and enhance motor improvement after stroke when administered in conjunction with motor rehabilitation. Finally, the fundamental behavioral and neural signals that drive motor map plasticity and improvements in motor function may also mediate enhancement of non-motor functions impaired after stroke such as memory or language processing. Thus, studies of motor map plasticity and motor improvement after stroke may provide important insights into potential therapies for overcoming various non-motor functional impairments such as cognitive deficits observed after stroke.

References

1. Hughlings Jackson J. Remarks on the relations of different divisions of the central nervous system to one another and to parts of the body. *Br Med J*. 1898;**1**:65–9.

2. Fritz G, Hitzig, E. Über die elektrische Erregbarkeit des Grosshirns. *Arch Anat Physiol wiss Med*. 1870;**37**:300–32.

3. Monti B, Berteotti C, Contestabile A. Subchronic rolipram delivery activates hippocampal CREB and arc, enhances retention and slows down extinction of conditioned fear. *Neuropsychopharmacology*. 2006;**31**:278–86.

4. Escudero JV, Sancho J, Bautista D, *et al*. Prognostic value of motor evoked potential obtained by transcranial magnetic brain stimulation in motor function recovery in patients with acute ischemic stroke. *Stroke*. 1998;**29**:1854–9.

5. Brouwer BJ, Schryburt-Brown K. Hand function and motor cortical output poststroke: are they related? *Arch Phys Med Rehabil*. 2006;**87**:627–34.

6. Wittenberg GF, Chen R, Ishii K, *et al*. Constraint-induced therapy in stroke: Magnetic-stimulation motor maps and cerebral activation. *Neurorehabil Neural Repair*. 2003;**17**:48–57.

7. Koski L, Mernar TJ, Dobkin BH. Immediate and long-term changes in corticomotor output in response to rehabilitation: Correlation with functional improvements in chronic stroke. *Neurorehabil Neural Repair*. 2004;**18**:230–49.

8. von Monakow C. *Die Lokalisation im Grosshirn und der Abbau der Funktion durch kortikale Herde*. Weisbaden: Bergmann; 1914.

9. Cramer SC. Repairing the human brain after stroke: I. Mechanisms of spontaneous recovery. *Ann Neurol.* 2008;**63**:272–87.

10. Duncan PW, Goldstein LB, Matchar D, *et al.* Measurement of motor recovery after stroke. Outcome assessment and sample size requirements. *Stroke.* 1992;**23**:1084–9.

11. Nudo RJ, Milliken GW. Reorganization of movement representations in primary motor cortex following focal ischemic infarcts in adult squirrel monkeys. *J Neurophysiol.* 1996;**75**:2144–9.

12. Talelli P, Rothwell J. Does brain stimulation after stroke have a future? *Curr Opin Neurol.* 2006;**19**:543–50.

13. Karni A, Meyer G, Jezzard P, *et al.* Functional MRI evidence for adult motor cortex plasticity during motor skill learning. *Nature.* 1995;**377**:155–8.

14. Franzini A, Ferroli P, Dones I, *et al.* Chronic motor cortex stimulation for movement disorders: A promising perspective. *Neurol Res.* 2003;**25**:123–6.

15. Frost SB, Barbay S, Friel KM, *et al.* Reorganization of remote cortical regions after ischemic brain injury: A potential substrate for stroke recovery. *J Neurophysiol.* 2003;**89**:3205–14.

16. Enzinger C, Johansen-Berg H, Dawes H, *et al.* Functional MRI correlates of lower limb function in stroke victims with gait impairment. *Stroke.* 2008;**39**:1507–13.

17. Zemke A, Heagerty P, Lee C, *et al.* Motor cortex organization after stroke is related to side of stroke and level of recovery. *Stroke.* 2003;**34**:E23–8.

18. Jankowska E, Edgley SA. How can corticospinal tract neurons contribute to ipsilateral movements? A question with implications for recovery of motor functions. *Neuroscientist.* 2006;**12**:67–79.

19. Gerloff C, Braun C, Staudt M, *et al.* Coherent corticomuscular oscillations originate from primary motor cortex: Evidence from patients with early brain lesions. *Hum Brain Mapp.* 2006;**27**:789–98.

20. Feydy A, Carlier R, Roby-Brami A, *et al.* Longitudinal study of motor recovery after stroke: recruitment and focusing of brain activation. *Stroke.* 2002;**33**:1610–7.

21. Lotze M, Cohen LG. Volition and imagery in neurorehabilitation. *Cogn Behav Neurol.* 2006;**19**:135–40.

22. Weiller C, Chollet F, Friston KJ, *et al.* Functional reorganization of the brain in recovery from striatocapsular infarction in man. *Ann Neurol.* 1992;**31**:463–72.

23. Fridman EA, Hanakawa T, Chung M, *et al.* Reorganization of the human ipsilesional premotor cortex after stroke. *Brain.* 2004;**127**:747–58.

24. Barbay S, Plautz EJ, Friel KM, *et al.* Behavioral and neurophysiological effects of delayed training following a small ischemic infarct in primary motor cortex of squirrel monkeys. *Exp Brain Res.* 2006;**169**:106–16.

25. Conner JM, Chiba AA, Tuszynski MH. The basal forebrain cholinergic system is essential for cortical plasticity and functional recovery following brain injury. *Neuron.* 2005;**46**:173–9.

26. Monfils MH, Plautz EJ, Kleim JA. In search of the motor engram: Motor map plasticity as a mechanism for encoding motor experience. *Neuroscientist.* 2005;**11**:471–83.

27. Mountcastle VB. The columnar organization of the neocortex. *Brain.* 1997;**120**:701–22.

28. Ghosh S, Porter R. Morphology of pyramidal neurones in monkey motor cortex and the synaptic actions of their intracortical axon collaterals. *J Physiol.* 1988;**400**:593–615.

29. Jankowska E, Padel Y, Tanaka R. The mode of activation of pyramidal tract cells by intracortical stimuli. *J Physiol.* 1975;**249**:617–36.

30. Stoney SD, Jr., Thompson WD, Asanuma H. Excitation of pyramidal tract cells by intracortical microstimulation: Effective extent of stimulating current. *J Neurophysiol.* 1968;**31**:659–69.

31. Cheney PD, Fetz EE, Palmer SS. Patterns of facilitation and suppression of antagonist forelimb muscles from motor cortex sites in the awake monkey. *J Neurophysiol.* 1985;**53**:805–20.

32. Monfils MH, Teskey GC. Skilled-learning-induced potentiation in rat sensorimotor cortex: A transient form of behavioural long-term potentiation. *Neuroscience.* 2004;**125**:329–36.

33. Teskey GC, Monfils MH, VandenBerg PM, *et al.* Motor map expansion following repeated cortical and limbic seizures is related to synaptic potentiation. *Cereb Cortex.* 2002;**12**:98–105.

34. Rioult-Pedotti MS, Friedman D, Hess G, *et al.* Strengthening of horizontal cortical connections following skill learning. *Nat Neurosci.* 1998;**1**:230–4.

35. Kleim JA, Barbay S, Nudo RJ. Functional reorganization of the rat motor cortex following motor skill learning. *J Neurophysiol.* 1998;**80**:3321–5.

36. Kleim JA, Barbay S, Cooper NR, *et al.* Motor learning-dependent synaptogenesis is localized to functionally reorganized motor cortex. *Neurobiol Learn Mem.* 2002;**77**:63–77.

37. Kleim JA, Hogg TM, VandenBerg PM, *et al.* Cortical synaptogenesis and motor map reorganization occur during late, but not early, phase of motor skill learning. *J Neurosci.* 2004;**24**:628–33.

38. MacDonald E, Van der Lee H, Pocock D, *et al.* A novel phosphodiesterase type 4 inhibitor, HT-0712, enhances rehabilitation-dependent motor recovery and cortical

reorganization after focal cortical ischemia. *Neurorehabil Neural Repair*. 2007;**21**:486–96.

39. Papadopoulos CM, Tsai SY, Cheatwood JL, *et al.* Dendritic plasticity in the adult rat following middle cerebral artery occlusion and Nogo-a neutralization. *Cereb Cortex*. 2006;**16**:529–36.

40. Kartje GL, Schulz MK, Lopez-Yunez A, *et al.* Corticostriatal plasticity is restricted by myelin-associated neurite growth inhibitors in the adult rat. *Ann Neurol*. 1999;**45**:778–86.

41. Wenk CA, Thallmair M, Kartje GL, *et al.* Increased corticofugal plasticity after unilateral cortical lesions combined with neutralization of the IN-1 antigen in adult rats. *J Comp Neurol*. 1999;**410**:143–57.

42. Emerick AJ, Neafsey EJ, Schwab ME, *et al.* Functional reorganization of the motor cortex in adult rats after cortical lesion and treatment with monoclonal antibody IN-1. *J Neurosci*. 2003;**23**:4826–30.

43. Fregni F, Pascual-Leone A. Hand motor recovery after stroke: Tuning the orchestra to improve hand motor function. *Cogn Behav Neurol*. 2006;**19**:21–33.

44. Tsubokawa T, Katayama Y, Yamamoto T, *et al.* Chronic motor cortex stimulation in patients with thalamic pain. *J Neurosurg*. 1993;**78**:393–401.

45. Katayama Y, Oshima H, Fukaya C, *et al.* Control of post-stroke movement disorders using chronic motor cortex stimulation. *Acta Neurochir Suppl*. 2002;**79**:89–92.

46. Garcia-Larrea L, Peyron R, Mertens P, *et al.* Electrical stimulation of motor cortex for pain control: A combined PET-scan and electrophysiological study. *Pain*. 1999;**83**:259–73.

47. Nguyen JP, Pollin B, Feve A, *et al.* Improvement of action tremor by chronic cortical stimulation. *Mov Disord*. 1998;**13**:84–8.

48. Kleim JA, Bruneau R, VandenBerg P, *et al.* Motor cortex stimulation enhances motor recovery and reduces peri-infarct dysfunction following ischemic insult. *Neurol Res*. 2003;**25**:789–93.

49. Adkins-Muir DL, Jones TA. Cortical electrical stimulation combined with rehabilitative training: enhanced functional recovery and dendritic plasticity following focal cortical ischemia in rats. *Neurol Res*. 2003;**25**:780–8.

50. Plautz EJ, Barbay S, Frost SB, *et al.* Post-infarct cortical plasticity and behavioral recovery using concurrent cortical stimulation and rehabilitative training: A feasibility study in primates. *Neurol Res*. 2003;**25**:801–10.

51. Teskey GC, Flynn C, Goertzen CD, *et al.* Cortical stimulation improves skilled forelimb use following a focal ischemic infarct in the rat. *Neurol Res*. 2003;**25**:794–800.

52. Yukimasa T, Yoshimura R, Tamagawa A, *et al.* High-frequency repetitive transcranial magnetic stimulation improves refractory depression by influencing catecholamine and brain-derived neurotrophic factors. *Pharmacopsychiatry*. 2006;**39**:52–9.

53. Kleim JA, Chan S, Pringle E, *et al.* BDNFval66met polymorphism is associated with modified experience-dependent plasticity of human motor cortex. *Nat Neurosci*. 2006;**9**:735–7.

54. Cheeran B, Talelli P, Mori F, *et al.* A common polymorphism in the brain-derived neurotrophic factor gene (BDNF) modulates human cortical plasticity and the response to rTMS. *J Physiol*. 2008;**586** (Pt 23):5717–25.

55. Siironen J, Juvela S, Kanarek K, *et al.* The Met allele of the BDNF Val66Met polymorphism predicts poor outcome among survivors of aneurysmal subarachnoid hemorrhage. *Stroke*. 2007;**38**:2858–60.

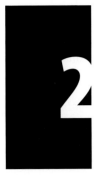

2 Molecular mechanisms of neural repair after stroke

S. Thomas Carmichael

Stroke induces a limited process of neuronal reorganization, repair and recovery. This reorganization includes axonal and dendritic sprouting in cortex ipsi- and contralateral to the stroke, formation of new patterns of short- and long-distance connections within sensorimotor cortical, striatal, brainstem and spinal circuits, and migration of newly born immature neurons into damaged tissue. From the formerly staid perspective of the adult brain, these processes are remarkable examples of structural plasticity. Within the past several years, some of the molecular systems that underlie these processes have been determined. With a better understanding of the molecular control of neural repair after stroke it may be possible to harness these processes to promote functional recovery. This chapter will describe axonal and dendritic sprouting and neurogenesis after stroke, and detail the molecular systems that may operate within defined cellular contexts to promote structural reorganization in the adult brain after stroke.

Cellular concepts of neural repair after stroke

Axonal and dendritic sprouting occur in cortex ipsilateral and contralateral to the infarct. Axonal sprouting in peri-infarct cortex in rodent models of focal stroke establishes new patterns of connections within sensorimotor maps [1]. As detected directly with high-resolution mapping of cortical connections, axonal sprouting occurs in a subset of the total cortical connections in sensory and motor areas. This sprouting is substantial enough that it re-maps the predominant pattern of cortical connections in, for example, the facial somatosensory map of the rat or mouse [1,2]. In non-human primates, small strokes in the motor cortex induce a remarkable long-distance sprouting in cortical connections from parietal to frontal cortex

within a system of motor to somatosensory connections [3]. These findings of axonal sprouting and reorganization of cortical connections after stroke are supported by similar reports of axonal sprouting in cortex after peripheral de-afferentation, such as retinal [4] and peripheral nerve lesions [5,6]. Axonal sprouting in the peri-infarct cortex occurs at a time of rapid dendritic plasticity and spine turnover in the peri-infarct cortex [7,8]. Post-stroke axonal and dendritic sprouting may account for the changes in receptive field maps in reorganizing sensorimotor representations in peri-infarct cortex [9]. However, the direct physiological significance of axonal and dendritic sprouting in peri-infarct cortex remains to be determined. Its timing is closely linked to the most dramatic periods of behavioral recovery and occurs in a region in which cortical re-mapping is closely associated with successful recovery of function [10].

Stroke also induces axonal sprouting from neurons in cortex contralateral to the infarct. After ischemic lesions, neurons in contralateral cortex sprout in their projections to the contralateral striatum, midbrain, and cervical spinal cord, and into the region of the peri-infarct cortex itself [11–14]. These regions that receive projections have been de-afferented as a result of the stroke and, from an anatomical perspective, the sprouting projections appear to elaborate a distal branch into the zone that was de-afferented. For example, axonal sprouting from contralateral (to the lesion) cortex into ipsilateral dorsal striatum establishes a projection into that region of the striatum that lost its projections as a result of the stroke [13,14]. In axonal sprouting into the red nucleus or cervical spinal cord, sprouting axons appear to take off from existing, normally present, projections to the red nucleus or cervical spinal cord ipsilateral to the stroke. These collateral sprouts then grow the short distances into the region of red nucleus and cervical spinal cord that

Brain Repair After Stroke, ed. S. C. Cramer and R. J. Nudo. Published by Cambridge University Press.
© Cambridge University Press 2010.

previously received a projection from the now-infarcted cortex. This sprouting from contralateral cortex can be increased by treatments that promote neuronal growth, such as inosine [1], or block myelin-associated growth inhibitors, such as NogoA [12]. The degree of axonal sprouting from contralateral cortex after stroke correlates with functional recovery. However, as with peri-infarct cortical sprouting after stroke, there have been no studies that have causally linked contralateral cortical sprouting with functional recovery.

Axonal sprouting in peri-infarct cortex and axonal sprouting from contralateral cortex after stroke differ in several important anatomical characteristics. Axonal sprouting from contralateral cortex after stroke into red nucleus and spinal cord, and possibly dorsolateral striatum, arises from normal, undamaged corticofugal axons into a brain region that is distant from the stroke site, but de-afferented or disconnected from it. There is no direct ischemic damage from the stroke at the site of the axonal sprouting, or at the site of origin of the cell bodies of the sprouting neurons. These areas that are de-afferented from a cortical or corticostriatal infarct do have microglial and astrocytic activation from the degenerating axons [15]. The activation of these two cell types as a result of Wallerian degeneration in distant projection zones of an infarct may play a role in axonal sprouting from contralateral cortex after stroke. However, this localized microglial and astrocytic reaction is a very different anatomical situation from the tissue reaction that occurs in the setting of peri-infarct axonal sprouting. In peri-infarct cortex neurons sprout new connections within cortical fields in which there is adjacent direct damage from the stroke, partial ischemic neuronal dropout, widespread activation of inflammatory cytokines and leukocyte infiltration, local angiogenesis, and distributed induction of glial growth-inhibitory proteins [16,17]. As will be discussed below, in developmental studies the molecular control of distal axonal branch formation can differ from the overall control of neuronal growth cone function [18]. By analogy, it may be that axonal sprouting from neurons within the peri-infarct cortex is under a different molecular control than distal axonal branch formation into midbrain and cervical spinal cord.

Stroke induces a process of neurogenesis and migration of immature neurons to areas of damage. In middle cerebral artery infarct models this post-stroke neurogenesis sends immature neurons into the striatum adjacent to the main neurogenic zone, the subventricular (or subependymal) zone (SVZ). In smaller cortical infarcts, immature neurons migrate long distances into peri-infarct cortex [19,20]. Immature neurons migrate with [21,22], or localize to [19] angiogenic blood vessels in peri-infarct cortex and striatum. Angiogenesis is causally linked to neurogenesis after stroke [19]. These findings suggest that there is a close molecular relationship between endothelial cells and immature neurons in a post-stroke neurovascular niche. However, astrocytes form a third cellular component to this niche [23], and are also activated during post-stroke neurogenesis [24]. Molecular signaling systems that might communicate among immature neurons, blood vessels and astrocytes in post-stroke neurogenesis will be discussed below.

Gene expression profiling and biological meaning

Gene expression profiling in a high throughput and massively parallel manner developed in the mid to late 1990s. Using microarray analysis or polymerase chain reaction (PCR)-based approaches it became possible to assay large gene pools and later the expression pattern of the entire genome in various time points or tissue locations after stroke. The biological interpretation of these data sets is limited because of the many variables that occur in the sampled time points or brain regions: angiogenesis, neurogenesis, astrocytosis, axonal sprouting, apoptosis, axonal degeneration and several distinct processes of inflammation. It is difficult to sort through the large tables of differentially regulated genes and ascribe these genes to specific biological events in repair and recovery. None the less, several important findings come out of these gene expression screens in terms of neural repair. Genes that have a prominent role in neuronal plasticity are upregulated in peri-infarct cortex at very early time points, such as *c-jun, SPRR1, NARP,* and *CPG21* activation 1 day after stroke in peri-infarct cortex [25,26]. There are substantial changes in gene expression in peri-infarct and contralateral cortex during late periods in reorganization and repair after stroke [27,28]. The pattern of gene expression in the brain in the first and second week after stroke differs with respect to age, and implicates several molecular pathways or cellular systems in the interplay of stroke repair with aging: several Notch-related genes, *TGFb1,* activin and the growth factor-related genes *FGF22, NGFb, IGF1* receptor, and *IGF2* are upregulated in the young adult and not aged brain after stroke [28,29]. Notch and TGFb pathways play a role in axonal sprouting and neurogenesis [30]. Insulin-like growth factors regulate axonal sprouting of cortical neurons during development [31] and neurogenesis both in the normal and post-stroke state [29]. This age effect in induction of these genes systems may relate to differences in recovery in the aged vs. young adult brain. In this chapter molecular events, including transcriptional changes, will be described not as lists of regulated genes but within the cellular context of neural repair and recovery.

Post-stroke neuronal sprouting: growth promoting molecular programs

Neuronal sprouting after stroke or other forms of CNS injury involves the interaction of two molecular programs that are both set in play within a broad region of peri-infarct tissue. Stroke activates a neuronal growth program in sprouting neurons and induces a set of glial inhibitory molecules. Cortical neurons are induced to sprout new connections over a broad zone, as these novel connections can be detected in the range of millimeters in the rodent to centimeters in the primate in peri-infarct cortex [1,3]. In counterpoint, axonal growth inhibitory molecules, produced in large part by activated astrocytes, are present not just in the local vicinity of the immediate stroke scar, but are upregulated throughout a range of peri-infarct tissue. The chondroitin sulfate proteoglycan neurocan is induced in a very broad region of peri-infarct cortex and striatum after stroke, well beyond the local glial scar [17,32]. NogoA is induced in neurons throughout the contralateral and ipsilateral cortex after stroke [33,34] and the developmentally regulated growth inhibitory molecules neuropilin 1 (semaphorin 3a receptor) and ephrin A5 are induced in cells extending well away from the glial scar in peri-infarct cortex [17,35]. Thus, in at least one area of post-stroke axonal sprouting, competing cellular programs of growth promotion and growth inhibition physically overlap within a region of active re-mapping and recovery of function. This overlap suggests that therapies that tip the balance toward axonal sprouting might improve recovery in peri-infarct cortex.

Axonal sprouting occurs across several temporal epochs of a neuronal growth program that is induced by stroke. The initial damage of the ischemic stimulus initiates an axonal growth response in adjacent or connected brain regions within the first week after stroke. Dendritic spine turnover in peri-infarct cortex accelerates 5–8-fold [8] and ultrastructural evidence of synapse number and axon terminals indicates axonal sprouting [7]. The timing of the ischemic stimulus for axonal sprouting is early after stroke and unique to the pathophysiology of acute, focal ischemia. Non-ischemic brain lesions induce a more limited axonal sprouting response than ischemic lesions [13,36,37]. Waves of highly correlated neuronal discharges within the first three days of the stroke induce axonal sprouting in at least one model of ischemic cortical damage [13]. During this early phase of axonal sprouting specific genes are activated that may initiate post-stroke axonal sprouting. These include the transcription factor c-jun, the growth cone phosphoproteins GAP43 and CAP23, and the cytoskeletal modifying protein SPRR1 [17,26,38,39]. These proteins have all been linked to the initiation of axonal outgrowth and regenerative axonal sprouting, through direct effects on growth cone signaling, transcriptional induction of a growth program or modification of the actin cytoskeleton [40–42]. During this early initiation period of axonal sprouting after stroke, neurons in peri-infarct cortex either express or become associated with VEGF1 and 2 in a region of cortex in which ischemia potentiates Hif1 signaling [43,44]. Hif1 induces VEGF and other genes that are linked to angiogenesis, such as erythropoietin, but also genes that play a potent role in neurite outgrowth (EPO and VEGF) and neurogenesis responses (EPO, VEGF, and SDF-1, reviewed in [45]).

At later phases in the axonal sprouting response cytoskeletal and cell adhesion molecules are induced. Tα1 tubulin, an embryonic tubulin isoform that is induced in regenerating neurons [46], is activated at day 14 after stroke. p21/waf1, a protein originally identified as a cyclin-dependent kinase inhibitor, is also induced at this time point. p21 inhibits Rho kinase to promote axonal outgrowth [47] and is induced by Hif1 [48], suggesting both a mechanistic role in peri-infarct neuronal sprouting and a link to the early induction of Hif1 after ischemia in this region. The axonal guidance molecule L1 and the growth cone phosphoprotein MARCKS are also induced in this intermediate period in post-stroke axonal sprouting. MARCKS, CAP23 and GAP43 mediate PI3 kinase signal transduction in the growth cone and promote actin-associated motility [49]. Over-expression of CAP23 and GAP43 act together to promote axonal sprouting into the spinal cord [40]. At one month after stroke new patterns of cortical connections can be detected neuroanatomically [1,2,13]. In axonal sprouting in the hippocampal system or after peripheral nerve lesion, this time period demarcates a termination phase of axonal sprouting. The exact period in which synaptogenesis occurs within post-stroke axonal sprouting is not established, but long-term changes in synaptic markers can be detected after this time [50] and so the one-month period after stroke has been identified as a termination or, possibly more accurately, a maturation phase of post-stroke axonal sprouting [10]. During this late phase of post-stroke axonal sprouting the stathmin family genes SCG10 and SCLIP are upregulated [17,27]. Stathmin family proteins interact with and destabilize microtubules to allow for the change and structural turnover necessary for axonal growth [51]. In contrast to their late induction in stroke, these genes are induced at early time points in peripheral nerve regeneration [52,53]. The late induction of MARCKS, SCG10 and SCLIP in post-stroke vs. peripheral nerve sprouting highlights important differences in the molecular underpinnings of central vs. peripheral axonal sprouting.

The induction of a neuronal growth state during an axonal sprouting response has been more completely analyzed in peripheral nerve and optic nerve injury models. The anatomy of these systems allows more selective (dorsal root ganglion, DRG) or nearly complete (retinal ganglion cell, RGC) isolation of the regenerating neurons. In comparison, the neurons that sprout new connections in the brain after stroke represent a relatively small subset of all neurons within a given region [1,3]. The tissue level of RNA isolation that has been reported for gene expression analysis in the post-stroke brain mixes the mRNA signals from this small population of cells that sprout after stroke with thousands of non-sprouting neurons (with diverse phenotypes), endothelial cells, inflammatory cells, and glia.

The gene expression studies from isolated regenerating DRGs and RGCs develop several important principles. Regeneration in peripheral nerve can be driven by transcription factors that control a cassette of expressed genes which mediate axonal outgrowth, possible "master switches" for nerve regeneration [52,54]. Stat3 and ATF3 are such transcription factors that are induced in regenerating DRG, and mediate peripheral nerve regeneration over inhibitory substrates [54,55]. An intrinsic growth program is likely

to involve an orchestrated response of adhesion, membrane-associated, and intracellular signaling molecules. Over-expressing a subset of growth-associated proteins, such as α7 integrin and GAP43, does not induce regeneration in poorly regenerating adult neurons [56]. Regenerating neurons activate a transcriptional profile that is overlapping with, but distinct from, developing neurons. Both RGCs and DRGs activate genes specific to regeneration, such as SPRR1a, galanin, GADD45, and moesin [42,57,58]. Further, in vitro studies suggest that axonal inhibitory molecules, such as the chondroitin sulfate proteoglycan aggrecan, activate regenerating DRG neurons in a way that is distinct from the predominant signaling form for axonal growth in development: Akt and ERK signaling are important second messenger signals in development whereas integrin-based systems are more important for regeneration [59]. In a phrase, regeneration does not fully recapitulate development. A full characterization of the molecular program that underlies post-stroke axonal sprouting will require selective isolation of the sprouting neurons after stroke, in a similar fashion to what has been done with DRG and RGC neurons.

Post-stroke neuronal sprouting: growth inhibitory molecular programs

The nature and role of proteins that inhibit axonal sprouting after CNS injury have been extensively reviewed [60,61]. These belong to three broad classes. Myelin-associated inhibitory proteins include myelin associated glycoprotein (MAG), oligodendrocyte myelin glycoprotein (OMgp), and NogoA. Extracellular matrix inhibitory proteins include chondroitin sulfate proteoglycans (CSPGs), heparin sulfate proteoglycans, NG2, and tenascin. Developmentally associated inhibitory proteins are termed this because their most prominent role is in regulation of axonal pathfinding in the developing CNS. These include ephrins, semaphorins, and slits. The role of many of these molecules in axonal growth inhibition is increasingly defined in spinal cord and optic nerve injury models [60,61]. Surprisingly, there has not been much study of these inhibitory systems in their normal, endogenous response to stroke. Instead, these have often been studied only in the context of a treatment, such as delivery of anti-Nogo, cytokine, or growth factor treatments, or stem/progenitor cell delivery. To determine the biology of growth inhibitory proteins after stroke and their relationship to the glial scar, and to more distant peri-infarct brain regions, recent studies have mapped candidate growth inhibitory proteins after strokes in specific relationship to the phases of axonal sprouting. The question in these studies is: who is in a position to block axonal sprouting after stroke when this process is just getting ramped up? The data suggest that, of the potentially broad number of candidate inhibitory proteins in CNS injury, only a small subset are active in the right place and the right time after stroke to be in a position to block axonal sprouting.

EphrinA5, EphB1, neurocan, MAG, and neuropilin 1 are induced early after stroke and persist for two weeks. These genes are induced near the infarct core, and extending away from the infarct core into peri-infarct striatum and cortex [17,32,35,62]. Semaphorin 3a, the ligand for neuropilin 1, and NG2, a proteoglycan, are induced at two weeks after stroke [17]. These data indicate that three very different molecular systems might mediate inhibition of post-stroke axonal sprouting: ephrinA5, neurocan, and semaphorin3a/neuropilin 1. Ephrin A5 and MAG are of interest because they are further induced in the aged brain after stroke, and may relate to the diminished axonal sprouting and functional recovery seen in some aged lesion models. CSPGs are secreted by reactive astrocytes, and some neurons, and play a prominent role in glial scar formation and axonal growth inhibition in spinal cord injury and penetrating brain trauma (stab wounds). The response of CSPGs after stroke differs with age. In young adult rats the expression of genes for phosphocan, brevican, versican, and aggrecan increases only late in the sprouting response, at day 28 [17]. In aged rats, phosphocan and brevican are induced early in the sprouting response – at days 3–14 post-stroke [62]. This gene expression profile suggests that aged animals may have a significant induction of CSPGs during the period of axonal sprouting, whereas young adult animals do not. This suggestion is supported by the fact that aged animals have an accelerated astrocytic reaction after stroke [63].

Axonal sprouting after stoke: a turf war

One important difference between axonal regeneration and developmental axonal outgrowth is the local environments that growing axons experience. Developmental axonal growth progresses through intermediate targeting stages in which growth cones are sensitized to attractive and repulsive molecules in a synchronized progression through space. The growth of commissural neurons across the ventral spinal cord uses what is now a paradigmatic sequence of responses to Slit and Robo proteins to both grow toward and then become repelled from the ventral midline [64]. In the optic nerve there is a sequential progression of an L1-expressing growth cone into a laminin substrate that controls growth cone collapse, attraction, or pausing when exposed to the inhibitory protein EphB2, through intracellular SCG10 microtubule control [65]. However, in axonal sprouting after stroke it is likely that there is no ordered presentation of guidance molecules to the regenerating growth cone. Neurocan, ephrinA5, semaphorin 3a, and MAG are all induced throughout peri-infarct cortex in the region of post-stroke axonal sprouting [17,35]. In axonal sprouting from the contralateral cortex to midbrain and spinal cord, activated microglia and astrocytes are also likely altering the zone of axonal sprouting in an inhomogeneous distribution. This suggests that rather than the orderly series of growth and re-direction points of neurodevelopment, the regenerative growth cone is fighting through a field of conflicting inhibitory signals, and responding to as yet uncharacterized attractive or positive signals. One such positive signal for post-stroke axonal and dendritic sprouting may be the reorganizing vasculature. In spinal cord injury axonal sprouting appears to directionally relate to reorganizing blood vessels near the lesion site [66]. In peri-infarct cortex after stroke, dendrites exhibit an orientation around radially projecting blood vessels that reorganize after the infarct [8]. Blood vessels provide both cell guidance molecules and cell adhesion substrates for axonal sprouting in the peripheral nervous system [67]. The reorganizing vasculature after stroke may play a similar role. Intermixed positive and negative cues for neuronal growth, in the setting of rapidly changing CNS tissue morphology after stroke, suggest a turf war in peri-infarct and other post-stroke axonal sprouting zones, in which regenerating axons confront hostile and friendly forces in the same field. The concept of such an axonal sprouting turf war also comes from the studies of DRG growth cones and spinal cord regeneration, in which axonal growth cones stall at inhibitory molecular boundaries, and attempt to digest their way through these zones [68].

Neuronal sprouting after stroke: the ischemic critical period

During neural development, the critical period (sometimes called the sensitive period) is a time zone in which changes in environmental stimulation can induce massive alterations in cortical organization and cortical sensory maps. The critical period is characterized by rapid shifts in cortical responses to visual, somatosensory, auditory, or other inputs and is accompanied by changes in dendritic and axonal structure within these regions. A classic example of critical period plasticity is the rapid shift in the response elements within the primary visual cortex to deprivation of one eye, termed ocular dominance plasticity [69]. In most cortical systems the critical period closes after the juvenile period. The critical period is a state of cortex likely set in place by a combination of several factors: protease activity that mediates breaking and re-forming of synapses [70], NMDA responses [71], extracellular matrix composition including a lack of perineuronal nets [72], lack of myelin-based axonal growth inhibitors [73], and a heightened expression of several key growth-related proteins, such as IGF-1 and CPG-15/neuritin [74,75]. The time course and action of tissue plasminogen activator (tPA) is essential for critical period plasticity, as it is in long-term potentiation (LTP), and appears to provide the mechanism for synaptic remodeling through proteolytic action [69,70]. Perineuronal nets are chondroitin sulfate proteoglycan and hyaluronan structures found in the adult cortex, prominently around interneurons but also more weakly stained around pyramidal neurons [76]. Perineuronal nets form at the end of the critical period, can be delayed by conditions that prolong the critical period, and digestion of perineuronal nets can re-open the critical period and provide substantial cortical plasticity [72]. The onset of Nogo expression appears to close the critical period, at least in mouse visual cortex [73].

These characteristics of the critical period in juvenile cortex are remarkably similar to features of the post-stroke peri-infarct cortex. Like the juvenile critical period, stroke or similar cortical lesions in the adult induce changes in cortical maps, dendritic and axonal plasticity, and a heightened response to altered peripheral stimulation [77,78]. Protease activity is upregulated in peri-infarct tissue after stroke through expression of matrix metalloproteinases 2 and 9 and ADAMTS 1 and 4 [79,80]. Perineuronal nets are reduced for at least one month in peri-infarct cortex

after stroke and have a long lag in re-synthesis after stroke, at least in the young adult [17,62,81]. NMDA responses are heightened in peri-infarct cortex, with a potentiation in LTP [82]. IGF-1 and CPG15/neuritin are induced in peri-infarct cortex [29,83]. These studies suggest a similarity in reorganization of cortical maps and structure between the juvenile critical period and a period of post-stroke brain plasticity, in terms of physiology, cellular structure, molecular expression profile, and extracellular matrix composition. It may be that stroke induces an "ischemic critical period" in peri-infarct and connected cortical areas for a brief interval, which in the rodent may be one month. There are limitations to this analogy. The juvenile critical period involves maturation changes in GABAergic signaling that do not appear to be present in the adult brain after stroke [84]. Similarly, the normal adult brain operates with different plasticity rules to the same inputs that induce juvenile critical period changes [85], and these "adult" plasticity rules likely influence the properties of post-stroke neuronal plasticity. And of course the cortical plasticity manifest in the post-stroke brain occurs in an environment of ischemic damage, myelin and neuronal debris, inflammation, angiogenesis, astrocytosis, and neurogenesis. These tissue responses will contribute directly to elements of cortical plasticity, but also limit neuronal responses and introduce an element of tissue chaos that is not present in the orderly progression of cortical plasticity seen in the juvenile animal after peripheral inputs are altered. Future experiments that explore the concept of an ischemic critical period may uncover molecular and cellular plasticity principles in the zones of synaptic connections affected by stroke, in an analogous manner to the way in which molecular and cellular principles have emerged through systematic study of the juvenile critical period.

Post-stroke neurogenesis

Stroke induces proliferation in the SVZ, migration of immature neurons to areas of ischemic damage, and survival of a very small number of newly born neurons in peri-infarct tissue. The endogenous molecular mechanisms that underlie post-stroke neurogenesis have not been studied extensively. Instead, many studies have delivered growth factors, cytokines, or stem/progenitor cells and assayed their effects on post-stroke neurogenesis. These studies have been reviewed recently [45,86]. Delivery of a cell therapy or a growth factor in pharmacological doses may indeed stimulate neurogenesis; however, it does not provide any information on the underlying pathophysiological events within the tissue that produce a neurogenic response after stroke. As one past mentor put it: "just because penicillin cures pneumonia does not mean that pneumonia is caused by a lack of penicillin" [Landau, personal communication, 1995].

The ischemic events in stroke initiate cell proliferation within the SVZ in the first detectable change in neurogenesis. Gene expression profiling of the SVZ of the mouse after middle cerebral artery occlusion indicates induction in specific gene sets within the TGFβ/ bone morphogenic protein family, fibroblast growth factor family, integrin and inflammatory/chemokine signaling systems, Notch and Wnt/catenin systems [87]. These data identify functional systems that may participate in post-stroke neurogenesis.

Inflammatory cytokine/chemokine signaling appears to play a critical role in post-stroke neurogenesis. The chemokine CCL2 is induced in the ischemic SVZ [87,88] and promotes migration of neural progenitor cells in culture. The chemokine MCP-1 is induced in peri-infarct cortex and striatum after stroke, where it is expressed in activated microglia and astrocytes, and induces migration of neural progenitor cells into peri-infarct tissues [89]. The chemokine SDF-1 is induced in peri-infarct blood vessels and is tropic for migrating neuroblasts into peri-infarct cortex [19]. Chemokines are specialized signaling molecules, which function as tropic factors within the immune system [90], and for neural progenitor cells during development [91]. It is likely that they are playing a similar role in post-stroke neurogenesis, and mediate a link between stroke-induced tissue reorganization (inflammation and angiogenesis) and neurogenesis [45]. Inflammation and inflammatory signaling can also inhibit neurogenesis, both in the normal brain [92] and after stroke [93], particularly via TNFα [94]. This potential "dual role" for inflammation in post-neurogenesis is incompletely understood and clearly warrants further study. However, it may be incorrect to classify chemokine upregulation and tropic function in post-stroke neurogenesis as "inflammatory". These proteins were first described in their role as tropic factors in the immune system, but in post-stroke neurogenesis they are functioning as astrocyte-to-neuroblast or blood vessel-to-neuroblast signaling and may be classified as simply "tropic" rather than "inflammatory".

Post-stroke neurogenesis occurs within a neurovascular niche. In models with small cortical strokes, migrating neuroblasts localize in peri-infarct cortex around angiogenic blood vessels. Blocking angiogenesis nearly completely eliminates neurogenesis [19]. In stroke models with large hemispheric or striatal damage, neuroblasts migrate along blood vessels into the peri-infarct striatum [21,22], a pattern reminiscent of their normal migration in the olfactory bulb [23]. The signaling molecules that mediate this migration are not known, but vascular angiopoietin 1 and SDF-1 are tropic for migrating neuroblasts after stroke [19]. Activated endothelial cells can secrete matrix metalloproteinases that induce neuroblast migration in vitro [95]. Protease activity is critical to migrating neuroblasts after stroke in vivo [96], and these cells may have to digest their way to the source of the tropic factor. This process is similar to growth cone function in an inhibitory environment (see above) and the migrating neuroblast and growth cone share similar cellular profiles and functions [45]. Overall, the concept of vascular–neuroblast associations in post-stroke neurogenesis provides a cellular framework for the future identification of key molecular signaling systems that communicate between these cells. For example, the cytokine erythropoietin has an endogenous role that both affects angiogenesis and promotes neuroblast migration after stroke [20]. The degree of angiogenesis after stroke has been linked to functional recovery in humans [97]. Because angiogenesis occurs well after any tissue might be salvaged from the initial ischemic event, it is likely that any role angiogenesis has in functional recovery is in its interaction with axonal sprouting (see above), neurogenesis or other aspects of tissue repair.

Conclusions

The molecular control of neural repair after stroke involves gene systems that support axonal and dendritic sprouting, cortical plasticity, neurogenesis and angiogenesis. Many of these molecular systems are also activated during development, but regeneration in the nervous system of the adult incorporates some molecular pathways that are distinct from those active in development. The brain after stroke shares molecular, cellular, and physiological similarities with the juvenile brain during the critical period. These findings suggest the concept of an ischemic critical period for neuroplasticity and neural repair after stroke. An important aspect of this ischemic critical period is that it occurs within the unique environment of the injured and reorganizing brain. Neural repair involves a communication among sprouting neurons, activated astrocytes, inflammatory cells, migrating neuroblasts and angiogenic blood vessels. The tissue environments that these cells form in the reorganizing brain hold the key to an integrated molecular view of neural repair. As research tools allow study of the adhesive, soluble, and cell membrane proteins that signal between these cell types, therapeutic targets can be developed that manipulate repair to promote recovery.

References

1. Carmichael ST, Wei L, Rovainen CM, *et al.* New patterns of intra-cortical connections after focal stroke. *Neurobiol Dis.* 2001;**8**:910–22.

2. Overman JJ, Kwok A, Willis D, *et al.* Post-stroke blockade of ephrinA5 increases axonal sprouting in layer IV of the mouse somatosensory cortex. *Soc Neurosci Abst.* 2007;**898**.22.

3. Dancause N, Barbay S, Frost SB, *et al.* Extensive cortical rewiring after brain injury. *J Neurosci.* 2005;**25**:10 167–79.

4. Darian-Smith C, Gilbert CD. Axonal sprouting accompanies functional reorganization in adult cat striate cortex. *Nature.* 1994;**368**:737–40.

5. Pons TP, Garraghty PE, Ommaya AK, *et al.* Massive cortical reorganization after sensory deafferentation in adult macaques. *Science.* 1991;**252**:1857–60.

6. Florence SL, Taub HB, Kaas JH. Large-scale sprouting of cortical connections after peripheral injury in adult macaque monkeys. *Science.* 1998;**282**:1117–21.

7. Ito U, Kuroiwa T, Nagasao J, *et al.* Temporal profiles of axon terminals, synapses and spines in the ischemic penumbra of the cerebral cortex: Ultrastructure of neuronal remodeling. *Stroke.* 2006;**37**:2134–9.

8. Brown CE, Li P, Boyd JD, *et al.* Extensive turnover of dendritic spines and vascular remodeling in cortical tissues recovering from stroke. *J Neurosci.* 2007;**27**:4101–09.

9. Winship IR, Murphy TH. In vivo calcium imaging reveals functional rewiring of single somatosensory neurons after stroke. *J Neurosci.* 2008;**28**:6592–606.

10. Carmichael ST. Cellular and molecular mechanisms of neural repair after stroke: Making waves. *Ann Neurol.* 2006;**59**:735–72.

11. Chen P, Goldberg DE, Kolb B, *et al.* Inosine induces axonal rewiring and improves behavioral outcome after stroke. *Proc Natl Acad Sci USA.* 2002;**99**:9031–6.

12. Papadopoulos CM, Tsai SY, Alsbiei T, *et al.* Functional recovery and neuroanatomical plasticity following middle cerebral artery occlusion and IN-1 antibody treatment in the adult rat. *Ann Neurol.* 2002;**51**:433–41.

13. Carmichael ST, Chesselet M-F. Synchronous neuronal activity is a signal for axonal sprouting after cortical lesions in the adult. *J Neurosci.* 2002;**22**:6062–70.

14. Riban V, Chesselet MF. Region-specific sprouting of crossed corticofugal fibers after unilateral cortical lesions in adult mice. *Exp Neurol.* 2006;**197**:451–7.

15. Aldskogius H, Liu L, Svensson M. Glial responses to synaptic damage and plasticity. *J Neurosci Res.* 1999;**58**:33–41.

16. Wei L, Erinjeri JP, Rovainen CM, *et al.* Collateral growth and angiogenesis around cortical stroke. *Stroke.* 2000;**32**:2179–84.

17. Carmichael ST, Archibeque I, Luke L, *et al.* Growth-associated gene expression after stroke: Evidence for a growth-promoting region in peri-infarct cortex. *Exp Neurol.* 2005;**193**:291–311.

18. Dent EW, Barnes AM, Tang F, *et al.* Netrin-1 and semaphorin 3A promote or inhibit cortical axon branching, respectively, by reorganization of the cytoskeleton. *J Neurosci.* 2004;**24**:3002–12.

19. Ohab JJ, Fleming S, Blesch A, *et al.* A neurovascular niche for neurogenesis after stroke. *J Neurosci.* 2006;**26**:13 007–16.

20. Tsai PT, Ohab JJ, Kertesz N, *et al.* A critical role of erythropoietin receptor in neurogenesis and post-stroke recovery. *J Neurosci.* 2006;**26**:1269–74.

21. Yamashita T, Ninomiya M, Hernandez Acosta P, *et al.* Subventricular zone-derived neuroblasts migrate and differentiate into mature neurons in the post-stroke adult striatum. *J Neurosci.* 2006;**26**:6627–36.

22. Thored P, Wood J, Arvidsson A, *et al.* Long-term neuroblast migration along blood vessels in an area with transient angiogenesis and increased vascularization after stroke. *Stroke.* 2007;**38**:3032–9.

23. Bovetti S, Hsieh YC, Bovolin P, *et al.* Blood vessels form a scaffold for neuroblast migration in the adult olfactory bulb. *J Neurosci.* 2007;**27**:5976–80.

24. Teramoto T, Qiu J, Plumier JC, *et al.* EGF amplifies the replacement of parvalbumin-expressing striatal interneurons after ischemia. *J Clin Invest.* 2004;**111**:1125–32.

25. Rao VL, Bowen KL, Dhodda VK, *et al.* Gene expression analysis of spontaneously hypertensive rat cerebral cortex following transient focal cerebral ischemia. *J Neurochem.* 2002;**83**:1072–86.

26. Lu A, Tang Y, Ran R, *et al.* Genomics of the periinfarction cortex after focal cerebral ischemia. *J Cereb Blood Flow Metab.* 2003;**23**:786–810.

27. Krüger C, Cira D, Sommer C, *et al.* Long-term gene expression changes in the cortex following cortical ischemia revealed by transcriptional profiling. *Exp Neurol.* 2006;**200**:135–52.

28. Buga AM, Dunoiu C, Bălşeanu A, *et al*. Cellular and molecular mechanisms underlying neurorehabilitation after stroke in aged subjects. *Rom J Morphol Embryol.* 2008;**49**:279–302.

29. Yan YP, Sailor KA, Vemuganti R, *et al*. Insulin-like growth factor-1 is an endogenous mediator of focal ischemia-induced neural progenitor proliferation. *Eur J Neurosci.* 2006;**24**:45–54.

30. Schölzke MN, Schwaninger M. Transcriptional regulation of neurogenesis: Potential mechanisms in cerebral ischemia. *J Mol Med.* 2007;**85**:577–88.

31. Arlotta P, Molyneaux BJ, Chen J, *et al*. Neuronal subtype-specific genes that control corticospinal motor neuron development in vivo. *Neuron.* 2005;**45**:207–21.

32. Deguchi K, Takaishi M, Hayashi T, *et al*. Expression of neurocan after transient middle cerebral artery occlusion in adult rat brain. *Brain Res.* 2005;**1037**:194–9.

33. Eslamboli A, Grundy RI, Irving EA. Time-dependent increase in Nogo-A expression after focal cerebral ischemia in marmoset monkeys. *Neurosci Lett.* 2006;**408**:89–93.

34. Cheatwood JL, Emerick AJ, Schwab ME, *et al*. Nogo-A expression after focal ischemic stroke in the adult rat. *Stroke.* 2008;**39**:2091–8.

35. Fujita H, Zhang B, Sato K, *et al*. Expressions of neuropilin-1, neuropilin-2 and semaphorin 3A mRNA in the rat brain after middle cerebral artery occlusion. *Brain Res.* 2001;**914**:1–14.

36. Kartje GL, Schulz MK, Lopez-Yunez A, *et al*. Corticostriatal plasticity is restricted by myelin-associated neurite growth inhibitors in the adult rat. *Ann Neurol.* 1999;**45**:778–86.

37. Napieralski JA, Butler AK, Chesselet MF. Anatomical and functional evidence for lesion-specific sprouting of corticostriatal input in the adult rat. *J Comp Neurol.* 1996;**373**:484–97.

38. Gregersen R, Christensen T, Lehrmann E, *et al*. Focal cerebral ischemia induces increased myelin basic protein and growth-associated protein-43 gene transcription in peri-infarct areas in the rat brain. *Exp Brain Res.* 2001;**138**:384–92.

39. Miyake K, Yamamoto W, Tadokoro M, *et al*. Alterations in hippocampal GAP-43, BDNF, and L1 following sustained cerebral ischemia. *Brain Res.* 2002;**935**:24–31.

40. Bomze HM, Bulsara KR, Iskandar BJ, *et al*. Spinal axon regeneration evoked by replacing two growth cone proteins in adult neurons. *Nat Neurosci.* 2001;**4**:38–43.

41. Bonilla IE, Tanabe K, Strittmatter SM. Small proline-rich repeat protein 1A is expressed by axotomized neurons and promotes axonal outgrowth. *J Neurosci.* 2002;**22**:1303–15.

42. Raivich G, Bohatschek M, Da Costa C, *et al*. The AP-1 transcription factor c-Jun is required for efficient axonal regeneration. *Neuron.* 2004;**43**:57–67.

43. Stowe AM, Plautz EJ, Eisner-Janowicz I, *et al*. VEGF protein associates to neurons in remote regions following cortical infarct. *J Cereb Blood Flow Metab.* 2007;**27**:76–85.

44. Stowe AM, Plautz EJ, Nguyen P, *et al*. Neuronal HIF-1 alpha protein and VEGFR-2 immunoreactivity in functionally related motor areas following a focal M1 infarct. *J Cereb Blood Flow Metab.* 2008;**28**:612–20.

45. Ohab JJ, Carmichael ST. Poststroke neurogenesis: Emerging principles of migration and localization of immature neurons. *Neuroscientist.* 2008;**14**:369–80.

46. Miller FD, Geddes JW. Increased expression of the major embryonic alpha-tubulin mRNA, T alpha 1, during neuronal regeneration, sprouting, and in Alzheimer's disease. *Prog Brain Res.* 1990;**86**:321–30.

47. Tanaka H, Yamashita T, Asada M, *et al*. Cytoplasmic p21(Cip1/WAF1) regulates neurite remodeling by inhibiting Rho-kinase activity. *J Cell Biol.* 2002;**58**:321–9.

48. Greijer AE, van der Groep P, Kemming D, *et al*. Up-regulation of gene expression by hypoxia is mediated predominantly by hypoxia-inducible factor 1 (HIF-1). *J Pathol.* 2005;**206**:291–304.

49. Laux T, Fukami K, Thelen M, *et al*. GAP43, MARCKS, and CAP23 modulate PI(4,5)P(2) at plasmalemmal rafts, and regulate cell cortex actin dynamics through a common mechanism. *J Cell Biol.* 2000;**149**:1455–72.

50. Stroemer RP, Kent TA, Hulsebosch CE. Neocortical neural sprouting, synaptogenesis, and behavioral recovery after neocortical infarction in rats. *Stroke.* 1995;**26**:2135–44.

51. Mori N, Morii H. SCG10-related neuronal growth-associated proteins in neural development, plasticity, degeneration, and aging. *J Neurosci Res.* 2002;**70**:264–73.

52. Costigan M, Befort K, Karchewski L, *et al*. Replicate high-density rat genome oligonucleotide microarrays reveal hundreds of regulated genes in the dorsal root ganglion after peripheral nerve injury. *BMC Neurosci.* 2002;**3**:16.

53. Mason MR, Lieberman AR, Grenningloh G, *et al*. Transcriptional upregulation of SCG10 and CAP-23 is correlated with regeneration of the axons of peripheral and central neurons in vivo. *Mol Cell Neurosci.* 2002;**20**:595–615.

54. Seijffers R, Mills CD, Woolf CJ. ATF3 increases the intrinsic growth state of DRG neurons to enhance peripheral nerve regeneration. *J Neurosci.* 2007;**27**:7911–20.

55. Qiu J, Cafferty WB, McMahon SB, *et al*. Conditioning injury-induced spinal axon regeneration requires signal

transducer and activator of transcription 3 activation. *J Neurosci.* 2005;**25**:1645–53.

56. Leclere PG, Norman E, Groutsi F, *et al.* Impaired axonal regeneration by isolectin B4-binding dorsal root ganglion neurons in vitro. *J Neurosci.* 2007;**27**:1190–9.

57. Fischer D, Petkova V, Thanos S, *et al.* Switching mature retinal ganglion cells to a robust growth state in vivo: Gene expression and synergy with RhoA inactivation. *J Neurosci.* 2004;**24**:8726–40.

58. Wang JT, Kunzevitzky NJ, Dugas JC, *et al.* Disease gene candidates revealed by expression profiling of retinal ganglion cell development. *J Neurosci.* 2007;**27**:8593–603.

59. Zhou FQ, Walzer M, Wu YH, *et al.* Neurotrophins support regenerative axon assembly over CSPGs by an ECM-integrin-independent mechanism. *J Cell Sci.* 2006;**119**:2787–96.

60. Liu BP, Cafferty WB, Budel SO, *et al.* Extracellular regulators of axonal growth in the adult central nervous system. *Phil Trans R Soc Lond B Biol Sci.* 2006;**361**:1593–610.

61. Busch SA, Silver J. The role of extracellular matrix in CNS regeneration. *Curr Opin Neurobiol.* 2007;**17**:120–7.

62. Li S, Carmichael ST. Growth-associated gene and protein expression in the region of axonal sprouting in the aged brain after stroke. *Neurobiol Dis.* 2006;**23**:362–73.

63. Popa-Wagner A, Carmichael ST, Kokaia Z, *et al.* The response of the aged brain to stroke: Too much, too soon? *Curr Neurovasc Res.* 2007;**4**:216–27.

64. Long H, Sabatier C, Ma L, *et al.* Conserved roles for Slit and Robo proteins in midline commissural axon guidance. *Neuron.* 2004;**42**:213–23.

65. Suh LH, Oster SF, Soehrman SS, *et al.* L1/Laminin modulation of growth cone response to EphB triggers growth pauses and regulates the microtubule destabilizing protein SCG10. *J Neurosci.* 2004;**24**:1976–86.

66. Richter MW, Fletcher PA, Liu J, *et al.* Lamina propria and olfactory bulb ensheathing cells exhibit differential integration and migration and promote differential axon sprouting in the lesioned spinal cord. *J Neurosci.* 2005;**25**:10 700–11.

67. Carmeliet P, Tessier-Lavigne M. Common mechanisms of nerve and blood vessel wiring. *Nature.* 2005;**436**:193–200.

68. Tom VJ, Steinmetz MP, Miller JH, *et al.* Studies on the development and behavior of the dystrophic growth cone, the hallmark of regeneration failure, in an in vitro model of the glial scar and after spinal cord injury. *J Neurosci.* 2004;**24**:6531–9.

69. Hooks BM, Chen C. Critical periods in the visual system: Changing views for a model of experience-dependent plasticity. *Neuron.* 2007;**56**:312–26.

70. Mataga N, Mizuguchi Y, Hensch TK. Experience-dependent pruning of dendritic spines in visual cortex by tissue plasminogen activator. *Neuron.* 2004;**44**:1031–41.

71. Kleinschmidt A, Bear MF, Singer W. Blockade of "NMDA" receptors disrupts experience-dependent plasticity of kitten striate cortex. *Science.* 1987;**238**:355–8.

72. Pizzorusso T, Medini P, Berardi N, *et al.* Reactivation of ocular dominance plasticity in the adult visual cortex. *Science.* 2002;**298**:1248–51.

73. McGee AW, Yang Y, Fischer QS, *et al.* Experience-driven plasticity of visual cortex limited by myelin and Nogo receptor. *Science.* 2005;**309**:2222–6.

74. Lee WC, Nedivi E. Extended plasticity of visual cortex in dark-reared animals may result from prolonged expression of cpg15-like genes. *J Neurosci.* 2002;**22**:1807–15.

75. Tropea D, Kreiman G, Lyckman A, *et al.* Gene expression changes and molecular pathways mediating activity-dependent plasticity in visual cortex. *Nat Neurosci.* 2006;**9**:660–8.

76. Alpár A, Gärtner U, Härtig W, *et al.* Distribution of pyramidal cells associated with perineuronal nets in the neocortex of rat. *Brain Res.* 2006;**1120**:13–22.

77. Biernaskie J, Chernenko G, Corbett D. Efficacy of rehabilitative experience declines with time after focal ischemic brain injury. *J Neurosci.* 2004;**24**:1245–54.

78. Ramanathan D, Conner JM, Tuszynski MH. A form of motor cortical plasticity that correlates with recovery of function after brain injury. *Proc Natl Acad Sci USA.* 2006;**103**:11 370–5.

79. Planas AM, Sole S, Justicia C. Expression and activation of matrix metalloproteinase-2 and -9 in rat brain after transient focal cerebral ischemia. *Neurobiol Dis.* 2001;**8**:834–46.

80. Cross AK, Haddock G, Stock CJ, *et al.* ADAMTS-1 and -4 are up-regulated following transient middle cerebral artery occlusion in the rat and their expression is modulated by TNF in cultured astrocytes. *Brain Res.* 2006;**1088**:19–30.

81. Hobohm C, Günther A, Grosche J, *et al.* Decomposition and long-lasting downregulation of extracellular matrix in perineuronal nets induced by focal cerebral ischemia in rats. *J Neurosci Res.* 2005;**80**:539–48.

82. Carmichael ST. Plasticity of cortical projections after stroke. *Neuroscientist.* 2003;**9**:64–75.

83. Rickhag M, Teilum M, Wieloch T. Rapid and long-term induction of effector immediate early genes (BDNF,

Neuritin and Arc) in peri-infarct cortex and dentate gyrus after ischemic injury in rat brain. *Brain Res.* 2007;**1151**:203–10.

84. Hensch TK. Critical period plasticity in local cortical circuits. *Nat Rev Neurosci.* 2005;**6**:877–88.

85. Sato M, Stryker MP. Distinctive features of adult ocular dominance plasticity. *J Neurosci.* 2008;**28**:10 278–86.

86. Greenberg DA, Jin K. Growth factors and stroke. *NeuroRx.* 2006;**3**:458–65.

87. Liu XS, Zhang ZG, Zhang RL, *et al.* Comparison of in vivo and in vitro gene expression profiles in subventricular zone neural progenitor cells from the adult mouse after middle cerebral artery occlusion. *Neuroscience.* 2007;**146**:1053–61.

88. Liu XS, Zhang ZG, Zhang RL, *et al.* Chemokine ligand 2 (CCL2) induces migration and differentiation of subventricular zone cells after stroke. *J Neurosci Res.* 2007;**85**:2120–5.

89. Yan YP, Sailor KA, Lang BT, *et al.* Monocyte chemoattractant protein-1 plays a critical role in neuroblast migration after focal cerebral ischemia. *J Cereb Blood Flow Metab.* 2007;**27**:1213–24.

90. Wells TN, Proudfoot AE, Power CA. Chemokine receptors and their role in leukocyte activation. *Immunol Lett.* 1999;**65**:35–40.

91. López-Bendito G, Sánchez-Alcañiz JA, Pla R, *et al.* Chemokine signaling controls intracortical migration and final distribution of GABAergic interneurons. *J Neurosci.* 2008;**28**:1613–24.

92. Monje ML, Toda H, Palmer TD. Inflammatory blockade restores adult hippocampal neurogenesis. *Science.* 2003;**302**:1760–65.

93. Hoehn BD, Palmer TD, Steinberg GK. Neurogenesis in rats after focal cerebral ischemia is enhanced by indomethacin. *Stroke.* 2005;**36**:2718–24.

94. Iosif RE, Ahlenius H, Ekdahl CT, *et al.* Suppression of stroke-induced progenitor proliferation in adult subventricular zone by tumor necrosis factor receptor 1. *J Cereb Blood Flow Metab.* 2008;**28**:1574–87.

95. Wang L, Zhang ZG, Zhang RL, *et al.* Matrix metalloproteinase 2 (MMP2) and MMP9 secreted by erythropoietin-activated endothelial cells promote neural progenitor cell migration. *J Neurosci.* 2006;**26**:5996–6003.

96. Lee SR, Kim HY, Rogowska J, *et al.* Involvement of matrix metalloproteinase in neuroblast cell migration from the subventricular zone after stroke. *J Neurosci.* 2006;**26**:3491–5.

97. Krupinski J, Kaluza J, Kumar P, *et al.* Role of angiogenesis in patients with cerebral ischemic stroke. *Stroke.* 1994;**25**:1794–8.

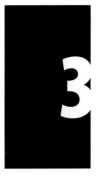

3 Behavioral influences on neuronal events after stroke

Theresa A. Jones & DeAnna L. Adkins

Introduction

Brain plasticity occurs in response to an ever-changing set of environmental and experiential demands, allowing animals, including humans, to adapt and learn. Experiences can modulate synaptic strengths, induce synapse formation and loss, alter glial–neuronal interactions, stimulate new brain vasculature and, sometimes, create new neurons [1,2]. These processes continue throughout the life span, even in stroke survivors. However, after stroke, the brain is also healing and reorganizing, and there is growing evidence that experience interacts with post-stroke degenerative and regenerative processes in a manner that significantly impacts functional outcome.

With a sufficient understanding of how experience alters the post-stroke brain, it should be possible to use behavioral manipulations to optimize brain reorganization. Why target experience for this purpose? Experience is a powerful means for driving *functionally* appropriate neural plasticity. While many promising avenues now exist for saving cells, facilitating neural plasticity, and modulating neural activity, there may be no more efficient way than to rely, at least in part, on this evolutionarily ancient means for placing new and stronger synapses (and possibly neurons) in just the right places within neural networks to improve function. Another consideration is that stroke itself results in diverse changes in behavioral experience. For example, stroke leads to disuse of impaired modalities (movements, language, memory, etc.) and compensatory strategies for coping with the impairments. Unless impeded by behavioral intervention, some of these post-stroke experiences may drive brain reorganization in detrimental directions.

Environmental enrichment and rehabilitative training have been found to induce robust restructuring in the brain and improve behavioral function in animal models of brain injury. However, not all behavioral manipulations improve function, and not all brain plasticity is adaptive. Here we review findings from animal models of experience–injury interactions and discuss how the manipulation of behavioral experience, either alone or in combination with other therapeutic approaches, can improve post-stroke function in adults.

Time-dependent post-stroke processes that are sensitive to experience

After stroke, there is a widespread and temporally evolving sequence of degenerative and regenerative responses. Stroke results in neurotoxic effects, including excitotoxicity, oxidative stress, mitochondrial injury, inflammation, and apoptosis that, in addition to fatally impacting the ischemic core, cause widespread neural and synaptic loss in the adjacent penumbra and connected areas [3] (Figure 3.1A–C). These degenerative events also act as signals to induce regenerative responses.

Growth and survival-promoting factors increase, glia react, neuronal cytoskeleton restructures, dendrites grow, axons sprout, synapses form, vasculature remodels, and newly generated cells migrate to the ischemic region [10–13]. Molecules that normally keep wayward axons at bay (presumably to reduce the formation of inappropriate neural connections) may be transiently inhibited, which contributes to a neuronal growth-permissive environment [10] (and see Chapter 2). Partially denervated neurons increase the expression of genes and molecules that help them survive the damage, and promote cytoskeletal restructuring, permitting dendrites and spines to grow or alter shape and

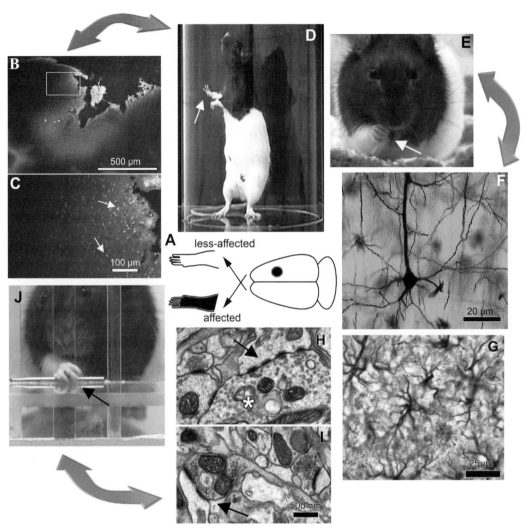

Figure 3.1 Illustration of the interconnected relationship between degenerative and regenerative processes after brain injury and behavioral experience. Unilateral sensorimotor cortical lesions (black oval) in rats result in impairments in the contralesional ("affected") forelimb (A). Degenerating neurons (fluorojade-B labeled) in the region of an ischemic lesion of the sensorimotor cortex (B,C). The white outline in B is the region viewed at higher magnification in C. The lesion leads to degeneration of transcallosal axonal projections to the contralesional sensorimotor cortex and a hyper-reliance upon the less-affected, ipsilesional, forelimb (arrows), e.g. as seen in a rat during exploration (D) and food handling behavior (E). In the contralesional sensorimotor cortex, the interaction of transcallosal degeneration and use of the less-affected forelimb induces dendritic growth (F, [4,5]), glial reactivity (G [6]), synaptogenesis [7] and an increase in the efficacious synapse subtypes, multisynaptic boutons (asterisk, H) and perforated synapses (arrows, H, I). Unilateral lesions also facilitate learning skill reaching with the less-affected limb (J [8]). In turn, this learning further enhances neural plasticity in the non-injured cortex while limiting the capacity for experience-driven changes in the injured cortex [9].

size in order to accommodate new synaptic connections from sprouting axons. The formation of new synapses may further help neurons survive by contributing survival molecules and by maintaining normal levels of cellular activity. As shown in Table 3.1, many components of these degenerative and regenerative responses are sensitive to manipulations of behavioral experience.

Injury also changes the fine structure of synapses in a manner that likely alters neural activity patterns. In cortical and striatal areas that have undergone reactive sprouting, there are more synapses that have ultrastructural characteristics of increased efficacy [31,32]. This includes perforated synapses (Figure 3.1H,I), an excitatory synapse subtype with abundant AMPA receptors that dominates

Table 3.1 Examples of behavioral influences on injury-induced brain changes

Injury-induced event	Direction	Finding
Tissue loss	+	Early forced use of the affected (contralesional) forelimb increased cortical damage after cortical lesions [14,15]. Restraint stress after motor cortical infarcts impeded recovery of forelimb function and exaggerated lesion size [16].
Tissue loss	–	Constraint-induced movement-like therapy decreased tissue loss after striatal hemorrhage [17].
Cell death	+	Early EC exaggerated post-ischemic hippocampal neuron death [18].
Cell death	–	Forced use of the affected forelimb decreased loss of dopamine neurons in a unilateral Parkinson's model [19]. EC after lesion of the ventral subiculum attenuated degeneration in hippocampus [20].
Growth factors	+	Delayed exercise increased brain derived neurotrophic factor (BDNF) after traumatic brain injury [21,22].
Growth factors	–	Too early exercise decreased BDNF and other plasticity-related proteins after traumatic brain injury [21,22].
Reactive astrocytes	+	Forced forelimb use increased astrocytic reactions to callosal denervation [6]. EC after cerebral ischemia increased astrocytic reactivity and fibroblast growth factor in hippocampus [23].
Axonal sprouting	+	EC increased axonal sprouting into deafferented superior colliculus after retinal lesion [24].
Axonal sprouting	–	Axonal sprouting was blocked by preventing behavioral asymmetries after unilateral nigrostriatal damage [25].
Dendritic growth	+	EC following cerebral ischemia increased dendritic density in hippocampus [26].
Dendritic growth	–	Dendritic growth contralateral to sensorimotor cortex lesions was blocked by constraint of the ipsilesional forelimb [4].
Synaptogenesis	+	Motor skills training increased cortical lesion-induced synaptogenesis in motor cortex [7]. EC after cerebral infarct increased synaptic density in hippocampus [26].
Neurogenesis	+	EC increased subventricular zone neurogenesis after cortical infarcts [27] (see Chapter 5). Skilled forelimb training increased hippocampal neurogenesis after sensorimotor cortical damage [28].
Neurogenesis	–	Exercise decreased subventricular zone neurogenesis after cortical infarct [27].
Cortical functional activity	+	Skilled reach training with the affected limb increased movement representations near cortical infarcts [29,30].

This table illustrates two points: (1) behavioral experiences can influence the degenerative and regenerative processes that follow brain injury; (2) the nature of the effect varies with dose, type, and timing of the behavioral experiences and with severity and type of injury. +, increased, –, decreased compared to control, EC, complex environment housing.

its simpler, typically smaller synaptic neighbors in its ability to depolarize the postsynaptic neuron [33]. Furthermore, multiple synapse complexes (Figure 3.1H), where a single bouton contacts more than one postsynaptic dendritic process, are more abundant than normal [31,34], suggesting that the re-utilization of boutons may be one means of re-innervating a brain region. At least in the cortex, the prevalence of these synapse subtypes is also sensitive to experience [7]. These synaptic changes may contribute to changes in neural activity and excitability that can be long lasting after the injury.

The degenerative–regenerative cascade occurs by varying degrees and on different time scales depending on whether one examines the perilesion or remote brain areas [10]. Sprouting patterns vary depending on injury locus and size, among other factors. New synapses formed in denervated regions tend to arise from the most proximal and prominent of the remaining pre-existing inputs [35]. Relative to the pre-injured state, the ultimate patterns of synaptic connectivity within and between brain regions may be dramatically altered after reorganization. The time course and extent of these processes can vary with age (older brains take longer, reviewed in [36]), and type of damage [37]. Although the most dramatic activity occurs earlier after the injury, degenerative and regenerative reactions continue for at least several months in rodent models and perhaps much longer [10,11].

Reorganization patterns can vary dramatically with injury extent. Dancause et al. [38] found that, in squirrel monkeys, ischemic lesions that destroy more than 50% of the forelimb representation region of the primary motor cortex (M1) induce extensive expansion of forelimb movement representations in the ipsilesional ventral premotor cortex (PMv). However, smaller lesions within M1 actually decrease the forelimb motor map in PMv. The expansion of PMv is associated with greater axonal sprouting from PMv into the penumbra of the M1 lesions and with improved rehabilitation-induced motor performance [39].

Sprouting is activity dependent. Brus-Ramer et al. [40] found that, after unilateral pyramidal tract lesions in adult rats, the sprouting of ipsilateral corticospinal projections into denervated regions of the spinal cord could be increased by electrical stimulation of this pathway. This indicates that there is a considerable capacity to refine sprouting patterns after injury by manipulating activity-dependent plasticity. It also supports that the developmental process of activity-dependent synaptic competition that is involved in establishing neural networks is also at play in reorganizing the CNS after damage.

Ischemia and other types of brain injury can increase the generation and migration of new glia and neurons (see Figure 3.1F) [41]. Molecules released by remodeling tissue appear to draw neural precursors to injured tissue [42]. However, in rats, few of the new neurons in the striatum and cortex survive for very long. Although new neurons are found near the cortical lesion core and penumbra, the overwhelming majority of newly generated cells develop into glia [43]. This injury-induced proliferation of glia may well play a critical role in neuronal plasticity after stroke. However, the sensitivity of neurogenesis to behavioral experience is also well established (see Chapter 5). Targeting post-stroke neurogenesis with behavioral manipulations provides another opportunity to manipulate brain reorganization with behavior.

Do the regenerative responses to stroke support better functional outcome? Functional recovery is greater following cortical ischemia, which induces major axonal sprouting in the striatum, compared to

injuries of the same size and location that result in little sprouting [37]. Treatments that reduce growth inhibitory substances, such as Nogo, and thus enhance neurite outgrowth, can also promote greater functional recovery [13]. Administration of substances, like neurotrophins, that promote neurogenesis and migration of immature neurons [42] also results in greater functional outcome after cortical infarcts. However, it should be expected that some examples of post-stroke plasticity are non-optimal or even maladaptive given that there are many examples of pathological neuroplasticity, such as that proposed to underlie the development of epilepsy, focal hand dystonia, and chronic pain. Experience-dependent neural plasticity can also have detrimental or mixed effects on functional outcome after stroke, as reviewed below.

Although many aspects of the degenerative–regenerative cascade have been found to be sensitive to behavioral experience, we currently know too little about how specifically to use this information to improve function after stroke. The problem is complex, considering that a single locus of damage instigates neural (and non-neural) reorganization in numerous brain areas. If examined in sufficient detail, the pattern of reorganization must be unique for every individual brain injury. Furthermore, it is clear that experience effects vary with timing and types of injury, among other factors (Table 3.1). Nevertheless, it is hoped that we will learn enough about the general principles of how experience influences these processes to be able to devise rehabilitative techniques that optimize brain remodeling and can be tailored for injuries that vary in type, locus, and extent.

Effects of "self-taught" behavioral change on brain reorganization

We have found that neural plasticity after unilateral cortical lesions is driven by the convergence of injury- and behaviorally induced pressures. After unilateral lesions of the sensorimotor cortex in rats, there is degeneration of transcallosal projections to the contralateral homotopic region of the motor cortex. This is followed by reactive astrocytic changes, growth of pyramidal neuron dendrites and synaptogenesis in the contralesional cortex [31,44,45]. Over time, the numbers and complexity of dendrites and synapses are increased relative to the same brain region of intact animals. Dendrites are overproduced and then partially eliminated, which is reminiscent of the dendritic overproduction and pruning found in studies of brain development.

The degeneration of transcallosal projections is one instigator of the contralesional glial and neural changes [5,6]. Another driver of the cellular changes is the animal's behavior. After the lesions, rats show impairments in the use of the contralesional forelimb. These changes are evident in forelimb movements used during exploration (Figure 3.1D) and in the dexterous way the animals handle food or other objects (Figure 3.1E). Much like humans [46], rats with these impairments begin to disuse the affected limb and rely on the ipsilesional forelimb more and in different ways to compensate [4,47]. When rats are prevented from using the ipsilesional forelimb (with limb-restricting vests), the dendritic growth does not occur [4]. Denervation and forelimb asymmetries, together, are sufficient variables to cause the dendritic outgrowth and astrocytic changes. They can be reproduced in animals by transecting the callosal fibers to the motor cortex and forcing use of one limb [4–6]. Together, these studies suggest that degeneration enhances the propensity of neurons in the contralateral cortex to grow new synapses and dendrites, and that behavioral pressures act on this sensitive neuronal environment to dramatically alter neuronal structure and connectivity.

This lesion–behavior interaction has functional consequences. After lesions of the sensorimotor cortex, rats have some impairments in the "less-affected" (ipsilesional) limb, but they are also able to better learn a new skilled motor task of manual dexterity (skilled reaching) with this limb than intact animals learning the same task with one limb (Figure 3.1J) [8,45]. The enhanced skill learning co-exists with impairments in ipsilesional forelimb skills that were established before the injury [48]. Thus, the lesions appear to impair existing motor engrams of the ipsilesional forelimb while enhancing some capacity to learn new skills with this limb.

This interaction between denervation-induced and experience-dependent neural plasticity may be considered adaptive if it permits the injured animal to rapidly learn compensatory behaviors. However, there are maladaptive consequences for the function of the affected limb. Training the ipsilesional forelimb in skilled reaching worsens motor performance of the affected limb and reduces the benefits of later rehabilitative training focused on the affected limb [45,49]. It also reduces experience-dependent activation of neurons in the peri-infarct motor cortex resulting from

affected limb training [9]. Bilateral training does not produce similar effects, suggesting that lateralized skill learning may be the culprit [9]. The peri-infarct motor cortex is important for functional recovery of the affected limb and for rehabilitative training efficacy (see the section on effects of training focused on impairments). As it already tends to have impaired experience-dependent plasticity [50] and undergoes a major loss of dendrites and spines [12], limiting its activity and plasticity even further may be particularly detrimental. The neural basis and behavioral parameters of this effect require much more investigation.

These findings are consistent with the idea that unilateral brain injury unbalances competitive interactions between the hemispheres [51], and indicate that behavioral experiences can contribute to this imbalance in a manner that limits functionally beneficial restructuring in the damaged hemisphere. They also suggest that the phenomenon of learned non-use, long studied by Taub and others [46], may be exacerbated by experience-dependent plasticity. Because maintenance of normal neuronal function is use-dependent, disuse of the affected body side may contribute to its dysfunction and limit opportunities for adaptive neural reorganization in the damaged hemisphere (reviewed in [2]). Behavioral interventions, such as extensive focused training of affected extremities (see the section on the effects of training focused on impairments) or combined therapeutic treatments (see the section on combining behavioral manipulation with other interventions), may be needed to counter the effect of learning with the less-affected, ipsilesional body side.

Another general implication of these findings is that post-injury regenerative processes sometimes cause brain regions to become more sensitive to experience-dependent plasticity. This could facilitate functionally beneficial neural plasticity, but could also be permissive of excessive and maladaptive plasticity. This leads to the question of how to capitalize on this process and steer it in an optimal direction through the use of specific behavioral manipulations. There is now a wealth of research indicating that manipulations of behavioral experience can influence post-injury neural plasticity and behavioral outcome.

Manipulating environmental complexity

A classic approach in animal models for studying the influence of behavioral experience is to compare rats housed in simple cages to those in complex, or "enriched" environments (EC). In a typical complex environment used for laboratory studies, rodents live in large social groups in cages with many objects that can be explored, traversed and manipulated. In the standard laboratory cage condition, one animal is housed alone or with one or two cagemates, and there are few or no objects with which to interact. Thus, EC simultaneously manipulates social, cognitive, sensory and motor experience. Compared to the standard cage condition, raising rats in EC increases neocortical thickness, dendritic arborization, synapse number, capillary volume, glial processes, hippocampal neurogenesis, and cerebellar Purkinje neuron dendritic arborization, and has myriad other brain effects, as reviewed previously [1]. Housing rats in EC in adulthood produces many of the same effects compared to standard housing, although the effect sizes tend to be smaller. Behaviorally, EC housed animals outperform rats from standard housing on many measures of learning, memory, and perceptual function.

As an experimental tool for understanding *whether* experience can influence post-injury recovery processes, there may be no more powerful manipulation. As reviewed in more detail in Chapter 5, many studies have found that EC promotes greater neural plasticity after brain damage and improves behavioral function. For example, EC influences post-injury synaptogenesis, astrocytic reactivity, and neurogenesis (Table 3.1).

What is improved by EC housing? Rose and colleagues found that EC promotes better behavioral compensation as opposed to true recovery of function [52]. For example, EC does not influence recovery on tests that are insensitive to practice, but it is very effective in improving performance on spatial memory tasks, which can be solved in a variety of ways. It is less useful for preserving memories of tasks learned before the injury than for enhancing post-injury learning. Thus, EC in animals with brain damage promotes the capacity for future learning and the capacity to switch between alternative strategies to perform tasks, as has long been proposed in intact animals [53].

What about EC leads to improvement in function? EC encourages physical activity, which may facilitate learning-related plasticity. Physical activity in intact animals, such as running, is associated with angiogenesis, neurogenesis, increases in neurotrophins, and other plastic changes in the hippocampus, cerebellum and neocortex [54]. The impetus to explore an environment that contains many obstacles may challenge animals to develop compensatory strategies for motor coordination and postural support. Motor coordination training alone has been found to improve motor function after unilateral cerebral injuries [7]. EC may promote a type of cognitive rehabilitation, because performances on some measures of cognitive function are also improved. Increased social interactions may have a major influence as well (see also the section on combining behavioral manipulation with other interventions). In intact rats, increasing the complexity of social interactions induces dendritic hypertrophy and synaptogenesis in the prefrontal cortex [55].

But what relevance do these findings have for human stroke survivors? After all, humans can be considered to normally live in an enriched environment. From the perspective that EC more closely resembles the human condition than standard laboratory cage conditions, these studies suggest that impoverishment of experience may limit plasticity and functional restoration after stroke and other types of injury. This seems highly relevant because, in humans, stroke can lead to reduced daily activities and social interactions [56], forms of impoverishment that animal studies suggest are likely to be detrimental to functional outcome.

EC manipulates many behavioral experiences at once, which increases the likelihood of detecting an effect on the brain, but limits the ability to know what type of experience led to the changes. For the purpose of understanding specific experience–injury interactions, and for targeting particular impairments, many researchers have investigated the post-injury effects of more focused training.

Effects of training focused on impairments

When animals are trained in an unfocused way, i.e. in a task that they can solve in a variety of ways, they tend to compensate with less-affected modalities. When rats are trained on a challenging obstacle course (the "acrobatic task") after unilateral sensorimotor cortical lesions, there is an overall improvement in a measure of locomotor skill. However, the training primarily improves the *less-affected* limb ipsilateral to the lesion, rather than the affected limb [7]. Furthermore, acrobatic training increased synaptogenesis in the contralesional motor cortex, but had no significant synaptogenic or dendritic growth effects in the residual motor cortex of the damaged hemisphere [57], a region which may be more important for affected limb function, at least after subtotal sensorimotor cortical damage [39]. Similarly, simply increasing physical activity (running), although it is well known to have many positive influences on brain function [54], had no beneficial effect for skilled motor function of the affected forelimb after unilateral ischemic sensorimotor cortex lesions [58].

In contrast to these effects of acrobatic training and exercise, motor skill training that focuses specifically on impaired extremities after brain injury seems to more readily improve those extremities' function and also induces reorganization and plasticity of neocortical areas [39]. Practice in skilled reaching (also known as "reach-to-grasp") has been extensively used in animal models of focused motor rehabilitative training (Figure 3.1J). This training approach is believed to capitalize upon neural mechanisms of motor skill learning to drive plasticity in regions relevant to the function of the affected limb. As intact animals learn reaching tasks, they undergo well-characterized and time-dependent neuroplastic changes in the primary motor cortex (see Chapter 1). Nudo *et al.* [29] found that, in squirrel monkeys, extensive practice in reaching with the affected forelimb following ischemic damage to the forelimb representation area of the primary motor cortex spared the tissue surrounding the lesion from a loss of movement representation, as measured with intracortical microstimulation mapping. Reaching practice has since been found also to enlarge forelimb motor map territory in ipsilesional ventral premotor areas [38]. Similarly, in rats, post-injury training in skilled reaching improves motor function and promotes reorganization of the remaining motor cortex [30]. Several studies in human stroke survivors support that focused training of the affected extremity can improve its function and promote activity in the remaining cortex of the injured hemisphere (see Chapter 21).

Although focused training improves skilled use of the affected limb, this hardly suggests that the functional improvements are due to "true recovery". Whishaw and others have found that improvements in skilled reaching are due to many subtle alterations in the movement sequences that animals use to perform the task with the affected limb [47,59]. Thus, even with directed training approaches, functional improvement may primarily reflect behavioral compensation, albeit of a more subtle type than that resulting from reliance on less-affected extremities or sensory systems. One must bear in mind, of course, the difficulty in instructing rats and monkeys in exactly how to move their limbs when performing these tasks.

Training has been found to be most beneficial if initiated early after a stroke. If training is delayed for one month after cortical infarcts, compared to training initiated within a week of injury, it is less effective in sparing movement representations in monkeys [60] and in improving motor function and enhancing dendritic growth in rats [61]. It is likely that time-dependent degenerative and regenerative processes make the brain more sensitive to behavioral changes that occur early after damage.

Aside from motor skills, there is sparse animal research on focused training of other impaired modalities. EC housing does enhance non-motor functions, but it manipulates multiple modalities at once so that it is difficult to know which experiences are important for a particular behavioral improvement. For rodent research, there are many tools available for measuring and manipulating cognitive, attentional, emotional, sensory, perceptual, social and other functions, and these present an opportunity to extend animal models of rehabilitative training to other functional modalities.

Combining behavioral manipulation with other interventions

The combination of post-injury pharmacological manipulations with behavioral training has been investigated for decades, as reviewed elsewhere [62] (see also Chapter 4). One adjunct to motor rehabilitative training that we have investigated is low-intensity cortical electrical stimulation (CS). In rats and monkeys with motor cortical infarcts, epi- or subdural CS delivered for 10–30 days over remaining regions of the motor cortex during daily practice in skilled reaching improves functional outcome compared with reach training alone [63]. A related approach under investigation in human stroke survivors is the use of non-invasive transcranial stimulation to modulate cortical activity [64]. CS-induced improvements in skilled motor performance are linked to several changes in the stimulated region of perilesion motor cortex, including increased density of dendrites [65], synapses and efficacious synapse subtypes [66], movement representation area [67], and stimulation-evoked potentials [68]. We found that rats with more severe post-lesion motor impairment benefit less from CS compared with rats with more moderate impairments [66]. However, the severely impaired rats were just beginning to attain levels of reaching performance equivalent to moderately impaired rats by the end of the treatment period and therefore might have benefited from a longer interval of CS and training [66].

As reviewed by Plow *et al.* [63], these animal studies were used to support the initiation of clinical trials in human stroke patients. Early phase studies were promising, indicating that CS was a safe and efficacious way to improve upper-extremity motor function in stroke survivors. However, the phase III, Everest, study failed to meet primary endpoints when the entire group of subjects was included in the analysis. Since this initial report, follow-up analysis has revealed that a subset of subjects showed major improvements. These subjects were ones in which the CS was delivered at intensity levels that were 50% of those needed to evoke movement, consistent with the parameters found to be effective in the smaller clinical trials and in the animal studies. In the other subjects, no movements could be evoked and therefore the CS was delivered at a predefined and probably insufficient intensity level. This may indicate that CS can be effective if descending motor pathways are sufficiently activated, which is likely to vary with different injuries and with stimulation location. This supports the need to better understand how to tailor treatment strategies for particular types of stroke.

Maladaptive behavioral experience

In an earlier section, we described how learning skills with the ipsilesional "less-affected" upper extremity may be detrimental to the outcome of the affected body side. Too much or too intense an experience with affected extremities early after a brain injury can also hinder recovery. If rats are forced to rely on their affected limb (by placing them in vests that restrict the less-affected limb) during the first week after sensorimotor cortical damage, motor impairments are worsened and there is greater degeneration of the perilesion cortex [14,69]. Tissue loss is further exaggerated in rats that are moved from group housing to social isolation at the time of the injury [70]. Furthermore, early forced *disuse* of the affected limb extends the time window of vulnerability to later overuse [69]. Early voluntary exercise after traumatic brain damage reduces the expression of plasticity-related molecules

in the hippocampus [21]. However, if voluntary exercise is delayed, animals show improved function and there is an enhanced expression of these molecules [21]. These effects vary with injury severity and type. Griesbach *et al.* [22] found that a longer delay is needed after more severe injuries for exercise to promote plasticity related proteins in the hippocampus. Tillerson *et al.* [19] found that early forced use of the affected forelimb reduces cell death and motor impairment in a rat model of unilateral Parkinson's degeneration, and this occurs only if it is initiated soon enough after the onset of neurodegeneration.

Intensely varied social experience may also impair recovery. Silasi, Hamilton, and Kolb [55] used a paradigm of increased social complexity in which male rats were exposed to a rotating set of cagemates of the same sex, all of which were familiar to them, but which were changed every 48 h. In intact animals, this experience promotes dendritic growth and synaptogenesis in the prefrontal cortex. However, when this regimen of social change is begun the day following ischemic motor cortex damage, it blocks spontaneous recovery of motor function. This, together with previous findings of the benefit of social housing after brain injury [70], suggests that, at least among adult male rats, *stable* social interaction may be optimal for outcome after brain injury. This study also provides another example of how experience-dependent plasticity interacts with injury in ways that can be maladaptive for functional outcome.

Conclusion

In some respects we may think of the adult post-stroke brain as similar to the developing brain in that it needs to be shaped by appropriate experiences. We are now faced with the challenge of understanding how best to do this. In this chapter, we overviewed findings from animal research on the significant interactions between injury and experience as the brain reorganizes following a stroke. Many aspects of the degenerative-regenerative cascade can be changed by behavioral manipulations, influencing post-stroke plasticity and improving behavioral outcome. However, experience has the capacity to worsen function, increase degeneration, and limit functionally beneficial plasticity. Not attempting to implement rehabilitative behavioral techniques is also risky, because non-directed experiences of the animal may drive neural reorganization in functionally maladaptive directions. This accentuates the urgency that we obtain more detailed and more clinically relevant knowledge about these processes. Because experience effects vary with injury severity, location and type, it seems important to investigate the many varieties of stroke that occur (see Chapter 8). There remain many other under-investigated stroke-related issues, including how age, gender, and modality of impairment interact with experience and degenerative processes. All of these issues are highly pertinent and suitable for investigation with animal models.

Acknowledgments

We thank Cole Husbands for editing, Soo Y. Kim for the fluorojade image and Dr. Rachel Allred for graphic design. Grant support: NS056839, NS06332 and NS064423.

References

1. Grossman AW, Churchill JD, Bates KE, *et al.* A brain adaptation view of plasticity: Is synaptic plasticity an overly limited concept? *Prog Brain Res.* 2002;**138**:91–108.

2. Kleim JA, Jones TA. Principles of experience-dependent neural plasticity: Implications for rehabilitation after brain damage. *J Speech Lang Hear Res.* 2008;**51**:S225–39.

3. Doyle KP, Simon RP, Stenzel-Poore MP. Mechanisms of ischemic brain damage. *Neuropharmacology.* 2008;**55**:310–8.

4. Jones TA, Schallert T. Use-dependent growth of pyramidal neurons after neocortical damage. *J Neurosci.* 1994;**14**:2140–52.

5. Adkins DL, Bury SD, Jones TA. Laminar-dependent dendritic spine alterations in the motor cortex of adult rats following callosal transection and forced forelimb use. *Neurobiol Learn Mem.* 2002;**78**:35–52.

6. Bury SD, Eichhorn AC, Kotzer CM, *et al.* Reactive astrocytic responses to denervation in the motor cortex of adult rats are sensitive to manipulations of behavioral experience. *Neuropharmacology.* 2000;**39**:743–55.

7. Jones TA, Chu CJ, Grande LA, *et al.* Motor skills training enhances lesion-induced structural plasticity in the motor cortex of adult rats. *J Neurosci.* 1999;**19**:10 153–63.

8. Bury SD, Jones TA. Unilateral sensorimotor cortex lesions in adult rats facilitate motor skill learning with the "unaffected" forelimb and training-induced dendritic structural plasticity in the motor cortex. *J Neurosci.* 2002;**22**:8597–606.

9. Allred RP, Jones TA. Maladaptive effects of learning with the less-affected forelimb after focal cortical infarcts in rats. *Exp Neurol.* 2008;**210**:172–81.

10. Carmichael ST. Cellular and molecular mechanisms of neural repair after stroke: Making waves. *Ann Neurol.* 2006;**59**:735–42.

11. Wieloch T, Nikolich K. Mechanisms of neural plasticity following brain injury. *Curr Opin Neurobiol.* 2006;**16**:258–64.

12. Brown CE, Murphy TH. Livin' on the edge: Imaging dendritic spine turnover in the peri-infarct zone during ischemic stroke and recovery. *Neuroscientist.* 2008;**14**:139–46.

13. Cheatwood JL, Emerick AJ, Kartje GL. Neuronal plasticity and functional recovery after ischemic stroke. *Top Stroke Rehabil.* 2008;**15**:42–50.

14. Kozlowski DA, James DC, Schallert T. Use-dependent exaggeration of neuronal injury after unilateral sensorimotor cortex lesions. *J Neurosci.* 1996;**16**:4776–86.

15. DeBow SB, McKenna JE, Kolb B, *et al.* Immediate constraint-induced movement therapy causes local hyperthermia that exacerbates cerebral cortical injury in rats. *Can J Physiol Pharmacol.* 2004;**82**:231–7.

16. Kirkland SW, Coma AK, Colwell KL, *et al.* Delayed recovery and exaggerated infarct size by post-lesion stress in a rat model of focal cerebral stroke. *Brain Res.* 2008;**1201**:151–60.

17. DeBow SB, Davies ML, Clarke HL, *et al.* Constraint-induced movement therapy and rehabilitation exercises lessen motor deficits and volume of brain injury after striatal hemorrhagic stroke in rats. *Stroke.* 2003;**34**:1021–6.

18. Farrell R, Evans S, Corbett D. Environmental enrichment enhances recovery of function but exacerbates ischemic cell death. *Neuroscience.* 2001;**107**:585–92.

19. Tillerson JL, Cohen AD, Philhower J, *et al.* Forced limb-use effects on the behavioral and neurochemical effects of 6-hydroxydopamine. *J Neurosci.* 2001;**21**:4427–35.

20. Dhanushkodi A, Bindu B, Raju TR, *et al.* Exposure to enriched environment improves spatial learning performances and enhances cell density but not choline acetyltransferase activity in the hippocampus of ventral subicular-lesioned rats. *Behav Neurosci.* 2007;**121**:491–500.

21. Griesbach GS, Gomez-Pinilla F, Hovda DA. The upregulation of plasticity-related proteins following TBI is disrupted with acute voluntary exercise. *Brain Res.* 2004;**1016**:154–62.

22. Griesbach GS, Gomez-Pinilla F, Hovda DA. Time window for voluntary exercise-induced increases in hippocampal neuroplasticity molecules after traumatic brain injury is severity dependent. *J Neurotrauma.* 2007;**24**:1161–71.

23. Briones TL, Woods J, Wadowska M, *et al.* Astrocytic changes in the hippocampus and functional recovery

after cerebral ischemia are facilitated by rehabilitation training. *Behav Brain Res.* 2006;**171**:17–25.

24. Caleo M, Tropea D, Rossi C, *et al.* Environmental enrichment promotes fiber sprouting after deafferentation of the superior colliculus in the adult rat brain. *Exp Neurol.* 2009;**21**:515–9.

25. Morgan S, Huston JP, Pritzel M. Effects of reducing sensory-motor feedback on the appearance of crossed nigro-thalamic projections and recovery from turning induced by unilateral substantia nigra lesions. *Brain Res Bull.* 1983;**11**:721–7.

26. Briones TL, Suh E, Jozsa L, *et al.* Behaviorally induced synaptogenesis and dendritic growth in the hippocampal region following transient global cerebral ischemia are accompanied by improvement in spatial learning. *Exp Neurol.* 2006;**198**:530–8.

27. Komitova M, Zhao LR, Gido G, *et al.* Postischemic exercise attenuates whereas enriched environment has certain enhancing effects on lesion-induced subventricular zone activation in the adult rat. *Eur J Neurosci.* 2005;**21**:2397–405.

28. Wurm F, Keiner S, Kunze A, *et al.* Effects of skilled forelimb training on hippocampal neurogenesis and spatial learning after focal cortical infarcts in the adult rat brain. *Stroke.* 2007;**38**:2833–40.

29. Nudo RJ, Wise BM, SiFuentes F, *et al.* Neural substrates for the effects of rehabilitative training on motor recovery after ischemic infarct. *Science.* 1996;**272**:1791–4.

30. Conner JM, Chiba AA, Tuszynski MH. The basal forebrain cholinergic system is essential for cortical plasticity and functional recovery following brain injury. *Neuron.* 2005;**46**:173–9.

31. Jones TA. Multiple synapse formation in the motor cortex opposite unilateral sensorimotor cortex lesions in adult rats. *J Comp Neurol.* 1999;**414**:57–66.

32. Meshul CK, Cogen JP, Cheng H-W, *et al.* Alterations in rat striatal glutamate synapses following a lesion of the cortico- and/or nigrostriatal pathway. *Exp Neurol.* 2000;**165**:191–206.

33. Ganeshina O, Berry RW, Petralia RS, *et al.* Synapses with a segmented, completely partitioned postsynaptic density express more AMPA receptors than other axospinous synaptic junctions. *Neuroscience.* 2004;**125**:615–23.

34. McNeill TH, Brown SA, Hogg E, *et al.* Synapse replacement in the striatum of the adult rat following unilateral cortex ablation. *J Comp Neurol.* 2003;**467**:32–43.

35. Raisman G, Field PM. Synapse formation in the adult brain after lesions and after transplantation of embryonic tissue. *J Exp Biol.* 1990;**153**:277–87.

36. Petcu EB, Sfredel V, Platt D, *et al.* Cellular and molecular events underlying the dysregulated response of the aged brain to stroke: A mini-review. *Gerontology.* 2008;**54**:6–17.

37. Carmichael ST, Chesselet MF. Synchronous neuronal activity is a signal for axonal sprouting after cortical lesions in the adult. *J Neurosci.* 2002;**22**:6062–70.

38. Dancause N, Barbay S, Frost SB, *et al.* Effects of small ischemic lesions in the primary motor cortex on neurophysiological organization in ventral premotor cortex. *J Neurophysiol.* 2006;**96**:3506–11.

39. Nudo RJ. Postinfarct cortical plasticity and behavioral recovery. *Stroke.* 2007;**38**:840–5.

40. Brus-Ramer M, Carmel JB, Chakrabarty S, *et al.* Electrical stimulation of spared corticospinal axons augments connections with ipsilateral spinal motor circuits after injury. *J Neurosci.* 2007;**27**:13 793–801.

41. Lichtenwalner RJ, Parent JM. Adult neurogenesis and the ischemic forebrain. *J Cereb Blood Flow Metab.* 2006;**26**:1–20.

42. Ohab JJ, Fleming S, Blesch A, *et al.* A neurovascular niche for neurogenesis after stroke. *J Neurosci.* 2006;**26**:13 007–16.

43. Gotts JE, Chesselet MF. Migration and fate of newly born cells after focal cortical ischemia in adult rats. *J Neurosci Res.* 2005;**80**:160–71.

44. Adkins DL, Voorhies AC, Jones TA. Behavioral and neuroplastic effects of focal endothelin-1 induced sensorimotor cortex lesions. *Neuroscience.* 2004;**128**:473–86.

45. Allred RP, Jones, TA. Experience – a double edged sword for restorative neural plasticity after brain damage. *Future Neurol.* 2008;**3**:189–98.

46. Taub E, Uswatte G, Mark VW, *et al.* The learned nonuse phenomenon: Implications for rehabilitation. *Eura Medicophys.* 2006;**42**:241–56.

47. Whishaw IQ. Loss of the innate cortical engram for action patterns used in skilled reaching and the development of behavioral compensation following motor cortex lesions in the rat. *Neuropharmacology.* 2000;**39**:788–805.

48. Hsu JE, Jones TA. Contralesional neural plasticity and functional changes in the less-affected forelimb after large and small cortical infarcts in rats. *Exp Neurol.* 2006;**201**:479–94.

49. Allred RP, Maldonado MA, Hsu And JE, *et al.* Training the "less-affected" forelimb after unilateral cortical infarcts interferes with functional recovery of the impaired forelimb in rats. *Restor Neurol Neurosci.* 2005;**23**:297–302.

50. Jablonka JA, Witte OW, Kossut M. Photothrombotic infarct impairs experience-dependent plasticity in neighboring cortex. *Neuroreport.* 2007;**18**:165–9.

51. Ward NS, Cohen LG. Mechanisms underlying recovery of motor function after stroke. *Arch Neurol.* 2004;**61**:1844–8.

52. Rose FD, Davey MJ, Attree EA. How does environmental enrichment aid performance following cortical injury in the rat? *Neuroreport.* 1993;**4**:163–6.

53. Greenough WT, Fass B, DeVoogd TJ. The influence of experience on recovery following brain damage in rodents: Hypotheses based on development research. In: Walsh RN, Greenough WT, editors. *Environments as therapy for brain dysfunction.* New York, NY: Plenum Press; 1976: pp. 10–50.

54. Vaynman S, Gomez-Pinilla F. License to run: Exercise impacts functional plasticity in the intact and injured central nervous system by using neurotrophins. *Neurorehabil Neural Repair.* 2005;**19**:283–95.

55. Silasi G, Hamilton DA, Kolb B. Social instability blocks functional restitution following motor cortex stroke in rats. *Behav Brain Res.* 2008;**188**:219–26.

56. Salter K, Hellings C, Foley N, *et al.* The experience of living with stroke: A qualitative meta-synthesis. *J Rehabil Med.* 2008;**40**:595–602.

57. Chu CJ, Jones TA. Experience-dependent structural plasticity in cortex heterotopic to focal sensorimotor cortical damage. *Exp Neurol.* 2000;**166**:403–14.

58. Maldonado MA, Allred RP, Felthauser EL, *et al.* Motor skill training, but not voluntary exercise, improves skilled reaching after unilateral ischemic lesions of the sensorimotor cortex in rats. *Neurorehabil Neural Repair.* 2008;**22**:250–61.

59. Alaverdashvili M, Foroud A, Lim DH, *et al.* "Learned baduse" limits recovery of skilled reaching for food after forelimb motor cortex stroke in rats: A new analysis of the effect of gestures on success. *Behav Brain Res.* 2008;**188**:281–90.

60. Barbay S, Plautz EJ, Friel KM, *et al.* Behavioral and neurophysiological effects of delayed training following a small ischemic infarct in primary motor cortex of squirrel monkeys. *Exp Brain Res.* 2005;**5**:1–11.

61. Biernaskie J, Chernenko G, Corbett D. Efficacy of rehabilitative experience declines with time after focal ischemic brain injury. *J Neurosci.* 2004;**24**:1245–54.

62. Goldstein LB. Neurotransmitters and motor activity: Effects on functional recovery after brain injury. *NeuroRx.* 2006;**3**:451–7.

63. Plow EB, Carey JR, Nudo RJ, *et al.* Cortical stimulation to promote recovery of function after stroke: A critical appraisal. *Stroke.* 2009;**40**:1926–31.

64. Edwards D, Fregni F. Modulating the healthy and affected motor cortex with repetitive transcranial magnetic stimulation in stroke: Development of new strategies for neurorehabilitation. *NeuroRehabilitation.* 2008;**23**:3–14.

65. Adkins-Muir DL, Jones TA. Cortical electrical stimulation combined with rehabilitative training: Enhanced functional recovery and dendritic plasticity following focal cortical ischemia in rats. *Neurol Res.* 2003;**25**:780–8.

66. Adkins DL, Hsu JE, Jones TA. Motor cortical stimulation promotes synaptic plasticity and behavioral improvements following sensorimotor cortex lesions. *Exp Neurol.* 2008;**212**:14–28.

67. Kleim JA, Bruneau R, VandenBerg P, *et al.* Motor cortex stimulation enhances motor recovery and reduces peri-infarct dysfunction following ischemic insult. *Neurol Res.* 2003;**25**:789–93.

68. Teskey GC, Flynn C, Goertzen CD, *et al.* Cortical stimulation improves skilled forelimb use following a focal ischemic infarct in the rat. *Neurol Res.* 2003;**25**:794–800.

69. Schallert T, Leasure JL, Kolb B. Experience-associated structural events, subependymal cellular proliferative activity, and functional recovery after injury to the central nervous system. *J Cereb Blood Flow Metab.* 2000;**20**:1513–28.

70. Woodlee MT, Schallert T. The impact of motor activity and inactivity on the brain. *Curr Directions Psychol Sci.* 2006;**15**:203–06.

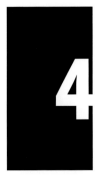

4 Post-stroke recovery therapies in animals

G. Campbell Teskey & Bryan Kolb

Introduction

One of the primary reasons scientists perform post-stroke recovery research on rodents is to determine the usefulness or efficacy of certain treatments or therapies. The foundation for the validity of animal research is the extended common history that other animals share with our species and the relatively conservative process by which evolutionary change takes place (Chapter 7). Thus there should be constancy in cerebral organization and function, both between and within mammalian species (Chapter 1). That said, the failure of clinical trials for certain treatments that were effective in animal models has raised an opposing view, expressed in its most extreme form as "animal research tells us nothing about whether a treatment will be effective in people." Whereas some postulated reasons for the failure of the clinical trials have been summarized elsewhere [1], here we offer a series of considerations that should be well contemplated when adopting an animal model to investigate whether a certain treatment or therapy will be effective and potentially translate to people that have sustained a stroke. The considerations fall into four broad categories: intervention issues, organismal factors, modeling stroke, and measurement. We also review four categories of treatments and therapies that are utilized in animal models to facilitate recovery: enrichment/experience, pharmacotherapy, cell-based therapies, and electrical stimulation.

Considerations (Table 4.1)

Timing and intensity of intervention

When a cerebral attack or stroke occurs there is a non-trivial interruption of the blood supply to one of the cerebral arteries. This sets off a domino-like cascade of neurodegenerative changes that develop over several timescales (Figure 4.1). The drop in oxygen concentration causes changes in the ionic balance of the affected regions over the first seconds to minutes, including changes in pH and properties of the cell membrane. These ionic changes result in a variety of pathological events, including the release of excessive amounts of glutamate and the prolonged opening of calcium channels. The open calcium channels allow high levels of calcium to enter the cell, which in turn leads to a number of toxic effects that result in cell death. The development of considerable edema (swelling) is a major complication over the first day following stroke. The swelling itself can cause neuronal injury, dysfunction, and death. These post-stroke changes in neuronal functioning lead to a drop in metabolic rate and/or glucose utilization in the injured hemisphere that may persist for days. Moreover, areas that receive synaptic input from the primarily damaged area suffer a sudden withdrawal of excitation or inhibition. Such sudden changes in input lead to a greater loss of function and secondary cell death that may be even more pronounced than the cell death resulting directly from the injury itself. Following cell death, inflammatory processes begin almost immediately. Microglia invade the damaged region via the vascular system and clear away degenerative debris, a process that may take months to complete. Astrocytes adjacent to the lesioned area enlarge and extend fibrous processes that serve to isolate the surfaces of the injury from the surrounding tissue. Stem cells may also be stimulated to increase division in the subventricular zone and to migrate to the injury, although we do not yet know what function these cells might have. Thus, when considering a treatment, the timing of the intervention in relation to the post-stroke neurodegenerative cascade must be evaluated.

Treatments for cerebral injury can be targeted at different aspects of the neurodegenerative cascade. Agents that are designed to protect neurons from the

Brain Repair After Stroke, ed. S. C. Cramer and R. J. Nudo. Published by Cambridge University Press.
© Cambridge University Press 2010.

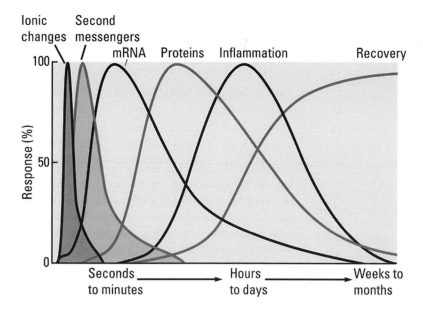

Figure 4.1 Time course of post-stroke events in the neurodegenerative cascade.

cascade of toxic events that follow an ischemic episode are called neuroprotectants. For example, drugs can be used to block calcium channels or prevent ionic imbalance. There are also new classes of drugs targeting novel channels. One example is the transient receptor potential (trp) channels that mediate the response of a cell to extracellular environmental changes by increasing or decreasing the selective permeability to particular ions. Lowering of temperature and thus slowing metabolism is another promising immediate post-stroke treatment [2]. Obviously the field of neuroprotection is critically important and should receive more inquiry.

Treatments that make use of plasticity, the endogenous ability to change the structure and function of the brain, are normally initiated some time after the ischemic insult. It is important to consider that if initiated in the immediate post-injury period, some types of activities might actually make cell death worse or interfere with beneficial plastic changes. During the course of studies investigating the promotion of functional recovery after injury, Schallert and his colleagues accidentally found that initiating intense therapy soon after a stroke worsened the damage [3] (see Chapter 8). In these studies, rats were fitted with a restraint harness that prevented them from using the forelimb ipsilateral to a sensorimotor cortex injury, thus forcing use of the impaired limb. Unfortunately, the rats that had continual forced use of the affected limb showed significantly enlarged lesion cavity and

worse functional outcome. Although few human stroke treatments would be this intense, the Schallert studies focus attention on the question of when therapy should commence and how intense it should be.

Related to the timing of the treatment or therapy is the intensity or amount of intervention. Our field is not sufficiently advanced to enable us to know a priori the amount of drug or intensity of therapy that will have the optimal effect. Similar to deriving a dose–response curve, researchers need to assess a series of different intensities of therapies for particular patient groups. Moreover, individual differences in responses should also be considered. There is growing evidence that patients who are placed in a dedicated stroke unit, rather than being treated on an outpatient basis, are likely to show a better outcome because they receive more intensive treatment from a variety of healthcare professionals.

Organismal factors

Age

Strokes can occur at any age with a relatively high incidence of cerebral attack in the young, usually at birth. However, most people that sustain and survive a stroke are aged. It has long been known that, on average, children seem to have a better outcome after injury than adults. Kolb has examined the behavior of adult rats that received focal injuries to the medial prefrontal, motor, temporal, posterior parietal, or posterior cingulate cortex on postnatal days 1, 4, 7, 10, or 90 (i.e., adult) [4]. The overall result was that regardless of the location of injury, the functional outcome was always best after injury sustained during the second week of life, which in the rat is a time of intense cerebral synaptogenesis and glial formation. The take-home message is that it is the stage of neural development, and not age per se, that is the important variable in recovery.

Injured young brains have been shown to compensate for lost tissue in three ways: (1) reorganization of existing neuronal networks; (2) development of novel networks; and (3) regeneration of the lost tissue (which is dealt with later in the chapter). Existing normal circuits are found to reorganize following unilateral damage to motor systems. When damage occurs to the cortex that normally gives rise to the corticobulbar and corticospinal pathways, the intact pathway on the opposite side sprouts both an enlarged ipsilateral corticospinal pathway as well as new connections to subcortical motor regions of the damaged hemisphere [5]. Similar findings are seen in sensory systems as novel pathways develop after damage [6]. Neuronal network remodeling in the form of changes to dendritic morphology have also been observed after early injuries. The overall result of these studies is that when functional outcome is positive, there is an increase in dendritic arborization and spine density in pyramidal neurons in the remaining cortex. When functional outcome is poor, however, there is an atrophy of dendritic arbor and spine density.

It is generally assumed that as animals age they become less plastic. Teuber reported that brain-injured soldiers also showed a benefit of younger age: 18-year-olds fared better than 25-year-olds, who in turn fared better than older soldiers [7]. Although it has been shown that older animals demonstrate less synaptic potentiation in response to high-frequency stimulation [8], even senescent animals can show considerable cortical plasticity [9]. Systematic studies of cerebral plasticity and behavior throughout the life span in both normal and brain-injured animals are still required. Moreover, the health status and life-history of experience rather than the age of the animal may be the predominant factor.

Comorbid conditions

Most people that survive a stroke often have a variety of other pre-existing medical conditions such as diabetes, arthritis, atherosclerosis, and hypertension that

need to be modeled by stroke researchers. For instance, a clinically relevant model of human stroke is the stroke-prone spontaneously hypertensive rat. This strain of rat has been shown to have a genetic predisposition to cerebral ischemia and exhibits hypertension and an increased sensitivity to experimentally induced stroke. Following stroke, these rats exhibit greater impaired functional recovery compared to a normotensive strain from which the hypertensive strain was derived [10]. The usage of animal models that replicate at least some of the more prevalent comorbid conditions in people that have had strokes will need to be more fully embraced by researchers.

Most stroke survivors take numerous medications for a variety of ailments and conditions. For instance, because clinical depression is found in the majority of stroke survivors (see Chapter 14), the prescription of specific serotonin reuptake inhibitors (SSRIs) has been almost universal where available. SSRIs have been shown to alter brain activity and modulate motor performance in stroke patients in a use-dependent fashion. Moreover, several antidepressants, including fluoxetine, increase growth factors and other proteins associated with plasticity, such as brain-derived neurotrophic factor (BDNF). In one study, however, the addition of fluoxetine treatment to rehabilitation therapy did not alter the degree or rate of recovery of function compared to non-treated animals [11]. In another study, fluoxetine did not affect sensorimotor or water-maze performance in aged rats after experimental stroke [12]. The ability of fluoxetine to alter brain activity and increase growth factors does not appear to be an effective pharmacological adjunct to rehabilitative therapy after ischemia in rats.

Seizures are observed following strokes in people and are also commonly observed following the creation of a stroke in animal models. Many investigators ignore the seizures and treat them as a nuisance. However, the duration and severity of seizures can dramatically affect stroke size and behavioral outcome, with long seizures associated with a negative outcome. Seizures can dramatically change the balance between excitation and inhibition, resulting in reorganized movement representations [13] and sensory function [14]. Moreover, seizures are known to reorganize circuits through Hebbian-like algorithms due to the coincident firing of pre- and postsynaptic neurons that occurs during an ictal event. Thus, seizures may "use up" plastic capacity, leaving the brain less responsive to treatments and therapies. Alternatively, brief and mild seizures are known to stimulate the production and release of growth factors, which in turn could support vulnerable neurons, prevent cell death and assist in the formation of new circuits. A common view in the medical community seems to be that all seizures are bad and should be treated with anticonvulsants. This leads to two problems: (1) not all seizures may be associated with negative outcomes and may in certain circumstances be beneficial or at least innocuous, and (2) anticonvulsant medications themselves are known to be associated with developmental delays and poorer functional recovery [15]. The take-home message on seizures is that they should not be ignored in experimental settings because they represent an important variable that needs to be understood.

Sex and hormonal status

Males and females have been shown to have different responses to brain injury and post-injury treatments. For example, the effect of frontal injury in both humans and rats is more severe in females than in males [4]. When rats with similar frontal injuries early in development were placed in complex environments, there was a greater benefit of the treatment on cognitive functions for male rats than for females, whereas the opposite pattern of results was found for motor functions [16]. Moreover, the cyclic nature of hormone levels and hormonal status (e.g. menopause) can also influence plasticity and, thus, recovery processes [17]. How the existing medical condition, medications and brain injury interact will likely be an extremely complex puzzle to untangle.

Modeling stroke

Occlusion of the middle cerebral artery (MCA), which is responsible for the majority of thrombotic strokes in humans, is the most widely employed model of stroke using rodents. This leads to a problem for those of us interested in functional recovery. The problem is that the infarct volume following MCA occlusion in rodents is proportionally very much larger than that found in humans, always involves both gray and white matter, and is devastating from a behavioral perspective. Thus, while the MCA occlusion has face validity, it is not a good choice for those interested in examining behavioral recovery. There are other methods to induce focal ischemic infarcts that can be fairly precisely localized to specific brain regions that leave

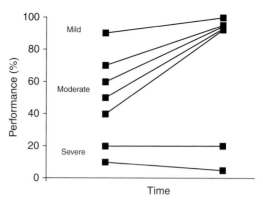

Figure 4.2 Amount of available recovery post-stroke. Animals with mild strokes recover fully but can only show small improvements. Animals with moderate strokes can show substantial recovery. Animals with severe strokes often do not recover and show progressive deterioration.

substantial tissue intact that will support functional recovery. These methods can also be used to lesion either gray or white matter (or both) and to target specific locations. The location of the stroke and type of impairment is also important, because this determines whether the infarct gives rise to sensory, motor, or cognitive impairment.

People who survive strokes vary in the degree of impairment from mild to catastrophic (see Figure 4.2). Those with mild impairments often make a full recovery to the point that they do not manifest obvious impairment of function. At the opposite end of the spectrum there are individuals who survive a stroke that will be maintained on artificial life support for the remainder of their life. In the laboratory, treatments are usually tested for efficacy in animals with moderate impairments, while severely and mildly impaired animals are removed from the study for ethical and practical reasons. Researchers should consider examining the amount of impairment on an individual animal basis to determine the relationship between the degree of impairment and the efficacy of the therapy. This is an important consideration from the perspective of industry, as they are interested in identifying individuals that will reap the most benefit from their treatment.

Measurement issues

Researchers routinely report quantitative end-point measures of the behaviors of their subjects. End-point measures, such as latency to initiate a movement or duration to complete a task, or percent success at

Table 4.1 Several considerations when modeling post-stroke treatment or therapy in animals.

Consideration category	Subcategories	Specifics
Intervention		
	Timing of intervention	How long after stroke
	Intensity of intervention	How much of the day and for how long
	Persistence of treatment effect	Duration of benefit
Organismal factors		
	Age at time of stroke	Newborn, young, adult, aged
	Comorbid conditions	Other medical conditions (atherosclerosis, coronary disease, diabetes, hypertension), medications, seizures
	Sex	Male, female
	Hormonal status	Juvenile, adult, post-menopausal
Modeling strokes		
	Type of stroke	Global, focal (thrombotic, hemorrhagic)
	Location of stroke	Gray matter, white matter, mixed
	Kind of impairment	Motor, sensory, cognitive, mixed
	Degree of impairment	Severe, moderate, mild
	Stroke induction methodology	Arterial occlusion, focal (pial strip, electrocautery, photothrombotic)
Measurement		
	Species	Size of brain (proportion of gray and white matter), available behavioral repertoire, practical (cost) and ethical (companion animals) concerns
	Measurement	End points of success, behavioral strategies (recovery or compensation)

retrieving a pellet, are three common examples. While end-point measures are important, they capture only a sliver of the whole behavior of the animal. Taking a more comprehensive approach to behavioral measurement can lead to important insights. For instance, Whishaw and colleagues developed a 10-point kinematic analysis of how rats use their forelimb when retrieving a food pellet [18]. Brain-injured rats often perform differently from controls on the task even though their end-point measures may be equivalent. Thus, a wealth of important data that are available to

the researcher should be utilized. Unfortunately, the measurement sophistication and detail in the clinic are often quite crude and are lagging behind those employed by animal researchers in the lab.

Each mammalian species has a behavioral repertoire available to it. The repertoire represents the whole range of behaviors supported by their brains and bodies. Rats in particular are highly skilled at reaching and performing fine and dexterous manipulations with their forelimbs [19]; thus, they provide wonderful models for behavioral study. However, there are important structural differences in the shoulder and wrist anatomy between rats and primates (including humans) and the differences must be accounted for when drawing parallels to humans. Simply put, species differences in sensory, cognitive, and motor function (e.g. bees have a visual range that includes the ultraviolet and dogs lack color vision) must be considered when examining and interpreting their behaviors.

Enrichment/experience

Studies of laboratory animals have consistently shown that the single most successful treatment strategy for optimizing functional recovery from a variety of forms of experimental brain injuries is placing animals in complex, stimulating environments [4,20]. Although the mechanisms responsible for the beneficial effects of complex housing are not fully known, it has been hypothesized that the treatment may increase the synthesis of neurotrophic factors, which in turn facilitate synaptic plasticity. Motor training has been shown to upregulate trophic factors such as BDNF and basic fibroblast growth factor (bFGF or FGF-2) [21], so we might anticipate that rehabilitative motor training after cerebral injury would also be beneficial. There is some evidence of benefits from repetitive motor training [22], and this type of training is often used by physiotherapists. Such treatments have not always been found to be beneficial, however, and the differences may be related to the details of the training.

Pharmacotherapy

Drug therapies can provide a relatively easy and cost-effective means of facilitating plastic changes in the injured brain that would support functional improvement. Psychomotor stimulants such as amphetamine or nicotine are known to stimulate changes in cortical and subcortical circuits in the normal brain. It is thus reasonable to suppose that these agents could stimulate plastic changes in the injured brain to facilitate recovery. Nicotine appears to facilitate recovery from strokes in motor regions and does so by supporting synaptic changes in spared motor regions [23]. These changes are correlated with both qualitative and quantitative changes in behavior. Amphetamine has also been shown to be beneficial in rats, but has had mixed clinical success. Kolb and colleagues have compared the effects of amphetamine on recovery from focal versus more extensive strokes [24]. Amphetamine

was effective in producing both synaptic change and behavioral improvement after focal cortical injuries, but showed little benefit after large middle cerebral occlusions. In contrast, nicotine still produced some benefit after larger strokes. One important difference between the drugs is that nicotine has more widespread effects on cortical circuitry than does amphetamine [25], a difference that may account for the added benefits of nicotine after cerebral injury. However, it should be recognized that the effect of nicotine was studied by giving rats nicotine alone and not in conjunction with smoke and other contaminants related to taking nicotine by smoking tobacco. It seems likely that post-injury smoking would not be the ideal treatment, especially after stroke. Moreover, the nicotine was delivered to naïve rats that did not have prior experience with nicotine. The beneficial effects of nicotine should not be assumed to occur in individuals with extensive experience with the drug.

Growth factors and their analogs form another class of compounds that hold promise in enhancing recovery after stroke. The first neurotrophic factor to be described was nerve growth factor (NGF), and later Kolb and colleagues showed that it produced about 20% increases in the dendritic arborization and spine density in cortical pyramidal neurons in otherwise normal animals [26]. A subsequent study showed that rats with large cortical strokes had about a 20% decrease in dendritic arborization in the remaining motor regions and that this loss was completely reversed by NGF [27]. Although the results of this study were compelling, the difficulty with NGF as a potential treatment is that it is expensive and does not pass the blood–brain barrier, a drawback that does not affect FGF-2. FGF-2 holds promise as a potential treatment because psychomotor stimulants also transiently increase FGF-2 [28]. There is evidence that administration of FGF-2 after stroke can stimulate functional improvement, although the effects were small and task-dependent [29]. A later study found that while FGF-2 alone had a minimal effect on recovery from motor cortex injury, FGF-2 was very effective in stimulating functional improvement when given in combination with rehabilitation training or complex housing. Furthermore, the functional improvement was correlated with increased synaptogenesis in the remaining motor regions. It may be the case that the endogenous production of neurotrophic factors is potentiated by experience [30]. Thus, it is possible that one mechanism whereby experience facilitates functional recovery is by increasing the endogenous production of neurotrophic factors, which in turn stimulate synaptic changes. For example, allowing animals to spontaneously run in running wheels or explore complex environments can increase levels of growth factors, stimulate neurogenesis, increase resistance to brain injury, and improve learning and mental performance [31]. Little is known, however, about the optimal timing or intensity of exercise needed to maximally enhance behavioral outcome or neuronal plasticity.

Cell-based therapies

The rapid progress in stem cell biology in recent years has led to an increasing interest in regeneration-based treatment strategies for damaged adult brain tissue. These novel tactics are based on two general approaches, namely replenishment of lost cells by transplantation, and enhanced activation of endogenous stem cells. Both approaches have their strengths and weaknesses with respect to practical and ethical considerations. A perfect scenario for recovery involving endogenous stem cells would at least involve the following general steps. Precursor cells are upregulated to sufficient levels to replace the cells lost due to the stroke. The cells then migrate to the site of injury and differentiate into the lost cell types (neurons, astrocytes, oligodendroglia, and others) and the uncounted myriad of subtypes (e.g. excitatory projection pyramidal cells and local inhibitory interneurons), in the correct, brain area-specific proportions. The neurons then form a working neural network with appropriate internal circuitry and correct synaptic connections with the spared tissue. In parallel, glial cells would provide their supportive and myelination roles. Finally, on the systems level the new tissue must operate correctly to restore function for the ultimate goal of regenerative medicine to be achieved. While at first this scenario may seem highly improbable, it should be remembered that during development most of this process occurs. The trick is to get the adult brain to recapitulate the normal developmental sequences within the lesioned area and then make proper contact with existing tissue. Thus, from a basic science perspective we need to fully understand the principles and specifics of brain development if we are to achieve brain tissue replacement.

A fortuitous observation that the medial prefrontal cortex can regenerate in postnatal rats provides a model of brain tissue replacement. Pioneering studies by Bryan Kolb demonstrated that neonatal rats that received medial frontal cortex lesions at 10 days of age exhibited spontaneous filling-in of the lesion cavity [32] and, when assessed as adults, these animals showed restitution of some behavioral abilities that are dependent on an intact medial frontal cortex [33]. Although the spontaneous regeneration that can occur after medial prefrontal cortex (mPFC) lesions is uncommon in other structures, it can be induced by infusion of FGF-2 after cortical injury on day 10 [34,35]. Richard Dyck confirmed the observations of spontaneous regeneration in mice lesioned at postnatal day 7 and extended this model to make use of transgenic technologies and thus identify molecular and genetic substrates that are necessary for regeneration. This understudied phenomenon could lead to enormous breakthroughs in the development of brain repair technologies.

The perfect scenario for recovery may be out of reach given our current limitations, but it is quite reasonable to propose a beneficial role of neuronal stem cells (see also Chapter 24). The exploitation of endogenous neural stem cells for therapeutic purposes has been investigated within a number of disease models including stroke. Experimental models of stroke induce proliferation of stem cells resident in the subventricular zone and/or dentate gyrus (Figure 4.3). Neuronal migration is rerouted from the rostral migratory stream to damaged cortex and striatum. Likewise, cells resident in the dentate gyrus will migrate to the lesion site within the hippocampus. Once at the lesion site, these new cells incorporate into the ischemic penumbra. Although most of these cells die within the first few weeks [36], those cells that do survive appear to differentiate into the predominant neuronal or glial phenotype and integrate into the existing circuitry. Unfortunately, this small number of surviving cells is not enough to support full functional recovery. As such, methods aimed at further increasing proliferation, differentiation, and survival are required to make optimal use of intrinsic stem cells. Singly and in combination, epidermal growth factor (EGF), FGF-2, and erythropoietin (EPO) have been shown to assist in the differentiation and survival of new neurons. Kolb and colleagues gave adult rats an ischemic lesion to the primary motor cortex and treated them three days later with EGF followed by EPO [27]. This treatment resulted in tissue regeneration concomitant with motor recovery. Importantly,

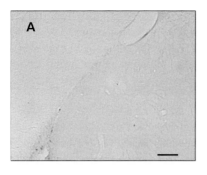
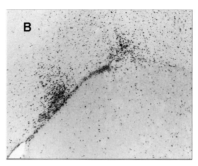
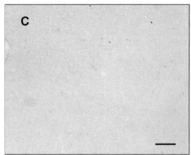
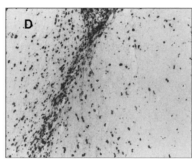

Figure 4.3 Bromodeoxyuridine (BrdU)-stained cells indicating cellular genesis after motor cortex lesion. Panels A (non-lesioned) and B (lesioned) indicate BrdU cells immediately dorsal to the lateral ventricle (bottom left in panels). Panels C (non-lesioned) and D (lesioned) indicate BrdU cells at cortical lesion sites. Cellular genesis is upregulated following lesion and cells migrate from the subventricular zone to the lesion sites. Scale bar in A is 300 μm and in C is 100 μm.

when this new tissue was removed following behavioral recovery the deficit re-emerged, demonstrating the importance of the new tissue to recovery. However, the exact role the new tissue plays in supporting recovery is not known. Two reasonable hypotheses are that the new area may be re-establishing lost connections, or playing an indirect role through enhancing cortical plasticity. One such possibility is that the new tissue secreted growth factors that increase plasticity of the adjacent tissue and thus promote functional improvement. The inappropriate migration, differentiation, and integration of numerous new neurons in the hippocampal dentate gyrus after prolonged and severe seizures brings home the point that the detection and prevention of status epilepticus in animal models is of paramount importance [37].

Importantly, adult neurogenesis is not the only self-repair mechanism of damaged CNS tissue. As the glial response and angiogenesis are active participants in repair mechanisms, the appropriate interactions among neurons, glial cells and vascular systems are crucial for functional CNS repair.

Astrocytes

The roles of reactive astrocytes in the repair of damaged CNS tissue have been controversial. Reactive astrocytes are thought to produce chondroitin sulfate proteoglycan, which inhibits axonal regeneration, thereby exerting a detrimental effect on CNS repair. However, reactive astrocytes also have beneficial effects on repair: they were shown to play a crucial role in wound healing and functional recovery before the completion of glial scar formation. Astrocytes surrounding the lesion undergo characteristic changes involving hypertrophy, process extension, and the increased expression of intermediate filaments. Astrocytes also migrate to the lesion area and compact inflammatory cells, thereby contracting the lesion area. Stat3, a principal mediator in a variety of biologic processes including cancer progression, wound healing, and the movement of various types of cells, is required for astrocyte migration. Thus, Stat3 signaling and reactive astrocytes may be potential new therapeutic targets for the treatment of CNS injury such as stroke.

Vascular system

Angiogenesis, the creation of new blood vessels, is known to occur following cerebral infarction. The expression of several angiogenesis-related genes is regulated in an orchestrated fashion in the brain after ischemia [38]. The role of the vascular system in CNS repair appears to be highly significant, and the potential roles of blood vessels as scaffolds for neuroblast migration in ischemic brain are intriguing. Palmer and colleagues speculated that neurogenesis was intimately associated with a process of active vascular recruitment and subsequent remodeling [39]. Adult neurogenesis occurs within an "angiogenic niche," which may provide an interface where mesenchyme-derived cells and circulating factors influence plasticity in the adult CNS [40]. Vascular endothelial cells released soluble factors that stimulated the self-renewal of neural stem cells, suggesting vascular endothelial cells to be a critical component of neural stem cell survival.

Our current knowledge base regarding the functions of newly generated cells must be expanded. Answering the question of the functional significance of adult cell genesis in intact animals is also of the utmost importance as we try to co-opt these mechanisms to repair damaged systems.

Electrical stimulation

Compared to other treatments and therapies, electrical stimulation has received much less attention. However, stimulating the surface of the brain as a means to modulate regional activity during motor performance is emerging as a promising approach for facilitating rehabilitative interventions after stroke. The premise is that cortical stimulation recruits neurons that may otherwise be insufficiently activated during task performance and that this enables activity-dependent synaptic plasticity that mediates recovery of skilled movements in the impaired forelimb. As a proof of principle, studies in rats with infarcts of the sensorimotor cortex indicate that the efficacy of rehabilitation can be enhanced by coupling it with cortical stimulation through electrodes positioned over peri-infarct areas (Figure 4.4). Thus cortical stimulation is really an adjunctive treatment to behavioral therapy. In this approach the minimum amount of current to elicit a forelimb movement is first determined. This also establishes that the electrode has been placed in the correct location and is capable of activating a movement – a practice that is, in our opinion, critical for translation into clinical trials. Then as the animals undergo daily training on a skilled reaching task they receive current at an intensity that is sub-threshold (usually 50%) to evoke movements. Several laboratories using different kinds of stroke induction methods (endothelin-1, pial strip, and electrocautery) have shown efficacy with bipolar or monopolar stimulation between 40 and 70% of initial movement thresholds and between 50 and 100 Hz.

Not all the neural mechanisms underlying these functional effects are known. However, cortical stimulation-induced improvements in reaching success

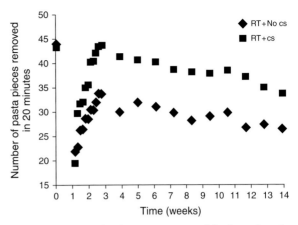

Figure 4.4 Enhanced and persistent recovery following unilateral focal ischemic infarct to sensorimotor neocortex. At baseline (0) rats demonstrate proficient use of a forelimb to retrieve pieces of pasta and then they undergo a focal ischemic infarct. One week post-stroke they demonstrate moderate impairment. Rats then receive two weeks of rehabilitative training (RT) on a motor task with (squares) or without (diamonds) electrical cortical stimulation (CS) using 100 Hz cathodal stimulation at 50% of movement threshold. Rats that received both the rehabilitative therapy and electrical stimulation show superior performance (weeks 2–3). Weekly follow-up testing without stimulation shows the enhanced performance persists (weeks 4–14).

[41] coincide with neuroplastic changes in the stimulated region of the sensorimotor cortex, including increased surface density of layer V dendritic processes [42], greater density of synapses with multisynaptic boutons and perforated post-synaptic densities that are presumed to be more efficacious [43], expansion of movement representations detected using intracortical microstimulation mapping in rats [44] as well as in monkeys [45], and enlargement of the polysynaptic component of motor cortical evoked potentials that is indicative of propagating neural activity through a network [46]. All of these enhancements were observed in comparison to animals receiving rehabilitation alone. The combination of task practice and cortical stimulation may aid in inducing greater structural and functional plasticity within adjacent cortical and, possibly, corticospinal pathways [47] leading to greater motor recovery following stroke. Elucidating the specific neural mechanisms mediating these functional improvements should assist with motor "re-learning" after brain damage [48].

Summary

When the brain is injured, there are both degenerative and reparative processes that occur over seconds to months. Degenerative processes produce the non-specific effects of the brain injury, such as the loss of cells and synapses in widespread brain regions. The reparative changes that follow use the brain's endogenous capacity to restructure, allowing compensatory behaviors to emerge and improve performance. Several treatments and therapies appear to facilitate the rate and extent of behavioral recovery, many of which work best when used in combination. There are many factors and issues that should be considered when selecting and implementing an animal model of stroke. Learning more about the brain's ability to relearn should help us improve recovery and quality of life for people who have had a stroke.

References

1. Gladstone DJ, Black SE, Hakim AM. Toward wisdom from failure: Lessons from neuroprotective stroke trials and new therapeutic directions. *Stroke*. 2002;**33**:2123–36.

2. Colbourne F, Sutherland G, Corbett D. Postischemic hypothermia. A critical appraisal with implications for clinical treatment. *Mol Neurobiol*. 1997;**14**:171–201.

3. Kozlowski DA, James DC, Schallert T. Use-dependent exaggeration of neuronal injury after unilateral sensorimotor cortex lesions. *J Neurosci*. 1996;**16**:4776–86.

4. Kolb B. *Brain plasticity and behavior*. Philadelphia, PA: Lawrence Erlbaum Associates; 1995.

5. Whishaw IQ, Kolb B. Sparing of skilled forelimb reaching and corticospinal projections after neonatal motor cortex removal or hemidecortication in the rat: Support for the Kennard doctrine. *Brain Res*. 1988;**451**:97–114.

6. Lomber S, Eggermont JJ. *Reprogramming the cerebral cortex*. London: Oxford University Press; 2006.

7. Teuber HL. Recovery of function after brain injury in man. *Ciba Found Symp*. 1975;**34**:159–90.

8. Barnes CA. Long-term potentiation and the ageing brain. *Phil Trans R Soc Lond B Biol Sci*. 2003;**358**:765–72.

9. Kolb B, Whishaw IQ. *Fundamentals of human neuropsychology*. 5th ed. New York: Worth; 2003.

10. McGill JK, Gallagher L, Carswell HV, *et al*. Impaired functional recovery after stroke in the stroke-prone spontaneously hypertensive rat. *Stroke* 2005;**36**:135–41.

11. Windle V, Corbett D. Fluoxetine and recovery of motor function after focal ischemia in rats. *Brain Res*. 2005;**1044**:25–32.

12. Zhao C, Puurunen K, Schallert T, *et al*. Behavioral and histological effects of chronic antipsychotic and antidepressant drug treatment in aged rats with focal ischemic brain injury. *Behav Brain Res*. 2005;**158**:211–20.

13. Teskey GC, Monfils M-H, VandenBerg P, *et al*. Motor map expansion following repeated cortical and limbic seizures is related to synaptic potentiation. *Cereb Cortex*. 2002;**12**:98–105.

14. Valentine PA, Teskey GC, Eggermont JJ. Kindling limits the inter-ictal neuronal temporal response properties in cat primary auditory cortex. *Epilepsia*. 2005;**46**:171–8.

15. Hernandez TD. Preventing post-traumatic epilepsy after brain injury: Weighing the costs and benefits of anticonvulsant prophylaxis. *Trends Pharmacol Sci*. 1997;**18**:59–62.

16. Kolb B, Gibb R, Gorny G. Experience-dependent changes in dendritic arbor and spine density in neocortex vary qualitatively with age and sex. *Neurobiol Learn Mem*. 2003;**79**:1–10.

17. Kolb B, Stewart J. Sex-related differences in dendritic branching of cells in the prefrontal cortex of rats. *J Neuroendocrinol*. 1991;**3**:95–9.

18. Whishaw IQ, Pellis SM, Gorny BP, *et al*. The impairments in reaching and the movements of compensation in rats with motor cortex lesions: an endpoint, videorecording, and movement notation analysis. *Behav Brain Res*. 1991;**42**:77–91.

19. Whishaw IQ, Kolb B. *The behaviour of the laboratory rat*. London: Oxford University Press; 2004.

20. Biernaskie J, Corbett D. Enriched rehabilitative training promotes improved forelimb motor function and enhanced dendritic growth after focal ischemic injury. *J Neurosci*. 2001;**21**:5272–80.

21. Kleim JA, Jones TA, Schallert T. Motor enrichment and the induction of plasticity before or after brain injury. *Neurochem Res*. 2003;**28**:1757–69.

22. Nudo RJ, Wise BM, SiFuentes F, *et al*. Neural substrates for the effects of rehabilitative training on motor recovery after ischemic infarct. *Science*. 1996;**272**:1791–4.

23. Gonzalez CLR, Gharbawie OA, Kolb B. Chronic low-dose administration of nicotine facilitates recovery and synaptic change after focal ischemia in rats. *Neuropharmacology*. 2006;**50**:777–87.

24. Kolb B, Gorny G, Li Y, *et al*. Amphetamine or cocaine limits the ability of later experience to promote structural plasticity in the neocortex and nucleus accumbens. *Proc Natl Acad Sci USA*. 2003;**100**:10 523–8.

25. Robinson TE, Kolb B. Structural plasticity associated with drugs of abuse. *Neuropharmacology*. 2004;**47** Suppl 1: 33–46.

26. Kolb B, Cote S, Ribeiro-da-Silva A, *et al*. Nerve growth factor treatment prevents dendritic atrophy and

promotes recovery of function after cortical injury. *Neuroscience*. 1997;**76**:1139–51.

27. Kolb B, Morshead C, Gonzalez C, *et al.* Growth factor-stimulated generation of new cortical tissue and functional recovery after stroke damage to the motor cortex of rats. *J Cereb Blood Flow Metab*. 2007;**27**:983–97.

28. Flores C, Stewart J. Changes in astrocytic basic fibroblast growth factor expression during and after prolonged exposure to escalating doses of amphetamine. *Neuroscience*. 2000;**98**:287–93.

29. Kawamata T, Speliotes EK, Finklestein SP. The role of polypeptide growth factors in recovery from stroke. *Adv Neurol*. 1997;**73**:377–82.

30. Kolb B, Forgie M, Gibb R, *et al.* Age, experience, and the changing brain. *Neurosci Biobehav Revs*. 1998;**22**:143–59.

31. Cotman CW, Berchtold NC. Exercise: A behavioral intervention to enhance brain health and plasticity. *Trends Neurosci*. 2002;**25**:295–301.

32. Kolb B. Animal models for human PFC-related disorders. *Prog Brain Res*. 1990;**85**:501–19.

33. Kolb B, Petrie B, Cioe J. Recovery from early cortical damage in rats: VII. Comparison of the behavioural and anatomical effects of medial prefrontal lesions at different ages of neural maturation. *Behav Brain Res*. 1996;**79**:1–14.

34. Monfils MH, Driscoll I, Vandenberg PM, *et al.* Basic fibroblast growth factor stimulates functional recovery after neonatal lesions of motor cortex in rats. *Neuroscience* 2005;**134**:1–8.

35. Monfils MH, Driscoll I, Kamitakahara H, *et al.* FGF-2-induced cell proliferation stimulates anatomical, neurophysiological and functional recovery from neonatal motor cortex injury. *Eur J Neurosci*. 2006;**24**:739–49.

36. Arvidsson A, Collin T, Kirik D, *et al.* Neuronal replacement from endogenous precursors in the adult brain after stroke. *Nat Med*. 2002;**8**:963–70.

37. Scharfman HE, Hen R. Is more neurogenesis always better? *Science*. 2007;**315**:336–8.

38. Hayashi T, Noshita N, Sugawara T, *et al.* Temporal profile of angiogenesis and expression of related genes in the brain after ischemia. *J Cereb Blood Flow Metab*. 2003;**23**:166–80.

39. Palmer TD, Willhoite AR, Gage FH. Vascular niche for adult hippocampal neurogenesis. *J Comp Neurol*. 2000;**425**:479–94.

40. Shen Q, Goderie SK, Jin L, *et al.* Endothelial cells stimulate self-renewal and expand neurogenesis of neural stem cells. *Science*. 2004;**304**:1338–40.

41. Adkins DL, Campos P, Quach D, *et al.* Epidural cortical stimulation enhances motor function after sensorimotor cortical infarcts in rats. *Exp Neurol*. 2006;**200**:356–70.

42. Adkins-Muir DL, Jones TA. Cortical electrical stimulation combined with rehabilitative training: Enhanced functional recovery and dendritic plasticity following focal cortical ischemia in rats. *Neurol Res*. 2003;**25**:780–8.

43. Adkins DL, Hsu JE, Jones TA. Motor cortical stimulation promotes synaptic plasticity and behavioral improvements following sensorimotor cortex lesions. *Exp Neurol*. 2008;**212**:14–28.

44. Kleim JA, Bruneau R, VandenBerg P, *et al.* Motor cortex stimulation enhances motor recovery and reduces peri-infarct dysfunction following ischemic insult. *Neurol Res*. 2003;**25**:789–93.

45. Plautz EJ, Barbay S, Frost SB, *et al.* Post-infarct cortical plasticity and behavioral recovery using concurrent cortical stimulation and rehabilitative training: A feasibility study in primates. *Neurol Res*. 2003;**25**:801–10.

46. Teskey GC, Flynn C, Goertzen CD, *et al.* Cortical stimulation improves skilled forelimb use following a focal ischemic infarct in the rat. *Neurol Res*. 2003;**25**:794–800.

47. Brown JA, Lutsep H, Cramer SC, *et al.* Motor cortex stimulation for enhancement of recovery after stroke: Case report. *Neurol Res*. 2003;**25**:815–8.

48. Cramer SC, Bastings EP. Mapping clinically relevant plasticity after stroke. *Neuropharmacology*. 2000;**39**:842–51.

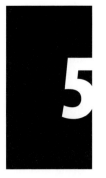

5 Environmental effects on functional outcome after stroke

Barbro B. Johansson

Introduction

Interaction between genes and environment is necessary for all life and has reached the highest level in the human cerebral cortex. The property of the brain to interact and adapt to environmental requirements and multisensory stimulation as well as to our activities, skill acquisitions, and thoughts is referred to as brain plasticity, and it occurs at many levels from molecules and cells to cortical networks [1,2]. Although the concept of plasticity had been proposed earlier, the first known experimental evidence that environment can influence behavior was provided by Donald Hebb in 1947, who reported that rats that were allowed to run around in his house had better memory and higher capacity to solve problems than rats housed in the laboratory [3]. In the 1960s, Rosenzweig and associates demonstrated that functional improvement induced by environmental enrichment was associated with morphological and biochemical changes [4]. Further experimental studies have verified that brain plasticity plays a role in the intact brain and after acute brain disorders [5–8], and there is accumulating evidence that environmental stimulation may have a beneficial influence in delaying the progress in degenerative disorders [9]. We usually talk about the positive aspects of plasticity, but it is important to realize that reduced sensory input and motor activity have the opposite, negative effects. The question dealt with here is what experimental and clinical evidence we have to support that environmental issues are important in stroke rehabilitation [10].

Environment, dendrites and dendritic spines

After a ligation of the middle cerebral artery (MCA), rats housed in an enriched environment during both the pre- and post-ischemic period improve earlier and slightly more than when housed in the enriched environment only during the post-ischemic period. Both groups perform significantly better in a variety of tests than rats housed in single cages, a condition that, in this review, is called deprived housing [11]. Environmental enrichment can also reduce the spatial memory deficit that is caused by cortical infarcts in the rat [12].

A consistent effect of environmental enrichment in intact animals has been on the morphology of dendrites and dendritic spines. It was shown 35 years ago that enriched housing increased the number of dendritic branches and dendritic spines in the intact rat brain [13,14] and many later studies have confirmed these observations [6]. Dendritic spines are the primary postsynaptic targets for excitatory glutaminergic synapses in the mature brain. The dendritic tree is covered with a variety of excitable synaptic channels operating on different timescales and with activity-dependent sensitivity enabling a sophisticated neuronal plasticity.

With a method that allows a three-dimensional view of dendritic spines and optimal quantification of dendrites, three weeks of enriched housing significantly increased the number of dendritic spines per unit length in pyramidal neurons in layers 2/3 and layer 5 compared with rats from the same litter housed in cages with 3–4 rats per cage. After a cortical infarct, the same effect was observed in layer 2/3 neurons in the homotopic contralateral somatosensory cortex (Figure 5.1) [15]. In contrast, the number of layer 5 pyramidal neurons was reduced in both groups with infarcts, most likely due to extensive reduction of connections from the corpus callosum in this model. The three-week postoperative time was chosen because at that time significant differences in functional outcome between enriched, standard (3–4 rats housed together), or deprived rats are well established.

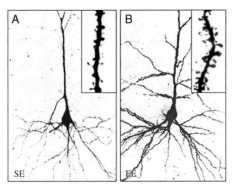

Figure 5.1 Dendritic morphology of pyramidal neurons in layer 2/3 in rats housed in standard (A), or in an enriched environment (B) as viewed in confocal laser scanning microscopy after microinjection of Lucifer yellow into the neurons. Based on data presented in [15].

Layer 2/3 pyramidal neurons are the most abundant cells of the neocortex. They have extensive horizontal connections with ipsilateral cortical regions that are strengthened following skill learning in the rat motor cortex [16]. The environmental effect on the number of dendritic spines in layers 2/3 in the somatosensory cortex is consistent with the better functional outcome, but does not prove a causal connection. To what extent changes in the contralateral cortex are essential for functional recovery is still debated.

Some studies on the effect of environmental enrichment suggest that environment may have some influence and sharpen the borders in somatosensory maps. Thus, the electrophysiological maps of the skin surfaces of the forepaw were compared in rats housed either in standard or enriched environments after weaning. In enriched rats the glabrous skin exhibited a significant representational expansion that occurred at the expense of responses to taps, pressure, or joints and the representation expansion favored the digit tips. In the standard environment condition, the phalanges were represented within a common finger area, whereas the phalanges were clearly separated and thus better defined in the stimulated rats [17]. A comparison between young adult (3.5–5 months), mature (6.5–8 months), and senescent (23–38 months) rats demonstrated that use-dependent remodeling of somatosensory maps occurs throughout life, and that environmental and social interaction can partially offset the age-related breakdown of somatosensory cortical maps [18]. Because a stimulating environment activates many muscles at the same time, the same competition between cortical regions as seen after specific motor training would not be expected [19].

With multiphoton confocal microscopy combined with 3D laser scanning, individual cells and cortical networks can be studied in vivo at a depth of up to 1 mm in the mouse cortex, enabling direct visualization of the behavior of cells in their natural environment and their response to manipulation over long periods of time [20]. The majority of spines are present during the entire imaging period (weeks), but some are transient, appearing and disappearing on a daily basis. Structural plasticity of axonal branches contributes to the remodeling of specific functional circuits. In a photothrombotic stroke model, peri-infarct dendrites were shown to be exceptionally plastic, manifested by a dramatic increase in the rate of spine formation that was maximal at 1–2 weeks (5–8-fold increase) and still evident 6 weeks after stroke [21]. In a longitudinal study of cortical reorganization after an infarct in the somatosensory cortex in mice combining 2 photon imaging with electrophysiology, autoradiography, and behavior, a marked transient increase in neuronal activity was observed in the intact contralateral cortex 2 days after an infarct, and followed by an increased turnover rate of synaptic spines at 1 week. At 4 weeks when functional recovery had occurred, a new pattern of electrical circuit activity in response to somatosensory stimuli was established, indicating that remodeling of neuronal circuits and establishment of new sensory processing in the contralateral hemisphere is possible in a mouse model [22]. So far no study with this in vivo technique has been specifically dedicated to environmental influences.

Gene expression, neurotrophic factors, and neurogenesis

In an enriched environment, animals have the opportunity for enhanced social interactions, and are exposed to multisensorial stimulation provided by the high level of physical activity and the frequent supply of new objects in the cages (Figure 5.2). To evaluate the relative importance of different factors, rats with focal cortical infarcts were housed in enriched, social (i.e. the same number of rats in a large cage but no equipment and objects) with individually housed rats with free access to a running wheel. The rats were tested in a variety of tasks from 2 to 13 weeks after the occlusion. Rats in the enriched environment performed significantly better than the other groups and the social group was better than runners [23]. The data are in agreement with earlier

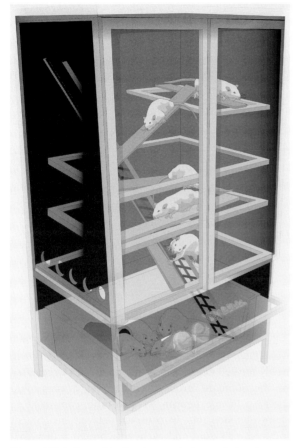

Figure 5.2 In the enriched environment rats can climb, swing, investigate, and handle a number of tools that are changed two or three times a week. The different levels were rearranged making it increasingly difficult to go from one place to another. Rats are particularly active climbing, swinging, and manipulating the tools and objects available in rather skilled ways. The highest activity is during the first hours of the night as shown with infrared video-registration during day and night. Illustration by Bengt Mattsson.

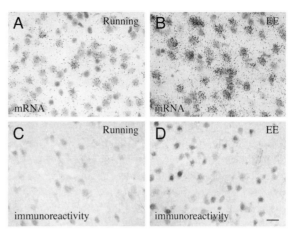

Figure 5.3 Sections showing *NGFI-A* mRNA (A and B) and immunoreactivity (C and D) in the same part of the contralateral parietal cortex one month after MCA occlusion from a rat housed with access to a running wheel (A and C) and a rat in an enriched environment (B and D). Note the higher mRNA and immunoreactivity levels of *NGFI-A* in the enriched rat compared with the running rat. Scale bar 20 µm. From [24], with permission.

data on intact rats demonstrating that social housing cannot explain the full effect of enriched environment and that running, although voluntary, might be stressful in rats with brain lesions [7]. A further study included the similar groups of enriched, social, and runners with the addition of a group of individually housed rats with no access to a running wheel. One month after the cortical infarct the mRNA expression of *NGFI-A* (nerve growth factor-induced gene A), and *NGFI-B* (nerve growth factor-induced gene B) was significantly higher in the enriched and social groups compared with rats in the running and individually housed groups. These higher expression levels were found in cortical regions in both hemispheres and in the hippocampus area CA1 [24], and correlated with

functional outcome. Rats that were housed in social or enriched environments did not differ from sham-operated control rats. The marked difference in mRNA protein and immune reactivity for NGFI-A in enriched rats and in runners is illustrated in Figure 5.3.

Data on the effect of enriched environment on brain-derived neurotrophic factor (BDNF), which is known to play an important role in brain plasticity, have been conflicting. Contrary to the hypothesis that enriched housing would enhance *BDNF* gene expression after cortical ischemia, a secondary increase in *BDNF* gene activation that was observed in rats in standard housing 2–12 days after the vascular occlusion in the peri-infarct cortex, hippocampus, and contralateral hemisphere was prevented in rats exposed to environmental enrichment. The BDNF protein level was reduced in the ipsilateral but not in the contralateral hemisphere 12 days after occlusion. An early downregulation of *NGFI-A* that has been shown to increase during environmental stimulation in intact rats was also noted. For reference and discussion of these studies see [7]. Focal ischemic lesions in BDNF +/– mice that have a decreased expression of BDNF was associated with enhanced recovery of motor performance and increased number of neuroblasts in the striatum with no difference between rats housed in enriched or standard environment following MCA occlusion [25]. Data on BDNF Val[66]Met polymorphism in human populations and its relation to brain plasticity in healthy individuals [26] raise the question of whether genetic differences in BDNF may occur also in rodents, an area that remains to be explored.

DNA microarray data have shown that environmental enrichment induces more changes in the hippocampus than in the sensorimotor cortex in intact rats. In contrast, 2 weeks after a cortical infarct, most changes in the injured brain occurred in the contralateral homotopic cortex reflecting increased susceptibility for injury-induced plastic changes in enriched rats [27]. Some of the genes detected corresponded to molecular pathways supposed to be involved in neuronal plasticity, but others provided new and hitherto unrecognized genes in relation to plasticity. In rats placed in an enriched environment for 1 month after MCA occlusion that had significantly improved spatial memory, microarray analysis suggested several differences in neuronal plasticity-related genes, but these changes could not be confirmed by quantitative real-time polymerase chain reaction (PCR) [28]. Molecular changes are often more evident during the dark phase when the rats have higher motor and exploratory activity. Diurnal variation may be absent in single-housed rats as shown for *NGFI-A* and some other genes in which an increase in mRNA expression was seen exclusively during the dark period [29]. This should be taken into account in studies of molecular mediators of experience-dependent neuronal plasticity.

Environment and neurogenesis

In the mammalian brain, neurogenesis persists in a subset of astrocytes in two distinct regions, the subgranular zone of the dentate gyrus (DG) in the hippocampus, and in the subventricular zone (SVZ). Cerebral ischemia enhances neurogenesis in the DG and newborn cells in the SVZ that, under normal conditions, migrate selectively to the olfactory bulb, or migrate to the site of the lesion. Environmental enrichment increases the survival of new neurons both in young and old rats. Neural, vascular, and stroma-derived growth factors participate in the process and in the striatum some new cells may develop into striatal neurons [30]. Whether cortical neurogenesis can be induced in the cortex remains a controversial question (see also Chapter 24).

Five weeks after occlusion of the MCA, a fivefold increase in surviving new cells was seen in the DG in 6-month-old rats housed either in standard cages or in

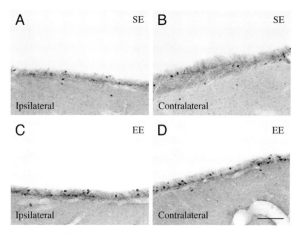

Figure 5.4 Mitotic cells in the subventricular zone 5 weeks after a cortical infarct in rats housed in standard (A and B) or enriched (C and D) environment. The marker for mitosis is phosphorylated histone H3. Photo: Mila Komitova.

an enriched environment. This was demonstrated by daily administration of BrdU, a marker for dividing cells, beginning 24 h post-occlusion and ending one week later [31]. Whereas there was no difference in newly formed neurons, very few astrocytes were noted in the standard group, resulting in a many-fold increase in the neuron to glia ratio compared to sham-operated rats. In contrast, delayed enrichment induced a fivefold and early enrichment a threefold increase in astrocytes compared to rats in standard housing. The neuron to glia ratio did not differ from sham-operated rats. The difference between the two enriched groups was not significant. The results suggest that post-ischemic environmental enrichment influenced the differentiation of the BrdU-labeled progenitor cells, steering them toward the astrocytic lineage. Astrocytes play an important role in neuronal plasticity including synaptogenesis, and the very low number of astrocytes in the standard group might not be an optimal environment for the long-term survival of new neurons.

Rats housed in an enriched environment either from the beginning or with a one-week delay had significantly more proliferating cells in the SVZ compared with animals in standard housing 5 weeks after the lesion (Figure 5.4), suggesting that environmental enrichment not only increased the number of progenitors in the SVZ, but also lengthened the survival of those cells [32].

Only a few neuroblasts were observed in the neocortex, and no newly formed mature neurons were identified. However, the number of newly generated reactive astrocytes was increased in the peri-infarct region in rats housed in the enriched environment, and post-ischemic environmental stimulation had widespread effects on another glial cell population [33]. The majority of BrdU-positive cells in intact ipsi- and contralateral cortex were BDNF immuno-reactive NG2-positive polydendrocytes that were located in close connection with neurons. NG2-positive polydendrocytes constitute the major cell type that proliferates constitutively in gray and white matter in intact brain. The origin and function of these cells is debated. They have earlier been presumed to be predominantly oligodendrocyte progenitors, but are now accepted to constitute a fourth class of neuroglia distinct from mature astrocytes, oligodendrocytes, and microglia that have been shown to have several roles in development and repair of the CNS [34]. It was proposed that they might act by providing trophic support to neurons and modulate extracellular matrix in the peri-infarct area.

In a photochemically induced focal ischemic infarct, enriched environment and reaching training both significantly improved functional recovery of the impaired forelimb and reduced the proliferation of microglia/macrophages in the perilesional zone [35]. NG2-positive cells were increased early in the enriched group. Daily training of the impaired forelimb significantly increased the survival of newly generated astrocytes.

During the first postoperative week, both standard and enriched housing increase cell proliferation in the SVZ, but running prevented the lesion-induced cell proliferation in [36]. Similarly, the survival of new-born cells in DG decreases in response to running after transient forebrain ischemia [37].

Interaction between environmental enrichment and other interventions

Baseline levels of neurotransmitters and growth factors are subject to environmental influences, and the difference in post-ischemic gene expression makes it reasonable to assume that the effect of therapeutic interventions could differ as a function of post-ischemic housing conditions. Thus, environmental influences can either enhance or cancel out the effect of drugs in rodents [7]. Forepaw training in combination with enriched housing increases the dendritic branching in layer 5 of the homotopic contralesional motor cortex when compared with standard housing

[38]. In this study, no controls with enriched environment without specific training were included, and dendritic spines were not quantified. Such a study remains to be performed. Considering the many studies on the effects of enriched environment on spine density, such a control group would most likely have differed from the standard groups. Possible differences between enriched environment and skill training could be associated with more spines, different turn-over rate of spines and synapses, or could be related to a larger area of motor representation for the trained muscles. Furthermore, there might be differences between somatosensory and motor cortex.

Fetal neocortical cell homogenate or tissue transplanted after the ischemic event survives and receives afferent connections from the ipsilateral and contralateral cortex, the thalamus, and other subcortical nuclei in the host brain. Although sensory stimulation of the rat vibrissae enhances the metabolic activity in grafts in standard environment, indicating that such connections can be functionally relevant, no effect on motor function was observed unless the rats were housed in an enriched environment. One week after a cortical infarct, 6-month-old rats received fetal rat cortical transplants (embryonic day 17) and were housed in a standard or enriched environment after the transplantation and followed for 20 weeks. One non-transplanted group was housed in an enriched environment. Repeated tests demonstrated more functional improvement in both groups of enriched rats than in transplanted rats in standard housing. The best outcome was seen after the combination of grafting, and enrichment also significantly reduced the thalamic atrophy that is normally seen after cortical infarct, presumably due to production of trophic factors in the transplant [39]. Afferent connections from the host brain developed more extensive connections within the graft in rats housed in enriched than in standard environments after grafting to infarct cavities, but not when the graft was placed in cavities induced by aspiration lesions [40], confirming earlier data on a favorable post-lesion environment after ischemic brain infarcts [40]. A beneficial effect of environmental enrichment on the effect of fetal transplantation is also documented in animal models of degenerative disorders [41].

The combination of spatial learning and enriched environment increased hippocampal neurogenesis in young rats, and the dentate gyrus neuronal progenitor cell pool increased after 4 and 8 but not after 2 weeks of enriched environment housing [42]. However, enriched environment and spatial learning were only studied together and their separate contributions were not evaluated.

Can we learn something from environmental enrichment in other brain disorders?

Studies on plasticity in a degenerative disease model and in the adult visual cortex have suggested a possible common mechanism for the effect of environmental enrichment on brain plasticity. In an Alzheimer mouse model that allows temporally and spatially restricted induction of neuronal loss, environmental enrichment reinstated learning behavior and re-established access to long-term memories after significant brain atrophy and neuronal loss had already occurred [43]. Chromatin is a DNA–protein complex in the nucleus. The effect of environmental enrichment was associated with modification of chromatin by histone acetylation, a process that is thought to underlie synaptic plasticity, memory formation, and learning. Increasing histone acetylation by inhibitors of histone deacetylase had the same effect as environmental enrichment on dendrites, synapses, learning behavior, and access to long-term memories. The levels of synaptic marker proteins and the Map-2 immunoreactivity were significantly higher in mice in a stimulating environment. Enriched environment restored both new learning and access to remote memories, suggesting that the effects were widespread within hippocampal and cortical areas. An important observation was that promoting histone acetylation restored function and learning and the access to long-term memories in a degenerated brain in the absence of neuronal regeneration.

Visual experience activates histone acetylation in the visual cortex during development, an effect that is downregulated in adult animals. Treatment that promotes histone acetylation enhances plasticity in the adult visual cortex. In rats made amblyopic by long-term monocular deprivation by suture of the eyelids, full visual acuity was restored after removing the suture only under enriched conditions, and it was associated with a marked local reduction of GABA [44,45]. The reduction of inhibition was paralleled by a lower density of the extracellular matrix molecules in perineuronal nets in the corresponding visual cortex and an increased expression of BDNF.

Restoration of plasticity was prevented by benzodiazepine.

That histone acetylation of chromatin enhances plasticity both in the visual cortex and in different learning and memory systems and that it can be induced by environmental enrichment has led to the proposal that chromatin remodeling may be the final gate environmental enrichment opens to enhance brain plasticity.

There are important differences between these two models and stroke. Ischemic lesions result in a permanent tissue loss with interruption of many networks, and the dynamic time-related molecular processes following acute stroke have presumably no correspondence in the other models. However, there may still be common components. Stroke rehabilitation is a relearning process that needs memory formation. The reduction of inhibition in the recovering visual cortex seems relevant at least for chronic stroke when the hand is usually more paretic than the upper arm. Significantly enhanced hand motor function can be obtained by reducing the intrahemispheric inhibition from less damaged regions by training the hand while the upper brachial plexus is anesthetized [46]. Furthermore, stroke is a risk factor for vascular dementia, and there is comorbidity between vascular dementia and Alzheimer disease [47]. However, to what extent epigenetic chromatin modification is associated with enriched environmental housing in stroke models remains to be shown.

Clinical comments and conclusions

There is substantial evidence that the aging processes are modulated by lifestyle and environmental factors. The two main components discussed are environmental stimulation and physical activity. Pre-stroke physical function predicts stroke outcome and pre-stroke social isolation is a predictor of poor outcome [48]. Similarly, early exposure to environmental enrichment prevents memory decline, increases synaptic plasticity markers, and increases the number of newly generated neurons during aging in the rat [49]. The studies on long-term molecular events after ischemic lesions have essentially been performed in rats housed in standard or deprived environments. To what extent and in what ways the post-ischemic molecular events excellently reviewed by Carmichael [50] (and see Chapter 2) would be modified in rats housed in enriched environment from weaning or young age remains to be shown. The evidence that environmental enrichment induces epigenetic changes that facilitate synaptogenesis and memory in other models of brain plasticity should stimulate more research on basic mechanisms underlying environmental influence on the recovery after stroke.

Stroke units may be the closest correspondence to an enriched environment for stroke patients. A stroke is a dramatic change for the patients and anything that can be done to optimize the hospital and rehabilitation environment should be beneficial. No study has shown to what extent the beneficial effect is due to specific rehabilitation strategies, to the time spent in physiotherapy and occupational therapy, and a non-specific effect of a more stimulating environment with competent staff that can encourage and support the patients and family members, but all these factors are likely to be important. The benefit of stroke units compared to general wards is most likely a combination of optimal medical and nursing care, task-oriented activities, and for the individual, meaningful training in an environment that gives them confidence, stimulation, and motivation. Mere admittance to a stroke unit with specially trained staff encouraging active participation in the rehabilitation process creates a positive and stimulating atmosphere. Also, cognitively impaired stroke patients do benefit from admission to an acute rehabilitation unit [51].

Patients with partial cortical infarcts and with capsular infarcts together constitute the major participants in chronic stroke trials, but have so far not been studied extensively in rodents, mainly due to the lack of good rodent models. The human brain has proportionally more white matter than all other species and the difference compared with rodents is enormous. The white matter tracts facilitate the spread of brain edema and make the consequences of complete occlusion of the MCA much more severe in human patients than in mice and rats. The models of striatal infarction after short-term MCA occlusion in mice and rats have told us much about post-ischemic neurogenesis. However, it has little correspondence to subcortical stroke in humans where the main functional deficits are related to the damage of the corticospinal tracts, and myelin inhibitor factors and modification of the extracellular matrix are likely to be more important.

Quality of life is not exclusively determined by the disability, but also by the patient's attitude and how the resulting handicap can be compensated for to enable the patient to take part in social and cultural activities.

Complex cognitive–emotional behavior emerges from dynamic interactions between brain networks. Memory problems, anxiety, mood disturbances, and persistent fatigue can remain despite minimal motor impairment. Patients with mild stroke may have subtle disabilities and difficulty with complex tasks that affect meaningful activity and life satisfaction [52]. Post-stroke physical and cognitive activities are essential to improve the quality of life and reduce the incidence of new vascular events, depression and dementia. Patient associations that arrange various physical and cultural activities for both patients and family caregivers can play a large role and should be actively supported by medical staff and members of the society. A stimulating environment is likely to be the optimal base from which to start specific training and other interventions as well as for continuous social and cognitive rehabilitation.

References

1. Pascual-Leone A, Amedi A, Fregni F, *et al*. The plastic human brain cortex. *Ann Rev Neurosci*. 2005;**28**:377–401.

2. Johansson BB. Brain plasticity in health and disease. *Keio J Med*. 2004;**53**:231–46.

3. Hebb DO. The effect of early experience on problem solving at maturity. *Am Psychol*. 1947;**2**:737–45.

4. Bennet EL, Diamond MC, Krech D, *et al*. Chemical and anatomical plasticity of brain. *Science*. 1964:**146**:610–19.

5. Mohammed AH, Zhu SW, Darmopil S, *et al*. Environmental enrichment and the brain. *Prog Brain Res*. 2002;**138**:109–33.

6. Will B, Galani R, Kelche C, *et al*. Recovery from brain injury in animals: Relative efficacy of environmental enrichment, physical exercise or formal training (1990–2002). *Prog Neurobiol*. 2004;**72**:167–82.

7. Johansson BB. Functional and cellular effects of environmental enrichment after experimental brain infarcts. *Restor Neurol Neurosci*. 2004;**22**:163–74.

8. Nilsson M, Pekny M. Enriched environment and astrocytes in central nervous system regeneration. *J Rehabil Med*. 2007;**39**:345–52.

9. Nithianantharajah J, Hannan AJ. Enriched environment, experience-dependent plasticity and disorders of the nervous system. *Nat Rev Neurosci*. 2006;7:697–709.

10. Johansson BB. Brain plasticity and stroke rehabilitation. The Willis lecture. *Stroke*. 2000;**31**:223–30.

11. Ohlsson A-L, Johansson BB. Environment influences functional outcome of cerebral infarction in rats. *Stroke*. 1995;**26**:644–9.

12. Dahlqvist P, Rönnbäck A, Bergström S-A, *et al.* Environmental enrichment reverses learning impairment in the Morris water maze after focal cerebral ischemia in rats. *Eur J Neurosci*. 2004;**19**:2288–98.

13. Globus A, Rosenzweig MR, Bennett EL, *et al.* Effect of differential experience on dendritic spine counts in rat cerebral cortex. *J Comp Physiol Psychol*. 1973;**82**:175–81.

14. Greenough WT, Volkmar FR, Juraska JM. Effects of rearing complexity on dendritic branching in frontolateral and temporal cortex of the rat. *Exp Neurol*. 1973;**41**:371–8.

15. Johansson BB, Belichenko PV. Neuronal plasticity and dendritic spines: Effect of environmental enrichment on intact and postischemic rat brain. *J Cereb Blood Flow Metab*. 2002;**22**:89–96.

16. Rioult-Pedotti MS, Friedman D, Hess G, *et al.* Strengthening of horizontal cortical connections following skill learning. *Nat Neurosci*. 1998;**1**:230–4.

17. Coq JO, Xerri C. Environmental enrichment alters organizational features of the forepaw representation in the primary somatocortex of adult rats. *Exp Brain Res*. 1998;**121**:191–204.

18. Coq JO, Xerri C. Sensorimotor experience modulates age-dependent alterations of the forepaw representation in the rat primary somatosensory cortex. *Neuroscience*. 2001;**104**:705–15.

19. Nudo RJ, Wise BM, SiFuentes F, *et al.* Neural substrates for the effects of rehabilitative training on motor recovery after ischemic infarct. *Science*. 1996;**272**:1791–4.

20. Holtmaat A, Svoboda K. Experience-dependent structural synaptic plasticity in the mammalian brain. *Nat Rev Neurosci*. 2009;**10**:647–58.

21. Brown CE, Li P, Boyd JD, *et al.* Extensive turnover of dendritic spines and vascular remodeling in cortical tissues recovering from stroke. *J Neurosci*. 2007;**27**:4101–09.

22. Takatsuru Y, Fukumoto D, Yoshitomo M, *et al.* Neuronal circuit remodeling in the contralateral cortical hemisphere during functional recovery from cerebral infarction. *J Neurosci*. 2009;**29**:10 061–6.

23. Johansson BB, Ohlsson A-L. Environment, social interaction, and physical activity as determinants of functional outcome after cerebral infarction in the rat. *Exp Neurol*. 2006;**139**:322–7.

24. Dahlqvist P, Rönnbäck A, Risedal A, *et al.* Effects of postischemic environment on transcription factor and serotonin receptor expression after permanent focal cortical ischemia in the rat. *Neuroscience*. 2003;**119**:643–52.

25. Nygren J, Kokaia M, Wieloch T. Decreased expression of brain-derived neurotrophic factor in BDNF(+/–) mice is associated with enhanced recovery of motor performance and increased neuroblast number following experimental stroke. *J Neurosci Res*. 2006;**84**:626–31.

26. Kleim JA, Chan S, Pringle E, *et al.* BDNF val66met polymorphism is associated with modified experience-dependent plasticity in human motor cortex. *Nat Neurosci*. 2006;**9**:735–7.

27. Keyvani K, Sachser N, Witte OW, *et al.* Gene expression profiling in the intact and injured brain following environmental enrichment. *J Neuropathol Exp Neurol*. 2004;**63**:598–609.

28. Rönnbäck A, Dahlqvist P, Svensson P-A, *et al.* Gene expression profiling of the rat hippocampus one month after focal ischemia followed by enriched environment. *Neurosci Lett*. 2005;**385**:173–8.

29. Rönnbäck A, Dahlqvist P, Bergström SA, *et al.* Diurnal effects of enriched environment on immediately early gene expression in the rat brain. *Brain Res*. 2005;**1046**:127–44.

30. Johansson BB. Regeneration and plasticity in the brain and spinal cord. *J Cerebr Blood Flow Metab*. 2007;**27**:1417–30.

31. Komitova M, Perfilieva E, Mattsson B, *et al.* Effects of cortical ischemia and postischemic environmental enrichment on hippocampal cell genesis and differentiation in the adult rat. *J Cereb Blood Flow Metab*. 2002;**22**:852–60.

32. Komitova M, Mattsson B, Johansson BB, *et al.* Enriched environment increases neural stem/progenitor cell proliferation and neurogenesis in the subventricular zone of stroke-lesioned adult rats. *Stroke*. 2005;**36**:1278–82.

33. Komitova M, Perfilieva E, Mattsson B, *et al.* Enriched environmental after focal cortical ischemia enhances the generation of astroglia and NG2 positive polydendrocytes in adult rat neocortex. *Exp Neurol*. 2006;**199**:113–21.

34. Nishiyama A. Polydendrocytes: NG2 cells with many roles in development and repair of the CNS. *Neuroscientist*. 2007;**13**:62–76.

35. Keiner S, Wurm F, Kunze A, *et al.* Rehabilitative therapies differentially alter proliferation and survival of glial cell populations in the perilesional zone of cortical infarcts. *Glia*. 2008;**56**:516–27.

36. Komitova M, Zhao LR, Gido G, *et al.* Postischemic exercise attenuates whereas enriched environment has certain enhancing effects on lesion-induced subventricular zone activation in the adult rat. *Eur J Neurol*. 2005;**21**:2397–405.

37. Yagita Y, Kitagawa K, Sasaki T, *et al.* Postischemic exercise decreases neurogenesis in the adult rat dentate gyrus. *Neurosci Lett.* 2006;**409**:24–9.

38. Biernaskie, Corbett D. Enriched rehabilitative training promotes improved forelimb motor function and enhanced dendritic growth after focal ischemic injury. *J Neurosci.* 2001;**21**:5272–80.

39. Mattsson B, Sorensen JC, Zimmer J, *et al.* Neural grafting to experimental neocortical infarcts improves behavioral outcome and reduces thalamic atrophy in rats housed in an enriched but not in standard environments. *Stroke.* 1997;**28**:1225–32.

40. Zeng J, Mattsson B, Schultz MK. Expression of zinc-positive cells and terminals in fetal neocortical homografts to adult rat depends on lesion type and rearing conditions. *Exp Neurol.* 2000;**164**:176–83.

41. Döbrössy MD, Dunnett SB. Optimizing plasticity: Environmental and training-associated brain repair. *Rev Neurosci.* 2005;**16**:1–21.

42. Matsumori Y, Hong SM, Fan Y, *et al.* Enriched environment and spatial learning enhance hippocampal neurogenesis and salvages ischemic penumbra after focal cerebral ischemia. *Neurobiol Dis.* 2006;**22**:187–98.

43. Fischer A, Sananbenesi F, Wang X, *et al.* Recovery of learning and memory is associated with chromatin remodeling. *Nature.* 2007;**447**:178–82.

44. Spolidoro M, Sale A, Berardi M, *et al.* Plasticity of the adult brain: Lesions from the visual system. *Exp Brain Res.* 2009;**192**:335–41.

45. Sale A, Maya Vetencourt JF, Medini P, *et al.* Environmental enrichment in adulthood promotes amblyopia recovery through a reduction of intracortical inhibition. *Nat Neurosci.* 2007;**10**:679–81.

46. Muellbacher W, Richards U, Ziemann U, *et al.* Improving hand function in chronic stroke. *Arch Neurol.* 2002;**59**:1278–82.

47. Jin YP, De Legge S, Ostbye T, *et al.* The reciprocal risk of stroke and cognitive impairment in an elderly population. *Alzheim Dementia* 2006;**2**:171–8.

48. Boden-Albala B, Litwak E, Elkind MS, *et al.* Social isolation and outcomes post stroke. *Neurology.* 2005;**64**:1888–92.

49. Leal-Galicia P, Castaneda-Bueno M, Quiroz-Baez R, *et al.* Long-term exposure to environmental enrichment since youth prevents recognition memory decline and increases synaptic plasticity markers in aging. *Neurobiol Learn Mem.* 2008;**90**:511–8.

50. Carmichael ST. Themes and strategies for studying the biology of stroke recovery in the poststroke epoch. *Stroke.* 2008;**39**:1380–5.

51. Rabadi MH, Rabadi FM, Edelstein L, *et al.* Cognitively impaired stroke patients do benefit from admission to an acute rehabilitation unit. *Arch Phys Med Rehabil.* 2008;**89**:441–8.

52. Edwards DF, Hahn M, Baum C, *et al.* The impact of mild stroke on meaningful activity and life satisfaction. *J Stroke Cerebrovasc Dis.* 2006;**14**:151–7.

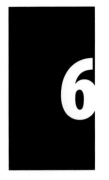

6

Functional and structural MR imaging of brain reorganization after stroke

Maurits P. A. van Meer & Rick M. Dijkhuizen

Introduction

Over the years, imaging methodologies have been applied increasingly to assess stroke pathophysiology for clinical diagnosis as well as for scientific research. The major neuroimaging modalities are computed tomography (CT), positron emission tomography (PET), and magnetic resonance imaging (MRI). In the clinic CT is the most commonly used technique and remains the standard for initial assessment on suspicion of stroke in most hospitals. It may rule out hemorrhage, visualize occluding thrombi, and identify early tissue changes and swelling. PET is less widely available than CT, but this modality enables unique measurements of the metabolic status of ischemic tissue. For example, PET-based calculation of the cerebral metabolic rate of oxygen ($CMRO_2$) after stroke may allow differentiation between partially viable and irreversibly damaged tissue [1]. In addition, PET has been applied in pioneering functional imaging studies to measure changes in brain activation patterns in stroke subjects [2]. However, the most versatile modality for stroke imaging is MRI, which relies on detection of MR signals from the highly abundant water protons in tissues. Its versatility stems from the ability to sensitize MRI acquisitions to distinct parameters, such as proton density, MR relaxation times (T_1, T_2), susceptibility contrast, diffusion, perfusion and flow. This enables multiparametric imaging studies on different pathological events as well as remodeling processes that are involved in the evolution of stroke-affected tissue. In particular, T_2-, diffusion-, and perfusion-weighted MRI are effective methods to detect early changes in brain tissue and perfusion status after stroke [3,4], and prospective MRI trials have shown that identification of a mismatch between the areas of diminished perfusion and reduced tissue water diffusion might provide a criterion for selection of patients who will benefit from recanalization therapies [5]. In recent years, MRI has also been applied to assess functional and structural reorganization in the brain in relation to recovery after stroke at later stages. A better understanding of long-term repair mechanisms can offer potential leads for therapeutic interventions. Earlier histological and electrophysiological experiments in animal stroke models have already provided considerable insights into post-stroke plasticity of neuronal circuitry in the brain [6]. MRI can add valuable information to this important research area as it allows repetitive in-vivo whole-brain measurements of both functional and anatomical changes in post-stroke brain. This chapter discusses different functional and structural MRI methods that may be used for studies on brain plasticity, with a focus on application in experimental stroke models.

Functional MRI

Functional MRI (fMRI) is based on detection of MR signals that are associated with neuronal activation. Typically, fMRI measures hemodynamic changes in response to increases in neuronal activity upon cognitive, visual, sensory, or motor stimulation. MRI methods that have been employed are blood oxygenation level-dependent (BOLD) MRI, which is susceptible to the magnetic properties of blood; arterial spin labeling (ASL) techniques, which are based on detection of the signal from magnetically labeled endogenous arterial water; and dynamic susceptibility contrast-enhanced and steady-state susceptibility contrast-enhanced MRI, which measure signal changes after intravascular injection of an exogenous paramagnetic contrast agent. These different MRI approaches can be utilized for detection of neuronal activation-induced changes in blood oxygenation (BOLD fMRI), cerebral blood flow (CBF) (ASL-based fMRI), or cerebral blood

Brain Repair After Stroke, ed. S. C. Cramer and R. J. Nudo. Published by Cambridge University Press.

volume (CBV) (contrast-enhanced fMRI) [7,8]. A detailed review of the principles of these distinct fMRI techniques can be found in a book chapter by Mandeville and Rosen [7].

The first reports on the use of fMRI to non-invasively investigate changes in activation patterns in stroke patients appeared in the mid to late 1990s (see Cramer and Bastings for a review [9]). Cramer et al. [10] and Cao et al. [11] conducted pioneering fMRI studies on stroke subjects who had recovered from hemiparesis. BOLD MRI acquisition during finger tapping revealed activation-induced signal increases in peri-infarct regions, secondary sensorimotor areas and the contralesional hemisphere, which were more extensive than in controls. From then on, numerous BOLD fMRI studies have demonstrated post-stroke rearrangement of ipsi- and contralesional functional brain fields in patients recovering from hemiparesis, aphasia, or hemianopia [9,12,13]. These patient fMRI studies have provided important details on changes in functional activation patterns. Yet variations in lesion size and location, comorbidities, differences in the post-stroke time of fMRI acquisition, head motion, and incomplete data sets complicate systematic examination of functional brain reorganization after stroke.

Contrary to most patient fMRI studies, fMRI experiments in animal stroke models can be performed under highly controllable and reproducible conditions. Furthermore, results from animal fMRI studies may be directly correlated with more invasive measurements, such as electrophysiological recordings and (immuno)histochemistry, which may aid in elucidation of the basis of normal and altered fMRI responses. A detailed overview of advantages and issues of fMRI in laboratory animals can be read in a review by Van der Linden et al. [14]. A number of studies have applied fMRI to analyze changes in functional brain activation in animal stroke models [15–22]. In general, the experimental protocol consisted of an electrical forelimb stimulation paradigm in rats, which under normal conditions gives rise to a robust response in the sensorimotor cortex (see Figure 6.1). Animal fMRI studies are often conducted at high magnetic field strengths (≥ 7 T) [20–22], and/or with contrast-enhanced CBV-weighted fMRI [15–21], which significantly improve sensitivity and specificity to detect activation responses [7,8]. Despite the common use of BOLD fMRI in human studies, BOLD signal intensity changes are typically on the order of only a few percent. Increased fMRI sensitivity can be achieved by acquisition at higher magnetic field strengths (horizontal bore MR systems for animal imaging up to field strengths of 14.1 T are available), or by enhancement with an exogenous contrast agent, as reviewed by Mandeville and Rosen [7] and Harel et al. [8]. Steady-state contrast-enhanced MRI requires the injection of a (super)paramagnetic blood pool contrast agent. Although this decreases the signal-to-noise ratio in brain MR images, the contrast-to-noise ratio for fMRI can be significantly increased as compared to BOLD techniques. The technique is largely CBV-dependent, since the relatively high concentration of the paramagnetic blood pool agent minimizes contribution of a BOLD effect to the CBV measurement, which also eliminates unwanted signal from large, remote vessels.

Consistent with patient fMRI papers, fMRI studies in experimental stroke models have reported diminished activation in the ipsilesional sensorimotor cortex [15–17,19,22], enhanced contralesional activation [16,17,19], and reinstatement of perilesional activity at later stages [17,19,22]. Figure 6.1 shows examples of shifts in cerebral responses to somatosensory stimulation in a rat stroke model detected with contrast-enhanced CBV-weighted fMRI.

Functional MRI studies in rats after permanent or transient unilateral middle cerebral artery (MCA) occlusion have shown that the fMRI-detected activation response to forelimb stimulation could be absent in the somatosensory cortex forelimb representation zone despite normal appearance on diffusion- and T_2-weighted MR images [15,17,19]. This indicates that intact structural integrity around a stroke lesion does not necessarily imply preservation of neuronal function, and demonstrates the significance of fMRI to detect tissue dysfunction in lesion border zones. Notably, it is possible that activation responses in perilesional cortical tissue recur. Dijkhuizen et al. [19] and Weber et al. [22] have shown that preservation or reinstatement of activation within the ipsilesional sensorimotor cortex is associated with functional recovery after transient MCA occlusion in rats, which agrees with results from fMRI studies in recovering hemiparetic stroke patients [13].

A rise in contralesional fMRI activity after unilateral cerebral ischemia has been demonstrated in some rat studies [16,17,19], and the relative degree of activation in the contralesional hemispheres corresponded with the extent of tissue injury in the

fMRI during forelimb stimulation in rats

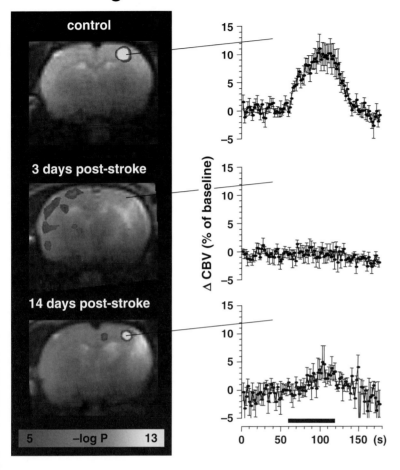

Figure 6.1 For the color version of this figure, see the Plate section. Left: T_2-weighted MR images of a rat brain slice overlaid by statistical activation maps calculated from contrast-enhanced CBV-weighted fMRI in combination with an electrical forelimb stimulation paradigm as described by Dijkhuizen *et al.* [17]. Right: Time-course of CBV changes in the right sensorimotor cortex in response to left forelimb stimulation (the stimulation period is indicated by the black bar) (mean ± SD, $n = 6$). Left forelimb stimulation induced significant activation responses in the right sensorimotor cortex in control rats. At 3 days after right-sided stroke, activation responses in the right, ipsilesional sensorimotor cortex were largely absent; however, responses were found in the left, contralesional hemisphere. After 14 days, partial restoration of activation was detected in the right, ipsilesional sensorimotor cortex. The unilateral stroke lesion is characterized by increased T_2-weighted signal intensity in the right somatosensory cortex and lateral striatum.

ipsilesional sensorimotor cortex [19]. Recruitment of contralateral counterparts of damaged functional fields may hypothetically contribute to functional recovery. On the other hand, contralesional activity may be a direct pathophysiological consequence (e.g. due to broad disinhibition). Thus the actual functional significance of enhanced activation in the unaffected hemisphere, which may be functionally nonspecific [17,19], remains unclear and requires further research (see also Chapter 3).

Although fMRI has become a well-established tool in neuroscience research, it is important to realize that the fMRI-based measurement of hemodynamic responses to neuronal activation relies on intact neurovascular coupling and cerebrovascular reactivity, which may be affected after cerebral ischemic injury. Moreover, fMRI studies in animals require the use of anesthetics that may influence neurovascular coupling. Nevertheless, fMRI is

certainly feasible with anesthesia protocols that preserve functional–metabolic coupling [14], and with the addition of tests to evaluate electrical activity and vascular responsiveness, the interpretation of fMRI data can be significantly improved. For example, Dijkhuizen *et al.* measured the hemodynamic response to a CO_2 inhalation challenge with CBV-weighted MRI and detected a significant vasodilatory effect in perilesional sensorimotor cortex where stimulus-induced fMRI responses were absent. This implies that the loss of fMRI-detected activation was not simply the result of local deficient vasoreactivity [17,19]. A tight coupling between the degree of fMRI responses and evoked potentials was observed by Weber *et al.* in a longitudinal fMRI study on rats recovering from stroke [22]. These authors demonstrated that re-emergence of fMRI activation in the intact ipsilesional somatosensory cortex was accompanied by restoration of electrical activity.

Besides elucidation of neural correlates of spontaneous functional recovery, fMRI may also provide a means to evaluate effects of treatment strategies on restoration of brain tissue function after stroke. Sauter *et al.* have demonstrated that prevention of ischemic damage to the primary somatosensory cortex by administration of a Ca^{2+} antagonist after permanent MCA occlusion in rats was accompanied by recovery of neuronal responses to electrical forelimb stimulation [18]. In studies on the therapeutic efficacy of late treatment with neuroprotective agents in a rat stroke model, Kim and colleagues reported enhanced fMRI activity in the perilesional somatosensory cortex in albumin- and lithium-treated animals, even though lesion size was not different from control animals [20,21]. Correspondingly, hyperactivity in the ipsilesional hemisphere, coinciding with improved motor performance, has been observed in a patient fMRI study after administration of fluoxetine [23].

Alternative functional MRI approaches

Traditional fMRI studies, as described above, focus on the brain's activation response to somatosensory stimuli or execution of a task. However, there are alternative fMRI approaches to study neuronal activity and excitability in the post-stroke brain.

Pharmacological MRI (phMRI), which measures hemodynamic changes associated with cerebral activity in response to centrally acting pharmacological agents [24], has been applied to detect functionally compromised brain tissue after stroke [25]. It was shown that the cerebral activation response to systemic administration of bicuculline, a $GABA_A$ antagonist, was strongly diminished after unilateral MCA occlusion in rats, as compared to controls. In theory, phMRI may allow evaluation of upregulation of specific neurotransmitter receptor systems associated with brain plasticity after stroke. However, to our knowledge this has not yet been demonstrated experimentally.

A method that computes changes in spatial functional correlations within various neural networks, without the need of stimulating a specific functional system, has been introduced as resting-state fMRI [26]. This technique aims to detect baseline brain activity related to ongoing neuronal signaling at 'rest' and is carried out by low-pass filtering of spontaneous BOLD MRI signals. Resting-state fMRI can identify temporal correlations of low-frequency BOLD signal fluctuations (< 0.1 Hz) between different brain areas, indicative of functional connectivity. In a pioneering resting-state fMRI study in neglect patients, He *et al.* illustrated dynamic changes in connectivity between attentional networks from acute to chronic stages after stroke [27]. We have recently conducted a pilot resting-state fMRI study in rats recovering from transient unilateral stroke. Functional connectivity maps were computed by voxel-wise calculation of correlations of spontaneous low-frequency BOLD signals between sensorimotor network regions. Figure 6.2 shows maps of mean functional connectivity between the contralesional forelimb region of the primary somatosensory cortex and the rest of the brain. Before stroke, there was a strong BOLD signal correlation particularly with the ipsi- and contralateral primary and secondary sensorimotor cortices. At 3 days after unilateral subcortical stroke, functional connectivity with the ipsilesional sensorimotor cortex was significantly reduced. After 10 weeks, however, interhemispheric functional connectivity was largely restored, which coincided with significant behavioral recovery.

The above-described phMRI and resting-state fMRI as well as other unconventional fMRI techniques, such as magnetic-source MRI [28] and activity-induced manganese-dependent MRI [29], are emergent functional imaging methods that, alongside traditional fMRI, might provide additional insights into reorganization of functional fields after cerebrovascular injury.

Structural MRI

The previous section describes MRI methods for measurement of brain activity, which can be applied to identify altered patterns of brain activation after stroke. Changes in functional brain responses are often closely linked to modification of neuronal, glial and endothelial structures. As a multiparametric imaging tool, MRI allows complementary assessment of structural changes that are associated with brain injury and repair after stroke, as will be discussed below.

Ischemic damage to brain tissue can be identified with T_2- and diffusion-weighted MRI, which are established imaging methods for detection of stroke lesions in the clinic and laboratory. Acute ischemia-induced cellular swelling, or cytotoxic edema, leads to significant reduction of the apparent diffusion coefficient (ADC) of tissue water, while vasogenic edema and chronic tissue degeneration combined with fluid accumulation result in T_2 prolongation and ADC increase [3,4]. The potential of MRI to assess structural

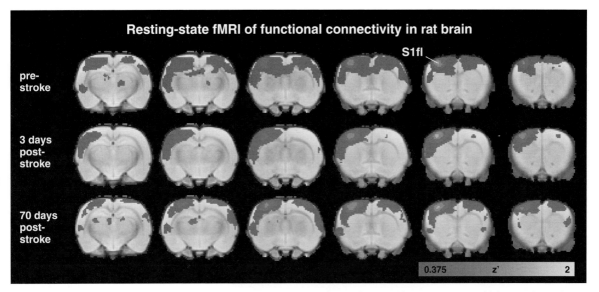

Figure 6.2 For the color version of this figure, see the Plate section. Maps of mean functional brain connectivity of left (contralesional after stroke) forelimb region of the primary somatosensory cortex (S1fl) in rats before, 3, and 70 days after a 90-min right MCA occlusion-induced subcortical lesion (n = 5). Functional connectivity maps are thresholded at a Fisher-transformed correlation coefficient (z') of 0.375, and overlaid on a T_2-weighted multislice anatomical rat brain template. Loss of functional connectivity with the ipsilesional sensorimotor cortex was evident at 3 days, while functional connectivity was restored at 10 weeks after stroke. Courtesy of Kajo van der Marel, Image Sciences Institute, University Medical Center Utrecht.

restorative changes related to post-stroke plasticity has been considerably less widely explored. In recent years, however, MRI methods such as diffusion tensor imaging (DTI) and manganese-enhanced MRI (MEMRI) have been successfully employed to investigate neuroanatomical reorganization after stroke.

Diffusion tensor imaging

DTI enables the assessment of the three-dimensional displacement of tissue water, mathematically characterized by an effective diffusion tensor consisting of nine matrix elements [30]. The principles of DTI have been described in many review papers; see, for example, Basser and Jones [31] and Mori and Zhang [32]. In brief, the diffusion tensor can be estimated by MRI with diffusion-weighting gradients in multiple directions. Computational diagonalization of the diffusion tensor yields three orthogonal principal diffusivities (eigenvalues) and its three principal coordinate directions (eigenvectors), which can be used to calculate scalar indices such as the direction-independent mean diffusivity and the fractional anisotropy (FA). The spatial characteristics of water diffusion in brain tissue are affected by anatomical barriers such as cell membranes and myelinated fibers. Consequently, the diffusion of water molecules will not be equal

in all directions or, in other words, anisotropic. Calculations of diffusion anisotropy and the principal diffusion direction can be used to model fiber architecture in the human or animal brain, visualized by orientation-based color-coded FA maps or three-dimensional fiber tractography images (see Figure 6.3) [32].

So far, specific issues in terms of data acquisition (long scan times; motion sensitivity; noise susceptibility) and analysis (non-Gaussian diffusion; tract reconstruction difficulties due to complex topography of fiber bundles) have limited the widespread exploitation of DTI in stroke studies. Nevertheless, DTI has the potential to assess particular pathological processes in gray and white matter areas, such as axonal degeneration and demyelination, that are not straightforwardly measured with more conventional (MR) imaging methods. Studies that have longitudinally conducted DTI in patients and animal models have reported elevated FA and reduced mean diffusivity acutely after stroke onset, pointing toward cytotoxic edema along with increased tortuosity of the swollen tissue, chronically followed by an increase in mean diffusivity and a decrease of FA, which was particularly prominent in affected white matter [33,34]. In a non-human primate stroke model, reduced FA was shown

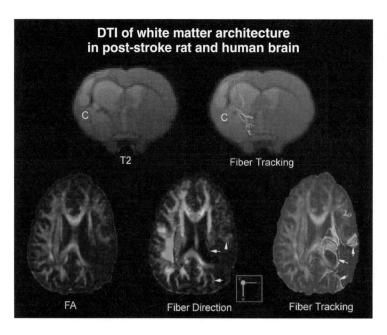

DTI of white matter architecture in post-stroke rat and human brain

T2

Fiber Tracking

FA

Fiber Direction

Fiber Tracking

Figure 6.3 For the color version of this figure, see the Plate section. Top row: T_2-weighted MR image and fiber-tracking image of a rat brain treated with neuroprogenitor cells after unilateral stroke, showing tracking of axonal projections in the lesion border zone. The marker **c** represents the ischemic core. Bottom row: FA, fiber direction, and fiber-tracking image of a horizontal brain slice from a stroke patient, illustrating orientation changes in the lesion boundary. Both fiber direction and fiber-tracking images show that tracking of axonal projections circumscribes the lesion boundary (white arrows). Red, green, and blue colors represent x, y, and z directions, respectively, on the fiber direction image. Details of the experimental protocols can be found in Jiang et al. [36]. Courtesy of Dr. Quan Jiang, Henry Ford Health Sciences Center.

to be correlated with the amount of myelin damage at chronic stages after transient or permanent MCA occlusion in non-human primates [34].

A growing amount of data suggest that DTI may also inform on alterations in brain connections associated with neuroplasticity. For instance, structural repair or remodeling of neuronal projections resulting in increased density of (myelinated) fibers would theoretically give rise to higher FA. In fact a progressive increase of FA in non-lesioned white matter has been found in patients during the first two years after stroke [35]. This was hypothesized to represent ongoing improvement of the integrity of normal-appearing white matter as a result of remyelination processes. Recent studies on neuronal repair after experimental cerebral ischemia have also shown an increase in FA in perilesional white matter at chronic time-points [36–38]. Jiang et al. [36] and Ding et al. [38] observed that FA rises progressively along the ischemic lesion boundary, which was significantly enhanced in rats treated with neural progenitor cells [36] (Figure 6.3) or sildenafil [38]. Histological examination in these studies revealed a high density of axons and myelin in areas with elevated FA. Van der Zijden et al. described a temporal profile of FA increase over a period of 9 weeks that followed an initial decline at 3 days after transient MCA occlusion in rats [37]. This particular pattern was specifically observed in areas consisting of white matter,

i.e. the internal capsule and corpus callosum. These data suggest that white matter integrity may improve after initial loss. However, other processes such as gliosis, i.e. proliferation of glial cells, may also occur in ischemic lesion border zones and could affect diffusion anisotropy. In the near future, additional experimental studies are required to establish to what extent diverse structural modifications in post-stroke brain, which include neuronal restructuring and glial scar formation, contribute to changes in DTI parameters.

Manganese-enhanced MRI

Besides DTI, MRI provides another interesting tool termed manganese-enhanced MRI (MEMRI) for assessment of neuronal networks. This method makes use of paramagnetic Mn^{2+} as a Ca^{2+} analog that can enter neurons through Ca^{2+} channels. In tissue, manganese shortens the local T_1, giving rise to an increase in signal intensity on T_1-weighted MR images. Under normal conditions endogenous manganese is present in only trace amounts, hence MEMRI typically involves application of exogenous manganese. The manganese-induced increase in longitudinal relaxation rate, R_1 ($1/T_1$), is proportional to the local manganese concentration [39], hence the amount of manganese accumulation after injection can be estimated from the difference between pre- and post-contrast R_1 (ΔR_1).

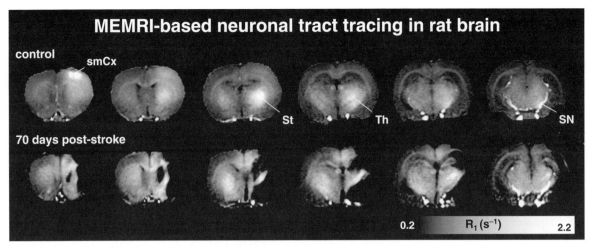

Figure 6.4 R_1 (= $1/T_1$) maps of consecutive coronal rat brain slices at 4 days after $MnCl_2$ injection in the right sensorimotor cortex (smCx) as described by van der Zijden et al. [44]. Top row: 4 weeks after sham-operation. Bottom row: 10 weeks after 90-min right MCA occlusion. Manganese-induced R_1 increase is evident in regions of the sensorimotor network, i.e. smCx, striatum (St), thalamus (Th) and substantia nigra (SN). At 10 weeks after stroke increased manganese accumulation is detectable in contralateral subcortical areas. The unilateral stroke lesion is characterized by reduced R_1.

Several variations of MEMRI have been introduced for experimental studies on the brain. First, enhanced cytoarchitectural information may be attained after systemic administration of manganese, which is selectively taken up in specific brain regions [39]. This approach may, for instance, enable identification of different cortical layers with MRI. Second, as briefly mentioned in the above section on fMRI, Mn^{2+} can be used to demonstrate Ca^{2+} influx upon neuronal activation, thereby providing an alternative tool for functional imaging [29]. This method, however, is hampered by the prerequisite to open the blood–brain barrier for sufficient manganese distribution to the brain. Third, MEMRI can be used to trace neuronal tracts, which has been the most commonly employed MEMRI technique [40], as will be discussed below.

In the late 1990s Pautler et al. were the first to demonstrate that injection of manganese into a specific neuroanatomical system is followed by neuronal uptake, axonal transport, and sometimes trans-synaptic transfer along connective pathways [41]. Since then, MEMRI has evolved into a unique in-vivo tract-tracing method to map neuronal network connections in laboratory animals [40]. Its success has also led to MEMRI-based tract-tracing studies for measurement of changes in neuronal connectivity in experimental stroke models [42–44]. Experiments by Van der Zijden et al. focused on characterization of the spatiotemporal pattern of manganese enhancement after

stereotaxic injection of $MnCl_2$ solution in perilesional tissue after transient unilateral MCA occlusion in rats [43,44] (see Figure 6.4). Compared to controls, $MnCl_2$ injection in the intact sensorimotor cortex at the border of a 2-week-old unilateral ischemic lesion was followed by delayed and diminished manganese-induced ΔR_1 in ipsilateral subcortical structures that are part of the sensorimotor network, i.e. the striatum, thalamus, and substantia nigra [43]. Yet when the same experiment was done at more chronic time points, i.e. 10 weeks after stroke, the degree of manganese accumulation in these regions was the same as in sham-operated animals [44]. Furthermore, significantly increased manganese build-up was detected in contralateral subcortical areas. These post-stroke time-dependent differences in manganese enhancement profiles within the sensorimotor network correlated with the accumulation pattern of a conventional neuroanatomical tract tracer as detected by immunohistochemistry [43,44]. This confirms that the MEMRI findings were associated with changes in neuronal connectivity. The initial reduction and subsequent increase of manganese enhancement in the ipsilateral striatum, thalamus, and substantia nigra suggest that a disturbed thalamocortical–corticothalamic circuit may restore or renew its connections at later stages. The enhanced manganese accumulation in the contralateral hemisphere probably reflects increased manganese transfer in crossing white matter tracts, pointing toward increased interhemispheric connectivity. These signs of structural plasticity as detected with in-vivo MEMRI-based neuroanatomical tract tracing correspond with histological evidence of unmasking or new formation of connections with perilesional areas in experimental stroke models [45].

Despite the exclusive opportunities for serial, three-dimensional, in-vivo neuronal tracing with MEMRI, there are some noteworthy limitations. First, spatial resolution of MEMRI is currently limited to about $100\,\mu m$, while much more detailed anatomical information can be achieved with microscopic analysis of conventional tracers. Second, although neuronal uptake and subsequent axonal transport likely represent the major mechanisms responsible for manganese enhancement in the brain, other processes such as passive diffusion in interstitial fluid, reabsorption in blood and cerebrospinal fluid, as well as glial uptake, may complicate the use of manganese as a pure neuronal tract tracer [46]. Third, the major drawback of manganese for brain studies is its neurotoxicity at high concentrations or after chronic exposure [39], which is the main reason why MEMRI-based neuronal tracing has not been applied in human studies. None the less, Canals et al. have recently shown that intracortical injection of a low dose of $MnCl_2$ at a very slow rate did not lead to neuronal and glial injury and improved the efficiency of tracing neuronal connections [47]. Without a doubt, such improvements in experimental protocols will further expand the prospects of in-vivo MEMRI-based neuronal tract-tracing experiments in a wide range of neuroscience research areas, including assessments of structural plasticity after stroke.

In conclusion, MRI offers a versatile tool to evaluate the spatiotemporal pattern of functional and structural changes after stroke in both clinical and experimental settings. The techniques discussed in this chapter demonstrate the ability of MRI to detect (changes in) brain activity and neuroanatomical connectivity, but its potential stretches even further. Recent experimental studies have shown that MR methods can also inform on angiogenesis (with T_2^*-weighted MRI [48] or steady-state contrast-enhanced MRI [49]) and metabolic alterations (with $^1H/^{13}C$ MR spectroscopic imaging [50]) in recovering post-stroke tissue. Thus in the coming years it is to be expected that various MR techniques will play an increasing role in the elucidation of structural and functional reorganization in the brain. The availability of MRI in experimental and clinical settings will further promote translational research on brain plasticity and may aid in monitoring of existing and novel therapeutic strategies to improve brain repair.

Acknowledgments

Part of the presented work was funded by the Alexandre Suerman program of the University Medical Center Utrecht and Utrecht University's High Potential program.

References

1. Baron JC. Mapping the ischaemic penumbra with PET: Implications for acute stroke treatment. *Cerebrovasc Dis*. 1999;**9**:193–201.

2. Chollet F, Weiller C. Imaging recovery of function following brain injury. *Curr Opin Neurobiol*. 1994;**4**:226–30.

3. Baird AE, Warach S. Magnetic resonance imaging of acute stroke. *J Cereb Blood Flow Metab*. 1998;**18**:583–609.

4. Dijkhuizen RM, Nicolay K. Magnetic resonance imaging in experimental models of brain disorders. *J Cereb Blood Flow Metab*. 2003;**23**:1383–402.

5. Neumann-Haefelin T, Steinmetz H. Time is brain: Is MRI the clock? *Curr Opin Neurol*. 2007;**20**:410–6.

6. Nudo RJ. Recovery after damage to motor cortical areas. *Curr Opin Neurobiol*. 1999;**9**:740–7.

7. Mandeville JB, Rosen BR. Functional MRI. In: Toga AW, Mazziotta JC, editors. *Brain mapping: the methods*. 2nd ed. New York, NY: Academic Press; 2002:315–49.

8. Harel N, Ugurbil K, Uludag K, et al. Frontiers of brain mapping using MRI. *J Magn Reson Imaging*. 2006;**23**:945–57.

9. Cramer SC, Bastings EP. Mapping clinically relevant plasticity after stroke. *Neuropharmacology*. 2000;**39**:842–51.

10. Cramer SC, Nelles G, Benson RR, et al. A functional MRI study of subjects recovered from hemiparetic stroke. *Stroke*. 1997;**28**:2518–27.

11. Cao Y, D'Olhaberriague L, Vikingstad EM, et al. Pilot study of functional MRI to assess cerebral activation of motor function after poststroke hemiparesis. *Stroke*. 1998;**29**:112–22.

12. Rijntjes M, Weiller C. Recovery of motor and language abilities after stroke: The contribution of functional imaging. *Prog Neurobiol*. 2002;**66**:109–22.

13. Calautti C, Baron JC. Functional neuroimaging studies of motor recovery after stroke in adults: A review. *Stroke*. 2003;**34**:1553–66.

14. Van der Linden A, Van Camp N, Ramos-Cabrer P, et al. Current status of functional MRI on small animals:

Application to physiology, pathophysiology and cognition. *NMR Biomed.* 2007;**20**:522–45.

15. Reese T, Porszasz R, Baumann D, *et al.* Cytoprotection does not preserve brain functionality in rats during the acute post-stroke phase despite evidence of non-infarction provided by MRI. *NMR Biomed.* 2000;**13**:361–70.

16. Abo M, Chen Z, Lai LJ, *et al.* Functional recovery after brain lesion–contralateral neuromodulation: An fMRI study. *Neuroreport.* 2001;**12**:1543–7.

17. Dijkhuizen RM, Ren J, Mandeville JB, *et al.* Functional magnetic resonance imaging of reorganization in rat brain after stroke. *Proc Natl Acad Sci USA.* 2001;**98**:12 766–71.

18. Sauter A, Reese T, Porszasz R, *et al.* Recovery of function in cytoprotected cerebral cortex in rat stroke model assessed by functional MRI. *Magn Reson Med.* 2002;**47**:759–65.

19. Dijkhuizen RM, Singhal AB, Mandeville JB, *et al.* Correlation between brain reorganization, ischemic damage, and neurologic status after transient focal cerebral ischemia in rats: A functional magnetic resonance imaging study. *J Neurosci.* 2003;**23**:510–7.

20. Kim YR, Van Meer MP, Mandeville JB, *et al.* fMRI of delayed albumin treatment during stroke recovery in rats: Implication for fast neuronal habituation in recovering brains. *J Cereb Blood Flow Metab.* 2007;**27**:142–53.

21. Kim YR, Van Meer MP, Tejima E, *et al.* Functional MRI of delayed chronic lithium treatment in rat focal cerebral ischemia. *Stroke.* 2008;**39**:439–47.

22. Weber R, Ramos-Cabrer P, Justicia C, *et al.* Early prediction of functional recovery after experimental stroke: Functional magnetic resonance imaging, electrophysiology, and behavioral testing in rats. *J Neurosci.* 2008;**28**:1022–9.

23. Pariente J, Loubinoux I, Carel C, *et al.* Fluoxetine modulates motor performance and cerebral activation of patients recovering from stroke. *Ann Neurol.* 2001;**50**:718–29.

24. Chen YC, Galpern WR, Brownell AL, *et al.* Detection of dopaminergic neurotransmitter activity using pharmacologic MRI: Correlation with PET, microdialysis, and behavioral data. *Magn Reson Med.* 1997;**38**:389–98.

25. Reese T, Bochelen D, Baumann D, *et al.* Impaired functionality of reperfused brain tissue following short transient focal ischemia in rats. *Magn Reson Imaging.* 2002;**20**:447–54.

26. Biswal B, Yetkin FZ, Haughton VM, *et al.* Functional connectivity in the motor cortex of resting human brain using echo-planar MRI. *Magn Reson Med.* 1995;**34**:537–41.

27. He BJ, Snyder AZ, Vincent JL, *et al.* Breakdown of functional connectivity in frontoparietal networks underlies behavioral deficits in spatial neglect. *Neuron.* 2007;**53**:905–18.

28. Xiong J, Fox PT, Gao JH. Directly mapping magnetic field effects of neuronal activity by magnetic resonance imaging. *Hum Brain Mapp.* 2003;**20**:41–9.

29. Lin YJ, Koretsky AP. Manganese ion enhances T1-weighted MRI during brain activation: An approach to direct imaging of brain function. *Magn Reson Med.* 1997;**38**:378–88.

30. Basser PJ, Mattiello J, LeBihan D. MR diffusion tensor spectroscopy and imaging. *Biophys J.* 1994;**66**:259–67.

31. Basser PJ, Jones DK. Diffusion-tensor MRI: Theory, experimental design and data analysis – A technical review. *NMR Biomed.* 2002;**15**:456–67.

32. Mori S, Zhang J. Principles of diffusion tensor imaging and its applications to basic neuroscience research. *Neuron.* 2006;**51**:527–39.

33. Sotak CH. The role of diffusion tensor imaging in the evaluation of ischemic brain injury – A review. *NMR Biomed.* 2002;**15**:561–9.

34. Liu Y, D'Arceuil HE, Westmoreland S, *et al.* Serial diffusion tensor MRI after transient and permanent cerebral ischemia in nonhuman primates. *Stroke.* 2007;**38**:138–45.

35. Wang C, Stebbins GT, Nyenhuis DL, *et al.* Longitudinal changes in white matter following ischemic stroke: A three-year follow-up study. *Neurobiol Aging.* 2006;**27**:1827–33.

36. Jiang Q, Zhang ZG, Ding GL, *et al.* MRI detects white matter reorganization after neural progenitor cell treatment of stroke. *Neuroimage.* 2006;**32**:1080–9.

37. Van der Zijden JP, Van der Toorn A, Van der Marel K, *et al.* Longitudinal in vivo MRI of alterations in perilesional tissue after transient ischemic stroke in rats. *Exp Neurol.* 2008;**212**:207–12.

38. Ding G, Jiang Q, Li L, *et al.* Magnetic resonance imaging investigation of axonal remodeling and angiogenesis after embolic stroke in sildenafil-treated rats. *J Cereb Blood Flow Metab.* 2008;**28**:1440–8.

39. Silva AC, Lee JH, Aoki I, *et al.* Manganese-enhanced magnetic resonance imaging (MEMRI): Methodological and practical considerations. *NMR Biomed.* 2004;**17**:532–43.

40. Pautler RG. In vivo, trans-synaptic tract-tracing utilizing manganese-enhanced magnetic resonance imaging (MEMRI). *NMR Biomed.* 2004;**17**:595–601.

41. Pautler RG, Silva AC, Koretsky AP. In vivo neuronal tract tracing using manganese-enhanced magnetic resonance imaging. *Magn Reson Med.* 1998;**40**:740–8.

42. Allegrini PR, Wiessner C. Three-dimensional MRI of cerebral projections in rat brain in vivo after

65

intracortical injection of MnCl2. *NMR Biomed.* 2003;**16**:252–6.

43. Van der Zijden JP, Wu O, Van der Toorn A, *et al.* Changes in neuronal connectivity after stroke in rats as studied by serial manganese-enhanced MRI. *Neuroimage.* 2007;**34**:1650–7.

44. Van der Zijden JP, Bouts MJ, Wu O, *et al.* Manganese-enhanced MRI of brain plasticity in relation to functional recovery after experimental stroke. *J Cereb Blood Flow Metab.* 2008;**28**:832–40.

45. Carmichael ST. Plasticity of cortical projections after stroke. *Neuroscientist.* 2003;**9**:64–75.

46. Watanabe T, Frahm J, Michaelis T. Functional mapping of neural pathways in rodent brain in vivo using manganese-enhanced three-dimensional magnetic resonance imaging. *NMR Biomed.* 2004;**17**:554–68.

47. Canals S, Beyerlein M, Keller AL, *et al.* Magnetic resonance imaging of cortical connectivity in vivo. *Neuroimage.* 2008;**40**:458–72.

48. Ding G, Jiang Q, Li L, *et al.* Angiogenesis detected after embolic stroke in rat brain using magnetic resonance T2*WI. *Stroke.* 2008;**39**:1563–8.

49. Lin CY, Chang C, Cheung WM, *et al.* Dynamic changes in vascular permeability, cerebral blood volume, vascular density, and size after transient focal cerebral ischemia in rats: Evaluation with contrast-enhanced magnetic resonance imaging. *J Cereb Blood Flow Metab.* 2008;**28**:1491–501.

50. Van der Zijden JP, Van Eijsden P, De Graaf RA, *et al.* 1H/13C MR spectroscopic imaging of regionally specific metabolic alterations after experimental stroke. *Brain.* 2008;**131**:2209–19.

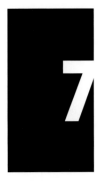

7

Stroke recovery in non-human primates: a comparative perspective

Randolph J. Nudo

Functional recovery following injury to motor cortex

Motor cortex lesions in humans result in weakness or paralysis in contralateral musculature and disruption of skilled limb use. However, gradual recovery of some motor abilities is commonly observed during the ensuing weeks. For example, within a few days following injury, tendon reflexes may again become active, and resistance to passive movement may increase. Limited recovery of voluntary movement often occurs. A gradual increase in muscle strength and coordination often follows. However, at least in humans, complete recovery of function in distal musculature, including independent control of digits, is uncommon.

Mechanistic bases to account for functional motor recovery following cortical injury have long been sought. Results as early as the 1950s by Glees and Cole using surface electrical stimulation techniques suggested that lost cortical functions are assumed by the adjacent cortical tissue [1]. Others have suggested that other cortical motor areas in the same or opposite hemisphere may play a role in recovery. Still others have suggested that subcortical structures are responsible. Over the past two decades, detailed examinations of neuroplasticity mechanisms in animal models of focal ischemia, as well as an explosion of neuroimaging data in human stroke survivors (see also Chapters 11–13), has provided a wealth of information that is beginning to shed light on critical questions. While we are still far from a complete understanding of the recovery process and the structures involved, it is now feasible to propose general principles regarding post-injury plasticity.

The use of non-human primates has contributed substantial information to this field. These species have great importance for translating new therapies to human stroke populations. The present review will focus principally on the unique role of non-human primates in stroke recovery research, primarily from an evolutionary perspective.

Non-human primates in studies of stroke recovery: practical and ethical issues

Evolution of primates

To understand the value of a particular model species for translation of neurological research, it is useful to consider phyletic relationships. It is reasonable to assume that the likelihood that a particular extant species will share common neuroanatomical and neurophysiological traits with humans is directly proportional to the recency of their common ancestors. Conversely, species that have been divergent in their phyletic histories will share relatively fewer features in common. In the past, evolutionary trees (or cladograms) were based entirely on morphological features of extant species and fossil records of presumed common ancestors. In the past decade, a revolution in evolutionary biology has taken place, as cladistic relationships are now derived on the basis of molecular genetic sequence analyses [2]. While there is still some discrepancy between molecular dates and the fossil record, and multiple hypotheses still exist regarding the relationships of a few higher-level lineages (e.g. colugos, tree shrews), there is general consensus that molecular data sets are rapidly becoming the gold standard for deciphering phyletic relationships among living mammals [3].

Four Superorders are now recognized within the mammalian Class. The Superorders Xenarthra (sloths, anteaters, armadillos, etc.) and Afrotheria (aardvarks, manatees, elephants, etc.) have their origins in the Southern Hemisphere (South America

Brain Repair After Stroke, ed. S. C. Cramer and R. J. Nudo. Published by Cambridge University Press.
© Cambridge University Press 2010.

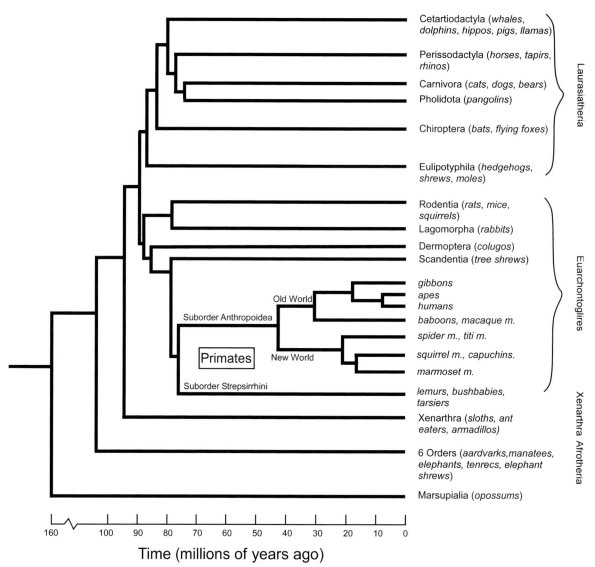

Figure 7.1 Cladogram of living mammals, with special emphasis on primates. Adapted from multiple sources (Janecka *et al.* [4]; Martin [3]).

and Africa, respectively). The Superorders Laurasiatheria (whales, hippos, horses, cats, dogs, bats, etc.) and Euarchontoglires (rodents, rabbits, lemurs, monkeys, apes, humans) are thought to have a Northern Hemisphere origin. New molecular data sets have radically altered our concepts of higher-level relationships. For example, based on morphological similarities, bats were once grouped with primates; tree shrews and colugos in the obsolete taxon Archonta. However, molecular evidence now puts bats in the Laurasiatheria Superorder with carnivores, ungulates, and cetaceans (Figure 7.1).

It is thought that the first primates emerged approximately 80 million years ago (mya), during the early Cretaceous period [4]. Probabilistic dating using molecular evidence estimates that the first divergence between the anthropoid primates (monkeys, apes, and humans) and strepsirrhine primates (lemurs, tarsiers, and bushbabies) occurred about 77.5 mya (range = 67.1–97.7 mya) [5]. About 43 mya, in the mid to late Eocene epoch (mid-Paleogene period), the Old World and New World monkey lineages diverged. Subsequently, the Cercopithecoidea (baboons, macaques) and Hominoidea (apes and humans) diverged about 30 mya, in the mid-Oligocene epoch (late Paleogene period). The last common ancestor of humans and gorillas was about 8.6 mya, while the last common ancestor of humans and chimps was about 6.6 mya, or during the late Miocene epoch (early Neogene period).

Returning to the hypothesis that morphological features become increasingly different between divergent taxa with increasing geological time, one can utilize the dates of last common ancestors as a quantitative gauge for their utility in translational studies. Thus, even for species currently used in stroke research that have diverged from the human lineage most recently (baboons, macaques), over 30 million years of brain evolution has occurred with different selective pressures in divergent taxa. If we search for the common ancestor of humans with New World monkeys (marmosets and squirrel monkeys), we need to trace back even further – over 40 million years. Carrying this logic back in geological time still further, one must retreat nearly 90 million years to find the last common ancestor of humans and rodents. Thus, even though primate and rodent species are members of the same Superorder (Euarchontoglires), they have not shared a common ancestor since the late Cretaceous period. Common ancestry for humans and other species used in neurological research (dogs, pigs, etc.) is a bit earlier than for rodents (88.8 versus 87.9 mya), although by only a small amount in geological time, since rapid divergence of mammalian lineages occurred during the late Cretaceous. Thus, from the standpoint of our hypothesis relating neurological diversity to phyletic relationships, rodents, carnivores, and ungulates are equally valid species.

It is primarily this phyletic rationale which makes non-human primates so valuable for understanding human brain function, and serving as models for stroke research. Undoubtedly there are other factors to consider when establishing an animal model. The brains of some mammalian species have become highly specialized, and probably do not closely resemble the brains of the common ancestors. Some brain properties of interest may be quite similar in widely divergent lineages due to convergent evolution. However, on a probabilistic basis, relative kinship is the principal determining factor in predicting genetic variance, and thus morphological variance, between the brains of different mammalian species.

Ethical and practical concerns

It is this very advantage of shared common ancestry that makes invasive research on non-human primates so controversial. For example, those opposed to invasive animal research generally point to the notion that some non-human organisms are sentient; that is, in its most literal sense, are capable of sensation and perception. With regard to invasive research, sentience is most controversial in the perception of pain and suffering. The fuzzy area is the affective component of any sensation or perception. The extreme view is to assume that any animal would perceive unpleasant events the same as a human would. But of course, this is a very anthropomorphic view, and is rejected by most scientists. None the less, if we accept that recency of common ancestry is a gauge of the degree of similarity in brain function among mammalian species, then one might conclude that non-human primates share more similarity in their awareness of pain and suffering than other mammalian species.

Additional factors that limit the use of certain primate species include the interrelated factors of availability and cost. Rapidly escalating costs even for primate species that currently exist in abundance in the wild or can be bred readily in captivity increasingly have limited the scope of non-human primate research.

Special characteristics of non-human primate brains for stroke recovery research

Several factors warrant the consideration of non-human primate species as models in stroke recovery research. First, from a theoretical standpoint, because of more recent shared common ancestry, non-human primate brains should respond to injury more similarly than rodents, especially with respect to behaviors that rely on specialized regions of cerebral cortex. Second, brain size may be an important factor in the penetration of pharmaceutical agents, although several larger-brained mammalian species, other than primates, can be used in stroke research including cats, dogs, pigs, and sheep. Third, white matter to gray matter ratio is significantly greater in primate brains than animals from other Orders, especially rodents. This fact may be critical in certain stroke models that target injury to descending pathways [6].

Finally, it is likely that several other structural and functional brain traits evolved in the primate lineage, especially with respect to the corticospinal (CS) tract. Primates uniquely have a spatially distinct concentration of CS neurons in a portion of the frontal cortex, corresponding to the ventral premotor cortex (PMv). This cortical field does not appear

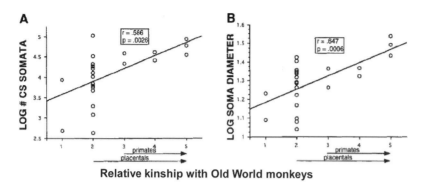

Figure 7.2 Relationship between CS neuron number/size and relative kinship with Old World primates (Nudo *et al.* [7]).

to exist in non-primate species. Further, primates have more corticospinal neurons concerned with control of the hand compared with other mammalian species (Figure 7.2). Still further, primates uniquely display larger and less concentrated CS cell bodies, indicative of increased neuropil. All of these changes occurred independent of any increase in body size [7].

The termination of CS neurons in the spinal cord also differs greatly across mammalian species, even within the primate Order. Specifically, the majority of CS neurons, regardless of species, terminate in intermediate lamina of the spinal cord. Only in select species do CS neurons terminate in deeper lamina, where motor neuron cell bodies are located. Thus, macaque monkeys, cebus monkeys, and humans have dense CS terminations in lamina IX. In contrast, squirrel monkeys, marmoset monkeys, and prosimian primates have sparse CS terminations in lamina IX [8]. Species variance in this particular trait is of prime importance in understanding the differences in behavioral response to cortical injury.

It has often been reported that one disadvantage of rodent models for stroke recovery studies is that spontaneous recovery proceeds too quickly, sometimes within days. This has especially been reported with focal cortical lesions. Non-human primates with similar lesions are thought to recover more slowly, more similar to humans. It is possible that the basis for this difference stems from an evolutionary principle called "encephalization of function." That is, the cerebral cortex assumes progressively more function in the primate lineage leading to humans, including functions once controlled at subcortical levels. This phenomenon was first studied systematically by Walker and Fulton who performed hemidecortication in several mammalian species [9]. Major differences were found in the ability of the different species to ambulate

on the first postoperative day. The primates, in particular, were much more debilitated. Furthermore, the degree of motor impairment appeared to be related to kinship with humans. For example, macaque monkeys could grasp the cage bars with the affected extremity while climbing within one week after the surgery. The recovery of grasp in the baboon required a month of recovery, while the chimpanzee never regained volitional grasp. Recovery of strength in the fingers and toes was incomplete in each of the primate species. In contrast, cats regained such strength within a few weeks.

Walker and Fulton also discussed spasticity following cortical injury, a hallmark of human stroke, which contributes to motor disability as well as the inability for stroke survivors to participate in rehabilitative therapy. Most animal models have failed to produce these same symptoms. Following hemidecortication in macaque monkeys, Walker and Fulton described the affected limbs as flaccid for about one week, followed by moderate spasticity. In the baboon, flaccidity was followed by more intense spasticity. In the chimpanzee, flaccidity lasted about three days, followed by even more intense spasticity. In chronic stages, some increased resistance to passive movement was observed in all animals, but substantial spasticity remained only in the chimpanzee.

Stroke models in non-human primates

Aspiration lesions

Historically, the most common lesion method in animals, especially for cortical lesions, has been aspiration, or suction ablation. These lesions have the advantage that they are highly reliable, since visual inspection of the cortical surface reveals the removed area. Obviously, this method does not mimic the clinical condition of stroke, except that a sizeable portion of cortical tissue is destroyed. They more closely mimic resection procedures that might be performed for removal of tumors or epileptic foci. There are disadvantages to this technique, since, unless the surgeon is highly skilled, inadvertent damage can be done to underlying white matter and adjacent gray matter. Further, fibers of passage are necessarily destroyed. Also, it is not clear what role necrotic tissue may play in subsequent inflammatory responses after injury. However, aspiration lesions have been very valuable in understanding the role of specific cortical areas in motor and sensory behavior.

Middle cerebral artery occlusion

One of the most common methods for creating a clinically relevant stroke in rodent models has been middle cerebral artery occlusion, or MCAo. This approach is attractive, since a large number of human strokes occur in the MCA, and this vessel supplies a wide swath of frontal and parietal cortex, affecting motor and somatosensory function. However, subtle vascular differences in the morphology of cerebral vessels exist across species, and such differences may result in wide variance in the resulting infarcted territory. For example, in the macaque, the anterior cerebral arteries join to form a single pericallosal artery in the midline, differing distinctly from the human cerebral vasculature pattern [10].

While surgical access to the MCA is relatively straightforward in rats, a much more invasive, transorbital surgical approach requiring enucleation is typically employed in non-human primate species. Usually, vessels are then occluded by microaneurysm clips [11], although photocoagulation using Rose Bengal has also been used [12]. Endovascular occlusion approaches would seem to be preferable, and some success has recently been reported using this method in macaque monkeys [13]. In this approach, a microcatheter is inserted into the femoral artery and guided fluoroscopically to occlude a branch of the MCA. However, substantial variability has been found in the outcomes. In the study by D'Arceuil et al. [13], in five macaque monkeys with MCAo for 3 h, stroke volume ranged from 0.1 to 4.5 ml. In four monkeys with permanent MCAo, stroke volume ranged from 2.9 to 20.5 ml. Animals with large lesions required extensive postoperative care, and survival was variable. Thus, while relatively non-invasive occlusion of the MCA is possible in non-human primates, the large variability in the outcome precludes its use in controlled therapeutic studies, since large numbers are required for adequate statistical power.

Another approach to modeling stroke is to inject emboli into the internal carotid artery (ICA). In one early study, emboli were formed within polyethylene tubing using silicone rubber compound, which primarily lodged in the M1 segment of the MCA [14]. In about 14% of the experiments, the embolus fractured, and lodged in multiple segmental locations affecting the distribution of the infarctions. In a variation on this technique, multiple silicone spheres were injected into the ICA of macaque monkeys [15]. In over 80% of the monkeys, the spheres were lodged at the junction of the ICA and the MCA. However, sometimes the distal embolus was located in the proximal anterior cerebral artery (ACA). In these early studies, only gross qualitative changes in cerebral morphology were described. In a more recent study, autologous blood clots were injected into the ICA in macaque monkeys [16]. This method resulted in extensive infarcts throughout the MCA territory in the cerebral cortex as well as extensive subcortical damage in the striatum and thalamus. Mean infarct volume as a percentage of the hemisphere was 28%, ranging from about 12 to 55% (based on scatterplot). This method has been subsequently used by this group to examine the effects of thrombolytic agents after stroke. While the infarct size range is somewhat broad, the variability is not unexpected given individual variation in the distribution of the MCA. Further development of cerebral vessel occlusion methods that do not require intracranial surgery will be extremely valuable to replicate the conditions of human stroke in non-human primate models.

Focal electrocoagulation

Several studies have employed more focal ischemia techniques, resulting in more restricted cortical injury than what is experienced in clinical stroke. This approach is used most often in conjunction with neurophysiological mapping techniques to determine details in the functional reorganization of the spared regions after injury. Since these techniques result in occlusion of the arterioles and venules of the entire vascular bed within a targeted region, there is little if any penumbra. Thus, they are not useful for neuroprotection studies, which generally have as a primary aim to salvage threatened penumbra. Also, focal coagulation techniques are most often used in lissencephalic brains such as owl monkeys or squirrel monkeys, since the somatosensory and motor hand areas are exposed over a flat, unfissured sector of cortex, allowing easy access to the vascular supply. The surface vessels can be seen to penetrate radially into the cortex, so that the infarcted territory closely matches the region of ischemia on the surface. Lesions as small as 2 mm in diameter on the surface of the cortex and penetrating throughout all six layers of cortex can be made reliably. Very large infarcts affecting much of the upper extremity representations in M1 and premotor areas are feasible [17]. It should also be noted that little, if any, direct necrosis of white matter occurs with this approach, although secondary degeneration of descending fibers necessarily occurs.

Organization of motor cortex in primates

In all primate species studied to date, multiple motor representations of the upper extremity have been found. The largest and most functionally important area is the primary motor cortex, or M1. This region lies anterior to the central sulcus, and has several anatomical and physiological properties which distinguish it from other motor areas. First, in either anesthetized or awake animals, specific joint movements can be elicited by small amounts of electrical stimulation within the deeper layers of all motor areas, but required currents are smallest in M1. M1 contains the largest proportion of CS neurons of any of the cortical motor areas. In addition, M1 contains the very large CS neurons, sometimes called Betz cells, especially in its posterior aspect.

Extensive neurophysiological and neuroanatomical studies have now revealed that individual muscles are not represented in discrete functional modules within M1. At its most elemental level, an individual CS neuron diverges to influence up to four or five motor neuron pools in the spinal cord. Further, CS neurons projecting to different subsets of motor neuron pools overlap substantially within M1. Hence, it is highly unlikely that stimulation of a small volume of cortical tissue in M1 with electrical current could elicit a contraction of only a single muscle, even if one could stimulate only a single neuron. Representations of disparate body parts, e.g. the arm and leg, are located in non-overlapping areas of M1. Thus, strict topographic organization based on the distribution of the skeletal musculature is maintained only on a global scale.

While a cortical motor field that is homologous to M1 is present in most mammalian species, premotor areas most likely evolved independently in the primate lineage [18]. These premotor areas include dorsal and ventral premotor cortex (PMd and PMv, respectively), the supplementary motor area (SMA), and the cingulate motor areas. By definition, each of the premotor areas is connected with M1 via reciprocal intracortical fibers. These areas are functionally distinct, and are thought to exert their influence on motor output primarily via M1. However, each of these areas also sends fibers to the spinal cord, and thus has the potential to participate in more direct control of spinal motor neurons in the absence of M1.

Plasticity of neurophysiological maps and their relationship to functional recovery

Neurophysiological maps can be derived in motor cortex using various stimulation techniques in experimental animals, even under anesthesia. Early studies using cortical surface stimulation techniques suggested that the hand representation in M1 of adult primates undergoes substantial remodeling following small lesions, and the cortical remodeling is correlated with functional recovery [1]. Using more modern intracortical microstimulation (ICMS) techniques, Nudo and Milliken found that movements represented in the infarcted zone did not reappear in the cortical sector surrounding the infarct. Instead, relatively small, subtotal lesions in representations of hand movements resulted in widespread reduction in the spared hand representations adjacent to the lesion, and apparent increases in adjacent proximal representations [19].

While the study cited above employed no post-infarct therapy, we have also examined consequences of motor training on the functional topography of motor cortex in uninjured squirrel monkeys [20]. The task required the monkeys to retrieve small food pellets from four wells on a Plexiglas board. The smallest well required the controlled insertion of only one or two digits to retrieve pellets. Retrieval skill was significantly improved by only a few days of intensive training, but then continued for 10–11 days. In each case, post-training maps revealed significant changes in the topographies of movement representation marked by expansion of the cortical sectors representing movements involved in the task. These experiments confirmed that the functional representations of primary motor cortex are remodeled by use, probably throughout life.

It was reasonable to hypothesize that these same training techniques could have an adaptive influence on motor representations after injury. In an initial experiment, small ischemic lesions were made in the M1 hand area, sparing a large portion of this area. Deficits in motor skill were apparent in the pellet retrieval task. Within about 5 days, the monkeys were able to participate in the task again, and repetitive training began, using a protocol much like that used for normal training. As monkeys gained proficiency at retrieval from large food wells, they advanced to progressively smaller wells. For most monkeys, pellet retrieval proficiency returned within about 2 weeks. At that point, the M1 hand area was explored with ICMS techniques once again. In monkeys receiving training, the spared M1 hand area was not statistically different from their baseline maps. That is, instead of a reduction in M1 hand area, the hand area was retained. In some cases, the hand area clearly expanded into former proximal representations [21].

Later experiments demonstrated that this effect of post-injury training was not related to the location of the focal infarct within the M1 hand area [22]. Regardless of whether the lesion was in the rostral or caudal portion, retention of the spared hand representation was observed after post-infarct rehabilitation. This is significant, since the rostral and caudal portions of the M1 hand area are functionally distinct. Both rostral and caudal portions of M1 receive input from the somatosensory cortex. However, the caudal M1 receives predominantly cutaneous input, and the rostral portion receives predominantly proprioceptive input. Behavioral deficits after restricted lesions in M1 reflect these differences in sensory input properties. Lesions in caudal M1 result in behavioral symptoms akin to sensory agnosia, in which the monkeys retrieve pellets, but appear not to know that the pellet is in their hand. They often open the hand, and look at the pellet, before bringing the hand to the mouth to eat the pellet. Conversely, lesions in rostral M1 do not result in sensory agnosia. In contrast, monkeys often overreach the target, dragging the hand back like a rake until the fingers enter the food well. The fact that the hand movement representations respond to rehabilitative training in the same way regardless of lesion location emphasizes that both cutaneous and proprioceptive cues are important in executing the motor task of pellet retrieval.

Focal lesions in a small portion of M1 have very different effects on remote hand representations in premotor cortex. Because of reciprocal connectivity of these areas with M1, if M1 is injured, there are inevitable effects in secondary motor areas. Using the PMv as a model for these remote effects, as early as a few days after M1 injury, neurons in PMv undergo substantial changes in expression of proteins thought to be involved in neuroprotection and angiogenesis [23].

In the chronic stage after M1 injury there is a linear relationship between the size of the M1 infarct and enlargement of the hand representation in PMv. After lesions in M1 that destroy less than 30% of the hand area, the PMv hand representation actually shrinks slightly. However, after progressively larger M1 injuries, the PMv representation expands in proportion to the M1 loss [24,25].

These remote effects of M1 lesions have now been extended to the hand representation in the SMA, again relating remote map expansion with M1 lesion size [17]. Movements can be evoked from these areas with relatively low amounts of electrical current even when the damage to M1 is extensive. While CS neurons from these secondary motor areas exist, their direct effects on spinal cord motor neurons are thought to be meager. However, at least in chronic stages after injury to M1, short latency responses can be elicited from these areas. The anatomical route underlying this effect is not yet clear. Possible pathways include cortico-rubro-spinal, cortico-reticulo-spinal, and direct CS pathways. Evidence for post-injury CS sprouting from the SMA has been established in macaque monkeys [26]. Thus, the intriguing possibility exists that areas remote from cortical injury adaptively reorganize to compensate for the loss of M1 CS output by sending larger numbers of CS axons to terminate on the denervated motor neurons.

Although remote areas expand, the functional significance of this change is still unclear. SMA may be an excellent model for understanding these effects, since it receives its blood supply from the ACA, and is often spared after MCA strokes. The SMAs of the two hemispheres are heavily interconnected, and share dense reciprocal projections with M1. It has also been estimated that 23% of SMA CS neurons project to the ipsilateral cord [27]. But a recent study in SMA after extensive ischemic lesions that extended across the M1, PMd, and PMv hand areas questions a direct functional relationship of map reorganization to recovery [17]. In this study, behavioral recovery was limited to the first three weeks post-injury. Behavioral performance remained relatively constant and suboptimal throughout the next 10 weeks. However, maps of the hand area in SMA actually contracted in the first three post-infarct weeks. They subsequently expanded over the next 10 weeks. This temporal mismatch is not easily explained by a simple relationship of remote reorganization in a single area, such as SMA, to behavioral recovery.

Another interesting aspect of SMA is that it has greater influence on motor neuron pools controlling proximal, rather than distal muscles [28]. In the Eisner-Janowicz study [17], the changes that were seen in the SMA hand representation after injury were attributed to wrist and forearm movement representations, not more distal, finger and thumb representations. In these chronic stages, monkeys were able to reach out and touch the pellet board, but were not able to retrieve pellets from the wells, or even insert their fingers into the wells. This is not unlike human stroke survivors who can use proximal musculature to propel the limb forward, but do not have distal control over hand movements. Thus, it is possible that SMA may contribute to the development of compensatory movement patterns that rely on more proximal musculature.

Neuroanatomical plasticity after injury

Due to a rich network of reciprocal intracortical connections, after focal injury to M1, remote areas are triggered to reorganize their axonal projection pathways. It is well known that in rats, after cortical injury, the cerebral cortex in the intact hemisphere sprouts crossed axonal projections to the striatum of the injured side of the brain. However, little is known regarding plasticity of intrinsic intracortical pathways interconnecting various cortical areas. Recently, using a squirrel monkey model of M1 infarct, Dancause *et al.* discovered that several months after an M1 infarct, PMv intracortical axons developed an aberrant trajectory [29]. Axons projecting toward the site of the lesion made sharp turns, and avoided the lesion zone. A substantial number of axons then turned more caudally, heading more lateral to circumvent the central sulcus, and finally terminated in a parietal area within the somatosensory cortex, area 1 (possibly both areas 1 and 2) [29]. This *de novo* cortical connection represented axonal growth of more than 1 cm, a very

long distance in the small squirrel monkey brain. Understanding the functional significance of injury-induced sprouting is an important topic for future research.

Studies of post-stroke interventions in non-human primates

Non-human primates have been used sporadically in preclinical investigations of new therapeutics for stroke recovery, including both pharmaceutical and device-oriented approaches. Impetus for non-human primate studies gained momentum after a large number of failed neuroprotection trials that did not translate from preclinical rodent studies to primates. As one of a large list of recommendations for preclinical drug development, the STAIR consensus conference recommended the increased use of non-human primates in stroke research [30]. It was thought that substantial species differences in drug metabolism, penetration of the drug into the brain, brain organization, and behavioral response to injury require that clinical trials be preceded by some level of assurance that the drug worked in a non-human primate model.

One study that has received considerable attention in this regard examined the effects of the free radical trapping agent, NXY-059, administered at 4 h after MCA branch occlusion in a marmoset monkey model [31]. NXY-059 reduced infarct volume by 28%, and resulted in attenuated motor and spatial neglect. However, clinical trials have had mixed results [32]. Discussions in the literature have questioned both the quality of preclinical study designs as well as adherence to preclinical protocols in the randomized clinical studies.

Conclusions

A full survey of the critical issues in successful translational research is well beyond the scope of this chapter. However, from the standpoint of comparative neurobiology, it should be kept in mind that humans and non-human primates do, indeed, have many neurological traits in common. Based on phyletic evidence, non-human primate models should approximate the response to ischemic injury better than other mammalian species. Likewise, a larger proportion of the variance in the effects of neuroprotective and restorative agents after stroke in humans can be predicted by examining their effects in non-human primate models in comparison with other mammalian

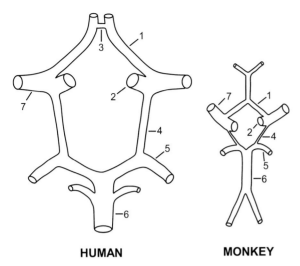

HUMAN　　　　　　**MONKEY**

Figure 7.3 Schematic representation of the cerebral arterial circle (of Willis) in human and monkey (*Macaca mulatta*). Arteries: 1, anterior cerebral; 2, internal carotid; 3, anterior communicating; 4, posterior communicating; 5, posterior cerebral; 6, basilar. Redrawn from Kapoor *et al.* [10].

models. However, even with optimal techniques for mimicking stroke, and strict adherence to high standards for study design, execution and reporting, tens of millions of years of brain evolution have occurred since the common ancestors of humans and most non-human primates. No single animal model, nor individual preclinical study, should be used as a litmus test for the predictability of a planned clinical trial. Resolution of reliability and validity (including construct, internal and external validity) for a particular therapeutic agent requires multiple replications under a variety of conditions before its predictive value in clinical trials can be estimated with accuracy. As the French physician/scientist Paul Broca said: "The least questioned assumptions are often the most questionable" [33].

References

1. Glees P, Cole J. Recovery of skilled motor functions after small repeated lesions in motor cortex in macaque. *J Neurophysiol.* 1950;**13**:137–48.

2. Murphy WJ, Eizirik E, O'Brien SJ, *et al.* Resolution of the early placental mammal radiation using Bayesian phylogenetics. *Science.* 2001;**294**(5550):2348–51.

3. Martin RD. Colugos: Obscure mammals glide into the evolutionary limelight. *J Biol.* 2008;**7**(4):13.

4. Janecka JE, Miller W, Pringle TH, *et al.* Molecular and genomic data identify the closest living relative of primates. *Science.* 2007;**318**(5851):792–4.

5. Steiper ME, Young NM. Primate molecular divergence dates. *Mol Phylogenet Evol.* 2006;**41**:384–94.

6. Frost SB, Barbay S, Mumert ML, *et al.* An animal model of capsular infarct: Endothelin-1 injections in the rat. *Behav Brain Res.* 2006;**169**:206–11.

7. Nudo RJ, Sutherland DP, Masterton RB, *et al.* Variation and evolution of mammalian corticospinal somata with special reference to primates. *J Comp Neurol.* 1995;**358**:181–205.

8. Lemon RN, Griffiths J. Comparing the function of the corticospinal system in different species: Organizational differences for motor specialization? *Muscle Nerve.* 2005;**32**:261–79.

9. Walker AE, Fulton JF. Hemidecortication in chimpanzee, baboon, macaque, potto, cat and coati: A study in encephalization. *J Nerv Ment Dis.* 1938;**87**:677–700.

10. Kapoor K, Kak VK, Singh B, *et al.* Morphology and comparative anatomy of circulus arteriosus cerebri in mammals. *Anat Histol Embryol.* 2003;**32**:347–55.

11. Fukuda S, del Zoppo GJ. Models of focal cerebral ischemia in the nonhuman primate. *ILAR J.* 2003;**44**:96–104.

12. Furuichi Y, Maeda M, Moriguchi A, *et al.* Tacrolimus, a potential neuroprotective agent, ameliorates ischemic brain damage and neurologic deficits after focal cerebral ischemia in nonhuman primates. *J Cereb Blood Flow Metab.* 2003;**23**:1183–94.

13. D'Arceuil HE, Duggan M, He J, *et al.* Middle cerebral artery occlusion in *Macaca fascicularis*: Acute and chronic stroke evolution. *J Med Primatol.* 2006;**35**:78–86.

14. Molinari GF, Moseley JI, Laurent JP, *et al.* Segmental middle cerebral artery occlusion in primates: An experimental method requiring minimal surgery and anesthesia. *Stroke.* 1974;**5**:334–9.

15. Watanabe O, Bremer AM, West CR, *et al.* Experimental regional cerebral ischemia in the middle cerebral artery territory in primates. Part 1: Angio-anatomy and description of an experimental model with selective embolization of the internal carotid artery bifurcation. *Stroke.* 1977;**8**:61–70.

16. Kito G, Nishimura A, Susumu T, *et al.* Experimental thromboembolic stroke in cynomolgus monkey. *J Neurosci Methods.* 2001;**105**:45–53.

17. Eisner-Janowicz I, Barbay S, Hoover E, *et al.* Early and late changes in the distal forelimb representation of the supplementary motor area after injury to frontal motor areas in the squirrel monkey. *J Neurophysiol.* 2008;**100**:1498–512.

18. Nudo RJ, Masterton RB. Descending pathways to the spinal cord, III: Sites of origin of the corticospinal tract. *J Comp Neurol.* 1990;**296**:559–83.

19. Nudo RJ, Milliken GW. Reorganization of movement representations in primary motor cortex following focal ischemic infarcts in adult squirrel monkeys. *J Neurophysiol*. 1996;75:2144–9.

20. Nudo RJ, Wise BM, SiFuentes F, *et al.* Neural substrates for the effects of rehabilitative training on motor recovery after ischemic infarct. *Science*. 1996; 272(5269):1791–4.

21. Nudo RJ, Milliken GW, Jenkins WM, *et al.* Use-dependent alterations of movement representations in primary motor cortex of adult squirrel monkeys. *J Neurosci*. 1996;16:785–807.

22. Friel KM, Barbay S, Frost SB, *et al.* Effects of a rostral motor cortex lesion on primary motor cortex hand representation topography in primates. *Neurorehabil Neural Rep*. 2007;21:51–61.

23. Stowe AM, Plautz EJ, Nguyen P, *et al.* Neuronal HIF-1 alpha protein and VEGFR-2 immunoreactivity in functionally related motor areas following a focal M1 infarct. *J Cereb Blood Flow Metab*. 2008;28:612–20.

24. Frost SB, Barbay S, Friel KM, *et al.* Reorganization of remote cortical regions after ischemic brain injury: A potential substrate for stroke recovery. *J Neurophysiol*. 2003;89:3205–14.

25. Dancause N, Barbay S, Frost SB, et al. Effects of small ischemic lesions in the primary motor cortex on neurophysiological organization in ventral premotor cortex. *J Neurophysiol*. 2006; 96: 3506–11.

26. McNeal DW, Darling WG, Pizzimenti M, *et al.* Long-term reorganization of the corticospinal projection from the supplementary motor cortex following brain injury is accompanied by motor recovery and prolonged microgliosis in the rhesus monkey. Program No. 77.4. 2007 *Neuroscience Meeting Planner*. San Diego, CA: Society for Neuroscience, 2007. Online.

27. Dum RP, Strick PL. Spinal cord terminations of the medial wall motor areas in macaque monkeys. *J Neurosci*. 1996;16:13–25.

28. Boudrias MH, Belhaj-Saif A, Park MC, *et al.* Contrasting properties of motor output from the supplementary motor area and primary motor cortex in rhesus macaques. *Cereb Cortex*. 2006;16:632–8.

29. Dancause N, Barbay S, Frost SB, *et al.* Extensive cortical rewiring after brain injury. *J Neurosci*. 2005;25:10 167–79.

30. Stroke Therapy Academic Industry Roundtable (STAIR). Recommendations for standards regarding preclinical neuroprotective and restorative drug development. *Stroke*. 1999;30: 2752–8.

31. Marshall JW, Cummings RM, Bowes LJ, *et al.* Functional and histological evidence for the protective effect of NXY-059 in a primate model of stroke when given 4 hours after occlusion. *Stroke*. 2003;34:2228–33.

32. Diener HC, Lees KR, Lydon P, *et al.* NXY-059 for the treatment of acute stroke: Pooled analysis of the SAINT I and II Trials. *Stroke*. 2008;39:1751–8.

33. Schiller F. *Paul Broca, explorer of the brain*. New York, NY: Oxford University Press; 1992.

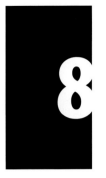

8 Issues in translating stroke recovery research from animals to humans

J. Leigh Leasure, Andreas Luft & Timothy Schallert

In Western nations the incidence of stroke and stroke fatalities is declining [1], but enhanced survival has resulted in a large population of individuals with long-term impairments and decreased quality of life. At present, there are no clearly effective treatments for these enduring deficits, despite a great deal of preclinical research directed at the problem. Yearly, a wealth of basic research is published on stroke recovery, cortical plasticity, and learning. So why are rehabilitation treatments at best of limited benefit and fail to provide a major advantage for the patient's life?

The problem may not be a lack of potential candidates, or a lack of clinical testing. Rather, the problem may be that candidates were not selected or optimized based on basic research information [2]. Many candidates are prematurely advanced into clinical trials. Using the wrong dose is a common reason why drug trials fail to show efficacy; dose estimation studies therefore have to be conducted before any Phase III trial is planned. For rehabilitation treatments, not only the dose but many other parameters have to be selected; among those are timing, concomitant treatments, psychological and social factors. We suggest that these and other factors discussed below contribute to the failure to translate research findings into viable treatments for human stroke patients.

Reason one: optimal timing and intensity of rehabilitation is uncertain

The mammalian brain actively attempts to repair itself after injury by inducing neuroplastic events in surviving perilesion and connected tissue, and homotopic areas in the intact hemisphere [3–15]. These restorative events are subject to modification by behavioral manipulation. Evidence for enhancement or inhibition of these processes comes from animal models in which behavior is characterized in relationship to

neuroanatomical events and then directly manipulated at different post-injury timepoints.

Injury to the forelimb representation area of the rat sensorimotor cortex (FL-SMC) causes limb use deficits in the contralateral forelimb [5,6,8]. There are transient deficits in forelimb placement reaching and grid-walking ability, as well as a long-lasting preference for the ipsilateral forelimb for lateral weight-supporting movements during wall exploration [3,13,16]. Taub and colleagues suggest that chronic reliance on the less-affected (ipsilateral) limb after unilateral brain injury is due in part to "learned non-use" of the affected (contralateral) limb [17]. That is, alternative motor strategies are developed with the ipsilateral limb in order to circumvent dysfunction in the affected extremity. If these strategies are effective, they encourage reliance upon the less-affected limb at the expense of the affected one. Thus, although restorative processes in surviving tissue may make effective use of the contralateral limb possible, use of it is rarely attempted and reliance on the ipsilateral limb persists. Taub and colleagues have demonstrated that the potential for substantial use of the affected extremity remains, however, and can be unmasked by restraint of the preferred limb [17], known as constraint-induced movement therapy (CIMT).

It is reasonable, therefore, to imagine that learned non-use could be avoided if reliance on the ipsilateral limb is not possible. Accordingly, we prevented use of the less-affected forelimb early after electrolytic lesions of the FL-SMC in rats by completely immobilizing it with a cast. This manipulation forced reliance on the contralateral forelimb for all motor activity. Surprisingly, early over-use of the affected forelimb did not enhance functional recovery. Rather, it exacerbated impairment of the contralateral forelimb and increased the extent of damage to perilesional tissue [18,19]. Yet CIMT, which also involves restraint of the

---

Brain Repair After Stroke, ed. S. C. Cramer and R. J. Nudo. Published by Cambridge University Press.
© Cambridge University Press 2010.

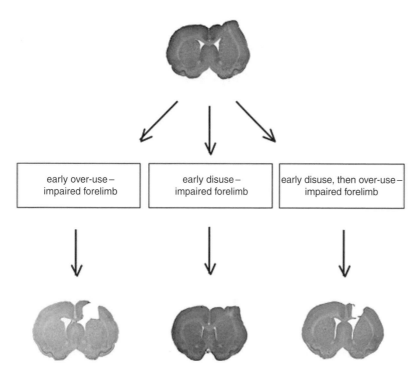

Figure 8.1 Schematic diagram showing the neural outcome of forelimb use manipulation after a focal cortical injury. A minimal amount of limb use may be necessary in order to maximize restorative processes in surviving tissue; however, extreme over-use increases the size of the lesion. Although complete disuse of the impaired forelimb does not, it interferes with functional recovery, and can increase the size of the lesion if it is followed by over-use.

less-affected limb, engenders detectable improvements in function of the impaired extremity [12]. Why, then, was early over-use of the impaired forelimb so disastrous?

Early post-traumatic neural events appear to be use-dependent, such that some minimal cognitive or motor activity is necessary to engender restorative processes in surviving tissue [4]. Early, vigorous rehabilitative measures likely exert their adverse effects by changing the course and magnitude of post-traumatic regenerative events. For example, excessive voluntary exercise early after cortical injury disrupts beneficial reactive protein expression [20] and can lead to excitotoxicity [21] and/or local peri-injury temperature increases [22]. Similarly, over-use of the forelimb impaired by a unilateral cortical lesion increases the reactive astrocytic response in surviving perilesional tissue [10], but limits use-dependent dendritic events in homotopic cortex [6]. In addition to being use-dependent, post-traumatic neural events are very likely time-dependent, characterized by definable phases in which the brain is differentially sensitive to behavioral modification [13]. We found that forced over-use of the affected limb during the first but not the second week after a lesion caused use-dependent exaggeration of injury [19]. Similarly, excessive voluntary exercise early, but not later, after cortical injury inhibits

recovery of function [20,23]. Collectively, the adverse effects of early over-use of the impaired forelimb can be explained by a window of time in which use-dependent restorative neural events can be disrupted by excessive behavioral pressure.

We reasoned that if over-use of an impaired limb could disrupt use-dependent neural events and functional recovery post-injury, *disuse* probably could as well. Accordingly, we used plaster of Paris casts to immobilize the affected forelimb of rats after unilateral injury to the FL-SMC [24]. This manipulation produced two effects with interesting clinical ramifications. First, it inhibited functional recovery and increased reliance on the ipsilateral limb after the cast had been removed. Second, it extended the window of vulnerability to the second post-injury week, which was previously shown to be a "safe" time in which to begin rehabilitative measures (Figure 8.1). In a clinical setting, it is not hard to imagine that a hemiplegic limb may be forcibly immobilized by sensory neglect or placement of an intravenous line. In such cases of early disuse, the window of vulnerability may be extended, and subsequent vigorous rehabilitative therapy may do more harm than good. We have also shown that immobilization of the affected forelimb reduced reactive expression of the neurotrophic factor FGF-2 in surviving tissue [13]. Thus, it seems

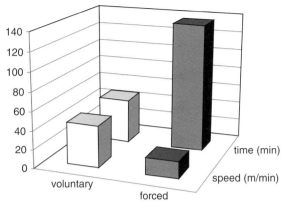

Figure 8.2 Forced and voluntary exercise in laboratory rats are fundamentally different. Assuming both groups run the same distance, rats that exercise voluntarily cover that distance at high speed (an average of 44 m/min) in a short period of time (about 47 min). In contrast, it is difficult to force rats to run faster than about 20 m/min for prolonged periods of time, so it takes much longer for forced exercisers to achieve the same distance.

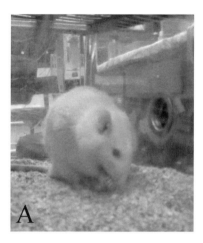

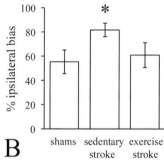

Figure 8.3 Rats with a unilateral stroke injury in the cortical forelimb area prefer to remove an adhesive stimulus from the ipsilateral limb [3], (A). Walking exercise, beginning a week after stroke, reduces this bias, (B) *$p < 0.05$ significantly different from shams.

that either extreme over-use or disuse of the affected forelimb may disrupt use-dependent neural events in remaining tissue, and inhibit functional recovery.

Although either extreme over-use or disuse can adversely affect recovery, less aggressive approaches may be more helpful. These may optimally exploit the capacity of the brain to undergo beneficial plastic changes, which is likely higher in the acute rather than later phases after stroke [25]. For example, gentle, focused, limb-specific interventions improve motor outcome [7,26] by encouraging functional reorganization of remaining tissue [7,27]. Indeed, along with timing, the intensity of post-injury rehabilitation may be an extremely important factor to consider when applying animal research results to post-stroke humans.

For example, exercise shows effectiveness preclinically as a preventative and restorative rehabilitative intervention for stroke. However, many of these studies are of constant-access voluntary wheel-running. Even early after brain injury, laboratory animals will run long distances in exercise wheels during a 24-h period. Since stroke-impaired humans have limited motor capacity and restricted access to exercise, the relevance of wheel-running studies to the post-stroke human condition is questionable, and forced exercise may represent a much more useful model. Forced exercise on a treadmill shows considerable benefit in chronic stroke survivors, affecting walking function and fitness [28,29].

When running distance is held constant in the animal model, forced exercise is characterized by extended, low-intensity exertion, whereas wheel-running is done in brief, high-intensity bouts (Figure 8.2) [30]. Forced treadmill exercise [31,32], but not voluntary wheel-running [31], is neuroprotective in animal models when begun prior to stroke. Perhaps wheel-running may be too high-intensity to be helpful. Indeed, early excessive voluntary running inhibits recovery after brain injury [20,23], but a more moderate voluntary exercise regimen has been reported to mildly enhance [33] or not inhibit recovery [26]. Furthermore, we have recently found that gentle, low-speed forced walking enhances recovery of sensorimotor function in aged rats following a stroke. As shown in Figure 8.3, aged rats that walked 5 days a week for 5 weeks (beginning 7 days post-injury) demonstrated less sensory bias towards the ipsilateral forelimb in the sensory asymmetry test.

Preclinical animal research studies indicate that early, vigorous physical rehabilitative efforts do not enhance functional recovery and can actually inhibit it. Yet determining when and how vigorously to institute rehabilitation in human stroke patients is very difficult. While CIMT can mitigate chronic stroke-induced impairments [12], CIMT was no better than traditional therapy when applied early in the course of stroke recovery [34]. It is possible that adverse effects of early training cancel or even counteract the beneficial effects. Recently, a study of human stroke patients found that forced rehabilitation immediately following stroke led to a worsening of outcome compared to untreated patients [35]. Furthermore, the effectiveness of rehabilitative measures may be "dose-dependent." A recent study of delayed therapy showed that patients on a 4 visits/week program improved more than those on a 1 or 3 visits/week regimen [36]. Animal studies that take into account the post-stroke human condition and clinical trials that are guided by the importance of timing and intensity of rehabilitation are necessary to pinpoint an effective treatment for chronic stroke-induced impairments.

Reason two: strokes are heterogeneous

Human strokes vary greatly in size, location and type. Most animal models are of ischemic injuries, produced by vessel occlusion, photothrombosis, thermocoagulation, pial vessel stripping, or vasoconstriction. Because the neural response to injury is lesion-dependent, each stroke model may have only a subset of neural responses and a unique behavioral impairment profile, and therefore be relevant only to a specific subset of human strokes.

Increasingly, it is being realized that recovery from brain injury is lesion-specific. For example, dendritic arborization occurs in the homotopic region following unilateral electrolytic [5,6] but not aspiration lesions [8] of the rat sensorimotor cortex. Axonal sprouting from the contralesional homotopic area is seen in the denervated striatum following unilateral cortical thermocoagulation of blood vessels but not aspiration lesions [9]. Furthermore, aspiration lesions decrease expression of GAP-43 in the striatum, but thermocoagulation lesions do not [37]. Finally, the neural response to hemorrhagic stroke is different from that to ischemia [38–43]. Therefore, it follows that functional impairment and recovery are also lesion-

dependent, and indeed, the severity and stability of post-injury motor impairments depend on whether they result from thermocoagulation or aspiration lesions [44].

Neural response and functional impairment are also dependent on the size of the lesion. This phenomenon is particularly obvious from study of middle cerebral artery occlusion (MCAo). MCAo for 2 h generated significantly more neurogenesis in the ipsilateral striatum compared to 30 min of MCAo [45], likely because 2 h of MCAo resulted in greater striatal damage. Furthermore, over-use of the forelimb impaired by MCAo confined to the cortex resulted in an increase in infarct volume, although when over-use followed a more severe MCAo that included the striatum, infarct size was not increased. Presumably, this was due to the fact that the more severe injury produced maximal damage that could not be exacerbated by post-stroke behavioral modification [13]. Behavioral recovery, too, is dependent on the type and size of the injury, and the degree of striatal involvement [3,46,47]. When there is minimal striatal damage, rats with a unilateral FL-SMC injury gradually begin to use the affected forelimb for some weight-supporting movements, such as landing from a rear. However, if striatal damage is significant, as it is when there is use-dependent exaggeration of injury, recovery of contralateral forelimb use is minimal or absent [18].

Finally, location of the lesion may also influence the neural response. Brain injury increases metabolic activity [48] and the proliferation of progenitor cells in neurogenic regions of the adult mammalian brain (for review see [14] and see Chapter 24). It has been suggested that in order to induce maximal proliferative response, an injury must be proximal to one of the two neurogenic regions, either the subependymal zone [49,50] or the dentate gyrus of the hippocampus [50]. To illustrate, lesions that are proximal to the dentate gyrus induce a more robust reactive response from progenitor cells than do more distal injuries [50]. However, introducing growth factors in the injured area may encourage tissue repair, functional recovery and generation of new tissue at the site of injury or in more remote areas [51].

Animal models offer the benefit of homogeneity of subject characteristics, lesion placement, and post-injury treatment, but information collected from them must be applied judiciously in order to maximize predictive validity. Findings from a specific animal model may be relevant to only a subset of human strokes. When testing the efficacy of a promising stroke treatment, it is important to match the brain insults to that of the animal model for which the treatment was tested. Of course, maintaining stroke homogeneity in patient trials is very difficult and often impractical. Therefore, before moving an experimental treatment forward to the clinic, the stroke diversity expected in patients should be replicated closely in the animal model [52], along with social and other environmental factors that can greatly influence outcome [53–55].

Reason three: preclinical stroke research is conducted in young animals

Despite the fact that stroke is far more common in the elderly than it is in the young [56–58], most preclinical stroke research is conducted in young animals [59]. This focus on young animals may account for why treatments that appeared promising preclinically failed to prove efficacious in clinical trials [60]. Structurally and chemically speaking, the aged brain represents a different environment than the young brain, and an important consideration is its reduced neuroplastic capacity. Rodents show age-related brain changes similar to those of humans, as well as associated cognitive and motor impairments, making them an excellent model in which to test potential stroke remedies.

Understandably, the cost of conducting stroke research in aged rodents is quite high. It is expensive to purchase aged animals, and the option of in-house breeding is not significantly more cost-effective, due to *per diem* care expenses. Yet it is essential to test promising therapies in an aged model before proceeding with clinical trials. It is possible, even likely, that a young brain would recover relatively well from a stroke in the absence of any treatment. Thus, the efficacy of a stroke treatment tested in young animals could easily be exaggerated.

Mortality is another issue when conducting stroke research in aged animals. Although it can be difficult to get aged animals to survive a massive stroke injury [61], focal lesions can be made in aged rats with low mortality rates [59,62,63]. In addition, these more restricted lesions produce significant and enduring motor deficits in aged animals, in contrast to the more minor and transient

deficits that would be observed in younger animals that sustained injury of comparable magnitude [59]. A model that produces long-standing and easily detectable deficits in aged animals therefore provides a useful way to test the efficacy of potential treatments in both the immediate post-injury phase and more chronic stages.

The increase in survival among stroke victims [1] has not been accompanied by a decrease in the severity of impairment [58,64]. The result is aging lesions within aging brains – a very difficult set of obstacles to surmount. Although they are not as robust as they are in young brains, neuroplastic mechanisms do persist into old age [65] and can be elicited by specific rehabilitation therapies in subjects > 60 years of age [66–68], and it is essential to pinpoint ways in which to harness them. Assessing potential therapies in the context of an aged model system will enhance the predictive validity of preclinical research.

Reason four: patients are on drugs, but research animals are not

Stroke is primarily an affliction of the aged, and is often linked to one or more of the other diseases associated with advancing age, such as hypertension, heart disease, or diabetes. An important consideration, therefore, is the extent to which medication for these diseases may affect stroke recovery, or interact with potential stroke treatments in clinical trials. Other common problems in the elderly, such as arthritis, while not directly related to stroke, also require medication that may influence post-stroke recovery. The elderly are therefore often taking one or more drugs on a regular basis, but research animals in which stroke is modeled are not. Thus, if any of the drugs being taken (or a combination of them) interacts with a potential stroke therapy, this interference would not be seen until clinical trials [69]. The treatment being tested, rather than the drugs, may be blamed.

Drugs commonly taken by the elderly could interfere with treatments being tested in a number of ways. They may disrupt attention, movement, or vision, thereby affecting the efficacy of motor rehabilitative strategies. Anticholinergic drugs could cause confusion or disorientation which may be difficult to counteract with a potential stroke therapy. Commonly used sleep aids or other psychoactive drugs, including anxiolytics, antipsychotics, and antidepressants, have all been found to influence recovery from stroke [69]. GABAergic agonists (such as many commonly used anxiolytics) disrupt recovery from head injury in rats if used repeatedly for a week or more after the first few post-injury days [70]. Polypharmacy is increasing in the elderly at risk of stroke, but based on their mechanisms of action, many of the drugs may either cancel efficacy or lead to adverse effects [69].

Taking patients off drugs is not realistic. Although statins have been shown to be beneficial early after brain injury [71–73], discontinuation of anticholesterol or antihypertension medications could increase the chances of future stroke. Taking patients off antidepressants may also be unwise, since depression contributes to poor post-stroke prognosis [74], while a positive attitude towards recovery is a predictor of improvement [75]; however, antidepressants increase the risk of future strokes [76], and one must carefully counterweigh risks and benefits before prescribing these medications. Taking stroke patients off their drugs may not be always possible, but putting research animals on them is. In particular, the new generation antipsychotics need to be examined with respect to stroke, especially since use of them is increasing in the elderly for the treatment of emotional and dementia-related behavioral issues, such as delusions and aggression [69]. Ideally, research animals should be put on the drugs prior to stroke injury, and maintained on them throughout the study.

Concluding remarks

It is becoming increasingly recognized that any single biological or behavioral therapeutic intervention is unlikely to provide all necessary components of an effective treatment for stroke. Furthermore, the characteristics required of a treatment change with time. In the case of ischemia, for example, an acute treatment should improve blood flow to the affected area and protect surviving tissue, whereas for chronic stages, restorative treatments should replace cells, re-myelinate, stimulate formation of appropriate new connectivity, enhance blood flow and metabolic capacity of the injured tissue, reduce barriers to axonal outgrowth, and reduce the extent of delayed degeneration. Pinpointing an effective stroke therapy therefore represents a major challenge. Addressing the problems outlined here, as well as other translational issues, may help overcome this challenge and unclog the basic research pipeline to optimal treatments for stroke [77–80].

References

1. Rautio A, Eliasson M, Stegmayr B. Favorable trends in the incidence and outcome in stroke in nondiabetic and diabetic subjects. Findings from the Northern Sweden MONICA stroke registry in 1985 to 2003. *Stroke*. 2008;**39**:3137–44.

2. Lindner MD. Clinical attrition due to biased preclinical assessments of potential efficacy. *Pharmacol Ther*. 2007;**115**:148–75.

3. Schallert T, Fleming SM, Leasure JL, *et al*. CNS plasticity and assessment of forelimb sensorimotor outcome in unilateral rat models of stroke, cortical ablation, parkinsonism and spinal cord injury. *Neuropharmacology*. 2000;**39**:777–87.

4. Schallert T, Jones TA. "Exuberant" neuronal growth after brain damage in adult rats: The essential role of behavioral experience. *J Neural Transplant Plast*. 1993;**4**:193–8.

5. Jones TA, Schallert T. Overgrowth and pruning of dendrites in adult rats recovering from neocortical damage. *Brain Res*. 1992;**581**:156–60.

6. Jones TA, Schallert T. Use-dependent growth of pyramidal neurons after neocortical damage. *J Neurosci*. 1994;**14**:2140–52.

7. Nudo RJ, Wise BM, SiFuentes F, *et al*. Neural substrates for the effects of rehabilitative training on motor recovery after ischemic infarct. *Science*. 1996; **272**(5269):1791–4.

8. Prusky G, Whishaw IQ. Morphology of identified corticospinal cells in the rat following motor cortex injury: Absence of use-dependent change. *Brain Res*. 1996;**714**:1–8.

9. Napieralski JA, Butler AK, Chesselet MF. Anatomical and functional evidence for lesion-specific sprouting of corticostriatal input in the adult rat. *J Comp Neurol*. 1996;**373**:484–97.

10. Bury SD, Eichhorn AC, Kotzer CM, *et al*. Reactive astrocytic responses to denervation in the motor cortex of adult rats are sensitive to manipulations of behavioral experience. *Neuropharmacology*. 2000;**39**:743–55.

11. Hsu JE, Jones TA. Time-sensitive enhancement of motor learning with the less-affected forelimb after unilateral sensorimotor cortex lesions in rats. *Eur J Neurosci*. 2005;**22**:2069–80.

12. Taub E, Uswatt G. Constraint-Induced Movement Therapy: Answers and questions after two decades of research. *NeuroRehabilitation*. 2006;**21**:93–5.

13. Schallert T, Humm JL, Bland ST, *et al*. Activity-associated growth factor expression and related neural events in recovery of function after brain injury. In: Choi D, Dacey RG, Hsu CY, Powers WJ, editors. *Cerebrovascular disease: Momentum at the end of the*

second millennium. Armonk, NY: Futura Publishing Comany, Inc.; 2002:**401**–26.

14. Schallert T, Leasure JL, Kolb B. Experience-associated structural events, subependymal cellular proliferative activity, and functional recovery after injury to the central nervous system. *J Cereb Blood Flow Metab*. 2000;**20**:1513–28.

15. Kleim, JA, Jones TA, Schallert T. Motor enrichment and the induction of plasticity before and after brain injury. *Neurochem Res*. 2003;**28**:1757–69.

16. Schubring-Giese M, Molina-Luna K, Hertler B, *et al.* Speed of motor re-learning after experimental stroke depends on prior skill. *Exp Brain Res*. 2007;**181**:359–65.

17. Taub E, Crago JE, Burgio LD, *et al.* An operant approach to rehabilitation medicine: Overcoming learned nonuse by shaping. *J Exp Anal Behav*. 1994;**61**:281–93.

18. Kozlowski DA, James DC, Schallert T. Use-dependent exaggeration of neuronal injury after unilateral sensorimotor cortex lesions. *J Neurosci*. 1996;**16**:4776–86.

19. Humm JL, Kozlowski DA, James DC, *et al.* Use-dependent exacerbation of brain damage occurs during an early post-lesion vulnerable period. *Brain Res*. 1998;**783**:286–92.

20. Griesbach GS, Hovda DA, Molteni R, *et al.* Voluntary exercise following traumatic brain injury: Brain-derived neurotrophic factor upregulation and recovery of function. *Neuroscience*. 2004;**125**:129–39.

21. Humm JL, Kozlowski DA, Bland ST, *et al.* Use-dependent exaggeration of brain injury: Is glutamate involved? *Exp Neurol*. 1999;**157**:349–58.

22. DeBow SB, McKenna JE, Kolb B, *et al.* Immediate constraint-induced movement therapy causes local hyperthermia and exacerbates cerebral cortical injury in rats. *Can J Physiol Pharmacol*. 2004;**82**:231–7.

23. Griesbach GS, Gomez-Pinilla F, Hovda DA. The upregulation of plasticity-related proteins following TBI is disrupted with acute voluntary exercise. *Brain Res*. 2004;**1016**:154–62.

24. Leasure JL, Schallert T. Consequences of forced disuse of the impaired forelimb after unilateral cortical injury. *Behav Brain Res*. 2004;**150**:83–91.

25. Carmichael ST. Cellular and molecular mechanisms of neural repair after stroke: Making waves. *Ann Neurol*. 2006;**59**:735–42.

26. Maldonado MA, Allred RP, Felthauser EL, *et al.* Motor skill training, but not voluntary exercise, improves skilled reaching after unilateral ischemic lesions of the sensorimotor cortex in rats. *Neurorehabil Neural Repair*. 2008;**22**:250–61.

27. Ro T, Noser E, Boake C, *et al.* Functional reorganization and recovery after constraint-induced movement

therapy in subacute stroke: Case reports. *Neurocase*. 2006;**12**:50–60.

28. Luft AR, Macko RF, Forrester LW, *et al.* Treadmill exercise activates subcortical neural networks and improves walking after stroke: A randomized controlled trial. *Stroke*. 2008;**39**:3341–50.

29. Macko RF, Ivey FM, Forrester LW, *et al.* Treadmill exercise rehabilitation improves ambulatory function and cardiovascular fitness in patients with chronic stroke: A randomized, controlled trial. *Stroke*. 2005;**36**:2206–11.

30. Leasure JL, Jones M. Forced and voluntary exercise differentially affect brain and behavior. *Neuroscience*. 2008;**156**:456–65.

31. Hayes K, Sprague S, Guo M, *et al.* Forced, not voluntary, exercise effectively induces neuroprotection in stroke. *Acta Neuropathol*. 2008;**115**:289–96.

32. Stummer W, Weber K, Tranmer B, *et al.* Reduced mortality and brain damage after locomotor activity in gerbil forebrain ischemia. *Stroke* 1994;**25**:1862–9.

33. Zhao X, Aronowski J, Liu SJ, *et al.* Wheel-running modestly promotes functional recovery after a unilateral cortical lesion in rats. *Behav Neurol*. 2005;**16**:41–9.

34. Boake C, Noser EA, Ro T, *et al.* Constraint-induced movement therapy during early stroke rehabilitation. *Neurorehabil Neural Repair*. 2007;**21**:14–24.

35. Dromerick AW, Lang CE, Powers WJ, *et al.* Very early constraint-induced movement therapy (VECTORS): Phase II trial results. *Stroke*. 2007;**38**:465.

36. Byl NN, Pitsch EA, Abrams GM. Functional outcomes can vary by dose: Learning-based sensorimotor training for patients stable poststroke. *Neurorehabil Neural Repair*. 2008;**22**:494–504.

37. Szele FG, Alexander C, Chesselet MF. Expression of molecules associated with neuronal plasticity in the striatum after aspiration and thermocoagulatory lesions of the cerebral cortex in adult rats. *J Neurosci*. 1995;**15**:4429–48.

38. Auriat AM, Grams JD, Yan RH, *et al.* Forced exercise does not improve recovery after hemorrhagic stroke in rats. *Brain Res*. 2006;**1109**:183–91.

39. Wu J, Hua Y, Keep RF, *et al.* Oxidative brain injury from extravasated erythrocytes after intracerebral hemorrhage. *Brain Res*. 2002;**953**:45–52.

40. Nakamura T, Keep RF, Hua Y, *et al.* Deferoxamine-induced attenuation of brain edema and neurological deficits in a rat model of intracerebral hemorrhage. *J Neurosurg*. 2004;**100**:672–8.

41. Nakamura T, Xi G, Hua Y, *et al.* Intracerebral hemorrhage in mice: Model characterization and application for genetically modified mice. *J Cereb Blood Flow Metab*. 2004;**24**:487–94.

42. Hua Y, Nakamura T, Keep RF, *et al.* Long-term effects of experimental intracerebral hemorrhage: The role of iron. *J Neurosurg.* 2006;**104**:305–12.

43. Shao J, Xi G, Hua Y, *et al.* Intracerebral hemorrhage in the iron deficient rat. *Stroke.* 2005;**36**:660–4.

44. Napieralski JA, Banks RJ, Chesselet MF. Motor and somatosensory deficits following uni- and bilateral lesions of the cortex induced by aspiration or thermocoagulation in the adult rat. *Exp Neurol.* 1998;**154**:80–8.

45. Thored P, Arvidsson A, Cacci E, *et al.* Persistent production of neurons from adult brain stem cells during recovery after stroke. *Stem Cells.* 2006;**24**:739–47.

46. Schallert T. Behavioral tests for preclinical intervention assessment. *NeuroRx.* 2006;**3**:497–504.

47. Hua Y, Schallert T, Keep RF, *et al.* Behavioral tests after intracerebral hemorrhage in the rat. *Stroke.* 2002;**33**:2478–84.

48. Valla J, Humm JL, Schallert T, *et al.* Metabolic activity increases in the subependymal zone following cortical injury. *NeuroReport.* 1999;**10**:2731–4.

49. Gotts JE, Chesselet MF. Migration and fate of newly born cells after focal cortical ischemia in adult rats. *J Neurosci Res.* 2005;**80**:160–71.

50. Kluska MM, Witte OW, Bolz J, *et al.* Neurogenesis in the adult dentate gyrus after cortical infarcts: effects of infarct location, N-methyl-D-aspartate receptor blockade and anti-inflammatory treatment. *Neuroscience.* 2005;**135**:723–35.

51. Kolb B, Morshead C, Gonzalez C, *et al.* Growth factor-stimulated generation of new cortical tissue and functional recovery after stroke damage to the motor cortex of rats. *J Cereb Blood Flow Metab.* 2007;**27**:983–97.

52. Adkins DL, Schallert T, Goldstein LB. Issues in pre-clinical and clinical research: Lost in translation. *Stroke.* 2008;**40**:8–9.

53. Silasi G, Hamilton DA, Kolb B. Social instability blocks functional restitution following motor cortex stroke in rats. *Behav Brain Res.* 2008;**188**:219–26.

54. Woodlee MT, Schallert T. The impact of motor activity and inactivity on the brain: implications for the prevention and treatment of nervous system disorders. *Curr Dir Psychol Sci.* 2006;**15**:203–06.

55. Craft TKS, Glasper ER, McCullough L, *et al.* Social interaction improves experimental stroke outcome. *Stroke.* 2006;**36**:2006–11.

56. Marini C, Triggiani L, Cimini N, *et al.* Proportion of older people in the community as a predictor of increasing stroke incidence. *Neuroepidemiology.* 2001;**20**:91–5.

57. Ramirez-Lassepas M. Stroke and the aging of the brain and the arteries. *Geriatrics.* 1998;**53**(Suppl 1):44–8.

58. Wyller TB. Prevalence of stroke and stroke-related disability. *Stroke.* 1998;**29**:866–7.

59. Lindner MD, Gribkoff VK, Donlan NA, *et al.* Long-lasting functional disabilities in middle-aged rats with small cerebral infarcts. *J Neurosci.* 2003;**23**:10 913–22.

60. Gladstone DJ, Black SE, Hakim AM. Toward wisdom from failure: Lessons from neuroprotective stroke trials and new therapeutic directions. *Stroke.* 2002;**33**:2123–36.

61. Wang RY, Wang PS, Yang YR. Effect of age in rats following middle cerebral artery occlusion. *Gerontology.* 2003;**49**:27–32.

62. Jin K, Minami M, Xie L, *et al.* Ischemia-induced neurogenesis is preserved but reduced in the aged rodent brain. *Aging Cell.* 2004;**3**:373–7.

63. Futrell N, Garcia JH, Peterson E, *et al.* Embolic stroke in aged rats. *Stroke.* 1991;**22**:1582–91.

64. Westling B, Norrving B, Thorngren M. Survival following stroke. A prospective population-based study of 438 hospitalized cases with prediction according to subtype, severity and age. *Acta Neurol Scand.* 1990;**81**:457–63.

65. Kramer AF, Bherer L, Colcombe SJ, *et al.* Environmental influences on cognitive and brain plasticity during aging. *J Gerontol A Biol Sci Med Sci.* 2004;**59**:M940–57.

66. Luft AR, McCombe-Waller S, Whitall J, *et al.* Repetitive bilateral arm training and motor cortex activation in chronic stroke: A randomized controlled trial. *JAMA.* 2004;**292**:1853–61.

67. Liepert J, Bauder H, Miltner WH, *et al.* Treatment-induced cortical reorganization after stroke in humans. *Stroke.* 2000;**31**:1210–6.

68. Luft AR, Macko RF, Forrester LW, *et al.* Treadmill exercise activates subcortical neural networks and improves walking after stroke: A randomized controlled trial. *Stroke.* 2008;**39**:3341–50.

69. Zhao CS, Hartikainen S, Schallert T, *et al.* CNS-active drugs in aging population at high risk of cerebrovascular events: Evidence from preclinical and clinical studies. *Neurosci Biobehav Rev.* 2008;**32**:56–71.

70. Schallert T, Hernandez TD, Barth TM. Recovery of function after brain damage: Severe and chronic disruption by diazepam. *Brain Res.* 1986;**379**:104–11.

71. Lu D, Mahmood A, Goussev A, *et al.* Atorvastatin reduces intravascular thrombosis, increases cerebral microvascular patency and integrity, and enhances spatial learning in rats subjected to traumatic brain injury. *J Neurosurg.* 2004;**101**:813–21.

72. Lu D, Qu C, Goussev A, *et al.* Statins increase neurogenesis in the dentate gyrus, reduce delayed neuronal death in the hippocampal CA3 region, and improve spatial learning in rat after traumatic brain injury. *J Neurotrauma.* 2007;**24**:1132–46.

73. Qu CS, Lu D, Goussev A, *et al.* Effect of atorvastatin on spatial memory, neuronal survival, and vascular density in female rats after traumatic brain injury. *J Neurosurg.* 2005;**103**:695–701.

74. Cole MG, Elie LM, McCusker J, *et al.* Feasibility and effectiveness of treatments for post-stroke depression in elderly inpatients: Systematic review. *J Geriatr Psychiatry Neurol.* 2001;**14**:37–41.

75. Hama S, Yamashita H, Kato T, *et al.* "Insistence on recovery" as a positive prognostic factor in Japanese stroke patients. *Psychiatry Clin Neurosci.* 2008;**62**:386–95.

76. Chen Y, Guo JJ, Li H, *et al.* Risk of cerebrovascular events associated with antidepressant use in patients with depression: A population-based, nested case-control study. *Ann Pharmacother.* 2008;**42**:177–84.

77. Cumberland Consensus Working Group: Cheeran B, Cohen L, Dobkin B, Ford G, Greenwood R, Howard D, Husain M, Macleod M, Nudo R, Rothwell J, Rudd A, Teo J, Ward N, Wolf S. The future of restorative neurosciences in stroke: Driving the translational research pipeline from basic science to rehabilitation of people after stroke. *Neurorehab Neural Repair.* 2009;**23**:97–107.

78. Ginsberg MD. Neuroprotection for ischemic stroke: Past, present and future. *Neuropharmacology.* 2008;**55**:363–89.

79. Keyvani K, Schallert T. Plasticity associated molecular and structural events in postlesional brain. *J Neuropathol Exper Neurol.* 2002;**61**:831–40.

80. Hicks A, Schallert T, Jolkkonen J. Cell-based therapies and functional outcome in experimental stroke. *Cell Stem Cell.* 2009;**7**:139–40.

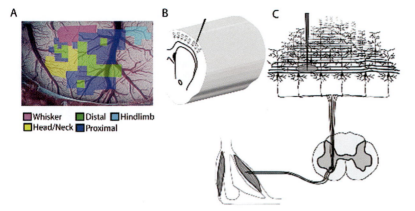

Whisker **Distal** **Hindlimb**
Head/Neck **Proximal**

Figure 1.2 Intracortical microstimulation (ICMS) technique used to derive maps of movement representation in rat motor cortex. **A**. Motor map showing areas of the cortex in which stimulation evoked movement. **B**. Movements are produced by lowering a stimulating electrode into layer V of the motor cortex and activating corticospinal neurons. **C**. Corticospinal neurons are activated trans-synaptically. These neurons then project to motor neurons in the spinal cord that in turn cause muscle contractions in the periphery.

fMRI during forelimb stimulation in rats

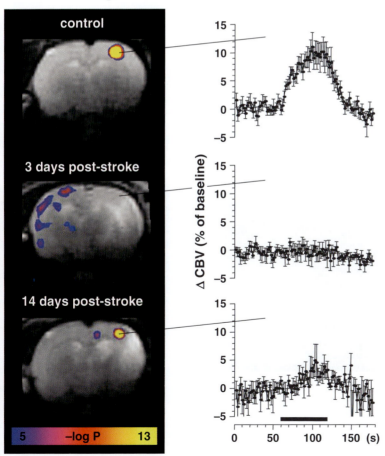

Figure 6.1 Left: T_2-weighted MR images of a rat brain slice overlaid by statistical activation maps calculated from contrast-enhanced CBV-weighted fMRI in combination with an electrical forelimb stimulation paradigm as described by Dijkhuizen et al. [17]. Right: Time-course of CBV changes in the right sensorimotor cortex in response to left forelimb stimulation (the stimulation period is indicated by the black bar) (mean ± SD, $n = 6$). Left forelimb stimulation induced significant activation responses in the right sensorimotor cortex in control rats. At 3 days after right-sided stroke, activation responses in the right, ipsilesional sensorimotor cortex were largely absent; however, responses were found in the left, contralesional hemisphere. After 14 days, partial restoration of activation was detected in the right, ipsilesional sensorimotor cortex. The unilateral stroke lesion is characterized by increased T_2-weighted signal intensity in the right somatosensory cortex and lateral striatum.

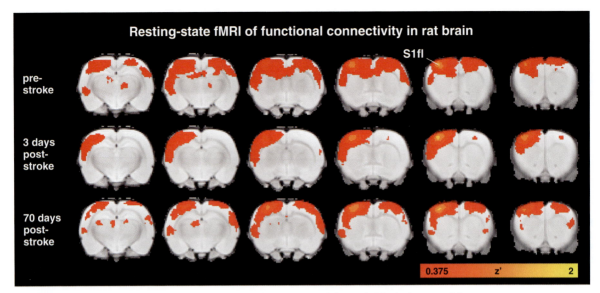

Figure 6.2 Maps of mean functional brain connectivity of left (contralesional after stroke) forelimb region of the primary somatosensory cortex (S1fl) in rats before, and 3 and 70 days after a 90-min right MCA occlusion-induced subcortical lesion ($n = 5$). Functional connectivity maps are thresholded at a Fisher-transformed correlation coefficient (z') of 0.375, and overlaid on a T_2-weighted multislice anatomical rat brain template. Loss of functional connectivity with the ipsilesional sensorimotor cortex was evident at 3 days, while functional connectivity was restored at 10 weeks after stroke. Courtesy of Kajo van der Marel, Image Sciences Institute, University Medical Center Utrecht.

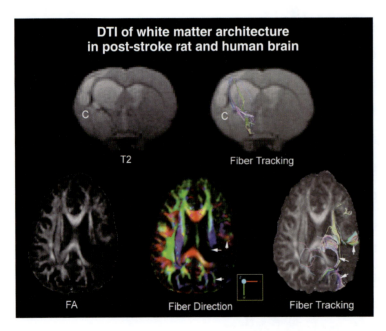

Figure 6.3 Top row: T_2-weighted MR image and fiber-tracking image of a rat brain treated with neuroprogenitor cells after unilateral stroke, showing tracking of axonal projections in the lesion border zone. The marker **c** represents the ischemic core. Bottom row: FA, fiber direction, and fiber-tracking image of a horizontal brain slice from a stroke patient, illustrating orientation changes in the lesion boundary. Both fiber direction and fiber-tracking images show that tracking of axonal projections circumscribes the lesion boundary (white arrows). Red, green, and blue colors represent x, y, and z directions, respectively, on the fiber direction image. Details of the experimental protocols can be found in Jiang et al. [36]. Courtesy of Dr. Quan Jiang, Henry Ford Health Sciences Center.

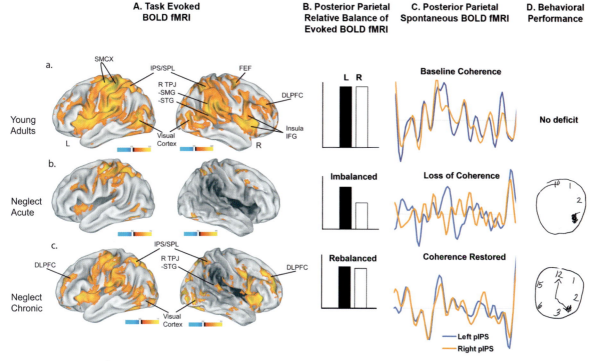

Figure 13.4 Acutely after stroke there is (A) a reduction of evoked BOLD activity in both hemispheres as compared to young adult controls, (B) a marked imbalance of evoked BOLD activity between the two hemispheres, (C) a loss of interhemispheric coherence of spontaneous BOLD activity between core regions of the attention network, and (D) impaired spatial performance. In the chronic state, there is a reactivation of evoked BOLD activity, rebalancing of relative activity between left and right posterior parietal cortex, return of spontaneous BOLD coherence, and behavioral improvement. A striking finding was that activity of the left dorso-parietal cortex was relatively stronger at the acute stage, but this imbalance decreased at the chronic stage when the right dorso-parietal cortex had reactivated. This "push–pull" pattern was detected in the IPS-SPL and visual cortex, but not in the FEF or TPJ. The relative contributions of interhemispheric imbalance versus loss of spontaneous BOLD coherence to behavioral deficits remain to be determined. Whether a similar pattern of recovery might apply to other bihemispherically represented systems is still unknown. (SMCX: somatomotor cortex; DLFPC: dorsolateral prefrontal cortex; IPS/SPL: intraparietal sulcus/superior parietal lobule; TPJ: temporo-parietal junction; SMG: supramarginal gyrus; STG: superior temporal gyrus; FEF: frontal eye fields; IFG: inferior frontal gyrus.)

Pre TDCS   Post TDCS

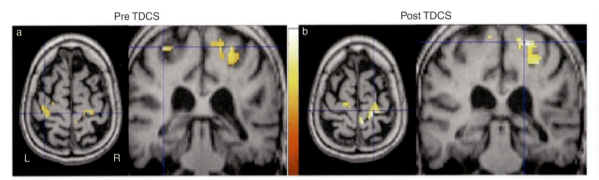

Figure 19.3 fMRI activation pattern in a stroke patient before and after tDCS. fMRI studies in patients recovering from a stroke have shown that the ipsilateral (to the moving hand) sensorimotor cortex can become active when a patient performs a movement with their recovering hand. Applying cathodal stimulation to the non-lesional motor cortex (the motor cortex that activated when the recovering wrist was moving) significantly decreased the activation on the ipsilateral site and was associated with an improvement in this patient's functional motor status. (This figure is reprinted from [73] with permission from Future Science Group.)

9 Brain events in the acute period of stroke in relation to subsequent repair

Rüdiger J. Seitz

Introduction

Brain ischemia results from a depression of the cerebral blood supply leading to disturbances of neural function and, in severe cases, ultimately manifesting as structural brain damage, e.g. infarction. Typically, stroke symptoms start abruptly, related to a cerebral artery occlusion [1]. Interruption of circulation due to cerebral artery occlusion induces immediate suppression of cerebral electrical activity causing peri-infarct depolarization with repeated episodes of metabolic stress and growth of the infarct lesion up to 24 h post-occlusion [2–6]. During ischemia, the thresholds for selective neuronal and tissue necrosis are a function of regional cerebral blood flow (rCBF) reduction [7]. Thus, critical determinants of acute stroke are the occlusion of a cerebral artery and the thereby induced local depression of cerebral blood flow and subsequent electrical, metabolic, and ionic changes [8]. Recent evidence in humans points to the occurrence of spreading depression in severe infarctions complicated by progressive expansion [9].

Stroke treatment should be initiated as early as possible in the acute period. However, it is not well established how long the acute period of stroke lasts. Does it last for 24 h of infarct manifestation when the majority of cerebral artery occlusion has been recanalized spontaneously [10,11]? Does the acute period last for 48 h, when emergency carotid surgery for carotid endarterectomy can be performed safely in acute stroke [12]? Does it last up to some 7 days, as long as stroke patients are treated on the stroke care units? Or does the acute period of stroke extend even further? For the purpose of this chapter we define the acute period of stroke operationally as the time the patients spend in the stroke care unit, which on average is 7 days after symptom onset. In this period, the patients receive acute stroke treatment such as thrombolysis, initiation of secondary prevention including anticoagulation, antiplatelet therapy as well as antihypertensive and antidiabetic medication, and dedicated physiotherapy or speech therapy. In fact, many patients enjoy a substantial recovery in this period, particularly when treated with thrombolysis [13].

Recovery from a brain lesion such as stroke comprises aspects of neural repair and functional reorganization. Since brain infarcts result in damage of gray and white matter, tissue repair resulting in replacement of the ischemic tissue debris by functional brain tissue would be optimal. Work in experimental models in laboratory animals suggests that stem cells in the subventricular germinal zone as well as neural progenitor cells proliferate in response to focal ischemia [14,15]. They seem to be regulated by a number of different factors, such as neurotrophic substances and inflammatory mediators [16,17]. However, it seems that neurons have only a limited capacity of regeneration and nerve fibers do not grow out across long distances, as they get stuck at the scars of central nervous tissue lesions [18]. Nevertheless, there is good evidence from animal experiments that nerve fibers of intact nerve cells in the perilesional cortex grow out even across considerable distances as well as that new synapses are formed from the outgrowing nerve fibers [19–21]. In fact, these reorganizational changes afford clinical recovery, which has been shown to be enhanced by dedicated rehabilitative training [22]. Such reorganizational processes are, however, slow and need many months to take place. Also, following stroke there is limited repair but mainly functional reorganization related to dedicated exercise and training. Notably, recovery commences early after the ischemic event. As will be described here, one of the major aspects of this spontaneous recovery is the rapid cerebral reperfusion. It determines the salvage of brain tissue threatened by

Brain Repair After Stroke, ed. S. C. Cramer and R. J. Nudo. Published by Cambridge University Press.
© Cambridge University Press 2010.

ischemia and limits the expansion of the ischemic brain lesion.

A major step in acute stroke treatment has been the advent of thrombolysis. It is targeted towards the rescue of brain tissue at the risk of ischemic damage by early recanalization. It has been shown to be effective when initiated within 4.5 h of stroke onset, with maximal efficacy within the first 90 min after symptom onset [23,24]. The beneficial role of early recanalization was shown by functional imaging [25,26] and monitoring with transcranial Doppler sonography [27,28]. If thrombolysis is not feasible, patients may develop severe infarctions with a disabling neurological deficit and little recovery, particularly in the advanced age group [29]. While the neurological deficit induced by ischemia resolves completely within 15 min after reperfusion as shown by artificial balloon occlusion of the human carotid artery [1], the evolution of a manifest brain infarct is more complex. The most important determinants of a brain infarct are the causes of ischemia (including its severity), the dimension and composition of the causal arterial emboli, the anatomy and the vascular changes of the cerebral arteries, and hyperglycemia in associated diabetes [30–32]. Beyond the acute time window of up to 24 h, secondary changes contribute to infarct manifestation, including vasogenic edema and inflammatory infiltration. These changes, however, have a smaller impact and regress spontaneously within 2 weeks after stroke. Although there is a large heterogeneity of spontaneous recovery over the first 3 months after stroke [33], the neurological state by day 4 is a powerful predictor of long-term neurological outcome [34,35]. Therefore, the brain events in the acute period of stroke are of great interest and will be discussed in this chapter. It will be shown that brain infarcts differ with respect to post-stroke recovery in terms of pathophysiology and important aspects of cerebral artery anatomy.

Perfusion–diffusion mismatch: relevance to prognosis and to repair

An occlusion of a cerebral artery results in a depression of cerebral perfusion, which if sustained will eventually result in the subsequent development of an infarct lesion. The depression of cerebral perfusion can be assessed non-invasively in the acute stroke patient with perfusion imaging using magnetic resonance imaging (MRI) and computed tomography (CT). The developing infarct lesion can be identified early by diffusion-weighted imaging (DWI) using MRI (Figure 9.1). DWI is sensitive to the development of cytotoxic brain edema which results in a depression of water perfusion through the affected brain tissue [36]. Since the changes of diffusion develop in a more protracted manner than the instantaneous depression of brain perfusion after an acute occlusion of a cerebral artery, perfusion abnormalities are supposed to exceed DWI changes resulting in a perfusion–diffusion mismatch [37–39]. In fact, a perfusion–diffusion mismatch is typical for the acute situation in an occlusion of a cerebral artery stem, while in an occlusion of a distal branch of a cerebral artery, the perfusion deficit area typically matches the DWI abnormality. In addition, blood oxygen level-dependent (BOLD) imaging can indicate the oxygen deprivation [40]. Nevertheless, these measures are affected by the dynamic growth of the DWI lesion volume and the regression of the perfusion deficit in relation to spontaneous or pharmacologically induced thrombus dissolution. Typically, the dynamic changes result in a spatial match of the perfusion deficit and the DWI lesion after 24 h [41].

Importantly, there is a close relationship between the volume of critically reduced cerebral perfusion and the neurological deficit [37,42]. It was found that in the first 3 h after symptom onset the most important

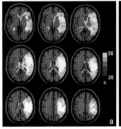 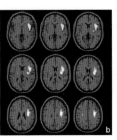 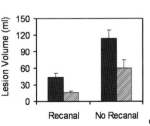

Figure 9.1 Perfusion–diffusion mismatch in acute MCA stroke before treatment onset. In a voxel-by-voxel analysis the area with a PWI delay (a) exceeded the area of DWI abnormality (b). The DWI changes involved the insula cortex and the adjacent hemispheric white matter [63]. (c) Volumetric data showed that the patients who showed recanalization ("Recanal") upon thrombolysis had smaller PWI (black columns) and DWI (hatched columns) lesion volumes than patients in whom thrombolysis failed ("No Recanal").

factor determining stroke evolution following the acute event is the volume of severe ischemia as assessed with perfusion imaging [43,44]. In fact, a perfusion delay of 6 s relative to the non-affected hemisphere before stroke treatment initiation predicted the T_2-lesion volume on day 8, irrespective of the treatment regimen. In contrast, neither the extent of the pretreatment DWI abnormalities nor the magnitude of the apparent diffusion coefficient were predictive or discriminating. This was probably due to the fact that DWI changes require longer than 3 h to develop. Moreover, it became evident that the abnormalities indicated by perfusion imaging before treatment onset were larger in patients lacking recanalization than in those with successful recanalization following thrombolysis [43]. Figure 9.1 shows, in addition, that the brain infarcts as visualized by MRI approximately 1 week after the stroke were larger in failed recanalization than in successful recanalization. Apparently, good leptomeningeal collaterals in addition to early recanalization of a middle cerebral arterial occlusion critically increase the chance of limited infarct growth and a favorable clinical outcome [45–47]. Importantly, survival of brain regions within brain areas of low perfusion can influence subsequent functional reorganization [48].

Altogether, the new recanalization strategies in acute stroke treatment have improved the prognosis of ischemic stroke for many patients and opened new windows for understanding the impact of focal ischemia on the resulting neurological deficit and the prospects of post-stroke recovery. Notably, the residual stroke lesion and the accompanying physiological changes deserve consideration, as they are critical for post-stroke recovery.

Types of stroke

It is well known that human stroke may affect each of the cerebral arteries, giving rise to different neurological deficit patterns that result from the brain areas affected. The pathogenesis of brain infarcts can vary substantially, for example, resulting from causes as diverse as a large artery embolism or hyalinosis of an arteriole [49,50]. Some patterns are instructive. For example, typically, infarcts in the territory of the posterior cerebral artery are embolic in origin and comprise the entire supply area of the affected artery [51]. In contrast, infarcts in the anterior cerebral artery typically are of atherosclerotic origin and more variable in lesion pattern and neurological deficit [52]. The

situation is more complicated in the middle cerebral artery (MCA) territory given the wide arborization of the artery, the large territory supplied by the artery, and the net-like anastomoses of the downstream arterial branches with the leptomeningeal arteries. Thus, an arterial obstruction in the MCA may have different consequences for the neurological deficit and infarct manifestation depending on the site of the occlusion [53]. This becomes even more diversified when one takes into account modern stroke therapy that aims at establishing rapid cerebral reperfusion [54,55].

In view of these complex spatiotemporal developments in MCA stroke, a refined schematic classification of stroke types is proposed building on the classification by Donnan and collaborators which originally was based on radiological findings [50]. This classification attains particular importance in the current context because type of stroke injury can influence features of post-stroke brain reorganization and repair.

Type I stroke

In this category, we deal with circumscribed territorial infarcts (Table 9.1). Depending on their size, either a distal or a more proximal branch of the MCA becomes occluded, giving rise to either small infarcts entirely limited to the cerebral cortex, or larger infarcts involving the cerebral cortex and the underlying white matter [56]. Typically, small emboli dissolve rapidly allowing for early reperfusion, while larger emboli tend to resist spontaneous or pharmacologically induced fibrinolysis [57,58]. Consequently, proximal branch occlusions may result in more long-standing ischemia and, thus, larger territorial brain infarctions typically affecting the cerebral white matter in addition to the cerebral cortex. Notably, small cortical infarctions may become apparent with mild or rapidly improving neurological symptoms [59], while larger cortical and cortico-subcortical infarcts may require 2–6 weeks for complete clinical recovery. Usually, such small territorial infarcts do not destroy the entire cortical respresentation area, nor the descending motor cortical output tract completely [60–62]. This leaves sufficient space for perilesional reorganization, as will be discussed below (also see Figure 9.2).

Type II stroke

This stroke type refers to infarcts affecting either large parts of or the entire striatocapsular region. They result from an embolic occlusion of the MCA stem (Table 9.1). In MCA stroke the perfusion is mainly

Table 9.1 Pathogenesis of cerebral stroke subtypes

Type	Infarct location	Size	Pathogenesis	Reperfusion
I	Territorial		Embolism into cerebral artery branch	
I.1	Cortical	Small	Distal branch	Early
I.2	Cortico-subcortical	Medium	Proximal branch	No or delayed
II	Striatocapsular		Embolism into MCA stem	
II.1	+/− Insula	Medium	Infarct core	Early
II.2	+ Periventricular white matter	Large	Complete infarct	No or delayed
III			Lacunar hyalinosis of arterioles	No or delayed
III.1	Fiber tracts			
III.2	Internal capsule (anterior choroidal artery)			
III.3	Basal ganglia, lateral thalamus			
III.4	Medial and anterior thalamus (perforating branches of posterior cerebral artery)			
IV			Chronic hemodynamic deficit + downstream emboli	
IV.1	Cortico-subcortical	Medium	Extracranial artery disease	No or delayed
			Intracranial large artery disease	Reactive
				Vasodilatation
IV.2	Arterial border zone	Medium	(Arterial dissection, arteriosclerosis)	

Understanding the pathogenesis of cerebral injury from stroke may be important to understanding and treating post-stroke brain repair.

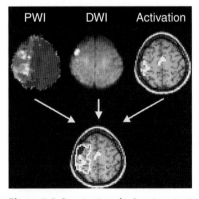

Figure 9.2 Reactivation of ischemic cortex in early post-stroke recovery. Coregistration of acute PWI, acute DWI, and subacute fMRI activation data related to sequential finger movements of the affected/recovered hand. Note that activation of sensorimotor cortex in the affected hemisphere is in a region of previous perfusion–diffusion mismatch [48].

reduced in the central portion of the MCA territory including the basal ganglia, insular cortex, and hemispheric white matter [63]. If reperfusion is achieved early, only the deep perforating arteries and the arteries that supply the insular cortex remain critically affected by ischemia-causing infarcts that are limited to the lentiform nucleus and insula (Figure 9.3). Such infarcts are more limited in impact, and thus afford a profound regression of the initial neurological deficit and marked recovery over the following weeks [64]. On the contrary, in the case of delayed or missing reperfusion of the MCA, the infarct becomes larger, also involving the adjacent periventricular white matter, in addition to the striatum and insula (Figure 9.3). This becomes an issue of great prognostic importance in patients with multiple vascular risk factors, since such patients often have widespread

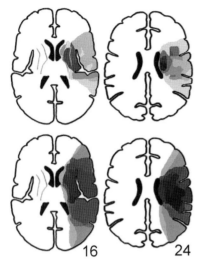

Figure 9.3 Strategic lesions in patients with MCA stem infarctions subjected to systemic thrombolysis. Upper row: The lesions were small and scattered in the patients who enjoyed rapid reperfusion. The area of maximal overlap was the middle portion of the periventricular white matter. Lower row: In the patients who showed delayed or no recanalization, the infarct lesions were larger, resulting in a large area of overlap in the insular cortex and the hemispheric white matter including the periventricular white matter. Displayed are axial Talairach stereotaxic space slices that are +16 and +24 mm dorsal to the intercommissural line.

atherosclerotic changes, such as large artery stenosis as well as poor leptomeningeal collaterals. Such patients experience particularly severe strokes with large areas of severely diminished perfusion and subsequent extensive brain damage, as well as limited recovery [43,65,66]. In fact, in addition to an acute MCA or ICA occlusion, the ischemic event appeared to result from widespread arterial changes such as vessel stenosis or occlusion in multiple cerebral arteries [43]. These observations suggest that the acute macrovascular occlusion of the MCA causing the acute neurological stroke syndrome can induce a particularly devastating perfusion deficit when a compensatory redistribution of arterial blood along collaterals is impaired. In accordance with this assumption, earlier findings with transcranial Doppler sonography [67], angiography [68], and positron emission tomography (PET) measurements of oxygen extraction [69] showed the importance of viable collaterals in the circle of Willis for a beneficial outcome after ischemia. Recently, the importance of viable collaterals was also shown for intra-arterial thrombolysis [70]. Nevertheless, using statistical parametric mapping, it was shown that in patients with more severe cerebral infarction, the hemispheric white matter is broadly affected, likely resulting in cortico-cortical and cortico-subcortical disconnections [63]. On this basis, white matter involvement is supposed to be the cause of neuropsychological disorders such as hemispatial neglect and conduction aphasia [71,72] (see Chapters 12 and 13). The larger injury of type II strokes means greater behavioral deficit, and less available tissue to contribute to post-stroke reorganization, compounded by disconnection due to white matter injury.

Type III stroke

These strokes result from a pathological change in the small cerebral arteries or even arterioles resulting in small-sized infarcts in the lacunar dimension (Table 9.1). They typically occur in the anterior choroidal artery, the deep perforating lenticular MCA branches, and thalamic branches of the posterior cerebral artery [73,74]. However, such lacunar infarcts may occur similarly also in brainstem structures and the pons. Typically, these strokes proceed to a completed infarct lesion, although of small spatial dimension. They result from local thrombosis subsequent to severe hyalinoid or microatheroma abnormalities of the small cerebral arteries in patients who tend to have poorly controlled arterial hypertension, diabetes mellitus, and hyperlipidemia [73–75]. Due to their strategic location, type III strokes are small in volume but large in behavioral impact. These strokes result in well-defined lacunar deficit syndromes including pure motor or pure sensory stroke. Accordingly, an occlusion of these arteries results in infarcts affecting subcortical gray and white matter structures including the internal capsule, the basal ganglia, and thalamus. When the posterior limb of the internal capsule is affected, loss of motor-evoked potentials and asymmetry of water diffusivity typically predict poor recovery [60,76]. Cortical reorganization has been extensively described with lacunar strokes and might contribute to a patient's recovery (see below).

Type IV strokes

These strokes occur in patients with long-standing cerebrovascular disease and chronic occlusion of extracranial cerebral arteries, and consist of embolic insults as well as hemodynamic border zone infarcts (Table 9.1). However, they may also occur in younger patients who suffer from dissection of the extracranial artery. In these patients, blood flow depression induces a reactive vasodilatation of the intracranial arteries.

This results in a sufficient supply with blood in the downstream cerebral artery territory, although the velocity of blood flow in the brain is reduced. Specifically, it was found that such patients exhibit a severe delay of brain perfusion, but have a normal cerebral blood volume corresponding to intact vascular autoregulation, and a normal neurological investigation [77,78]. In moyamoya disease, characterized by an intracranial occlusion of the carotid artery, small cerebral arteries proliferate, giving the angiographic finding that gives the name to the disease. These patients may become symptomatic upon progressive carotid artery occlusion, or when an embolus forms distally to the chronic arterial occlusion and obstructs a downstream cerebral artery. Again, the interval until successful reperfusion determines the severity of the neurological deficit, the subsequent infarct volume, and the capacity for recovery [79]. Less is known regarding how abnormalities of brain perfusion per se influence post-stroke brain reorganization and repair.

Origin and composition of arterial emboli

Arterial emboli typically consist of blood cells, platelets, and fibrin bonds between them. They may originate from arteriosclerotic plaques in the extracranial cerebral arteries, in particular from the bifurcation area of the carotid artery. Also, they may be of cardiac origin as in atrial fibrillation or patent foramen ovale. Thrombolysis using recombinant tissue plasminogen activator (rtPA) aims to dissolve the fibrin bonds between the platelets. In fact, early reopening of occluded arteries is supposed to be brought about by this action [23,24]. However, it is important to realize that platelets have become activated by thrombus formation being prone to ongoing fibrinogen binding, which may be the cause for secondary vessel occlusion after initial successful thrombolysis [80]. Here, antagonists against platelet glycoprotein receptors have been observed to be beneficial, as they antagonize activated platelets and are able to keep the re-opened cerebral arteries patent [81].

Nevertheless, thrombolysis may fail altogether, which is frequently the case after cardiac emboli. Recently, it was found that thrombo-emboli in acute stroke may contain endothelial components and calcifications [32]. Also, emboli removed from acutely occluded cerebral arteries by endovascular catheters were found to consist of old thrombotic material corresponding to a so-called organized thrombus. In such

a situation, fibrin is no longer soluble, which precludes successful thrombolysis with rtPA. In vivo this becomes manifest by the so-called "dense artery sign" in CT scanning which, in some patients, can be detected over a couple of days despite acute stroke treatment. In consequence, such a patient may develop a full-blown infarction of stroke type II, which may turn into a malignant brain infarct requiring hemicraniectomy as a life-saving intervention [82].

Neuroprotective agents

The development of a cerebral infarct is a highly dynamic process that is the expression of a cascade of biochemical events initiated by the ischemic event [8]. Evidence from MRI shows that the area of the perfusion deficit generally exceeds the manifest stroke lesion as defined in DWI within the first hours after stroke onset [37,64,83]. Accordingly, there seems to be a great opportunity for the action of neuroprotective agents in the early period after stroke onset. Over the last 30 years, countless experimental studies have been performed for the purpose of identifying suitable neuroprotective agents. However, none has yet proven to be effective in human stroke patients [84,85].

As a neuroprotective action, hypothermia has been advocated to reduce hypoxic brain damage and infarct growth and, thus, improve clinical outcome after stroke [86–88]. This complicated medical procedure is now being investigated in a multicenter trial [89].

The reasons for overall failure of neuroprotective strategies are probably multifold and include inadequate experimental design, small sample size, lack of blinding of the experimenters, and use of young rather than aged animals. Proper experimentation in animal models according to guidelines used in clinical trials has been proposed as a further means to identify substances that may work in human stroke in the future. The limited progress of neuroprotective agents in human stroke emphasizes the potential importance of examining parallel interventions, such as those related to brain repair.

Reperfusion injury

A critical issue is whether early reperfusion induces a secondary reperfusion injury. In analogy to animal experiments, reperfusion injury was supposed to result in an enlargement of the infarct volume due to a number of secondary processes. Such processes may include oxygen radical formation, hyperglycemia, leukocyte infiltration, cortical spreading depression, platelet and complement activation, post-ischemic hyperperfusion, and breakdown of the blood–brain barrier [9,90,91]. Conversely, chaperones have been found to exert a protective action on brain tissue following post-ischemic reperfusion [92]. It is important to note, however, that the final infarct volume is typically predicted by the volume of the initial deprivation of perfusion [43,93]. Specifically, these studies showed that the resulting infarct volume occupied the total initial perfusion deficit in permanent MCA occlusion, particularly when there was a persistent carotid artery occlusion. Again, in such a situation the ischemic event may lead to the life-threatening condition of a malignant MCA infarct.

Nevertheless, in successful early recanalization there is a considerable local heterogeneity of lesion evolution. While there is evidence for the no-reflow phenomenon [94], recent evidence from DWI shows that portions of the ischemic area may show a prolonged abnormality of diffusion for many weeks, which might suggest regions with prolonged ischemia [95]. Since such long-standing DWI lesions were found preferentially in the hemispheric white matter, they may have become manifest by chronic hemodynamic compromise subsequent to cerebral artery occlusion.

Furthermore, there are a few patients with MCA stem occlusions and rapid recanalization who develop secondary hemorrhages within the ischemic territory. Probably, such patients have suffered severe damage to the cerebral arteries in the ischemic area which rendered the vascular endothelium particularly vulnerable for reperfusion injury, leading to increased blood cell penetration upon recanalization [96,97]. Importantly, these secondary hemorrhages are relatively limited and occur preferentially in the infarct core.

These factors, and their variation across patients, attain increased significance given the potential contribution of inflammation to brain repair, as noted below.

Post-ischemic inflammatory infiltration

Inflammation might be a key trigger of many of the brain repair processes [98,99]. Thus, many of the inflammatory processes that contribute to injury early after stroke can contribute to repair days later. A better understanding of these inflammatory events in humans might therefore be of value to advancing brain repair therapeutics.

One inflammatory process that has been studied in humans is the early phase of macrophage brain activity post-stroke. Approximately 6 days after a cerebral infarction, lymphocytes and macrophages have been shown by MRI to accumulate in a perivascular distribution in infarcted brain tissue. These cells were labeled by uptake of iron by macrophages after intravenous injection [100–102]. A similar approach employed tracers against the peripheral GABA receptor which is located on macrophages using PET for imaging the distribution of inflammatory infiltrates [103]. Neuropathology has assumed that these infiltrating cells mediate the removal of post-ischemic debris. Interestingly, such cells were also found in remote locations corresponding to the notion of post-ischemic nerve fiber degeneration [104]. Recently, however, it was observed that the areas with inflammatory infiltration are heterogeneously distributed within the infarct area (Figure 9.4). It was speculated that due to their immunological competence these cells augment the infarct lesion. This raises the interesting hypothesis that immunosuppression

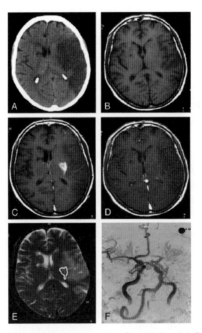

Figure 9.4 Heterogeneity of post-ischemic inflammation in a patient with a large MCA infarction as evident from (A) CT and (E) T2-MRI due to a MCA stem occlusion as evident from (F) magnetic resonance angiography. The infarct was not evident in a (B) T1-MRI and there was no breakdown of the blood–brain barrier as shown by (D) a lack of gadolinium enhancement. Note the detection (C) of labeled macrophages in the striatocapsular compartment (see C and E), which was at the border of the infarct [102].

may limit lesion growth in stroke. However, the infiltrates may also promote repair processes and, thus, may limit the infarct growth and, thereby, be beneficial for post-stroke recovery [105]. Thus, the role of inflammatory infiltration following stroke is still unresolved at present.

Changes of functional representations

Animal experiments have shown that there is synaptic plasticity related to spontaneous recovery after stroke when animals are kept in an enriched environment or subjected to dedicated training [19,22] (see also Chapters 2, 3, and 5). These plastic changes have been shown to result in structural changes such as growing of axons and formation of new synapses. These changes occur in the perilesional vicinity and in remote locations in functionally related areas in the affected and contralesional non-affected hemisphere [19,20]. At the molecular level, there are changes in the expression of glutamate and GABA as well as of neurotrophic mediators [106–108]. Notably, Heiss and collaborators were able to show in the human that the expression of the GABA benzodiazepine receptor is downregulated in ischemic brain tissue, suggesting extensive neuronal damage [109].

Functional imaging studies

Most functional imaging studies of cerebral changes related to recovery of motor functions, speech, and attention were performed in the chronic stage many weeks after the infarction [see Chapter 11]. Since there is a variable amount of spontaneous recovery in the acute and subacute stage after stroke which levels out after about 6 months after stroke [34,110], the majority of studies focused on the chronic stage to investigate the effect of rehabilitative training.

Patients with small cortical lesions typically show a fast recovery of their initial neurological deficits, often with complete return of function. This early recovery steadily evolves over weeks, leveling out over the subsequent months [34,110,111]. Notably in the first 4 weeks there is a perilesional activation in such patients which seems to be localized in the vicinity of the infarct lesion such that it harbors those portions of the motor cortical area that are not affected [112]. On longer follow-up of some 2 years it was possible to show that cortical activations related to finger movements moved into a

more dorsal location [113,114]. Recently, it was shown by transcranial magnetic stimulation (TMS) that the spots of activation moved in the direction of maximal cortical disinhibition [115]. In large ischemic lesions, salvage of brain tissue by rapid recanalization of the supplying artery and reperfusion are the most important determinants of early recovery. In such instances the former functional representation can become reactivated within the former perfusion deficit area, which can support neurological recovery [48]. Thus, an area of ischemia has the potential to harbor a large hemispheric stroke lesion (type II stroke), but can alter its appearance with early and sufficient recanalization and, thereby, be reduced to a focal cortical stroke (type I stroke), which can support recovery. Most likely, patients with such extensive areas of hypoperfusion suffer from a transient electrical–hemodynamic decoupling which was shown to occur in the subacute phase after stroke. In fact, in such patients clinical recovery began to occur in parallel with elicitation of motor-evoked potentials (MEPs), while a hemodynamic response related to brain activation was absent in the hemodynamically affected cortex [112].

Patients who recover from an infarct lesion tend to show a progressively normal activation pattern [116,117]. Nevertheless, even well-recovered patients often show a bilateral activation pattern after stroke [118,119]. In some patients with limited restitution of the affected muscles, as evidenced from an abnormal electromyographic activity pattern, the bilateral activation pattern was shown to be due to associated movements of the non-affected hand involving the intact motor cortex in the contralesional hemisphere (Figure 9.5). However, well-recovered patients also can show contralesional activations which were not present in healthy subjects performing the same movements. These abnormal activities involved premotor and motor cortical areas, and probably relate to motor learning (Figure 9.5). The latter has been interpreted to reflect active inhibition of the intact motor cortex, which is more excitable than normally [119]. The enhanced cortical excitability is probably the cause for the mirror movements frequently observed initially after stroke [120]. Apart from local activations, network types of fMRI data analysis can reveal abnormalities in the intra- and interhemispheric coupling between cortical areas. With such an approach it was shown that the coupling of the ipsilesional SMA and

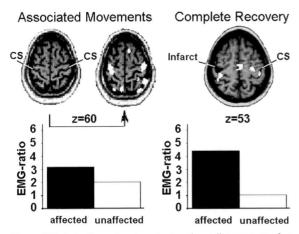

Figure 9.5 Activation pattern in patients with excellent recovery after stroke. In a patient with associated movements, a bilateral activation pattern was apparent. Note too the low level of electromyographic activity in the affected hand of this subject. Without EMG-guided analysis of the fMRI data, cerebral activation was not apparent (the left brain slice under "Associated Movements"), but with EMG-guided fMRI analysis, activation become apparent (the right brain slice). In a patient with complete recovery, note activation bilaterally in motor cortex and premotor cortex contralesional to the infarct. Here, the electromyographic activity (ratio is presented, movement divided by rest) in the unaffected hand did not increase, and so the EMG ratio was approximately 1. It was argued that the contralesional fMRI activity was due to active suppression of output from the non-affected motor cortex, which is under enhanced excitatory drive due to the cortical lesion in the opposite hemisphere [119].

contralesional MI was reduced after striatocapsular stroke, which correlated with impaired bimanual performance [121].

Transcranial magnetic stimulation

Transcranial magnetic stimulation (TMS) allows stimulation of the brain to study physiological properties of neural populations. There are different approaches to using TMS for elucidating abnormalities of the motor cortical output system after stroke. Typically single-pulse TMS is used to investigate the integrity of the motor cortex and the corticospinal tract. It was shown that the presence of MEPs and somatosensory evoked potentials predicts recovery [122]. Specifically, normal MEPs at 1 day after stroke predicted good recovery, reduced MEPs indicated prolonged recovery lasting for up to a year, while lacking MEPs indicated poor recovery [76,123].

Following the electrophysiologic period of an MEP, there is electrical silence in the stimulated muscle, which has been termed the silent period, and is considered related to inhibitory tone. If cortical areas projecting to the motor cortex are damaged by ischemia, an enhanced duration of the silent period as an expression of inhibition was observed. Such an enhanced inhibition was shown to occur after extensive ischemia of premotor or parietal cortex resulting in hemiparesis [124,125]. This inhibition regressed in parallel to the spontaneous clinical recovery in the subsequent weeks. These observations are supported by experimental studies in rats showing that transient ischemia impairs synaptic transmission, while the direct wave of the MEPs and the early potential of the somatosensory-evoked potentials promptly recovered [126]. Conversely, disinhibition occurs after circumscribed infarction of motor cortex as was demonstrated by a shortened silent period following the MEP [124,127]. In such patients, paired TMS revealed disinhibition of the cerebral cortex and was associated with rapid clinical recovery [128].

Using paired-pulse TMS, intracortical inhibition as probably mediated by GABAergic neurotransmission can be investigated. It was found that within the first 7 days after a brain infarct there is an enhanced cortical excitability in the cortex adjacent to the brain lesion but also in the contralateral hemisphere [129–131]. Notably, the enhanced perilesional excitability was secondary to the infarct lesion and not due to an abnormality of interhemispheric inhibition, while the lesion-induced enhanced excitability was also transmitted to the intact motor cortex in the contralesional hemisphere [132]. Interestingly, the enhanced excitability decreased in the contralesional hemisphere in the patients who showed a good recovery within the 90 days, while it persisted in those patients with poor recovery [129,132]. The enhanced cortical excitability probably corresponded to the changed pattern of the GABA receptor in the perilesional vicinity after experimental ischemia [133]. Further data about the changes of cortical excitability in relation to recovery in the chronic stage after stroke are described in Chapter 10. Together, these insights into changes in functional maps may link acute injury with elements of brain repair and reorganization that are important to return of function.

Early commencement of stroke rehabilitation

There are numerous reports about rehabilitative approaches to improve the neurological deficit following stroke [134]. However, in the acute phase, data are largely missing. Typically, a hemiparetic stroke patient stays in bed, since he/she cannot move by him/herself. In addition, the early medical situation after stroke is often so grave that the patients are bedridden. There is, however, the notion that early mobilization will facilitate cerebral reorganization and will enhance the patient's insight that he/she can move, counteracting psychological regression and secondary immobilization [135]. There is a large trial ongoing to address this question and to investigate if very early onset of mobilization and stroke rehabilitation will be beneficial. Notably, some data suggest that the intensity of the training in the early weeks following a stroke, rather than the type of training, appears to be the greatest determinant of long-term motor improvement [136]. Also, constraint-induced therapy has been shown to be effective in enhancing recovery after stroke. Interestingly, these therapeutic approaches result in a widespread recruitment of motor representations in the affected hemisphere during the learning period as observed with fMRI and TMS [137,138]. Based on the evidence from fMRI and TMS studies, a number of strategies that capitalize on pathophysiological mechanisms have been proposed to promote motor recovery after stroke [122]. These include modulations that target the altered excitability in the affected and contralesional hemisphere and are applied as cortical stimulation directly onto the brain or as anaesthesia of the peripheral nerves [139–142]. Future work needs to evaluate how the combination of dedicated training and these external stimulations result in sustained neurological improvements. It should be noted, however, that infarct lesions do not only induce sensorimotor deficits, but are known to induce neuropsychological disturbances such as aphasia, apraxia, and neglect depending on the infarct locations within the brain. In addition, cortical and cortico-subcortical infarcts can induce dementia [143]. Particularly with respect to these post-stroke cognitive impairments, it is unclear whether repetitive or cognitive training approaches based on motor imagery are useful in the acute phase after stroke.

References

1. Reivich M. (1992) Crossed cerebellar diaschisis. *Am J Neuroradiol.* 1992;**13**:62–4.

2. Heiss WD, Huber M, Fink GR, *et al.* Progressive derangement of periinfarct viable tissue in ischemic stroke. *J Cereb Blood Flow Metab.* 1992;**12**:193–203.

3. Hossmann KA, Fischer M, Bockhorst K, *et al.* NMR imaging of the apparent diffusion coefficient (ADC) for the evaluation of metabolic suppression and recovery after prolonged cerebral ischemia. *J Cereb Blood Flow Metab.* 1994;**14**:723–31.

4. Lee LJ, Kidwell CS, Alger J, *et al.* Impact on stroke subtype diagnosis of early diffusion-weighted magnetic resonance imaging and magnetic resonance angiography. *Stroke.* 2000;**31**:1081–9.

5. Li F, Liu KF, Silva MD, *et al.* Transient and permanent resolution of ischemic lesions on diffusion-weighted imaging after brief periods of focal ischemia in rats: Correlation with histopathology. *Stroke.* 2000;**31**:946–54.

6. Mohr JP, Foulkes MA, Polis AT, *et al.* Infarct topography and hemiparesis profiles with cerebral convexity infarction: The Stroke Data Bank. *J Neurol Neurosurg Psychiatry.* 1993;**56**:344–51.

7. Hossmann KA. Viability thresholds and the penumbra of focal ischemia. *Ann Neurol.* 1994;**36**:557–65.

8. Dirnagl U, Iadecola C, Moskowitz MA. Pathobiology of ischaemic stroke: An integrated view. *Trends Neurosci.* 1999;**22**:391–7.

9. Dohmen C, Sakowitz OW, Fabricius M, *et al.* Spreading depolarizations occur in human ischemic stroke with high incidence. *Ann Neurol.* 2008;**63**:720–8.

10. Ringelstein EB, Biniek R, Weiller C, *et al.* Type and extent of hemispheric brain infarctions and clinical outcome in early and delayed middle cerebral artery recanalization. *Neurology.* 1992;**42**:289–98.

11. Wunderlich MT, Goertler M, Postert T, *et al.* Recanalization after intravenous thrombolysis: Does a recanalization time window exist? *Neurology.* 2007;**68**:1364–8.

12. Huber R, Muller BT, Seitz RJ, *et al.* Carotid surgery in acute symptomatic patients. *Eur J Vasc Endovasc Surg.* 2003;**25**:60–7.

13. Veronel D, Ringelstein A, Cohnen M, *et al.* Systemic thrombolysis based on CT or MRI stroke imaging. *J Neuroimag.* 2008;**18**:381–7.

14. Kokaia Z, Thored P, Arvidsson A, *et al.* Regulation of stroke-induced neurogenesis in adult brain – Recent scientific progress. *Cereb Cortex.* 2006;**16**:162–7.

15. Ohab JJ, Fleming S, Blesch A, *et al.* A vascular niche for neurogenesis after stroke. *J Neurosci.* 2006;**26**:13 007–16.

16. Schäbitz WR, Steigleder T, Cooper-Kuhn CM, *et al.* Intravenous brain-derived neurotrophic factor enhances poststroke sensorimotor recovery and stimulates neurogenesis. *Stroke.* 2007;**38**:2165–72.

17. Pluchino S, Muzio L, Imitola J, *et al.* Persistent inflammation alters the function of the endogenous brain stem cell compartment. *Brain.* 2008;**131**:2564–78.

18. Hermanns S, Klapka N, Müller HW. The collagenous lesion scar – An obstacle for axonal regeneration in

brain and spinal cord injury. *Restor Neurol Neurosci.* 2001;**19**:139–48.

19. Biernaskie, Corbett D. Enriched rehabilitative training promotes improved forelimb motor function and enhanced dendritic growth after focal ischemic injury. *J Neurosci.* 2001;**21**:5272–80.

20. Frost SB, Barbay S, Friel KM, *et al.* Reorganization of remote cortical regions after ischemic brain injury: A potential substrate for stroke recovery. *J Neurophysiol.* 2003;**89**:3205–14.

21. Dancause N, Barbay S, Frost SB, *et al.* Extensive cortical rewiring after brain injury. *J Neurosci.* 2005;**25**:10 167–79.

22. Nudo R, Wise B, SiFuentes F, *et al.* Neural substrates for the effects of rehabilitative training on motor recovery after ischemic infarct. *Science.* 1996;**272**:1791–4.

23. Hacke W, Donnan G, Fieschi C, *et al.* Association of outcome with early stroke treatment: Pooled analysis of ATLANTIS, ECASS, and NINDS rt-PA stroke trials. *Lancet.* 2004;**363**:768–74.

24. Hacke W, Kaste M, Bluhmki E, *et al.* Thrombolysis with alteplase 3 to 4.5 hours after acute ischemic stroke. *N Engl J Med.* 2008;**359**:1317–29.

25. Heiss WD, Grond M, Thiel A, *et al.* Tissue at risk of infarction rescued by early reperfusion: A positron emission tomography study in systemic recombinant tissue plasminogen activator thrombolysis of acute stroke. *J Cereb Blood Flow Metab.* 1998;**18**:1298–307.

26. Kidwell CS, Saver JL, Starkman S, *et al.* Late secondary ischemic injury in patients receiving intraarterial thrombolysis. *Ann Neurol.* 2002;**52**:698–703.

27. Alexandrov AV, Demchuk AM, Felberg RA, *et al.* High rate of complete recanalization and dramatic clinical recovery during tPA infusion when continuously monitored with 2-MHz transcranial Doppler monitoring. *Stroke.* 2000;**31**:610–4.

28. Alexandrov AV, Burgin WS, Demchuk AM, *et al.* Speed of intracranial clot lysis with intravenous tissue plasminogen activator therapy: Sonographic classification and short-term improvement. *Circulation.* 2001;**103**:2897–902.

29. Jorgensen HS, Reith J, Nakayama H, *et al.* What determines good recovery in patients with the most severe strokes? The Copenhagen Stroke Study. *Stroke.* 1999;**30**:2008–12.

30. Els T, Klisch J, Orszagh M, *et al.* Hyperglycemia in patients with focal cerebral ischemia after intravenous thrombolysis: Influence on clinical outcome and infarct size. *Cerebrovasc Dis.* 2002;**13**:89–94.

31. Parsons MW, Barber PA, Desmond PM, *et al.* Acute hyperglycemia adversely affects stroke outcome: A magnetic resonance imaging and spectroscopy study. *Ann Neurol.* 2002;**52**:20–8.

32. Alekhlafi MA, Hu WY, Hill MD, *et al.* Calcification and endothelialisation of thrombi in acute stroke. *Ann Neurol.* 2008;**64**:344–52.

33. Cramer SC. Repairing the human brain after stroke: I. Mechanisms of spontaneous recovery. *Ann Neurol.* 2008;**63**:272–87.

34. Kwakkel G, Kollen BJ, van der Grond J, *et al.* Probability of regaining dexterity in the flaccid upper limb: Impact of severity of paresis and time since onset in acute stroke. *Stroke.* 2003;**34**:2181–6.

35. Sprigg N, Gray LJ, Bath PM, *et al.* Early recovery and functional outcome are related with causal stroke subtype: Data from the tinzaparin in acute ischemic stroke trial. *J Stroke Cerebrovasc Dis.* 2007;**16**:180–4.

36. Kim D, Liebeskind DS. Neuroimaging advances and the transformation of acute stroke care. *Semin Neurol.* 2005;**25**:345–61.

37. Neumann-Haefelin T, Wittsack H-J, Wenserski F, *et al.* Diffusion- and perfusion-weighted MRI. The DWI/ PWI mismatch region in acute stroke. *Stroke.* 1999;**30**:1591–7.

38. Rohl L, Ostergaard L, Simonsen CZ, *et al.* Viability thresholds of ischemic penumbra of hyperacute stroke defined by perfusion-weighted MRI and apparent diffusion coefficient. *Stroke.* 2001;**32**:1140–6.

39. Sobesky J, Weber OZ, Lehnhardt F-G, *et al.* Which time-to-peak threshold best identifies penumbral flow? A comparison of perfusion-weighted magnetic resonance imaging and positron emission tomography in acute ischemic stroke. *Stroke.* 2004;**35**:2843–7.

40. Geisler BS, Brandhoff F, Fiehler J, *et al.* Blood-oxygen-level-dependent MRI allows metabolic description of tissue at risk in acute stroke patients. *Stroke.* 2006;**37**:1778–84.

41. Wittsack HJ, Ritzl A, Fink GR, *et al.* MR imaging in acute stroke: diffusion-weighted and perfusion imaging parameters for predicting infarct size. *Radiology.* 2002;**222**: 397–403.

42. Beaulieu C, de Crespigny A, Tong DC, *et al.* Longitudinal magnetic resonance imaging study of perfusion and diffusion in stroke: Evolution of lesion volume and correlation with clinical outcome. *Ann Neurol.* 1999;**46**:568–78.

43. Seitz RJ, Meisel S, Weller P, *et al.* The initial ischemic event: PWI and ADC for stroke evolution. *Radiology.* 2005;**237**:1020–8.

44. Weller P, Wittsack H-J, Siebler M, *et al.* Motor recovery as assessed with isometric finger movements and perfusion MRI after acute ischemic stroke. *Neurorehab Neural Rep.* 2006;**20**:390–7.

45. Toni D, Fiorelli M, Bastianello S, *et al.* Acute ischemic strokes improving during the first 48 hours of onset: Predictability, outcome, and possible mechanisms.

A comparison with early deteriorating strokes. *Stroke.* 1997;**28**:10–4.

46. Toni D, Fiorelli M, Zanette EM, *et al.* Early spontaneous improvement and deterioration of ischemic stroke patients. A serial study with transcranial Doppler ultrasonography. *Stroke.* 1998;**29**:1144–8.

47. Wildermuth S, Knauth M, Brandt T, *et al.* Role of CT angiography in patient selection for thrombolytic therapy in acute hemispheric stroke. *Stroke.* 1998;**29**:935–8.

48. Kleiser R, Wittsack H-J, Bütefisch CM, *et al.* Functional activation within the PI-DWI mismatch region in recovery from hemiparetic stroke: Preliminary observations. *Neuroimage.* 2005;**24**:515–23.

49. Thrift AG, Dewey HM, MacDonnell RA, *et al.* Incidence of the major stroke subtypes: Initial findings from the North East Melbourne stroke incidence study (NEMESIS). *Stroke.* 2001;**32**:1732–8.

50. Dewey HM, Sturm J, Donnan GA, *et al.* Incidence and outcome of subtypes of ischaemic stroke: Initial results from the North East Melbourne stroke incidence study (NEMESIS). *Cerebrovasc Dis.* 2003;**15**:133–9.

51. Finelli PF. Neuroimaging in acute posterior cerebral artery infarction. *Neurologist.* 2008;**14**:170–80.

52. Kang SY, Kim JS. Anterior cerebral artery infarction. Stroke mechanism and clinical-imaging study in 100 patients. *Neurology.* 2008;**70**:2386–93.

53. Bang OY, Lee PH, Heo KG, *et al.* Stroke specific DWI lesion patterns predict prognosis after acute ischaemic stroke within the MCA territory. *J Neurol Neurosurg Psychiatry.* 2005;**76**:1222–8.

54. Delgado-Mederos R, Rovira A, Alvarez-Sabín J, *et al.* Speed of tPA-induced clot lysis predicts DWI lesion evolution in acute stroke. *Stroke.* 2007;**38**:955–60.

55. von Kummer R, Meyding-Lamadé U, Forsting M, *et al.* Sensitivity and prognostic value of early CT in occlusion of the middle cerebral artery trunk. *Am J Neuroradiol.* 1994;**15**:9–15.

56. Wang X, Lam WW, Fan YH, *et al.* Topographic patterns of small subcortical infarcts associated with MCA stenosis: A diffusion-weighted MRI study. *J Neuroimaging.* 2006;**16**:266–71.

57. Derex L, Hermier M, Adeleine P, *et al.* Influence of the site of arterial occlusion on multiple baseline hemodynamic MRI parameters and post-thrombolytic recanalization in acute stroke. *Neuroradiology.* 2004;**46**:883–7.

58. Gadda D, Vannucchi L, Niccolai F, *et al.* Multidetector computed tomography of the head in acute stroke: Predictive value of different patterns of dense artery sign revealed by maximum intensity projection reformations for location and extent of the infarcted area. *Eur Radiol.* 2005;**15**:2387–95.

59. Coutts SB, Simon Je, Eliasiw M, *et al.* Triaging transient ischemic attack and minor stroke patients using acute magnetic resonance imaging. *Ann Neurol.* 2005;**57**:848–54.

60. Binkofski F, Seitz RJ, Arnold S, *et al.* Thalamic metabolism and integrity of the pyramidal tract determine motor recovery in stroke. *Ann Neurol.* 1996;**39**:460–70.

61. Crafton KR, Mark AN, Cramer SC. Improved understanding of cortical injury by incorporating measures of functional anatomy. *Brain.* 2003;**126**:1650–9.

62. Rey B, Frischknecht R, Maeder P, *et al.* Patterns of recovery following focal hemispheric lesions: Relationship between lasting deficit and damage to specialized networks. *Restor Neurol Neurosci.* 2007;**25**:285–94.

63. Stoeckel MC, Meisel S, Wittsack HJ, *et al.* Pattern of cortex and white matter involvement in severe middle cerebral artery ischemia. *J Neuroimag.* 2007;**17**:131–40.

64. Neumann-Haefelin T, du Mesnil de Rochemont R, Fiebach JB, *et al.* Effect of incomplete (spontaneous and postthrombolytic) recanalization after middle cerebral artery occlusion: A magnetic resonance imaging study. *Stroke.* 2004;**35**:109–14.

65. Bozzao A, Floris R, Gaudiello F, *et al.* Hemodynamic modifications in patients with symptomatic unilateral stenosis of the internal carotid artery: Evaluation with MR imaging perfusion sequences. *Am J Neuroradiol.* 2002;**23**:1342–5.

66. Bang OY, Saver JL, Buck BH, *et al.* Impact of collateral flow on tissue fate in acute ischaemic stroke. *J Neurol Neurosurg Psychiatry.* 2008;**79**:625–9.

67. van Everdingen KJ, Visser GH, Klijn CJ, *et al.* Role of collateral flow on cerebral hemodynamics in patients with unilateral internal carotid artery occlusion. *Ann Neurol.* 1998;**44**:167–76.

68. Mull M, Schwarz M, Thron A. Cerebral hemispheric low-flow infarcts in arterial occlusive disease. Lesion patterns and angiomorphological conditions. *Stroke.* 1997;**28**:118–23.

69. Furlan M, Marchal G, Viader F, *et al.* Spontaneous neurological recovery after stroke and the fate of the ischemic penumbra. *Ann Neurol.* 1996;**40**:216–26.

70. Arnold M, Nedeltchev K, Mattle HP, *et al.* Intra-arterial thrombolysis in 24 consecutive patients with internal carotid artery T occlusions. *J Neurol Neurosurg Psychiatry.* 2003;**74**:739–42.

71. Karnath HO, Fruhmann Berger M, Kuker W, *et al.* The anatomy of spatial neglect based on voxelwise statistical analysis: A study of 140 patients. *Cereb Cortex.* 2004;**14**:1164–72.

72. Saur D, Lange R, Baumgaertner A, *et al.* Dynamics of language reorganization after stroke. *Brain.* 2006;**129**:1371–84.

73. Fisher CM. Lacunar strokes and infarcts: A review. *Neurology.* 1982;**32**:871–6.

74. Boiten J, Lodder J. Lacunar infarcts. Pathogenesis and validity of the clinical syndromes. *Stroke.* 1991;**22**:1374–8.

75. Chen X, Wen W, Anstey KJ, *et al.* Prevalence, incidence, and risk factors of lacunar infarcts in a community sample. *Neurology.* 2009;**73**:266–72.

76. Stinear CM, Barber PA, Smale PR, *et al.* Functional potential in chronic stroke patients depends on corticospinal tract integrity. *Brain.* 2007;**130**:170–80.

77. Surikova I, Meisel S, Siebler M, *et al.* Significance of the perfusion–diffusion mismatch area in chronic cerebral ischemia. *J Magn Reson Imaging.* 2006;**24**:771–8.

78. Blondin D, Seitz RJ, Rusch O, *et al.* Clinical impact of MRI perfusion disturbances and normal diffusion in acute stroke patients. *Eur J Radiol.* 2009;**71**:1–10.

79. Kurada S, Houkin K. Moyamoya disease: Current concepts and future perspectives. *Lancet Neurol.* 2008;**7**:1056–66.

80. Alexandrov AV, Felberg RA, Demchuk AM, *et al.* Deterioration following spontaneous improvement: Sonographic findings in patients with acutely resolving symptoms of cerebral ischemia. *Stroke.* 2000;**31**:915–9.

81. Seitz RJ, Siebler M. Platelet GPIIb/IIIa receptor antagonists in human ischemic brain disease. *Curr Vasc Pharmacol.* 2008;**6**:29–36.

82. Jüttler E, Schwab S, Schmiedek P, *et al.* Decompressive surgery for the treatment of malignant infarction of the middle cerebral artery (DESTINY): Randomized, controlled trial. *Stroke.* 2007;**38**:2518–25.

83. Kidwell CS, Saver JL, Mattiello J, *et al.* Thrombolytic reversal of acute human cerebral ischemic injury shown by diffusion/perfusion magnetic resonance imaging. *Ann Neurol.* 2000;**47**:462–9.

84. Sena E, Bart van der Worp H, Howells D, *et al.* How can we improve the pre-clinical development of drugs for stroke? *TINS.* 2007;**30**:433–9.

85. Dirnagl U. Bench to bedside: the quest for quality in experimental stroke research. *J Cereb Blood Flow Metab.* 2006;**26**:1465–78.

86. Keller E, Steiner T, Fandino J, *et al.* Changes in cerebral blood flow and oxygen metabolism during moderate hypothermia in patients with severe middle cerebral artery infarction. *Neurosurg Focus.* 2000;**8**:e4.

87. DeGeorgia MA, Krieger DW, Abou-Chebi A, *et al.* Cooling for acute ischemic brain damage (COOL AID): A feasibility trial of endovascular cooling. *Neurology.* 2004;**63**:312–7.

88. Ramani R. Hypothermia for brain protection and resuscitation. *Curr Opin Anaesthesiol.* 2006;**19**:487–91.

89. Kollmer R, Schwab S. Ischaemic stroke: Acute management, intensive care, and future perspectives. *Br J Anaesth.* 2007;**99**:95–101.

90. Kent TA, Soukup VM, Fabian RH. Heterogeneity affecting outcome from acute stroke therapy: Making reperfusion worse. *Stroke.* 2001;**32**:2318–27.

91. Pan J, Konstas AA, Bateman B, *et al.* Reperfusion injury following cerebral ischemia: Pathophysiology, MR imaging, and potential therapies. *Neuroradiology.* 2007;**49**:93–102.

92. Giffard RG, Xu L, Carrico W, *et al.* Chaperones, protein aggregation, and brain protection from hypoxic/ischemic injury. *J Exp Biol.* 2004;**207**:3213–20.

93. Murphy BD, Fox AJ, Lee DH, *et al.* Identification of penumbra and infarct in acute ischemic stroke using computed tomography perfusion-derived blood flow and blood volume measurements. *Stroke.* 2006;**37**:1771–7.

94. Nadasy GL, Greenberg JH, Reivich M, *et al.* Local cerebral blood flow during and after bilateral carotid artery occlusion in unanesthetized gerbils. *Stroke.* 1990;**21**:901–17.

95. Rivers CS, Wardlaw JM, Armitage PA, *et al.* Persistent infarct hyperintensity on diffusion-weighted imaging late after stroke indicates heterogeneous, delayed, infarct evolution. *Stroke.* 2006;**37**:1418–23.

96. Bang OY, Buck BH, Saver JL, *et al.* Prediction of hemorrhagic transformation after recanalization therapy using T2*-permeability magnetic resonance imaging. *Ann Neurol.* 2007;**62**:170–6.

97. Kastrup A, Gröschel K, Ringer TM, *et al.* Early disruption of the blood–brain barrier after thrombolytic therapy predicts hemorrhage in patients with acute stroke. *Stroke.* 2008;**39**:2385–7.

98. Feuerstein G, Wang X, Barone F. Inflammatory gene expression in cerebral ischemia and trauma. Potential new therapeutic targets. *Ann NY Acad Sci.* 1997;**825**:179–93.

99. Lucas SM, Rothwell NJ, Gibson RM. The role of inflammation in CNS injury and disease. *Br J Pharmacol.* 2006;**147**(Suppl 1):S232–40.

100. Schroeter M, Saleh A, Wiedermann D, *et al.* Histochemical detection of ultrasmall superparamagnetic iron oxide (USPIO) contrast medium uptake in experimental brain ischemia. *Magn Reson Med.* 2004;**52**:403–06.

101. Saleh A, Schroeter M, Jonkmanns C, *et al.* In vivo MRI of brain inflammation in human ischaemic stroke. *Brain.* 2004;**127**:1670–7.

102. Saleh A, Schroeter M, Ringelstein A, *et al.* Iron oxide particle-enhanced MRI suggests variability of brain

inflammation at early stages after ischemic stroke. *Stroke.* 2007;**38**:2733–7.

103. Price CJ, Wang D, Menon DK, *et al.* Intrinsic activated microglia map to the peri-infarct zone in the subacute phase of ischemic stroke. *Stroke* 2006;**37**:1749–53.

104. Gerhard A, Schwarz J, Myers R, *et al.* Evolution of microglial activation in patients after ischemic stroke: A [11C](R)-PK11195 PET study. *Neuroimage.* 2005;**24**:591–5.

105. McCombe PA, Read SJ. Immune and inflammatory responses to stroke: Good or bad? *Int J Stroke.* 2008;**3**:254–65.

106. Witte OW, Bidmon H-J, Schiene K, *et al.* Functional differentiation of multiple perilesional zones after focal cerebral ischemia. *J Cereb Blood Flow Metab.* 2000;**20**:1149–65.

107. Carmichael ST, Wei L, Rovainen CM, *et al.* Growth-associated gene expression after stroke: Evidence for a growth-promoting region in the peri-infarct cortex. *Exp Neurol.* 2005;**193**:291–311.

108. Centonze D, Rossi S, Tortiglione A, *et al.* Synaptic plasticity during recovery from permanent occlusion of the middle cerebral artery. *Neurobiol Dis.* 2007;**27**:44–53.

109. Heiss WD, Sobeski J, Smekal U, *et al.* Probability of cortical infarction predicted by flumazenil binding and diffusion-weighted imaging signal intensity: A comparative positron emission tomography/ magnetic resonance imaging study in early ischemic stroke. *Stroke.* 2004;**35**:1892–8.

110. Duncan PW, Lai SM, Keighley J. Defining post-stroke recovery: Implications for design and interpretation of drug trials. *Neuropharmacology.* 2000;**39**:835–41.

111. Binkofski F, Seitz RJ, Hackländer T, *et al.* The recovery of motor functions following hemiparetic stroke: A clinical and MR-morphometric study. *Cerebrovasc Dis.* 2001;**11**:273–81.

112. Binkofski F, Seitz RJ. Modulation of the BOLD-response in early recovery from sensorimotor stroke. *Neurology.* 2004;**63**:1223–9.

113. Hamzei F, Knab R, Weiller C, *et al.* The influence of extra- and intracranial artery disease on the BOLD signal in fMRI. *Neuroimage.* 2003;**20**:1393–9.

114. Jaillard A, Martin CD, Garambois K, *et al.* Vicarious function within the human primary motor cortex? A longitudinal fMRI stroke study. *Brain.* 2005;**128**:1122–38.

115. Liepert J, Haevernick K, Weiller C, *et al.* The surround inhibition determines therapy-induced cortical reorganization. *Neuroimage.* 2006;**32**:1216–20.

116. Marshall RS, Perera GM, Lazar RM, *et al.* Evolution of cortical activation during recovery from corticospinal tract infarction. *Stroke.* 2000;**31**:656–61.

117. Nhan H, Barquist K, Bell K, *et al.* Brain function early after stroke in relation to subsequent recovery. *J Cereb Blood Flow Metab.* 2004;**24**:756–63.

118. Foltys H, Krings T, Meister IG, *et al.* Motor representation in patients rapidly recovering after stroke: A functional magnetic resonance imaging and transcranial magnetic stimulation study. *Clin Neurophysiol.* 2003;**114**:2404–15.

119. Bütefisch CM, Kleiser R, Körber B, *et al.* Recruitment of contralesional motor cortex in stroke patients with recovery of hand function. *Neurology.* 2005;**64**:1067–9.

120. Nelles G, Cramer S, Schaechter J, *et al.* Quantitative assessment of mirror movements after stroke. *Stroke.* 1998;**29**:1182–7.

121. Grefkes C, Nowak AD, Eickhoff SB, *et al.* Cortical connectivity after subcortical stroke assessed with functional magnetic resonance imaging. *Ann Neurol.* 2008;**63**:236–46.

122. Seitz RJ, Buetefisch CM. Recovery from ischemic stroke: A translational research perspective for neurology. *Future Neurol.* 2006;**1**:571–86.

123. Delvaux V, Alagona G, Gérard P, *et al.* Post-stroke reorganization of hand motor area: A 1-year prospective follow-up with focal transcranial magnetic stimulation. *Clin Neurophysiol.* 2003;**114**:1217–25.

124. von Giesen HJ, Roick H, Benecke R. Inhibitory actions of motor cortex following unilateral brain lesions as studied by magnetic brain stimulation. *Exp Brain Res.* 1994;**99**:84–96.

125. Classen J, Schnitzler A, Binkofski F, *et al.* The motor syndrome associated with exaggerated inhibition within the primary motor cortex of patients with hemiparetic stroke. *Brain.* 1997;**120**:605–19.

126. Bolay H, Dalkara T. Mechanisms of motor dysfunction after transient MCA occlusion: Persistent transmission failure in cortical synapses is a major determinant. *Stroke.* 1998;**29**:1988–93.

127. Schnitzler A, Benecke R. The silent period after transcranial magnetic stimulation is of exclusive cortical origin: Evidence from isolated cortical ischemic lesions in man. *Neurosci Lett.* 1994;**180**:41–5.

128. Liepert J, Hamzei F, Weiller C. Motor cortex disinhibition of the unaffected hemisphere after acute stroke. *Muscle Nerve.* 2000;**23**:1761–3.

129. Bütefisch CM, Netz J, Wessling M, *et al.* Remote changes in cortical excitability after stroke. *Brain.* 2003;**126**:470–81.

130. Cincenelli P, Pascualetti P, Zaccagnini M, *et al.* Interhemispheric asymmetries of motor cortex excitability in the postacute stroke stage: A paired-pulse transcranial magnetic stimulation study. *Stroke.* 2003;**34**:2653–8.

131. Manganotti P, Acler M, Zanette GP, *et al.* Motor cortical disinhibition during early and late recovery after stroke. *Neurorehab Neural Repair.* 2008;**22**:396–403.

132. Bütefisch CM, Wessling M, Netz J, *et al.* Excitability and of ipsi- and contralesional motor cortices and their relationship in stroke patients. *Neurorehab Neural Repair.* 2008;**22**:4–21.

133. Redecker C, Luhmann HJ, Hagemann G, *et al.* Differential downregulation of GABA-A receptor subunits in widespread brain regions in the freeze-lesion model of focal cortical malformations. *J Neurosci.* 2000;**20**:5045–53.

134. Cramer SC. Repairing the human brain after stroke: II. Restorative therapies. *Ann Neurol.* 2008;**63**:549–60.

135. Bernhardt J, Dewey H, Thrift A, *et al.* A very early rehabilitation trial for stroke (AVERT): Phase II safety and feasibility. *Stroke.* 2008;**39**:390–6.

136. Kwakkel G, Wagenaar RC, Twisk JW, *et al.* Intensity of leg and arm training after primary middle-cerebral-artery stroke: A randomised trial. *Lancet.* 1999;**354**:191–6.

137. Boake C, Noser EA, Baraniuk S, *et al.* Constraint-induced movement therapy during early stroke rehabilitation. *Neurorehabil Neural Repair.* 2008;**21**:14–24.

138. Wittenberg GF, Chen R, Ishii K, *et al.* Constraint-induced therapy in stroke: Magnetic-stimulation motor maps and cerebral activation. *Neurorehabil Neural Repair.* 2003;**16**:1–10.

139. Muehlbacher W, Richards C, Ziemann U, *et al.* Improving hand function in chronic stroke. *Arch Neurol.* 2002;**59**:1278–82.

140. Floel A, Nagorsen U, Werhahn KJ, *et al.* Influence of somatosensory input on motor function in patients with chronic stroke. *Ann Neurol.* 2004;**56**:206–12.

141. Fregni F, Boggio PS, Mansur CG, *et al.* Transcranial direct current stimulation of the unaffected hemisphere in stroke patients. *Neuroreport.* 2005;**16**:1551–5.

142. Hummel F, Celnik P, Giraux P, *et al.* Effects of non-invasive cortical stimulation on skilled motor function in chronic stroke. *Brain.* 2005;**128**:490–9.

143. Troncoso JC, Zonderman AB, Resnick SM, *et al.* Effect of infarcts on dementia in the Baltimore longitudinal study of aging. *Ann Neurol.* 2008;**64**:168–76.

10 Changes in cortical excitability and interhemispheric interactions after stroke

P. Talelli, O. Swayne & J. C. Rothwell

Animal models of stroke have provided essential insights into the neural mechanisms that contribute to recovery of function. These involve not only synaptic plasticity but also growth of new connections within and between cortical areas. Recent work in humans has been directed to developing non-invasive methods of testing whether similar changes occur in patients after stroke. If successful, they would give us methods of following changes in neural organization during recovery and of using this knowledge to guide treatment. Tools presently available for this include functional brain imaging, electroencephalography, magnetoencephalography, and transcranial magnetic stimulation (TMS). This chapter will focus on knowledge obtained from TMS measures of cortical excitability in the hemisphere damaged by stroke as well as in the non-stroke hemisphere. We concentrate on motor function, since this forms the basis of the majority of studies in this area, and since this is among the most commonly affected domains of behavior affected by stroke.

Using TMS to quantify the damage resulting from a stroke

Single pulses of TMS over the motor cortex evoke twitches in contralateral muscles of the body that can be recorded electrophysiologically by placing surface electrodes over the muscle of interest (motor-evoked potential, MEP) [1]. A series of basic physiological studies, including recordings of descending corticospinal activity from electrodes implanted into the spinal epidural space for treatment of chronic pain, have shown the following sequence of events [2,3]. Each stimulus activates the axons of interneurons in the cortex that in turn have excitatory synapses onto corticospinal pyramidal cells. When these discharge, the action potential travels in rapidly conducting corticospinal projections to the spinal cord where there are monosynaptic connections onto spinal motoneurons. Discharge of the latter leads to the MEP. In resting subjects, a single descending volley in the corticospinal tract fails to discharge any spinal motoneurons because the synaptic depolarization is insufficient to bring the neural membrane to threshold. However, a single TMS pulse to the cortex actually results in repetitive discharge of corticospinal neurons at high frequency (600 Hz: I-waves) due to reverberation of activity in intracortical circuits. Receipt of two or more of these descending volleys brings resting spinal motoneurons to threshold.

Given this sequence of events, it is evident that MEPs ought to be able to provide some estimate of the functional integrity of the corticospinal tract after stroke [4]. However, it should also be clear that since MEPs rely on a rather complex sequence of events, involving not only corticospinal conduction but also synaptic transmission at cortex and cord, the interpretation of changes can sometimes be complex.

Two main measures have been used to quantify corticospinal function after stroke: (a) the motor threshold (MT) for generating an MEP response, and (b) the relationship between the intensity of the TMS at suprathreshold levels and the amplitude of the evoked MEP. When the TMS intensity is increased gradually, in steps commonly expressed as percentage of the MT, an input–output (I/O) curve can be generated. In practice, many researchers have measured the MEP amplitude at a single point of the I/O curve. As detailed below, threshold depends on the excitability of cortical axons and synapses [5], whereas the slope of the I/O curve depends on the distribution of

Brain Repair After Stroke, ed. S. C. Cramer and R. J. Nudo. Published by Cambridge University Press.

excitability in the corticospinal projection as well as the total number of available fibers in that connection [6]. A more detailed description of the principles of TMS appears in this chapter's Appendix.

Three main factors can change the threshold, for stimulation, and the contribution of each will depend on the lesion location and load. (1) Changes in the ionic composition of extracellular fluid: at a cortical level, these can increase the threshold for activating axons; in capsular strokes they may reduce or block conduction in corticospinal axons. These effects should resolve relatively quickly after the stroke [7]. (2) Altered excitability of synaptic connections at both cortex and spinal cord: in the cortex, there may be disconnection from peripheral afferent inputs in the case of a subcortical lesion, and also from cortico-cortical inputs in the case of pure cortical strokes. In both cases, this will affect the excitability of postsynaptic neurons and increase thresholds. At the spinal cord, loss of any tonic descending facilitation will also reduce spinal motoneuron excitability and again increase thresholds. (3) Related to both these considerations is the fact that multiple descending volleys are necessary to activate spinal motoneurons, especially with the target muscle at rest. The system may fail to produce these because of changes in the excitability of intracortical circuits or in the membrane properties of corticospinal neurons. In addition, any compromise of axonal conduction in the internal capsule may cause conduction block of repetitive transmission to the cord.

Similarly, the amplitude of the MEP may be reduced for a number of reasons. One possibility is that there are not enough working connections available to generate the full response to a standard suprathreshold TMS pulse. Indeed, failure to produce repetitive firing and dysynchronization of the descending impulses at the spinal level could also result in smaller multiphasic MEPs commonly seen in stroke patients. In theory, however, the same could be seen if the remaining connections were adequate in numbers but the distribution of excitability was skewed towards higher values. In this situation, threshold measurements could even remain relatively normal, but typical increments in stimulation intensity might not be enough to recruit additional fibers. In this case the slope of the I/O curve would be reduced. If the stimulator's output was enough to activate all the available connections, the plateau of the curve, i.e. the maximum available output, should not be affected. On the contrary, a critical reduction in the number of

fibers would additionally affect the plateau level. Obviously, the plateau level is a major determinant of the gradient of the curve, thus such interpretations are really informative when a plateau has been reached. Finally, as with threshold assessments, I/O curves are subject to excitability changes in the spinal cord. In most instances, mainly in terms of threshold and MEP amplitude, both active and resting measures show similar trends, which suggests that the cause of the abnormalities cannot be placed solely at spinal level [8–12]. Additional support comes from studying spinal reflex arcs, such as H-reflexes and F-waves, which do not appear to be changed, at least within the first few months after the stroke [13,14].

Given the complexity of the events following a TMS pulse, it is not surprising that the results reported in the literature have been relatively variable (see Talelli et al. for review [4]). As a general rule, TMS often fails to elicit responses in the affected hand muscles [8,11,13,15–20]. When responses are present, increased threshold and reduced MEP amplitudes can be expected. The slope of the I/O curves has been also shown to be reduced [21]. In most instances, measures improve with time after stroke, tending to reach a plateau after about 3–6 months, paralleling the usual time course of improvement of motor symptoms [9,12,14,21,22]. Often this improvement is incomplete and abnormal TMS values persist in the chronic stage even when clinical recovery is good [23–25].

There are, however, interesting details that may be explicable given the complex mechanisms of the MEP outlined above. For example, some researchers have found that patients with cortical lesions may have relatively normal thresholds as early as the first post-stroke day [20], although the amplitude of the MEP was significantly reduced. This could suggest a patchy ischemia pattern sparing some of the low-threshold connections that are preferentially activated by TMS. In fact increased extracellular K^+ concentration could even tend to depolarize neural membranes and reduce thresholds. In one study, repeated measures of active thresholds (AMT) in the acute post-stroke period revealed an initial tendency for AMTs to increase before starting to steadily decline [21]. Whether these variations are relevant to the long-term evolution in electrophysiology and/or recovery remains unclear. They should, however, be kept in mind, since threshold calculations are used to deliver most TMS protocols, both observational, such as I/O curves, and interventional, such as repetitive TMS.

Another interesting point is the pattern in which TMS measures improve over time. Most reports tend to agree that most of the change is seen within the first 90 days. Thresholds appear to be the first measure to reach a plateau [14], which can sometimes lie within the normal range [21]. The amplitude of the MEP and the gradient of the I/O curve may continue to change in the next 2–3 months [21]. It also appears more common for these values to remain abnormal in the long term [14,20,23–25]. It is possible that the I/O relationship, depending both on the distribution of excitability and on the availability of corticospinal connections, is more difficult to normalize.

An important question that is usually posed by TMS measures is their relationship to an individual patient's clinical status. Early recovery is most probably related to reperfusion of the ischemic penumbra and resolution of edema resulting in reinstitution of connections that have been malfunctioning but not critically damaged [7] (see also Chapter 9). These events could also be the cause of the electrophysiological amelioration seen within the first few weeks, at which point the lesion load should be final. Indeed, many authors suggest that during this stage both thresholds [19,22] and amplitude of the MEP [14] show some association with severity of symptoms. In one report, 56% of the variability in the function of the affected hand could be explained by either MTs or the gradient of the I/O curve [21]. Interestingly, the correlation between the slope of I/O curve and clinical measures became weaker over time. Similarly, correlations between TMS measures and clinical scores in cross-sectional studies in chronic patients have been less consistent. Several reasons may contribute to that. Some of these must relate to the way we measure clinical recovery. For example, when functional tests are used, it is possible that what we measure early after the stroke is "closer" to the core deficits. With time, patients may perform tasks using compensatory strategies and score higher in clinical tests without necessarily improving their core deficits. Whether these compensatory phenomena would be reflected in measures of corticospinal excitability/connectivity is questionable. On the other hand, clinical tests may be inadequate to record improvements in the quality of motor control. This is particularly problematic when dealing with a group of patients of variable severity. However, other issues are also worthy of consideration. For example, a gradually weakening correlation between I/O curves and clinical scores could suggest

that these measures are not adequate to quantify long-term improvements in corticospinal connectivity, or that other mechanisms or pathways may gradually become more relevant to the recovery process. These possibilities are discussed below.

Using TMS to explore mechanisms of recovery

As detailed in other chapters, animal models of stroke have provided many insights into the mechanisms that may underlie the improvement in motor function commonly seen after stroke. While it is not possible to obtain the equivalent information in human patients, non-invasive techniques have recently begun to make a positive contribution by allowing aspects of cortical physiology to be measured in real time during the recovery phase. As described above, single-pulse TMS can be used to assess the excitability of the corticospinal projection. Using pairs of pulses separated by a few milliseconds, information can also be gained about the activity in regulatory intracortical circuits within the motor cortex (see Table 10.1 for details) – the use of a second coil can even allow the functional connections between two separate regions to be tested. If such parameters can be related to clinical measures in groups of patients, then conclusions can be drawn about the relevance of physiological changes for recovery.

The affected hemisphere

There is evidence from animal models that changes occur in cortical motor maps – the areas of cortex from which movements may be evoked – in the regions surrounding but not directly involved in an area of cortical infarction. It seems reasonable that such a process may prove helpful to recovery, either by recruiting adjacent intact cortex (in the case of a cortical lesion) or by providing access to an intact corticospinal outflow tract (in the case of a subcortical lesion). In support of this, cross-sectional and longitudinal TMS mapping studies in conscious stroke patients comparing the motor hand representations of the affected and unaffected hemispheres have shown that the "center of gravity" of such representations may shift in the ipsilesional side often by several centimeters [20,26]. These shifts are not usually present early after the stroke, suggesting that they may occur by means of a gradual cortical process similar to that seen in non-human primates [20,23,25–27]. Some

Table 10.1 Commonly used TMS techniques: what are they and what do they measure?

Measure	Definition and application
Resting and active motor threshold (RMT/AMT)	The minimum stimulation intensity that can produce a predefined recordable level of EMG response (motor evoked potential, MEP) in the target muscle at rest (RMT) or during a low-strength active muscle contraction (AMT). This is the most basic measure of cortical excitability. It is also used to set the stimulation intensity for other measures.
Input/output curve (I/O curve)	Plots the increase in the amplitude of the MEP ("output") with increasing stimulation intensity ("input"). Typically S-shaped, the curve reaches a plateau at 140–160% MT. Used for detailed assessment of corticospinal output. The plateau level gives information about the maximum output available; the gradient of the middle, linear part of the curve, on the distribution of excitability in the corticospinal projections, i.e. how many of the projections available are closer to threshold.
Short intracortical inhibition (SICI)	Paired-pulse stimulation protocol. Measures the reduction of the MEP elicited by a standard suprathreshold pulse when this is preceded by a subthreshold pulse by 1–4 ms. Assesses the function of mainly $GABA_A$ (inhibitory) interneurons that synapse onto pyramidal cells.
Intracortical facilitation (ICF)	As with SICI, but using a time between pulses (interstimulus interval) that is longer, i.e. 7–15 ms. Assesses facilitatory interneurons that are thought to be primarily glutamatergic.
Long intracortical inhibition (LICI)	As above, but both pulses are suprathreshold and separated by 100–200 ms. Assesses probably $GABA_B$ (inhibitory) interneurons that synapse onto pyramidal cells.
Interhemispheric inhibition (IHI)	Paired-pulse stimulation protocol. Measures the reduction of the MEP elicited by a standard suprathreshold pulse when a pulse of similar intensity is given to the contralateral motor cortex 7–40 ms earlier. Assesses the function of callosal projections, but other pathways involving subcortical structures could also be involved. Both $GABA_A$ and $GABA_B$ circuits may be implicated.

GABA, gamma amino butyric acid.

have suggested that the greatest shifts tend to be seen after dense subcortical strokes, which often disconnect a significant area of cortex [9]. Although results have been variable, a positive correlation has been reported between the magnitude of map shift and motor recovery in a group of patients with intact corticospinal excitability [28], suggesting that such a phenomenon may represent a constructive adaptive response to injury.

How do such changes in motor representations occur? Animal studies have pointed to the importance of horizontal cortical connecting fibers as potential candidates. There is evidence that cortical reorganization depends on the removal of GABAergic intracortical inhibition, being enhanced or blocked by GABA antagonists or agonists, respectively. A form of intracortical inhibition (short-interval intracortical inhibition, SICI) which is GABA-dependent can readily be measured using paired pulse TMS, and is known to be reduced in the context of normal motor learning, which is widely used as an analogy for recovery following stroke [29]. A number of studies have therefore

investigated whether such a release from GABAergic inhibition may play a role in allowing the reorganization of motor representations after stroke.

Reduced SICI in the affected hemisphere has been widely reported in the acute period after stroke [10,13,30] and in some investigations in the chronic stage [31]. The spatial distribution of SICI might influence patterns of shift in the centre of gravity that arise with treatment-induced plasticity [32]. A reduction in a second form of GABAergic inhibition, termed long-interval intracortical inhibition (LICI), has also been described after stroke [21], while intracortical facilitation (a possible glutamatergic phenomenon) has been consistently reported as being normal. The presence of clear disinhibition would be consistent with reduced GABAergic activity and would favor reorganization according to animal models. However, without more invasive tests, it is not possible to be certain whether this represents a constructive "response" to injury or an epiphenomenon. Finally, when interpreting the results of paired-pulse TMS experiments, it is worth bearing in mind that while certain parameters

(SICI, LICI, etc.) are commonly ascribed to specific intracortical populations, the reality may be more complex. The investigator can simply measure the effect of the conditioning pulse on the test pulse, which may reflect the overlapping influences of several neuronal populations. Recent studies in healthy subjects have begun to tease out these contributions by using a variety of intensities and orientations of conditioning and test pulses, but these have yet to be applied to patient groups.

The contralesional hemisphere

There has been considerable interest in studying physiological changes in cortical motor areas in the "intact", or contralesional, hemisphere. This has stemmed from the finding of altered contralesional cortical excitability in animal models of stroke, and also from the demonstration of increased activity in contralesional cortical regions during use of the affected hand using functional imaging in humans.

The unaffected hemisphere is in many ways more amenable to study by TMS than the affected hemisphere, with motor thresholds that are normal and stable. Although one group reported abnormally increased MEP amplitudes early on after stroke [20], it is now generally accepted that corticospinal excitability probably remains within normal limits. Some groups [33,34] reported a higher than normal probability of evoking an ipsilateral (uncrossed) MEP from the unaffected hemisphere in the affected limb, but this phenomenon was only seen in severely affected patients, and it is not thought that uncrossed projections play any significant role in recovery of hand function. However, the situation may be different in more proximal muscles; for example, recovery of swallowing in dysphagic patients after hemispheric stroke appears to rely mostly on expansion of control from the unaffected hemisphere.

As with other TMS measures, investigations of GABAergic inhibition in the unaffected hemisphere have yielded a variety of results with the majority of reports finding normal or reduced inhibition. Interestingly, the situation may change over time. In one longitudinal study, unaffected hemisphere SICI was measured at two early time points; only patients who recovered well showed reduced inhibition suggesting that it may have positive role in promoting change after damage [13]. A second longitudinal study showed that clinical correlations with a number of paired pulse TMS parameters, including SICI in the unaffected hemisphere, only became strong around the 3 month time point and weakened again with time after that [21]. Such a relationship was not observed when SICI was tested within the first few weeks [35], or across a wide range of later time points [31], and it may well be that the clinical relevance of activity in intracortical circuits changes dynamically during recovery.

The rise in the correlation of paired-pulse TMS measures with clinical state seems to occur at the same time as there is a gradual decline in the correlations with measures of corticospinal excitability in the affected hemisphere. One interpretation of this is that function immediately after stroke is limited by the extent of damage to the original corticospinal projection. However, over time, disinhibition allows cortical areas to reorganize in order to maximize function in the remaining pathways and improve movement. This would be consistent with functional imaging studies of motor activation patterns after stroke that show secondary and contralesional motor cortical regions are recruited in a "step-wise" manner in the face of increasing severe disruption of the corticospinal tract [36].

Interhemispheric interactions

TMS can be used to measure interhemispheric interactions, most commonly between the two motor cortices, by using a paired-pulse interaction delivered via two coils. At rest, the predominant effect is inhibition, but prior to movement there is a reduction in inhibition from the inactive to the active hemisphere, which then becomes facilitatory just before EMG onset. After stroke, interhemispheric inhibition (IHI) from the unaffected to the affected hemisphere (UH–AH) is normal at rest, but that in the other direction (AH–UH) is thought to be deficient [37,38]. This is not necessarily due to direct damage to the transcallosal projections [39], since it is also seen when the stroke is more caudal. A relationship has been demonstrated in such patients between reduced IHI (AH–UH) and loss of SICI within the unaffected hemisphere, suggesting that the latter may be a result of transcallosal disinhibition.

The switch to facilitation normally observed just prior to movement onset does not occur when patients move their paretic hand (i.e. measuring IHI from UH to AH) [37]. This is consistent with the hypothesis that the unaffected hemisphere suppresses excitability of the affected hemisphere, thus doubly disabling its residual motor function. This has led to the idea that reducing the excitability of the unaffected motor cortex may improve recovery, and has provided the rationale for a number of therapeutic studies. It has not been clearly established which hemisphere is responsible for the failure to "switch off" IHI; it could reside within the unaffected hemisphere, or it could equally well result from an abnormality in circuits mediating IHI within the affected hemisphere. In favor of the first interpretation, a study of experimental anesthesia of the healthy arm produced improved motor function in the paretic arm while also reducing premovement IHI [40]. However, not all evidence supports the idea that the non-stroke hemisphere interferes with function of the damaged side. The performance of complex movements with the paretic hand is degraded by a disruptive train of TMS pulses given to the contralesional primary motor cortex [41], suggesting a positive contribution from this region. In summary, the significance of IHI targeting the lesioned hemisphere after stroke is yet to be resolved. This question may turn out to be important since individual differences in the presence of excessive IHI may determine whether or not interventions that are designed to reduce contralesional excitability are successful.

TMS has been used to characterize a number of inter-regional interactions from non-primary motor regions targeting the motor cortex in healthy humans, and their roles in relation to different aspects of movement (see Reis *et al.* for review [42]). Although a number of the cortical regions involved in these interactions show greater than normal hemodynamic activity during hand movement after stroke [43], almost nothing is known about what role, if any, such activity may play in recovered motor function. One exception is the dorsal premotor cortex (PMd), which in healthy humans is involved in movement selection. Imaging studies have suggested that, depending on the extent of damage, either the ipsilesional or contralesional PMd may be an important contributor to recovered arm movement following stroke [44]. Two "virtual lesion" TMS studies have shown that disruption of activity in this area increases reaction times of the paretic hand in stroke patients, whereas no effect is seen in healthy subjects [41,45]. Unpublished data from this group have also demonstrated a loss or reversal of the normal inhibitory interhemispheric influence of the contralesional PMd on the primary motor cortex of the lesioned hemisphere, and have suggested that this

region may help to support recovered function via such an interaction.

Conclusions

TMS has made it possible for the physiology of the motor system to be examined in some detail after stroke, providing information in two broad categories. First, single-pulse TMS measures have been used to quantify the damage to the corticospinal tract as reflected in raised motor thresholds and impaired MEP. Second, changes in cortical motor maps and paired-pulse measures of intracortical activity have provided insights into the mechanisms by which reorganization at the cortical level may assist motor recovery. There has been considerable variability between studies with respect to the pathophysiological changes reported. Some of this may relate to methodological differences, patient heterogeneity, or to the range of time points after stroke at which such measures have been made. It is also likely that some of this variability may reflect physiological differences between individual patients which are not yet understood. Such between-patient differences may relate to the degree of corticospinal disruption, to the location of the lesion, to genetic factors, or even to other factors which are not yet clear. A better understanding of what determines the pattern of physiological changes is likely to be important if such measurements are to inform rehabilitation strategies.

Current approaches to rehabilitation usually aim either to increase the excitability of the primary motor cortex in the stroke hemisphere or to reduce the excitability of the intact hemisphere, based largely on evidence suggesting an "imbalance" between the respective contributions of the two hemispheres [46]. The methods by which this has been achieved have included repetitive TMS, direct current stimulation, increasing afferent input from the affected limb, or reducing afferent input from the contralateral limb [47–50]. These approaches have often proved successful in small patient groups, but it has frequently been found that patients respond to such interventions to a variable degree: at present there is no way to predict who will or will not respond. Given the between-subject variability of physiological changes seen after stroke, it seems important to explore methods that might predict the response to a given therapeutic intervention and guide the choice of treatment.

The idea of physiological measures guiding treatment strategies in individual patients is not a new one, and one might foresee two different approaches. First, virtual lesion TMS could be used to identify cortical regions that contribute to movement of the paretic hand and these regions could be "primed" by techniques such as repetitive TMS prior to physical therapy. Second, it may be that certain physiological abnormalities are associated with a good response to a given therapeutic strategy. A number of investigators have identified physiological changes that occurred in response to a successful treatment approach, such as improvements in motor cortical representations [51], an increase in SICI [51], or a reduction in IHI targeting the stroke hemisphere [40]. However, there is so far little information as to which baseline physiological abnormalities may predict a good response to treatment [52], and such an approach may only prove fruitful once the pathophysiological changes are better understood. To use such information to create rational rehabilitation strategies in individual patients is the ultimate aim of this work.

Appendix

Understanding the basic principles of TMS function

TMS is delivered via a coil held tangentially on the scalp over the targeted brain area. The coil consists of an insulated copper wire and is connected to the stimulator, a capacitor that can generate electrical currents up to 8000 mA in 50 μs. TMS is based on the principle of electromagnetic induction. The current running through the coil induces a perpendicular magnetic field of 1.5–2.5 Tesla lasting for less than 1 ms. The magnetic field is attenuated to a minimal degree, depending mainly on the thickness of the scalp and the distance to the brain surface [53]. The rapidly changing magnetic field in turn induces a perpendicular electrical field at the brain surface which runs parallel to the current in the coil, i.e. tangentially to the brain surface. This current activates the neuronal axons. Maximal activation occurs when the axon turns away from the current at approximately 90°. It is thought that the first elements to be activated are interneurons [54,55], which in turn activate the pyramidal cells trans-synaptically. However, direct activation of pyramidal cells is possible with higher stimulation intensities [3]. Once the pyramidal cells fire, the resulting impulses travel down the corticospinal tract (CST), depolarize the α spinal motoneurons and a motor-evoked potential

(MEP) can be recorded from the target muscle. With increasing stimulation intensity more motor units are activated and the size of the MEP increases, reaching a plateau at 140–160% of the threshold. It should be noted that the depolarization of the α motoneurons depends on the temporal synchronization of the descending impulses, which partially explains why MEPs are so variable, and on the level of activation of the a motoneurons themselves, which explains why MEPs are facilitated by pre-activating the target muscle.

The area and the depth of cortical activation depend on several parameters whose details are beyond the scope of this chapter. In short, the area of activation is smaller – i.e. TMS is more focal – with figure-of-eight coils compared to circular coils and with lower stimulation intensities. With this type of "flat" coil the depth of activation is generally limited to 2–4 cm below the surface, such that TMS is thought not to activate subcortical structures directly. However, with higher intensities and special "bent" coils, the shape of the induced field can change and the depth of the activation increase, for example enough to reach the bottom of the motor homunculus and elicit responses from the small foot muscles.

TMS measures of corticospinal excitability

Several TMS measures can be used to assess corticospinal excitability. The motor threshold (MT), defined as the minimal intensity required to elicit a response from the target muscle, is thought mainly to reflect the excitability of the axonal membrane and is markedly increased by membrane stabilizing drugs, e.g. carbamazepine. At suprathreshold intensities the MEP latency can be recorded; subsequent TMS over the spinal roots allows the calculation of the central motor conduction time, simply by deducting the peripheral latency from the central latency. The MEP amplitude can also be measured at a standard suprathreshold intensity, typically defined relative to the MT. Perhaps a more informative approach is to produce a recruitment curve (RC) plotting the MEP amplitude against the stimulating intensity, gradually increasing from subthreshold to "plateau" intensities. The maximal MEP recorded can be used as a measure of the maximal available output, while the gradient of the RC additionally reflects the relative excitability of the whole neuronal population: the more neurons are closer to firing threshold the steeper the curve will be.

TMS maps may be derived by recording all scalp areas from which an MEP can be elicited at a standard suprathreshold intensity; the total map area and/or volume can be computed, but perhaps the most reliable measure is the map's "center of gravity" (TMS map CoG), which is often close to the the spot consistently producing the largest MEPs. TMS motor maps show good spatial accuracy, as evaluated by PET, fMRI, and direct stimulation of the exposed cortex [56,57]. Apart from quantifying the available corticospinal output, this method also allows the identification of significant shifts in the cortical representation of the target muscles that may reflect acute or chronic plastic reorganization.

Most of these TMS parameters are measured with the target muscle at rest, but for some the target muscle is slightly pre-activated (e.g. active MTs). When a standard amount of tonic activation is generated, some of the α motoneurons are expected to be at firing level when the TMS pulse arrives, making such measures less susceptible to changes in spinal excitability. Thus the "active" TMS measures are thought to be better markers of supraspinal excitability; however, their reliance on voluntary activation makes them prone to greater variability.

TMS measures of intracortical excitability and inter-regional interactions

Short-interval intracortical inhibition (SICI) is measured using a paired-pulse protocol: when a suprathreshold (test) pulse is preceded by a subthreshold (conditioning) pulse given 1–4 ms earlier, the resulting MEP is reduced and the extent of this reduction can be quantified as SICI. Conversely, intracortical facilitation (ICF) can be measured as the increase seen in the test MEP when the conditioning pulse is given 7–20 ms beforehand. Long-interval intracortical inhibition (LICI) is seen when the conditioning pulse is suprathreshold and given 100–200 ms beforehand. These paired-pulse protocols are usually performed at rest. There is evidence to suggest that each measure reflects the function of a particular intracortical circuit. SICI has been strongly associated with GABA$_A$ circuits, cortical silent period (CSP) and LICI with GABA$_B$, while ICF appears at least partly to reflect glutamatergic activity.

The use of two TMS coils allows the conditioning and test pulses to be delivered to separate cortical regions. Such an approach can be used to test specific physiological interactions, both cortico-cortical,

between remote cortical regions and the primary motor cortex, and interhemispheric [42]. The interaction between the two primary motor cortices, as assessed by TMS, is mainly inhibitory, and it is commonly referred to as interhemispheric inhibition (IHI). This is mostly done with the subject at rest, but by employing a reaction time paradigm, dynamic changes in IHI can be demonstrated in relation to the onset of a voluntary movement. In both intracortical and inter-regional paired-pulse protocols, the interactions measured depend critically on the intensity of both the conditioning and the test pulse.

References

1. Rothwell JC, Thompson PD, Day BL, *et al*. Motor cortex stimulation in intact man. 1. General characteristics of EMG responses in different muscles. *Brain.* 1987;**110**:1173–90.

2. Day BL, Rothwell JC, Thompson PD, *et al*. Delay in the execution of voluntary movement by electrical or magnetic brain stimulation in intact man. Evidence for the storage of motor programs in the brain. *Brain.* 1989;**112**:649–63.

3. Di Lazzaro, V, Oliviero A, Pilato F, *et al*. Corticospinal volleys evoked by transcranial stimulation of the brain in conscious humans. *Neurol Res.* 2003;**25**:143–50.

4. Talelli P, Greenwood RJ, Rothwell JC. Arm function after stroke: Neurophysiological correlates and recovery mechanisms assessed by transcranial magnetic stimulation. *Clin Neurophysiol.* 2006;**117**:1641–59.

5. Ziemann U, Lonnecker S, Steinhoff BJ, *et al*. Effects of antiepileptic drugs on motor cortex excitability in humans: A transcranial magnetic stimulation study. *Ann Neurol.* 1996;**40**:367–78.

6. Devanne H, Lavoie BA, Capaday C. Input–output properties and gain changes in the human corticospinal pathway. *Exp Brain Res.* 1997;**114**:329–38.

7. Furlan M, Marchal G, Viader F, *et al*. Spontaneous neurological recovery after stroke and the fate of the ischemic penumbra. *Ann Neurol.* 1996;**40**:216–26.

8. Catano A, Houa M, Caroyer JM, *et al*. Magnetic transcranial stimulation in non-haemorrhagic sylvian strokes: Interest of facilitation for early functional prognosis. *Electroencephalogr Clin Neurophysiol.* 1995;**97**:349–54.

9. Cicinelli P, Traversa R, Rossini PM. Post-stroke reorganization of brain motor output to the hand: A 2–4 month follow-up with focal magnetic transcranial stimulation. *Electroencephalogr Clin Neurophysiol.* 1997;**105**:438–50.

10. Cicinelli P, Pasqualetti P, Zaccagnini M, *et al*. Interhemispheric asymmetries of motor cortex excitability in the postacute stroke stage: A paired-pulse

transcranial magnetic stimulation study. *Stroke*. 2003;**34**:2653–8.

11. Cruz-Martinez A, Tejada J, Diez TE. Motor hand recovery after stroke. Prognostic yield of early transcranial magnetic stimulation. *Electromyogr Clin Neurophysiol*. 1999;**39**:405–10.

12. Traversa R, Cicinelli P, Pasqualetti P, *et al.* Follow-up of interhemispheric differences of motor evoked potentials from the 'affected' and 'unaffected' hemispheres in human stroke. *Brain Res*. 1998;**803**:1–8.

13. Manganotti P, Patuzzo S, Cortese F, *et al.* Motor disinhibition in affected and unaffected hemisphere in the early period of recovery after stroke. *Clin Neurophysiol*. 2002;**113**:936–43.

14. Traversa R, Cicinelli P, Oliveri M, *et al.* Neurophysiological follow-up of motor cortical output in stroke patients. *Clin Neurophysiol*. 2000;**111**:1695–703.

15. Berardelli A, Inghilleri M, Manfredi M, *et al.* Cortical and cervical stimulation after hemispheric infarction. *J Neurol Neurosurg Psychiatry*. 1987;**50**:861–5.

16. Pennisi G, Rapisarda G, Bella R, *et al.* Absence of response to early transcranial magnetic stimulation in ischemic stroke patients: Prognostic value for hand motor recovery. *Stroke*. 1999;**30**:2666–70.

17. Trompetto C, Assini A, Buccolieri A, *et al.* Motor recovery following stroke: A transcranial magnetic stimulation study. *Clin Neurophysiol*. 2000;**111**:1860–7.

18. Alagona G, Delvaux V, Gerard P, *et al.* Ipsilateral motor responses to focal transcranial magnetic stimulation in healthy subjects and acute-stroke patients. *Stroke*. 2001;**32**:1304–09.

19. Nardone R, Tezzon F. Inhibitory and excitatory circuits of cerebral cortex after ischaemic stroke: Prognostic value of the transcranial magnetic stimulation. *Electromyogr Clin Neurophysiol*. 2002;**42**:131–6.

20. Delvaux V, Alagona G, Gerard P, *et al.* Post-stroke reorganization of hand motor area: A 1-year prospective follow-up with focal transcranial magnetic stimulation. *Clin Neurophysiol*. 2003;**114**:1217–25.

21. Swayne OB, Rothwell JC, Ward NS, *et al.* Stages of motor output reorganization after hemispheric stroke suggested by longitudinal studies of cortical physiology. *Cereb Cortex*. 2008;**18**:1909–22.

22. Catano A, Houa M, Caroyer JM, *et al.* Magnetic transcranial stimulation in acute stroke: Early excitation threshold and functional prognosis. *Electroencephalogr Clin Neurophysiol*. 1996;**101**:233–9.

23. Byrnes ML, Thickbroom GW, Phillips BA, *et al.* Long-term changes in motor cortical organisation after recovery from subcortical stroke. *Brain Res*. 2001;**889**:278–87.

24. Pennisi G, Alagona G, Rapisarda G, *et al.* Transcranial magnetic stimulation after pure motor stroke. *Clin Neurophysiol*. 2002;**113**:1536–43.

25. Thickbroom GW, Byrnes ML, Archer SA, *et al.* Motor outcome after subcortical stroke: MEPs correlate with hand strength but not dexterity. *Clin Neurophysiol*. 2002;**113**:2025–9.

26. Bastings EP, Greenberg JP, Good DC. Hand motor recovery after stroke: A transcranial magnetic stimulation mapping study of motor output areas and their relation to functional status. *Neurorehabil Neural Repair*. 2002;**16**:275–82.

27. Liepert J, Bauder H, Wolfgang HR, *et al.* Treatment-induced cortical reorganization after stroke in humans. *Stroke*. 2000;**31**:1210–6.

28. Thickbroom GW, Byrnes ML, Archer SA, *et al.* Motor outcome after subcortical stroke correlates with the degree of cortical reorganization. *Clin Neurophysiol*. 2004;**115**:2144–50.

29. Liepert J, Classen J, Cohen LG, *et al.* Task-dependent changes of intracortical inhibition. *Exp Brain Res*. 1998;**118**:421–6.

30. Liepert J, Storch P, Fritsch A, *et al.* Motor cortex disinhibition in acute stroke. *Clin Neurophysiol*. 2000;**111**:671–6.

31. Shimizu T, Hosaki A, Hino T, *et al.* Motor cortical disinhibition in the unaffected hemisphere after unilateral cortical stroke. *Brain*, 2002;**125**:1896–907.

32. Liepert J, Haevernick K, Weiller C, *et al.* The surround inhibition determines therapy-induced cortical reorganization. *Neuroimage*. 2006;**32**:1216–20.

33. Turton A, Wroe S, Trepte N, *et al.* Contralateral and ipsilateral EMG responses to transcranial magnetic stimulation during recovery of arm and hand function after stroke. *Electroenceph Clin Neurophys*. 1996;**101**:316–28.

34. Netz J, Lammers T, Homberg V. Reorganization of motor output in the non-affected hemisphere after stroke. *Brain*. 1997;**120**:1579–86.

35. Butefisch CM, Netz J, Wessling M, *et al.* Remote changes in cortical excitability after stroke. *Brain*. 2003;**126**:470–81.

36. Ward NS, Newton JM, Swayne OB, *et al.* Motor system activation after subcortical stroke depends on corticospinal system integrity. *Brain*. 2006;**129**:809–19.

37. Murase N, Duque J, Mazzocchio R, *et al.* Influence of interhemispheric interactions on motor function in chronic stroke. *Ann Neurol*. 2004;**55**:400–09.

38. Butefisch CM, Wessling M, Netz J, *et al.* Relationship between interhemispheric inhibition and motor cortex excitability in subacute stroke patients. *Neurorehabil Neural Repair*. 2008;**22**:4–21.

39. Boroojerdi B, Diefenbach K, Ferbert A. Transcallosal inhibition in cortical and subcortical cerebral vascular lesions. *J Neurol Sci.* 1996;**144**:160–70.

40. Floel A, Hummel F, Duque J, *et al.* Influence of somatosensory input on interhemispheric interactions in patients with chronic stroke. *Neurorehabil Neural Repair.* 2008;**22**:477–85.

41. Lotze M, Markert J, Sauseng P, *et al.* The role of multiple contralesional motor areas for complex hand movements after internal capsular lesion. *J Neurosci.* 2006;**26**:6096–102.

42. Reis J, Swayne OB, Vandermeeren Y, *et al.* Contribution of transcranial magnetic stimulation to the understanding of cortical mechanisms involved in motor control. *J Physiol.* 2008;**586**:325–51.

43. Ward NS, Brown MM, Thompson AJ, *et al.* Neural correlates of motor recovery after stroke: A longitudinal fMRI study. *Brain.* 2003;**126**:2476–96.

44. Ward NS, Newton JM, Swayne OB, *et al.* The relationship between brain activity and peak grip force is modulated by corticospinal system integrity after subcortical stroke. *Eur J Neurosci.* 2007;**25**:1865–73.

45. Johansen-Berg H, Rushworth MF, Bogdanovic MD, *et al.* The role of ipsilateral premotor cortex in hand movement after stroke. *Proc Natl Acad Sci USA.* 2002;**99**:14 518–23.

46. Talelli P, Rothwell J. Does brain stimulation after stroke have a future? *Curr Opin Neurol.* 2006;**19**:543–50.

47. Celnik P, Hummel F, Harris-Love M, *et al.* Somatosensory stimulation enhances the effects of training functional hand tasks in patients with chronic stroke. *Arch Phys Med Rehabil.* 2007;**88**:1369–76.

48. Floel A, Nagorsen U, Werhahn KJ, *et al.* Influence of somatosensory input on motor function in patients with chronic stroke. *Ann Neurol.* 2004;**56**:206–12.

49. Fregni F, Boggio PS, Valle AC, *et al.* A sham-controlled trial of a 5-day course of repetitive transcranial magnetic stimulation of the unaffected hemisphere in stroke patients. *Stroke.* 2006;**37**:2115–22.

50. Talelli P, Greenwood RJ, Rothwell JC. Exploring theta burst stimulation as an intervention to improve motor recovery in chronic stroke. *Clin Neurophysiol.* 2007;**118**:333–42.

51. Stinear CM, Barber PA, Coxon JP, *et al.* Priming the motor system enhances the effects of upper limb therapy in chronic stroke. *Brain.* 2008;**131**:1381–90.

52. Stinear CM, Barber PA, Smale PR, *et al.* Functional potential in chronic stroke patients depends on corticospinal tract integrity. *Brain.* 2007;**130**:170–80.

53. Stokes MG, Chambers CD, Gould IC, *et al.* Simple metric for scaling motor threshold based on scalp-cortex distance: Application to studies using transcranial magnetic stimulation. *J Neurophysiol.* 2005;**94**:4520–7.

54. Day BL, Thompson PD, Dick JP, *et al.* Different sites of action of electrical and magnetic stimulation of the human brain. *Neurosci Lett.* 1987;**75**:101–06.

55. Day BL, Dressler D, Maertens de Noordhout A, *et al.* Electric and magnetic stimulation of human motor cortex: Surface EMG and single motor unit responses. *J Physiol.* 1989;**412**:449–73.

56. Classen J, Knorr U, Werhahn KJ, *et al.* Multimodal output mapping of human central motor representation on different spatial scales. *J Physiol.* 1998;**512**:163–79.

57. Krings T, Buchbinder BR, Butler WE, *et al.* Stereotactic transcranial magnetic stimulation: Correlation with direct electrical cortical stimulation. *Neurosurgery.* 1997;**4**:1319–25.

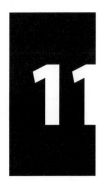

Human brain mapping of the motor system after stroke

Nick S. Ward

Introduction

After stroke, recovery of useful upper-limb function occurs in only 50% of those with significant early paresis, leading to dramatically impaired quality of life and sense of well-being [1,2]. For most patients, the term "rehabilitation" refers to approaches designed to improve societal participation and quality of life. In this sense, rehabilitation is often successful, but on its own may not take full advantage of the enormous potential for plastic change in the adult human brain, even after focal injury [3]. We have learned much from studying animal models of focal brain injury, but the tools available for studying the working human brain are different to those used in animal models. In human subjects, experiments are performed at the level of neural systems rather than single cells or molecules. Both approaches have something to learn from the other, and it is likely that for a complete understanding of the way the brain responds to injury, both will be helpful. This chapter will concentrate on the ways that functional brain imaging has contributed to our understanding of how the brain responds to injury, and how it might be used in the future to help improve therapeutic approaches to stroke patients with persistent impairment.

BOLD signal in cerebrovascular disease

Most functional imaging studies performed in stroke patients have used functional magnetic resonance imaging (fMRI), which relies on the blood oxygen level-dependent (BOLD) signal. The BOLD signal relies on the close coupling between blood flow and metabolism. During an increase in neuronal activation, the most significant change is an increase in local cerebral blood flow. Only a small proportion of the greater amount of oxygen delivered locally to the tissue is used, and so the net result is an increase in the tissue ratio of oxyhemoglobin and deoxyhemoglobin in the local capillary bed. The magnetic properties of hemoglobin depend on its level of oxygenation so that this change in balance results in an change in local magnetic field, increasing tissue-derived signal intensity on T_2^*-weighted MR images [4].

The mechanism of neurovascular coupling is still unclear, although it is likely to involve metabolic [5] and neurochemical [6] mechanisms. The generation of the BOLD signal is influenced by other parameters such as venous blood volume, blood flow, blood oxygenation, and oxygen consumption, and any disease state that changes these parameters may modify the BOLD signal. It is therefore reasonable to consider whether the BOLD signal is reliable in patients who have suffered stroke and in subjects with evidence of both large- and small-vessel atherosclerosis.

In most forms of analysis, the BOLD signal is assumed to have the same shape in all subjects and in all brain regions [7], but this might not always be the case after stroke. Newton *et al.* demonstrated a greater time to peak BOLD response in primary motor cortex (M1) contralateral to the moving hand compared to ipsilateral M1 in healthy controls [8]. However, in three chronic stroke patients the time to peak BOLD response in contralesional M1 was equivalent or less than that for ipsilesional M1, representing a finding opposite to that seen in healthy controls. Pineiro *et al.* [9] also described a slower time to peak BOLD response in sensorimotor cortex bilaterally in 12 chronic stroke patients with lacunar infarcts; therefore modeling the BOLD response with a canonical hemodynamic response function (HRF) might be less efficient in stroke patients. It is worth considering how the results of a standard functional imaging analysis using the general linear model approach would be affected. If

Brain Repair After Stroke, ed. S. C. Cramer and R. J. Nudo. Published by Cambridge University Press.
© Cambridge University Press 2010.

the canonical HRF was a poor fit for the true response, the residual error of the analytical model would be greater (than if the fit was good), thus lowering t-and Z-scores and reducing sensitivity to detection of differences. In general, most studies of stroke patients have found increased activation in a number of brain regions over and above healthy controls, as will be described below. It is unlikely that altered hemodynamics can account for these results and in fact it is possible that these overactivations have been underestimated.

In addition to temporal changes, the BOLD signal may be reduced, or even become negative, in patients with impaired cerebrovascular reserve or advanced narrowing of the cerebral arteries [10–12]. Röther et al. [13] describe a single patient who was found to have bilateral occluded internal carotid arteries and an occluded vertebral artery. The cerebrovascular reactivity, as determined by reduced change in T_2^*-signal during hypercapnia, was severely impaired in the left hemisphere and the local BOLD response was negative for the duration of the task. This suggests that the initial dip in BOLD signal, due to a relative decrease in oxyhemoglobin, was not followed by the normal vascular response. This subject had previously suffered from a transient ischemic attack involving the right arm. It is likely that these symptoms were related to hemodynamic insufficiency and it is interesting to speculate that the presence of a prolonged negative dip in BOLD signal represents a marker for those at risk from such symptoms. Several studies have now suggested that impairment of normal vasodilatation in response to hypercapnia is associated with diminished magnitude of BOLD signal [11,12,14,15]. Thus in patients with severely impaired cerebrovascular reactivity, neuronal activation may not translate into a BOLD response in the conventional sense, and standard models using the canonical HRF may not be sufficient.

Although these results suggest that the BOLD signal may have shortcomings as an investigative tool for studying selected stroke patients, the scale of the problem is not yet clear. For example, the cerebrovascular reactivity in the right hemisphere of the patient studied by Röther et al. [13] was moderately impaired and the BOLD response during a motor task with the left hand was entirely normal. Patients with hemodynamic symptoms are relatively uncommon, and are likely to be excluded from many fMRI studies. In addition, patients with severe stenosis of ipsilesional

internal carotid arteries are usually also excluded, although it is not clear that this is necessary. It may also be the case that small-vessel disease may also make a significant contribution to impaired cerebrovascular reactivity.

There is no evidence that the BOLD signal is erroneously detected in patients with impaired cerebrovascular reactivity, i.e. this is largely a problem of false negative results, which is unlikely to explain the common finding of overactivity in patients compared to controls. Several studies have begun to use a correlation approach rather than categorical comparison of control subjects and stroke patients. This is based on the idea that stroke patients are different by virtue of severity and lesion location in particular, and so averaging across a group of stroke patients who are not a-priori selected as homogeneous is not useful. Correlation approaches attempt to explain variability in the task-related BOLD signal with some other parameter such as a measure of impairment [16] or corticospinal tract integrity [17,18], for example. It is unlikely that changes in cerebrovascular responsiveness will correlate with these measures and so differences in cerebrovascular reactivity cannot account for the results from these studies. Ultimately, to address specific hypotheses about BOLD signal alterations will require a multimodal approach using different imaging techniques (BOLD, perfusion, hypercapnic challenge) and concurrent neurophysiological methods (EEG, MEG, TMS).

The effect of increasing age on cerebrovascular hemodynamics has also been examined. This is relevant to the discussion given that stroke is more common with advancing age, and that often age-matched controls are used in studies of stroke patients. D'Esposito et al. examined the effect of age on the BOLD signal generated during a button press task using a sparse event-related design [19]. Four times the number of suprathreshold voxels were present in the younger compared to the older subjects. However, there was no difference in the magnitude of task-related signal change in primary motor cortex between the older and younger subjects. The main difference accounting for the reduced number of suprathreshold voxels is a reduced signal to noise ratio (SNR) in elderly subjects. Results from single subject or group fixed effects analyses of functional imaging data are generally presented as t-statistics for each voxel (volume element) of the brain. The result is therefore dependent on both the magnitude of the signal change and the residual variance. Thus an increased SNR will lead to a lower *t*-statistic, and therefore fewer suprathreshold voxels.

The problem of reduced SNR can be effectively dealt with by employing a random-effects analysis rather than a fixed-effects analysis. Random-effects analysis of functional imaging data treats each subject as a random variable. The experimental variance is dominated by between-subjects variability (as opposed to within-subject variability in the case of fixed-effects models). The data for each subject comprise the voxel-wise parameter estimate for the task under consideration, which reflects the magnitude of the signal change in each voxel. Appropriate statistics can be performed on these data, which are less likely to be influenced by differences in SNR [19]. Using a random effects analysis, and employing both temporal and dispersion derivatives of the HRF, Ward et al. [20] demonstrated no change in the shape of the hemodynamic response during a hand grip task with advancing age, in keeping with the findings described above.

Patterns of reorganization in the motor system after stroke

The first studies of stroke patients using functional imaging were exploratory and designed simply to establish whether the cortical motor system was organized differently after subcortical stroke. Investigators chose to study chronic stroke patients with good recovery so that all subjects would be able to perform the same task. Differences in activation between the patients and healthy volunteers would then provide some clue about how these patients were able to move previously paretic limbs despite the persistence of anatomical damage. In general, group studies of stroke patients with subcortical lesions found greater activation within a number of motor-related cortical regions compared to controls during a finger tapping task, first using positron emission tomography (PET) [21–25] and subsequently with fMRI [26,27]. Specifically, task-related increases in brain activity were seen in cortical regions such as premotor cortex (both ventral and dorsal), supplementary motor area, cingulate motor areas, as well as prefrontal and parietal cortices, and was often bilateral.

Furthermore, there was evidence to suggest that the site of representations of body parts, in particular the hand, had shifted in these patients. Cramer et al. reported shifts in cortical maps in two patients with

good recovery following mild cortical strokes involving either pre- or post-central gyrus [28]. Weiller et al. [25] described a ventral shift in peak sensorimotor cortex activation and others have reported an overall caudal shift in a group of recovered stroke patients [9]. Rossini et al. [29] also reported this shift of cortical hand representation using fMRI, magnetoencephalography, and TMS, in a patient with recovered hand function following cortical stroke. There appears to be no consistent direction of this shift, and the observation has not been clearly linked to recovery, although it may be influenced by the pattern of injury, and furthermore might reflect the finding that the hand, for example, has several spatially distinct representations in primary motor cortex [30].

There are also data to support the notion that surviving peri-infarct cortical tissue may be helpful to the recovering patient. Cao et al. [31] studied teenage patients who had suffered a perinatal infarct, each with only moderate recovery. Sequential finger movements of the affected hand were associated with bilateral activations, as well as peri-infarct cortical rim activations. Peri-infarct cortical rim activations in recovered stroke patients were seen by Cramer et al. during similar tasks [27]. Taken together, these studies indicated that there had been reorganization both within and between regions in a distributed motor-related network, and highlighted that functionally relevant reorganization was possible after stroke.

Anatomical substrate of recovered motor function

These results must be viewed in the context of the known anatomical structures and pathways of the motor system. The cortical motor system is made up of four main regions: primary motor cortex (M1), premotor cortex, supplementary motor area, and cingulate motor area [32]. Premotor cortex has dorsal (PMd) and ventral (PMv) regions, each with different anatomical connectivity profiles [33]. These cortical motor regions can be further subdivided based on topographic organization and the demands of the task. For example, primary motor cortex is divided into anterior (Brodmann area 4a) and posterior (Brodmann area 4p) regions, with activity in BA 4p modulated by attention to the task [34]. Many of these areas contribute fibers to the descending corticofugal motor pathways, some of which project to the ventral horn of the spinal cord (corticospinal pathway) [35–37] and others which project to brainstem nuclei.

Cortical regions including the primary sensory cortex (S1), posterior parietal cortex and insula also contribute to these pathways. Although descending motor pathways from M1 are of critical importance, it is clear that several structures contribute to motor control and may potentially be useful in supporting recovery of movement after stroke [38]. The pathways through which secondary cortical motor regions might generate this motor output are not clear. In primates, projections from secondary motor areas to spinal cord motor neurons are less numerous and less efficient at exciting spinal cord motoneurons than those from M1 [39,40]. Moreover, unlike M1, facilitation of distal muscles from SMA, PMd, and PMv is not significantly stronger than facilitation of proximal muscles. Another possibility is that signals descend via the reticulospinal projections to cervical propriospinal premotoneurons [41,42]. Propriospinal projections have divergent projections to muscle groups operating at multiple joints [43,44]. This solution might account for the multijoint "associated" movements such as the synergistic flexion seen when patients with only poor and moderate recovery attempt isolated hand movements. The fact that descending pathways from secondary motor areas are thought not to be able to efficiently generate distal limb movements suggests that cortico-cortical interactions, presumably with surviving primary motor cortex output, play an important role. Indeed, several secondary motor areas have bilateral projections to cortical motor regions, in particular M1 [45,46]. Overall, it is feasible that a number of motor networks acting in parallel could generate an output to the spinal cord necessary for movement, and that damage in one of these networks could be at least partially compensated for by activity in another [47,48].

Relationship to recovery

Many of the first functional imaging studies after stroke were performed in well-recovered patients. The conclusion drawn from the studies described above was that there were a number of mechanisms responsible for recovery, including recruitment of parallel descending motor pathways originating from secondary cortical motor areas. However, this conclusion would be less compelling if the same results were also found in patients with greater impairment. Addressing this issue required that a cross-sectional cohort of patients with a wide variety of outcomes be studied. Alternatively, longitudinal studies in single patients

could be performed. In the first such cross-sectional study, a group of chronic stroke patients with infarcts sparing primary motor cortex were scanned during a hand grip with visual feedback task using fMRI [16]. Using the hand grip allowed patients without return of fractionated finger movements to be studied. The target forces used were always a proportion of each subject's own maximum grip force, so that any differences were unlikely to be due to differences in effort. There were no differences between the activation maps of control subjects and patients without residual impairment. However, patients with more marked impairment showed relative overactivations in a number of secondary motor areas bilaterally [16]. Thus, a negative correlation was found between the magnitude of brain activation and outcome in these brain regions, almost all of them part of the normal motor network. Patients with greater motor impairment had increased task-related activity in secondary motor regions in both affected and unaffected hemispheres, whereas patients with little residual impairment had activation patterns that were no different from those in healthy age-matched volunteers. A similar result was observed in a group of patients studied at earlier time points after stroke, i.e. approximately 10 days post-stroke [49]. It was hypothesized that secondary motor areas are recruited in response to damage to corticospinal output and are available to participate in the generation of a simple movement (if required) as early as 10 days post-stroke. A subsequent study demonstrated a strong positive correlation between secondary motor area recruitment in both hemispheres and corticospinal system damage as assessed with transcranial magnetic stimulation (TMS) [17]. A more injured corticospinal system was associated with greater task-related activity in contralesional M1 (hand area) compared to those with less corticospinal system damage. Together these results suggest a progressive shift away from primary to secondary motor areas with increasing disruption to corticospinal system (Figure 11.1), presumably because ipsilesional M1 is less able to influence motor output in these patients.

Another way to explore the relationship between reorganization and recovery is to follow individual patients over time. Longitudinal fMRI studies have shed further light on the process [21,50–53], although only a few have studied patients on more than two occasions. One study scanned subcortical stroke patients on average eight times over the first 6 months after stroke [53], and demonstrated an early overactivation

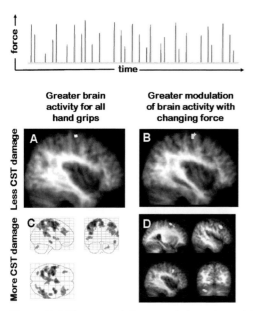

Figure 11.1 The top panel shows a typical experimental time line for an fMRI experiment over approximately 6 min. Each "spike" represents a single isometric hand squeeze performed by a stroke patient with the affected hand. The bottom trace represents force from the resting hand in order to look for mirror movements, which in this case are absent. Target forces are set at either 15%, 30%, or 45% of the force generated during each subject's own maximum voluntary contraction.

Varying the target forces enables us to measure two parameter estimates for each voxel representing (i) the magnitude of signal change during all hand squeezes irrespective of force, and (ii) how much the signal covaries with peak force. These two measurements provide information about different aspects of motor activation and are independent of one another.

The results are taken from [17,18]. Patients underwent fMRI using the isometric hand squeeze paradigm described above, and also underwent TMS assessment outside the scanner to measure the functional integrity of the corticospinal tract (CST). The images illustrate how the two parameters of motor activation vary as a function of CST integrity. Ipsilesional primary motor cortex (M1) is more active in patients with less CST damage, and (B) ipsilesional M1 activity also covaries with peak force in patients with less CST damage, exactly as occurs in healthy volunteers. (C) This "glass brain" is shown (clockwise from top left) from the right side, from the front so that the left side of the brain is on the left, and from above with the front of the brain to the right. In these images, left is contralesional. They show a number of secondary motor areas (particularly contralesional) that become increasingly active during affected hand squeeze in patients with greater CST damage. (D) Lastly, activity in a number of premotor regions (clockwise from top left, contralesional dorsal premotor cortex, contralesional ventral premotor cortex, ipsilesional ventral premotor cortex) and in contralesional superior cerebellum covaries with peak force in patients with greater damage to CST.

in primary and many non-primary motor regions. Thereafter functional recovery was associated with a focusing of task-related brain activation patterns towards a "normal" lateralized pattern. These patients had variable degrees of motor impairment early after

stroke, but all made excellent recoveries. Whether this pattern of longitudinal change occurs in all patients is still not clear. In general, longitudinal studies have demonstrated a focusing of activity towards the lesioned hemisphere motor regions that is associated with improvement in motor function [21,51]. However, this is not always the case, with examples of patients showing persistent bilateral recruitment [50]. Considering that cross-sectional studies have reported patients with persistent contralesional activation, it seems unlikely that all patients will follow this same longitudinal evolution of changes in task-related brain activation. Indeed in some patients it is possible that it will be activity in the contralesional hemisphere that will become more organized [54]. A number of studies have examined changes in brain activity before and after therapeutic intervention in chronic stroke patients [55]. Many studies found treatment-associated increases in ipsilesional activity in keeping with the previous longitudinal studies, but some saw a shift in the balance of activation in the opposite direction [56,57]. The evidence suggests that the contribution of contralesional motor regions varies, but it is not clear what baseline characteristics or features of injury might predict such shifts.

Changing hemispheric balance?

Understanding how the post-stroke brain is organized is important when thinking about restorative treatments. Strategies to "normalize" the more bilateral post-stroke motor cortex activity towards the ipsilesional hemisphere (as in healthy brains) have become a major focus of attempts to reduce upper limb impairment after stroke [58]. These approaches are based on the finding that in the studies described so far, patients with minimal impairment tend to have a more normal activation pattern. In addition, data from both TMS [59] and fMRI [60] studies suggest that in some subcortical stroke patents, contralesional M1, although "active", may exert an abnormally high degree of interhemispheric inhibitory drive towards ipsilesional M1 during attempted voluntary movement of the affected hand. This led to suggestions that contralesional M1 overactivity hinders recovery, although another interpretation is that it has adopted the characteristics of the dominant motor cortex in the face of ipsilesional M1 disconnection and hypofunction.

Although these studies were performed in small homogeneous groups and are therefore not representative of all patients, there are empirical data to support the idea that increased contralesional M1 activity is often maladaptive. Several studies have used this concept to transiently improve motor function after stroke by suppressing excitability in contralesional M1 [61–66]. Proof-of-principal studies in chronic mild impairment subcortical stroke patients are encouraging [67], but a critical question remains whether this normalization is appropriate for all patients. However, the question of whether contralesional M1 is a help or a hindrance in supporting recovered function is not yet answered. Many functional imaging studies have observed motor task-related brain activity in contralesional M1 in stroke patients as described earlier [8,16,17,25–27], probably more so in patients with residual impairment [16,49]. Contralesional hemisphere activity has also been demonstrated in stroke patients using EEG [68]. The fine temporal resolution of EEG was able to detect that this activity occurred *after* the motor response had been made, suggesting that it was not related to movement initiation in these patients. However, because EEG lacks fine spatial resolution, it is not certain that this result related to contralesional M1 and not to premotor cortex, for example. A similar approach using an event-related fMRI design has demonstrated that contralesional M1 activity peaked seconds before ipsilesional M1 in stroke patients, in comparison to controls in whom the opposite relationship was observed [8]. This change in the characteristics of motor system activation might point to a change of role in different patients, but does not prove a functional role during movement nor exclude the possibility that contralesional M1 activity is hindering recovery.

In studies involving adult patients with small subcortical infarcts, the effect of disruption of contralesional M1 function by TMS depends on whether the motor task is a simple react time task (no disruption) [69,70], or involves pressing sequences of buttons (disruption of timing) [71], supporting a role for contralesional M1 in some patients and in some tasks. Serrien and colleagues used directed EEG coherence to investigate whether there is increased informational flow from the contralesional motor cortex following motor stroke [72]. They found that in less well-recovered patients, most task-related flow of information between the sensorimotor cortices in the low beta band of the EEG came from the contralesional hemisphere (i.e. ipsilateral to movement) during grip with the affected hand. This was not the case in recovered patients nor in controls, among whom cortical activity was driven from the contralateral sensorimotor cortex. These findings again suggest a functional role for the contralesional hemisphere in organizing movement of the impaired, ipsilateral limb following stroke, but only in those patients that do not make a good functional recovery. Patients making a fuller recovery, however, continue to organize movement-related cortical activity from the hemisphere contralateral to movement.

In addition, there is evidence that non-M1 secondary motor areas in the contralesional hemisphere contribute to recovered function. First, experiments in which TMS transiently disrupts activity in either ipsilesional or contralesional PMd, or contralesional M1, demonstrate worsening of recovered motor behaviors in some chronic subcortical stroke patients with no effect on healthy volunteers [69,71,73]. Furthermore, TMS to contralesional PMd is more disruptive in patients with greater impairment [69], whereas TMS to ipsilesional PMd is more disruptive in less impaired patients [73], implying a contralesional shift in the balance of functionally relevant activity with greater impairment.

Another approach is to measure how task-related activity covaries with modulation of task parameters. In healthy humans, for example, increasing force production is associated with linear increases in BOLD signal in contralateral M1 and medial motor regions, implying that they have a functional role in force production [74–76]. A recent study examined specifically for regional changes in the control of force modulation after stroke [18]. In patients with greater corticospinal system damage, force-related signal changes were seen mainly in contralesional dorsolateral premotor cortex, bilateral ventrolateral premotor cortices, and contralesional cerebellum, but not ipsilesional primary motor cortex (Figure 11.1). Interestingly, a qualitatively similar result was found in healthy volunteers with increasing age, suggesting that this "reorganization" might be a generic property of the cortical motor system in response to a variety of insults [20]. Thus not only do premotor cortices become increasingly active as corticospinal system integrity diminishes [17], but they can take on a new "M1-like" role during modulation of force output, which implies a new and functionally relevant role in motor control.

These results are important because they tell us that the response to focal injury does not involve simple up- or downregulation of the motor network as a whole. It is clear that nodes within remaining motor networks can take on new functional roles and that the post-stroke motor system is organized differently to that in the normal brain. However, there are now several lines of evidence to suggest that the mechanisms of reorganization are lesion-specific. If restoration of function is dependent on the interaction of the treatment and the residual motor network, it therefore follows that treatments will have different effects in different patients. Furthermore, individual patients may require different rehabilitative strategies in order to "interact" with motor systems which are organized differently. An interesting line of research to emerge from this line of thinking is whether it is possible to predict the likelihood of improving with a particular treatment, based on a careful study of the residual post-stroke structural and functional anatomy.

Predicting recovery

How does this help us to understand how best to treat the impairment suffered by patients after stroke? Clearly, the anatomy of the damage will introduce constraints. For example, Stinear and colleagues [77] set out to determine whether characterizing the state of the motor system of a series of chronic stroke patients would help in predicting the functional gains made in a subsequent motor practice programme. A variety of tools were used, including TMS, structural MRI, and functional MRI. The presence or absence of MEPs to TMS in the affected upper limb, and fractional anisotropy values were both used to assess the structural integrity of the descending white matter pathways in the posterior limb of the internal capsules. In addition, fMRI was used to assess the degree of lateralization of activity during a motor task. Not surprisingly, in patients with MEPs, meaningful gains with motor practice were still possible three years after stroke. The situation in patients without MEPs has never been clear-cut, as this is often taken as a poor prognostic sign [78]. In this study, the functional potential of patients without MEPs declined with increasing corticospinal pathway disruption. Disappointingly, the degree of lateralization of brain activity as measured with fMRI could not predict future functional gains through motor practice. The task used during scanning was a self paced opening and closing of the hand, and so it is possible that variations in performance of the task (to which the magnitude of activation is sensitive) introduced additional variability into the fMRI data. A task that probed for a measure of motor system plasticity in the context of motor practice might have provided different results. Nevertheless, this study illustrates how multimodal imaging and neurophysiological data can be used to assess the state of the motor system which might in turn predict response to therapeutic interventions and lead to treatment algorithms for clinical practice.

In a similar approach, Cramer et al. [79] assessed which of 13 baseline clinical/radiological measures were able to predict subsequent gains made during 6 weeks of rehabilitation therapy. Of all these measures only greater clinical status and lower motor cortex activation during fMRI at baseline remained significant and independent predictors of clinical improvement. This is an interesting finding, because in general, patients with greater impairment are more likely to have less task-related ipsilesional M1 activity, although this is an inconsistent finding. This result tells us that there is something in the imaging data which is independent of baseline clinical impairment which predicts improvements. Lower baseline motor cortex activation was also associated with larger increases in motor cortex activation after treatment, so perhaps in some patients, low baseline cortical activity represents underuse of surviving cortical resources. A measure of brain function might be important for optimal clinical decision-making in the context of a restorative intervention.

A separate study attempted to use fMRI data acquired in the first few days after stroke to determine a subsequent change in motor performance over and above initial stroke severity and lesion volume [80]. They found a pattern of brain activation which was highly predictive of clinical change. Although the multivariate analysis used did not allow anatomical inference to be made, it is clear that there is something about the way the function of the brain responds to injury, over and above the anatomy of the damage, that holds clues about future clinical progression. The pattern was distributed and certainly not confined to the motor system, even though clinical improvement was measured in the motor domain. The idea that motor improvement may not be solely related to the integrity of the corticospinal system, but also with other characteristics of the post-stroke brain is supported by the finding that motor performance at 3 months correlated only weakly with a measure of corticospinal tract integrity (using TMS) but strongly with a measure of intracortical excitability [81]. These findings suggest that the anatomy of the damage may set a limit on the extent of recovery, but that at least in some patients, other parameters, perhaps preserved cortico-cortical connectivity, might be important when considering whether a patient has the capacity or potential to improve.

Summary

After focal brain damage, there is a reconfiguration of the cerebral motor system. This does not appear to be a simple up- or downregulation of motor networks in their entirety, but the residual functional networks seem to operate in a different way, with some brain regions adopting the characteristics of damaged or disconnected regions. This reorganization varies across chronic stroke patients, but does so in a way that appears to be predictable, which gives us hope that a deeper understanding of these processes will allow us to treat patients with impairments more effectively. It is important to stress that this reorganization is often not successful in returning motor function to normal. It is less effective than that in the intact brain, but will nevertheless support what recovered function there is. The exact configuration of this new motor system will be determined most obviously by the extent of the anatomical damage. This includes the extent to which the damage affects cortical motor regions, white matter pathways [82], and even which hemisphere is affected [83]. In patients with damage to primary sensorimotor cortex, for example, tests of fractionated finger movement correlated more strongly with the proportion of surviving "normal" sensorimotor cortex (as defined by functional activation maps in normal controls) than with total infarct volume [84]. The potential for functionally relevant change to occur will depend on a number of other factors, not least the biologic age of the subject and the premorbid state of their brain [20], but also current drug treatments [85]. Furthermore, levels of neurotransmitters and growth factors which are able to influence the ability of the brain to respond to afferent input (i.e. how plastic it is) might be determined by their genetic status [86]. The basis of impairment-based treatment is likely to be the promotion of activity-dependent change within these surviving networks, and so understanding the factors that shape it – possibly at the level of the individual patient – will be critical [87]. Functional brain imaging will play a central role in achieving this goal.

References

1. Nichols-Larsen DS, Clark PC, Zeringue A, *et al.* Factors influencing stroke survivors' quality of life during subacute recovery. *Stroke.* 2005;**36**:1480–4.

2. Wyller TB, Sveen U, Sodring KM, *et al.* Subjective well-being one year after stroke. *Clin Rehabil.* 1997;**11**:139–45.

3. Cramer SC, Chopp M. Recovery recapitulates ontogeny. *Trends Neurosci.* 2000;**23**:265–71.

4. Buxton RB. *An introduction to functional magnetic resonance imaging: principles and techniques.* Cambridge: Cambridge University Press; 2002.

5. Magistretti PJ, Pellerin L. Cellular mechanisms of brain energy metabolism and their relevance to functional brain imaging. *Phil Trans R Soc Lond B Biol Sci.* 1999;**354**:1155–63.

6. Attwell D, Iadecola C. The neural basis of functional brain imaging signals. *Trends Neurosci.* 2002;**25**:621–5.

7. Friston KJ, Josephs O, Rees G, *et al.* Nonlinear event-related responses in fMRI. *Magn Reson Med.* 1998;**39**:41–52.

8. Newton J, Sunderland A, Butterworth SE, *et al.* A pilot study of event-related functional magnetic resonance imaging of monitored wrist movements in patients with partial recovery. *Stroke.* 2002;**33**:2881–7.

9. Pineiro R, Pendlebury S, Johansen-Berg H, *et al.* Functional MRI detects posterior shifts in primary sensorimotor cortex activation after stroke: Evidence of local adaptive reorganization? *Stroke.* 2001;**32**:1134–9.

10. Carusone LM, Srinivasan J, Gitelman DR, *et al.* Hemodynamic response changes in cerebrovascular disease: Implications for functional MR imaging. *Am J Neuroradiol.* 2002;**23**:1222–8.

11. Hamzei F, Knab R, Weiller C, *et al.* The influence of extra- and intracranial artery disease on the BOLD signal in fMRI. *Neuroimage.* 2003;**20**:1393–9.

12. Rossini PM, Altamura C, Ferretti A, *et al.* Does cerebrovascular disease affect the coupling between neuronal activity and local haemodynamics? *Brain.* 2004;**127**:99–110.

13. Röther J, Knab R, Hamzei F, *et al.* Negative dip in BOLD fMRI is caused by blood flow–oxygen consumption uncoupling in humans. *Neuroimage.* 2002;**15**:98–102.

14. Krainik A, Hund-Georgiadis M, Zysset S, *et al.* Regional impairment of cerebrovascular reactivity and BOLD signal in adults after stroke. *Stroke.* 2005;**36**:1146–52.

15. Murata Y, Sakatani K, Hoshino T, *et al.* Effects of cerebral ischemia on evoked cerebral blood oxygenation responses and BOLD contrast functional MRI in stroke patients. *Stroke.* 2006;**37**:2514–20.

16. Ward NS, Brown MM, Thompson AJ, *et al.* Neural correlates of outcome after stroke: A cross-sectional fMRI study. *Brain.* 2003;**126**:1430–48.

17. Ward NS, Newton JM, Swayne OB, *et al.* Motor system activation after subcortical stroke depends on corticospinal system integrity. *Brain.* 2006;**129**:809–19.

18. Ward NS, Newton JM, Swayne OB, *et al.* The relationship between brain activity and peak grip force is modulated by corticospinal system integrity after subcortical stroke. *Eur J Neurosci.* 2007;**25**:1865–73.

19. D'Esposito M, Zarahn E, Aguirre GK, *et al.* The effect of normal aging on the coupling of neural activity to the bold hemodynamic response. *Neuroimage.* 1999;**10**:6–14.

20. Ward NS, Swayne OB, Newton JM. Age-dependent changes in the neural correlates of force modulation: An fMRI study. *Neurobiol Aging.* 2008;**29**:1434–46.

21. Calautti C, Leroy F, Guincestre JY, *et al.* Dynamics of motor network overactivation after striatocapsular stroke: A longitudinal PET study using a fixed-performance paradigm. *Stroke.* 2001;**32**:2534–42.

22. Chollet F, DiPiero V, Wise RJ, *et al.* The functional anatomy of motor recovery after stroke in humans: A study with positron emission tomography. *Ann Neurol.* 1991;**29**:63–71.

23. Seitz RJ, Hoflich P, Binkofski F, *et al.* Role of the premotor cortex in recovery from middle cerebral artery infarction. *Arch Neurol.* 1998;**55**:1081–8.

24. Weiller C, Chollet F, Friston KJ, *et al.* Functional reorganization of the brain in recovery from striatocapsular infarction in man. *Ann Neurol.* 1992;**31**:463–72.

25. Weiller C, Ramsay SC, Wise RJ, *et al.* Individual patterns of functional reorganization in the human cerebral cortex after capsular infarction. *Ann Neurol.* 1993;**33**:181–9.

26. Cao Y, D'Olhaberriague L, Vikingstad EM, *et al.* Pilot study of functional MRI to assess cerebral activation of motor function after poststroke hemiparesis. *Stroke.* 1998;**29**:112–22.

27. Cramer SC, Nelles G, Benson RR, *et al.* A functional MRI study of subjects recovered from hemiparetic stroke. *Stroke.* 1997;**28**:2518–27.

28. Cramer SC, Moore CI, Finklestein SP, *et al.* A pilot study of somatotopic mapping after cortical infarct. *Stroke.* 2000;**31**:668–71.

29. Rossini PM, Caltagirone C, Castriota-Scanderbeg A, *et al.* Hand motor cortical area reorganization in stroke: A study with fMRI, MEG and TCS maps. *Neuroreport.* 1998;**9**:2141–6.

30. Sanes JN, Donoghue JP. Plasticity and primary motor cortex. *Ann Rev Neurosci.* 2000;**23**:393–415.

31. Cao Y, Vikingstad EM, Huttenlocher PR, *et al.* Functional magnetic resonance studies of the reorganization of the human hand sensorimotor area after unilateral brain injury in the perinatal period. *Proc Natl Acad Sci USA* 1994;**91**:9612–6.

32. Porter R, Lemon RN. *Corticospinal function and voluntary movement.* Oxford: Oxford University Press; 1993.

33. Tomassini V, Jbabdi S, Klein JC, *et al.* Diffusion-weighted imaging tractography-based parcellation of the human lateral premotor cortex identifies dorsal and ventral subregions with anatomical and functional specializations. *J Neurosci.* 2007;**27**:10 259–69.

34. Johansen-Berg H, Matthews PM. Attention to movement modulates activity in sensori-motor areas, including primary motor cortex. *Exp Brain Res.* 2002;**142**:13–24.

35. Dum RP, Strick PL. The origin of corticospinal projections from the premotor areas in the frontal lobe. *J Neurosci.* 1991;**11**:667–89.

36. He SQ, Dum RP, Strick PL. Topographic organization of corticospinal projections from the frontal lobe: Motor areas on the lateral surface of the hemisphere. *J Neurosci.* 1993;**13**:952–80.

37. He SQ, Dum RP, Strick PL. Topographic organization of corticospinal projections from the frontal lobe: Motor areas on the medial surface of the hemisphere. *J Neurosci.* 1995;**15**:3284–306.

38. Strick PL. Anatomical organization of multiple motor areas in the frontal lobe: Implications for recovery of function. *Adv Neurol.* 1988;**47**:293–312.

39. Boudrias MH, Belhaj-Saif A, Park MC, *et al.* Contrasting properties of motor output from the supplementary motor area and primary motor cortex in rhesus macaques. *Cereb Cortex.* 2006;**16**:632–8.

40. Maier MA, Armand J, Kirkwood PA, *et al.* Differences in the corticospinal projection from primary motor cortex and supplementary motor area to macaque upper limb motoneurons: An anatomical and electrophysiological study. *Cereb Cortex.* 2002;**12**:281–96.

41. Mazevet D, Meunier S, Pradat-Diehl P, *et al.* Changes in propriospinally mediated excitation of upper limb motoneurons in stroke patients. *Brain.* 2003;**126**:988–1000.

42. Stinear JW, Byblow WD. The contribution of cervical propriospinal premotoneurons in recovering hemiparetic stroke patients. *J Clin Neurophysiol.* 2004;**21**:426–34.

43. Mazevet D, Pierrot-Deseilligny E. Pattern of descending excitation of presumed propriospinal neurones at the onset of voluntary movement in humans. *Acta Physiol Scand.* 1994;**150**:27–38.

44. Pierrot-Deseilligny E. Transmission of the cortical command for human voluntary movement through cervical propriospinal premotoneurons. *Prog Neurobiol*. 1996;**48**:489–517.

45. Dancause N, Barbay S, Frost SB, *et al*. Ipsilateral connections of the ventral premotor cortex in a new world primate. *J Comp Neurol*. 2006;**495**:374–90.

46. Dancause N, Barbay S, Frost SB, *et al*. Interhemispheric connections of the ventral premotor cortex in a new world primate. *J Comp Neurol*. 2007;**505**:701–15.

47. Dum RP, Strick PL. Spinal cord terminations of the medial wall motor areas in macaque monkeys. *J Neurosci*. 1996;**16**:6513–25.

48. Rouiller EM, Moret V, Tanne J, *et al*. Evidence for direct connections between the hand region of the supplementary motor area and cervical motoneurons in the macaque monkey. *Eur J Neurosci*. 1996;**8**:1055–9.

49. Ward NS, Brown MM, Thompson AJ, *et al*. The influence of time after stroke on brain activations during a motor task. *Ann Neurol*. 2004;**55**:829–34.

50. Feydy A, Carlier R, Roby-Brami A, *et al*. Longitudinal study of motor recovery after stroke: Recruitment and focusing of brain activation. *Stroke*. 2002;**33**:1610–7.

51. Marshall RS, Perera GM, Lazar RM, *et al*. Evolution of cortical activation during recovery from corticospinal tract infarction. *Stroke*. 2000;**31**:656–61.

52. Small SL, Hlustik P, Noll DC, *et al*. Cerebellar hemispheric activation ipsilateral to the paretic hand correlates with functional recovery after stroke. *Brain*. 2002;**125**:1544–57.

53. Ward NS, Brown MM, Thompson AJ, *et al*. Neural correlates of motor recovery after stroke: A longitudinal fMRI study. *Brain*. 2003;**126**:2476–96.

54. Luft AR, Waller S, Forrester L, *et al*. Lesion location alters brain activation in chronically impaired stroke survivors. *Neuroimage*. 2004;**21**:924–35.

55. Hodics T, Cohen LG, Cramer SC. Functional imaging of intervention effects in stroke motor rehabilitation. *Arch Phys Med Rehabil*. 2006;**87**(12 Suppl 2):S36–42.

56. Luft AR, McCombe-Waller S, Whitall J, *et al*. Repetitive bilateral arm training and motor cortex activation in chronic stroke: A randomized controlled trial. *JAMA*. 2004;**292**:1853–61.

57. Schaechter JD, Kraft E, Hilliard TS, *et al*. Motor recovery and cortical reorganization after constraint-induced movement therapy in stroke patients: A preliminary study. *Neurorehabil Neural Repair*. 2002;**16**:326–38.

58. Ward NS, Cohen LG. Mechanisms underlying recovery of motor function after stroke. *Arch Neurol*. 2004;**61**:1844–8.

59. Murase N, Duque J, Mazzocchio R, *et al*. Influence of interhemispheric interactions on motor function in chronic stroke. *Ann Neurol*. 2004;**55**:400–09.

60. Grefkes C, Nowak DA, Eickhoff SB, *et al*. Cortical connectivity after subcortical stroke assessed with functional magnetic resonance imaging. *Ann Neurol*. 2008;**63**:236–46.

61. Mansur CG, Fregni F, Boggio PS, *et al*. A sham stimulation-controlled trial of rTMS of the unaffected hemisphere in stroke patients. *Neurology*. 2005;**64**:1802–04.

62. Liepert J, Zittel S, Weiller C. Improvement of dexterity by single session low-frequency repetitive transcranial magnetic stimulation over the contralesional motor cortex in acute stroke: A double-blind placebo-controlled crossover trial. *Restor Neurol Neurosci*. 2007;**25**:461–5.

63. Takeuchi N, Chuma T, Matsuo Y, *et al*. Repetitive transcranial magnetic stimulation of contralesional primary motor cortex improves hand function after stroke. *Stroke*. 2005;**36**:2681–6.

64. Nowak DA, Grefkes C, Dafotakis M, *et al*. Effects of low-frequency repetitive transcranial magnetic stimulation of the contralesional primary motor cortex on movement kinematics and neural activity in subcortical stroke. *Arch Neurol*. 2008;**65**:741–7.

65. Fregni F, Boggio PS, Mansur CG, *et al*. Transcranial direct current stimulation of the unaffected hemisphere in stroke patients. *Neuroreport*. 2005;**16**:1551–5.

66. Fregni F, Boggio PS, Valle AC, *et al*. A sham-controlled trial of a 5-day course of repetitive transcranial magnetic stimulation of the unaffected hemisphere in stroke patients. *Stroke*. 2006;**37**:2115–22.

67. Talelli P, Rothwell J. Does brain stimulation after stroke have a future? *Curr Opin Neurol*. 2006;**19**:543–50.

68. Verleger R, Adam S, Rose M, *et al*. Control of hand movements after striatocapsular stroke: High-resolution temporal analysis of the function of ipsilateral activation. *Clin Neurophysiol*. 2003;**114**:1468–76.

69. Johansen-Berg H, Rushworth MF, Bogdanovic MD, *et al*. The role of ipsilateral premotor cortex in hand movement after stroke. *Proc Natl Acad Sci USA*. 2002;**99**:14 518–23.

70. Werhahn KJ, Conforto AB, Kadom N, *et al*. Contribution of the ipsilateral motor cortex to recovery after chronic stroke. *Ann Neurol*. 2003;**54**:464–72.

71. Lotze M, Markert J, Sauseng P, *et al*. The role of multiple contralesional motor areas for complex hand movements after internal capsular lesion. *J Neurosci*. 2006;**26**:6096–102.

72. Serrien DJ, Strens LH, Cassidy MJ, *et al*. Functional significance of the ipsilateral hemisphere during

movement of the affected hand after stroke. *Exp Neurol.* 2004;**190**:425–32.

73. Fridman EA, Hanakawa T, Chung M, *et al.* Reorganization of the human ipsilesional premotor cortex after stroke. *Brain.* 2004;**127**:747–58.

74. Dettmers C, Fink GR, Lemon RN, *et al.* Relation between cerebral activity and force in the motor areas of the human brain. *J Neurophysiol.* 1995;**74**:802–15.

75. Thickbroom GW, Phillips BA, Morris I, *et al.* Differences in functional magnetic resonance imaging of sensorimotor cortex during static and dynamic finger flexion. *Exp Brain Res.* 1999;**126**:431–8.

76. Ward NS, Frackowiak RS. Age-related changes in the neural correlates of motor performance. *Brain.* 2003;**126**:873–88.

77. Stinear CM, Barber PA, Smale PR, *et al.* Functional potential in chronic stroke patients depends on corticospinal tract integrity. *Brain.* 2007;**130**:170–80.

78. Heald A, Bates D, Cartlidge NE, *et al.* Longitudinal study of central motor conduction time following stroke. 2. Central motor conduction measured within 72 h after stroke as a predictor of functional outcome at 12 months. *Brain.* 1993;**116**:1371–85.

79. Cramer SC, Parrish TB, Levy RM, *et al.* Predicting functional gains in a stroke trial. *Stroke.* 2007;**38**:2108–14.

80. Marshall RS, Zarahn E, Alon L, *et al.* Early imaging correlates of subsequent motor recovery after stroke. *Ann Neurol.* 2009;**65**:596–602.

81. Swayne OB, Rothwell JC, Ward NS, *et al.* Stages of motor output reorganization after hemispheric stroke suggested by longitudinal studies of cortical physiology. *Cereb Cortex.* 2008;**18**:1909–22.

82. Newton JM, Ward NS, Parker GJ, *et al.* Non-invasive mapping of corticofugal fibres from multiple motor areas – Relevance to stroke recovery. *Brain.* 2006;**129**:1844–58.

83. Zemke AC, Heagerty PJ, Lee C, *et al.* Motor cortex organization after stroke is related to side of stroke and level of recovery. *Stroke.* 2003;**34**:e23–8.

84. Crafton KR, Mark AN, Cramer SC. Improved understanding of cortical injury by incorporating measures of functional anatomy. *Brain.* 2003;**126**:1650–9.

85. Goldstein LB. Pharmacology of recovery after stroke. *Stroke.* 1990;**21**(Suppl):III139–42.

86. Kleim JA, Chan S, Pringle E, *et al.* BDNF val66met polymorphism is associated with modified experience-dependent plasticity in human motor cortex. *Nat Neurosci.* 2006;**9**:735–7.

87. Ward NS. Getting lost in translation. *Curr Opin Neurol.* 2008;**21**:625–7.

12 Recovery from aphasia: lessons from imaging studies

Cornelius Weiller & Dorothee Saur

During the last 20 years, application of functional brain imaging to stroke patients has brought a new momentum into rehabilitation [1]. We understand better what happens in the brain of patients: we "see an active ipsilateral motor cortex" when we notice mirror movements of the healthy hand during the ward rounds (see also Chapter 11), or assume a resolution of diaschisis when language performance improves abruptly from one day to the other within the first week after a stroke (see also Chapter 9). This chapter highlights recent findings from neuroimaging studies of aphasia, focusing on the dynamic process of reorganization from acute to chronic stroke and points to recent developments, which enable the investigation of language reorganization within a framework of interconnected brain regions.

Imaging the acute phase

Imaging the acute phase of recovery from aphasia, i.e. the first days after stroke onset, offers the opportunity for unique insights into the function and dysfunction of the language network.

As displayed in Figure 12.1a, loss of function can be explained in terms of direct or indirect consequences of ischemia. On the one hand, the ischemic lesion may directly affect language-relevant gray (A) and white matter (B) structures due to either critical hypoperfusion with incomplete infarction, or to parenchymal damage (complete infarction) [2]. Ischemia may also cause a dysfunction in remote, non-infarcted areas (C, D). The idea of "diaschisis" was introduced by von Monakow [3]. Diaschisis is explained by a functional disconnection. The observed language impairment reflects the result of both direct local and indirect remote effects. Taken together, the lesion of a critical network component may result in an acute global network breakdown. In this situation, we typically observe a severe aphasia.

In this hyperacute phase the lesion may be unstable, resulting in sometimes rapid fluctuations in language performance. This mainly includes changes in cerebral perfusion and extension of the peri-infarct edema. Reperfusion of left posterior middle temporal and frontal areas may be associated with acute improvement in picture naming [4]. Von Monakow [3] introduced the term "diaschisis" to explain acute language improvements after stroke. Figure 12.1b–d displays an example of early functional MRI (fMRI) activation in a patient with acute global aphasia due to a left temporal middle cerebral artery (MCA) infarction. In an auditory language comprehension task, the patient listened to three sentences of intelligible speech (SP), and also listened to sentences of reversed speech (REV). Extraction of condition-wise effect sizes (Figure 12.1c and d) showed that in the hyperacute phase about 10 h after onset, remote L and R inferior frontal gyrus (IFG) were dysfunctional. Although a strong effect for both the SP and REV conditions was observed, both areas did not distinguish between intelligible SP and unintelligible REV – activation was the same for both tasks. However, three and seven days later, in parallel with improvement of language behavior, a clear differentiation between both conditions returned to both brain areas, indicating functional recovery of these remote areas, which is most likely explained by a resolution of diaschisis. That is, injury to left temporal language areas produced diaschisis in bilateral IFG which produced dysfunction and inability to distinguish SP from REV; with resolution of this diaschisis, bilateral IFG function returned, and these language network areas were able to restart function and thereby contribute to effective language behavior and thus compensation for the deficit [5].

Another lesson that may be learned from imaging the acute phase of aphasia relates to the understanding of subcortical aphasia. Combining the findings from

Brain Repair After Stroke, ed. S. C. Cramer and R. J. Nudo. Published by Cambridge University Press.
© Cambridge University Press 2010.

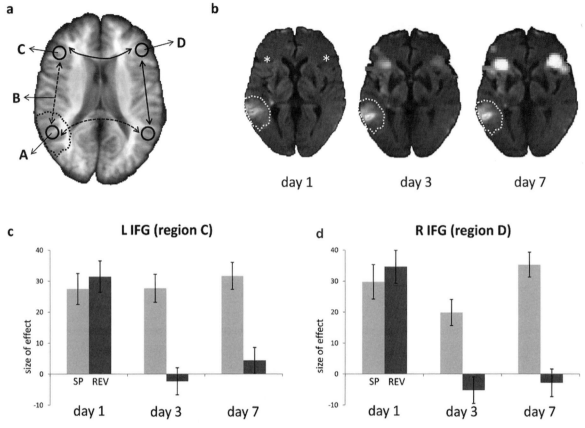

Figure 12.1 (a) Schematic diagram of direct and indirect consequences of focal ischemia on the language network. The dotted line indicates ischemic area in the left temporal cortex; black circles indicate candidate language areas in both hemispheres. Ischemia may cause direct damage of language-relevant gray (A) and white (B) matter (dashed lines), resulting in a functional and anatomical disconnection of remote areas C and D due to missing functional input (diaschisis). (b) fMRI activation is presented for a patient with a left (dominant) temporal infarction performing two auditory language comprehension tasks, one being listening to speech and the other being listening to speech presented in reverse. The fMRI analysis that contrasts speech with reversed speech is displayed ($p< 0.05$, corrected for multiple comparisons). The infarct is outlined with a dashed line. At day 1, no language-specific activation was detectable, i.e. there was no significant difference in language area activation when the language task (speech) was contrasted with the non-language task (reversed speech). At this time, the patient presented with acute global aphasia. Follow-up examinations at days 3 and 7 revealed strong, increased language-specific activation in language areas (bilateral inferior frontal gyrus (IFG)), which was paralleled by an improvement of behavioral language function. (c, d) Effect sizes for fMRI activation, extracted from left (region C) and right (region D) IFG. Notably, at day 1, there is a strong effect for both the language task (speech, "SP") and the non-language (reversed speech, "REV") tasks. However, L and R IFG did not distinguish between these two conditions, indicating an acute dysfunction of preserved, remote areas in terms of diaschisis. This ability to distinguish between speech and reversed speech is recovered at days 3 and 7, indicating a resolution of diaschisis, in parallel with language behavioral gains.

structural MRI and cerebral angiography, Weiller *et al.* [6] demonstrated that aphasia in striatocapsular infarction was related to the cortical hypoperfusion caused by an occlusion of the proximal segment of the MCA rather than the subcortical infarction itself, and this cortical hypoperfusion led to a subsequent cortical atrophy one year later, interpreted as selective neuronal loss [2], which is typically invisible on conventional MRI but detectable with Iomazenil-single-photon computed tomography [7]. This observation was later confirmed by a perfusion imaging study by

Hillis *et al.* [8], who demonstrated that aphasia due to acute, subcortical infarction can be largely explained by concurrent cortical hypoperfusion. These findings underline the importance of an accurate characterization of the acute ischemia including registration of hypoperfused tissue by performing multiparametric MRI sequences.

Imaging dynamics of reorganization

Neural reorganization of language functions may be better understood by imaging the recovery process

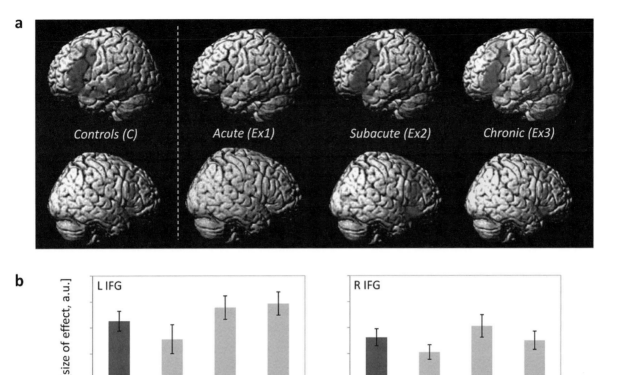

Figure 12.2 (a) Dynamics of language-specific (SP contrasted with REV) fMRI activation in healthy control subjects (first column, a single fMRI exam) and in 14 patients with acute aphasia (columns 2–4, representing the three exams). Activation is shown for the left hemisphere in the top row, and for the right hemisphere in the bottom row. Note that in patients there is little or no left hemisphere activation in the acute stage. This is followed by a strong bilateral increase in activation in the subacute stage, peaking in the right hemisphere homolog of Broca's area. In the chronic phase, a consolidation and gradual normalization emerged, with a "re-shift" to the left hemisphere. (b) Parameter estimates extracted in left and right IFG, indicating a continuous increase of activation in left IFG over time but a biphasic course in right IFG. Modified from [42].

throughout all phases after stroke, which allows one to relate changes in language performance to changes in language-related brain activation. Saur *et al.* [5] performed the same auditory comprehension task as described above for the single subject study on a heterogeneous group of 14 aphasic patients suffering from a left MCA stroke affecting temporal, frontal, and subcortical brain regions. fMRI data were collected in the acute (< 4 days after stroke, Exam 1), subacute (about 2 weeks after stroke, Exam 2), and chronic (4–12 months after stroke, Exam 3) phases of recovery. Across these three fMRI exams, patients recovered from aphasia. Group analysis of the fMRI data (Figure 12.2a) revealed no or little left hemisphere (top row) activation in the acute stage followed by a strong bilateral increase in activation in the subacute stage, peaking in the right hemisphere (bottom row) homolog of Broca's area. In the chronic phase, a consolidation and gradual normalization emerged, with a "re-shift" to the left hemisphere. Language-specific

effect sizes (Figure 12.2b, which presents SP contrasted with REV) showed a continuous increase throughout all phases in left IFG, while in the right hemisphere homolog, a more biphasic course with a temporary increase in the subacute stage was observed. Importantly, the early increase of activation in the right hemisphere homolog of Broca's area correlated with early improvement of language function.

Since in this study an overall pattern of reorganization was derived from a heterogeneous group of stroke patients, a relation of the group activation to the lesion site was not possible. Consequently, Saur *et al.* [9] investigated a homogeneous group of eight patients who all suffered from a left temporal infarction. The strongest lesion overlap in this group was found in the anterior temporal lobe. The longitudinal study design was the same as described above. Again, in the acute phase, strongly reduced activation in the entire language network was found, including within preserved (spared by stroke) left frontal cortex. Since in all patients left IFG was intact, reduced activation in this area can be best interpreted in terms of diaschisis. That is, in the acute phase, the left IFG lacks functional input from left temporal areas. In the subacute phase, a strong increase in bilateral IFG was observed; however, in contrast to the mixed group, the highest activation remained in the left hemisphere. Notably, activation in left and right IFG emerged simultaneously. This is of particular interest since right hemisphere activation in recovery from aphasia is interpreted to reflect disinhibition caused by dysfunctional left language areas, which are unable to inhibit their homologs in the right hemisphere. If this is the case, we would expect that right hemisphere activation reveals a reciprocal rather than a parallel course of activation. However, a reciprocal pattern is not always observed. In fact, simultaneous increase of activation in bilateral IFG could also be interpreted in terms of a functional dependency of right homolog language areas on their left hemisphere counterparts. Finally, in the chronic phase, perilesional activation in posterior temporal areas emerged. This perilesional activation was also found in areas activated in healthy subjects, indicating a reactivation of temporarily dysfunctional tissue rather than a true recruitment of novel brain areas. Importantly, in this perilesional tissue, high correlation between language performance and language activation over time was found. This further supports the high functional relevance of left hemisphere areas for long-term language recovery.

Taken together, we postulated a model of language recovery, which proceeds in three phases [1,5]. In a first period during which near-complete abolishment of language function is seen, there is little if any activation in brain regions which later can be activated by the language task. In this acute phase a global network breakdown, in which "diaschisis", or ischemic stunning [10], is the key factor. A second, "hyperactive" stage of brain activation follows, in which the altered function recovers at a rapid pace. It is characterized by a sudden return of activation in left and often a hyper-activation of homolog right hemisphere areas. In the third stage, a consolidation of activation resembling the patterns in healthy controls is observed.

These patterns of reorganization are derived from a highly selected group of patients. In fact, Saur et al. [5] screened a total of 198 consecutively admitted aphasic patients to find 14 to match the inclusion criteria. Most patients were excluded since they were not able to perform early fMRI due to poor general

medical condition. Thus, the results are somewhat biased by a selection of the best patients, and further studies might clarify how these findings extend to the broader spectrum of stroke patients.

Imaging the chronic phase

The majority of imaging studies on language recovery were performed in the chronic phase after stroke. In these studies, patients who recovered from aphasia to various degrees were examined once or sequentially with PET or fMRI to identify the pattern of the language activation in the lesioned brain. In sum, as in the motor system (see Chapter 11), these studies with very heterogeneous designs, methods, and patients have shown that post-stroke language system reorganization of function involves undamaged areas in the left hemisphere, perilesional tissue, and homologous areas in the right hemisphere [11–18]. Depending on site and size of the lesion and the residual language impairment, portions of these three areas are more activated as compared to healthy control subjects [17]. More specific conclusions can be drawn by correlating the proficiency of a particular language function with task-related activation in a cross-sectional design. For instance, Crinion et al. [19] demonstrated in a group of 17 patients with left temporal stroke that performance in auditory sentence comprehension was positively correlated with activation in the right lateral superior temporal gyrus (STG). These results underline that in the chronic phase, too, right hemisphere activation might be beneficial. More sustained evidence comes from a dynamic challenge in which repetitive behavioral studies are performed. Musso et al. showed that after repeated 8-min sessions of language comprehension training, subsequent behavioral improvement correlated with an increase of activation in the right temporal cortex [12], supporting a role for right hemisphere language homolog areas in language function after stroke.

When discussing the functional role of right hemisphere activation in chronic aphasia, we have to think about the potential factors influencing the amount of right hemisphere involvement. First, the premorbid degree of language lateralization seems to be an important factor. Although impossible to control, it is likely that patients with a more bilateral premorbid language representation are more likely to utilize the homolog right areas after left hemisphere damage. Second, the more complete the damage of left core language areas and the more severe the associated residual language deficit, the more likely a permanent involvement of the right hemisphere homolog areas will be observed (see also below regarding the concept of critical lesions). This might lead to the conclusion that right hemisphere activation is disadvantageous or maladaptive rather than functionally beneficial, assuming a negative influence of right hemisphere (in particular right frontal) activation which prevents recovery. In support of this logic, note that studies using repetitive transcranial magnetic stimulation (rTMS) to inhibit function of right hemisphere language regions in chronic stroke patients have described improvement of language functions [20]. However, a deterioration of language functions after rTMS application to right frontal areas has also been observed [21]. A final judgment of this issue is difficult, as neither transcallosal interaction nor the mechanisms of rTMS are anywhere near to completely understood.

Impact of therapy on reorganization

Several studies have shown task-related activation changes from pre- to post-treatment scans. Even studies providing short-term treatment influence the neural basis of language processing, such as the one by Musso *et al.* [12]. Blasi *et al.* [22] demonstrated increased activity in the right frontal cortex associated with learning a word retrieval task. Studies performing long-term training found either left [23–26], or right [27,28], or bilateral activation to be associated with treatment-induced improvement [29–31]. In contrast, Richter *et al.* [32] found no significant changes of fMRI activation at all after 2 weeks of "constraint-induced aphasia therapy". This heterogeneity of results is best explained by differences in treatment strategies, language impairments, as well as differences in lesion sites and sizes. In post-stroke brain reorganization, as with many aspects of acute stroke, many factors can contribute to differences between patients. However, these studies do clearly demonstrate that remodeling of cortical functions is possible even years after the stroke, and typically occurs in both left and right as well as perilesional language zones, similar to what has been described in the motor system [33] (see also Chapter 11).

Summary and outlook: the network approach

Most brain functions are organized in distributed, segregated and interconnected networks, and brain reorganization due to lesions or interventions mainly takes place within the framework of these networks [1,34]. Language is a brain function, which is especially suited to assess a network approach on recovery, as it is represented in a widespread, bilateral brain network. Recent combinations of fMRI with probabilistic fiber tracking, integrating pairwise point-to-point anatomical connections along with measurements of functional connectivity, resulted in a relatively complete network description of language processing around the Sylvian fissure [35,36]. In contrast to classical diagrams, which suppose speech comprehension to be localized in the temporal lobe and speech production in the inferior frontal lobe and both regions connected through the arcuate fascicle, the modern anatomical view sees the left temporal lobe connected to most of the frontal lobe along two segregated and integrating large association tracts [35,37–39] (Figure 12.3): a dorsal route along the arcuate fasciculus/superior longitudinal fasciculus mainly projects to premotor cortices and renders automated sensory-motor mapping, while several aspects of language comprehension utilize a ventral route via the extreme capsule mainly projecting to the prefrontal cortex. These new findings not only require a new description of anatomical correlation of language functions and dysfunctions, but also imply various routes of compensation after stroke.

The network view addresses another frequent misconception: the assumption of functional independence of brain "centers". As an example, conduction aphasia, which is often defined as an isolated repetition failure with preserved comprehension and spontaneous speech, is supposed to result from a destruction of the pathway (i.e. the arcuate fascicle) connecting the sensory and the motor speech center, which are both intact. Such a conclusion assumes that the temporal lobe suffices for comprehension and the inferior frontal cortex

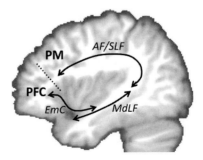

Figure 12.3 Schematic diagram of ventral and dorsal language pathways projecting to the prefrontal (PFC) and premotor (PM) cortex. MdlF=middle longitudinal fascicle, EmC=extreme capsule, AF=arcuate fasciculus, SLF=superior longitudinal fasciculus.

for language production and that a disruption of the connecting pathway does not affect the function of either area. We know from imaging experiments that this is not true: semantic tasks activate Broca's area and propositional speech also the temporal lobe [40]. The various constituents of the language circuitry are not independent from each other; interruption of the network has an impact on the remaining parts of the network. In other words, the functions of Broca's or Wernicke's area with an intact arcuate fascicle may not be the same as after that fascicle's destruction. The network view takes this into account when interpreting symptoms and activations in patients with aphasia.

If the individual nodes of the network influence each other through their connections, the importance of a network node might be determined by the number of its connections used for a certain task. This leads directly to the concept of critical lesions. The more important a network node is to a behavior, the more behavioral effects its lesioning will have. Using a combination of functional and anatomical connectivity to identify networks subserving auditory language comprehension within a temporofrontal network, the posterior part of the middle temporal gyrus and the inferior frontal gyrus in the left hemisphere were identified to have the most functional relevant connections [36]. Therefore both regions are especially important in comprehension. One question posed was, how much of the left hemisphere network must be spared to prevent right hemisphere recruitment [1]? The network approach above would focus this question to critical lesions of the left hemisphere, i.e. those that affect the regions with most connections. For example, in patients with temporal lesions sparing the posterior temporal region, it is exactly this posterior region which shows the best correlation with language performance over time [9]. In contrast, if this posterior region is involved, the contralateral hemisphere comes into play [15]. However, there is also a clear hierarchy between the nodes of a network, such as Broca's area, which is indispensible for grammar [41].

Combining functional and structural network identification procedures is a promising approach to improve our understanding of loss and recovery of brain functions. However, beyond this more theoretical interest, we suggest that a precise description of the lesioned network might be useful to guide the application of focal brain stimulation techniques such as transcranial direct current stimulation or rTMS (see also Chapter 19). In future settings, patients will be investigated with fMRI and diffusion tensor imaging prior to brain stimulation. Processing of the impaired language function will be analyzed with the above-mentioned network identification procedures. Subsequent brain stimulation and adjuvant therapies might then be applied to the identified central processing nodes to support behavioral training.

The study of brain adaptation after stroke and during recovery still poses one of the most intriguing aspects of neurological research. While an ever more detailed description of such complex issues as brain and language is needed (e.g. various functions for Broca's area, BOLD versus electrical signals, functional definition of tracts, cytochemical mapping down to synapses, proteins, and DNA), a complete explanation remains evasive. However, the better our understanding of brain reorganization will be, including with respect to normal connections and patterns of network activity, the better that restorative treatments can effectively be used.

References

1. Rijntjes M, Weiller C. Recovery of motor and language abilities after stroke: The contribution of functional imaging. *Prog Neurobiol*. 2002;**66**:109–22.

2. Weiller C, Willmes K, Reiche W, *et al*. The case of aphasia of neglect after striatocapsular infarction. *Brain*. 1993;**116**:1509–25.

3. Monakow C von. Aphasie und Diaschisis. *Neurologisches Centralblatt*. 1906;**25**:1026–38.

4. Hillis AE, Kleinman JT, Newhart M, *et al*. Restoring cerebral blood flow reveals neural regions critical for naming. *J Neurosci*. 2006;**26**:8069–73.

5. Saur D, Lange R, Baumgaetner A, *et al*. Dynamics of language reorganization after stroke. *Brain*. 2006;**129**:1371–84.

6. Weiller C, Ringelstein EB, Reiche W, *et al*. The large striatocapsular infarct. *Arch Neurol*. 1990;**47**:1085–91.

7. Saur D, Buchert R, Knab R, *et al*. Iomazenil-single-photon emission computed tomography reveals selective neuronal loss in magnetic resonance-defined mismatch areas. *Stroke*. 2006;**37**:2713–9.

8. Hillis AE, Wityk RJ, Barker PB, *et al*. Subcortical aphasia and neglect in acute stroke: The role of cortical hypoperfusion. *Brain*. 2002;**125**:1094–104.

9. Saur D, Kummerer D, Kellmeyer P, *et al.*, editors. Dynamics of language reorganization in left temporal stroke. *15th Annual Meeting of the Organization for Human Brain Mapping*; 2009; San Francisco, CA: NeuroImage: in press.

10. Alexandrov AV, Hall CE, Labiche LA, *et al*. Ischemic stunning of the brain: Early recanalization without

immediate clinical improvement in acute ischemic stroke. *Stroke.* 2004;**35**:449–52.

11. Heiss WD, Kessler J, Thiel A, *et al.* Differential capacity of left and right hemispheric areas for compensation of poststroke aphasia. *Ann Neurol.* 1999;**45**:430–8.

12. Musso M, Weiller C, Kiebel S, *et al.* Training-induced brain plasticity in aphasia. *Brain.* 1999;**122**:1781–90.

13. Rosen HJ, Petersen SE, Linenweber MR, *et al.* Neural correlates of recovery from aphasia after damage to left inferior frontal cortex. *Neurology.* 2000;**55**:1883–94.

14. Warburton E, Price CJ, Swinburn K, *et al.* Mechanisms of recovery from aphasia: Evidence from positron emission tomography studies. *J Neurol Neurosurg Psychiatry.* 1999;**66**:155–61.

15. Weiller C, Isensee C, Rijntjes M, *et al.* Recovery from Wernicke's aphasia: A positron emission tomographic study. *Ann Neurol.* 1995;**37**:723–32.

16. Zahn R, Schwarz M, Huber W. Functional activation studies of word processing in the recovery from aphasia. *J Physiol Paris.* 2006;**99**:370–85.

17. Leff A, Crinion J, Scott S, *et al.* A physiological change in the homotopic cortex following left posterior temporal lobe infarction. *Ann Neurol.* 2002;**51**:553–8.

18. Sharp DJ, Scott SK, Wise RJ. Retrieving meaning after temporal lobe infarction: The role of the basal language area. *Ann Neurol.* 2004;**56**:836–46.

19. Crinion J, Price CJ. Right anterior superior temporal activation predicts auditory sentence comprehension following aphasic stroke. *Brain.* 2005;**128**:2858–71.

20. Naeser MA, Martin PI, Nicholas M, *et al.* Improved picture naming in chronic aphasia after TMS to part of right Broca's area: An open-protocol study. *Brain Lang.* 2005;**93**:95–105.

21. Winhuisen L, Thiel A, Schumacher B, *et al.* Role of the contralateral inferior frontal gyrus in recovery of language function in poststroke aphasia: A combined repetitive transcranial magnetic stimulation and positron emission tomography study. *Stroke.* 2005;**36**:1759–63.

22. Blasi V, Young AC, Tansy AP, *et al.* Word retrieval learning modulates right frontal cortex in patients with left frontal damage. *Neuron.* 2002;**36**:159–70.

23. Cornelissen K, Laine M, Tarkiainen A, *et al.* Adult brain plasticity elicited by anomia treatment. *J Cogn Neurosci.* 2003;**15**:444–61.

24. Leger A, Demonet JF, Ruff S, *et al.* Neural substrates of spoken language rehabilitation in an aphasic patient: An fMRI study. *Neuroimage.* 2002;**17**:174–83.

25. Meinzer M, Flaisch T, Breitenstein C, *et al.* Functional rerecruitment of dysfunctional brain areas predicts language recovery in chronic aphasia. *Neuroimage.* 2008;**39**:2038–46.

26. Vitali P, Abutalebi J, Tettamanti M, *et al.* Training-induced brain remapping in chronic aphasia: A pilot study. *Neurorehabil Neural Repair.* 2007;**21**:152–60.

27. Crosson B, Moore AB, Gopinath K, *et al.* Role of the right and left hemispheres in recovery of function during treatment of intention in aphasia. *J Cogn Neurosci.* 2005;**17**:392–406.

28. Raboyeau G, De Boissezon X, Marie N, *et al.* Right hemisphere activation in recovery from aphasia: Lesion effect or function recruitment? *Neurology.* 2008;**70**:290–8.

29. Fridriksson J, Morrow-Odom L, Moser D, *et al.* Neural recruitment associated with anomia treatment in aphasia. *Neuroimage.* 2006;**32**:1403–12.

30. Fridriksson J, Moser D, Bonilha L, *et al.* Neural correlates of phonological and semantic-based anomia treatment in aphasia. *Neuropsychologia.* 2007;**45**:1812–22.

31. Meinzer M, Obleser J, Flaisch T, *et al.* Recovery from aphasia as a function of language therapy in an early bilingual patient demonstrated by fMRI. *Neuropsychologia.* 2007;**45**:1247–56.

32. Richter M, Miltner WH, Straube T. Association between therapy outcome and right hemispheric activation in chronic aphasia. *Brain.* 2008;**131**:1391–401.

33. Liepert L, Bauder H, Miltner WHR, *et al.* Treatment-induced cortical reorganisation after stroke in humans. *Stroke.* 2000;**31**:1210–6.

34. Weiller C, Rijntjes M. Learning, plasticity, and recovery in the central nervous system. *Exp Brain Res.* 1999;**128**:134–8.

35. Saur D, Kreher BW, Schnell S, *et al.* Ventral and dorsal pathways for language. *Proc Natl Acad Sci USA.* 2008;**105**:18 035–40.

36. Saur D, Mader W, Schnell S, *et al.* Combining functional and anatomical connectivity reveals brain networks for auditory comprehension. *NeuroImage.* 2010. In press.

37. Anwander A, Tittgemeyer M, von Cramon DY, *et al.* Connectivity-based parcellation of Broca's area. *Cereb Cortex.* 2007;**17**:816–25.

38. Frey S, Campbell JS, Pike GB, *et al.* Dissociating the human language pathways with high angular resolution diffusion fiber tractography. *J Neurosci.* 2008;**28**:11 435–44.

39. Makris N, Pandya DN. The extreme capsule in humans and rethinking of the language circuitry. *Brain Struct Funct.* 2009;**213**:343–58.

40. Vigneau M, Beaucousin V, Herve PY, *et al.* Meta-analyzing left hemisphere language areas: Phonology, semantics, and sentence processing. *Neuroimage.* 2006;**30**:1414–32.

41. Musso M, Moro A, Glauche V, *et al.* Broca's area and the language instinct. *Nat Neurosci.* 2003;**6**:774–81.

42. Saur D, Lange R, Baumgaertner A, *et al.* Dynamics of language reorganization after stroke. *Brain.* 2006;**129**:1371–84.

13 Brain mapping of attention and neglect after stroke

Alex R. Carter, Gordon L. Shulman & Maurizio Corbetta

The psychology of attention

"Selective attention" broadly refers to a set of mechanisms that allow people to perceive and respond to events that are behaviorally relevant. Selection is important to maintain behavioral coherence in the face of multiple stimuli and thoughts that may call for contradictory actions, and to address the limited processing capacity of the brain.

Spatial attention, the most commonly investigated form of attention, is defined as the ability to select information from one or multiple locations in the environment. Selection is based on internal knowledge (top-down or goal-driven) as well as salient sensory information (bottom-up or stimulus-driven) [1], which may be integrated in a common "saliency" map [2]. Selection of environmental stimuli amplifies the neural responses to those stimuli and suppresses neural responses to stimuli in unattended regions [3]. Hence lesions in the brain can disrupt selective processing of stimuli by affecting associative regions that direct spatial attention and/or by affecting sensory regions in which selection modulates neural activity.

Once sensory stimuli are selected, they must be linked with the appropriate motor action (e.g. looking or reaching). As multiple motor responses are potentially available, the process of "stimulus–response mapping" is also selective. Visual stimuli are coded in visual cortex based on their retinal location, while movements are coded in motor cortex in directional coordinates, such as centered on the arm. This is the well-known problem of frames of reference in sensory-to-motor transformations. The brain's solution is to first integrate retinal information with eye position, and then integrate this eye-centered representation with other inputs (such as vestibular, proprioceptive, or auditory) to create a viewer-centered map of the environment that is used by the motor system to plan actions. Different spatial maps may be used to guide different kinds of actions (looking, reaching, grasping). For example, information about "far" space may be used to optimize goal-directed behavior for directing the eyes or turning the head toward a salient feature in the environment, while information about "near" space may be used for reaching with a hand toward a desired object [4].

Spatial neglect: a model of attention deficits after brain injury

Hemispatial neglect is the prototypical spatial attention deficit after focal brain injury. Patients with neglect present with deficits in perceiving, responding to, moving toward, visualizing, remembering, and even conceiving of stimuli in the contralesional field [5,6]. Patients with neglect may have difficulty visualizing the left side of a well-known mental image, although the memory for both sides of that image is preserved. These deficits point to a bias in sensory and motor processing that favors stimuli on the right side of the environment or of mental images (Figure 13.1).

Several subtypes of neglect have been proposed based on the modality or frame of reference that is impaired. We recently found that only 9 of 43 patients with acute neglect showed clear signs of directional hypokinesia, a difficulty in reaching toward contralesional stimuli, the hallmark deficit of motor neglect [7]. In a longitudinal analysis of neglect symptoms (n=61), deficits of lateralized attention were far more severe than motor deficits and tended to improve more in time [8]. Therefore, lateralized deficits of attention/perception are the most important for tracking recovery of neglect.

Neglect occurs in multiple reference frames. There is strong evidence for deficits of attending/responding to stimuli in both *allocentric*, i.e. with respect to the environment, and *egocentric*, i.e. with respect to the

Brain Repair After Stroke, ed. S. C. Cramer and R. J. Nudo. Published by Cambridge University Press.
© Cambridge University Press 2010.

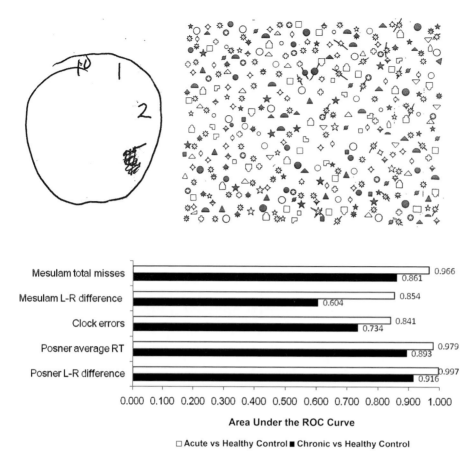

Figure 13.1 The left upper panel shows performance of a patient with a right hemispheric lesion on a clock drawing task, where the patient with left neglect draws more numbers on the right side of the clock than the left. The right panel illustrates performance on the Mesulam target cancellation task, where the patient with left neglect cancels many more symbols on the right than left side of the page. The bottom panel shows that not all tests are equally sensitive to the presence of spatial neglect. Here, clock drawing and the Mesulam test are compared with a computerized Posner task. In the Posner task, the patient fixates on a central cross that is flanked by two boxes. At the beginning of every trial an arrow pointing left or right transiently replaces the fixation cross to indicate where the target will appear. After a variable interval, the target appears either to the right or the left of fixation at which time the patient must make a button press. In persons with left spatial neglect, reaction times are increased when the target appears in the left visual field. An analysis of the receiver operating characteristics of these tests reveals that while all the tests were reasonably good at detecting the non-lateralized component of impaired attention, the computerized Posner task was best at detecting the lateralized component of neglect, especially at the chronic stage [8].

observer, frames of reference [9]. Interestingly, deficits are not mapped in retinal coordinates, the most common reference frame found in visual sensory areas, consistent with the notion that core deficits of neglect reflect intermediate representations, in which viewer-centered coding is important, rather than sensory representations [10].

A second cluster of deficits in neglect that are clinically relevant have been termed "non-lateralized" deficits of attention [11], including deficits of vigilance/arousal and spatial/temporal capacity that generalize across the entire visual field. Many authors have suggested that the alerting/arousal component of attention is right hemisphere dominant, both when an alert state is endogenously maintained and when it is transiently increased by a warning signal [12]. Clinically, non-lateralized deficits are seen especially in right hemisphere injured patients, who have lower arousal and wider fluctuations in arousal than left hemisphere patients. Heilman and colleagues suggested the lateralization of arousal is related to the lateralization of neglect, i.e. the observation that contralesional neglect is more sustained and severe after right than left hemisphere lesions [13]. In subjects with spatial neglect after right hemispheric strokes, auditory cues known to produce a change in phasic arousal cause a significant, albeit transient, improvement of spatial neglect [14].

Anatomical basis of neglect and related models

Neglect can arise from lesions in many cortical and subcortical regions. An interesting study that compared superior parietal and inferior parietal (or temporo-parietal junction, TPJ) cortex damage on tasks designed to measure shifts of spatial attention to sensory stimuli reported problems only for TPJ damage [15]. Other studies have reported neglect following lesions of inferior frontal cortex [16], middle temporal gyrus and/or the temporo-parietal periventricular white matter [17], parietal and anterior cingulate cortex and posterior white matter [18], superior temporal gyrus [19], as well as subcortical regions such as basal ganglia and thalamus [20] (Figure 13.2). Overall, anatomical studies indicate that the most frequently damaged cortical regions in unilateral spatial neglect correspond to the ventral portion of the parietal and frontal lobes and the superior temporal gyrus.

Several groups have attempted to identify the anatomy of different neglect subtypes [8,21,22]. The distinction between perceptual/attention vs. motor/intentional neglect, for example, has been mapped onto parietal and frontal cortex, respectively [23–25], although this distinction is variable at the behavioral level and has not been tested using modern voxel-based mapping methods.

Damage to white matter tracts connecting temporal, parietal, and frontal cortex may be critical to the genesis of neglect (Figure 13.2B). A CT/SPECT study by Leibovitch [18] implicated lesions in the white matter connecting the parietal and temporal lobes and the parietal and frontal lobes, while Doricchi [26] reported that lesions in 21 neglect patients showed a region of maximal overlap in the superior longitudinal fasciculus (SLF) beneath the supramarginal gyrus (SMG). He et al. [27] reported that the SLF was damaged in patients with more severe neglect, and electrical stimulation of the SLF shifted the subjective midline during line bisection [28]. It has also been proposed that previous studies such as those of Committeri et al. [21] and Karnath et al. [18] may have overlooked a significant contribution from SLF damage [29]. This evidence has led some authors to re-cast spatial neglect as a disconnection syndrome [29–31], in which a focal lesion results in the functional isolation of cortical modules and dysfunctional activity in regions that are structurally intact. Damage to several distinct long-range fronto-parietal paths, including the arcuate fasciculus (AF), SLF, inferior longitudinal fasciculus (ILF), and fronto-occipital fasciculus (FOF) has been proposed to underlie different types of neglect.

Several influential models based on anatomical information have been proposed to account for the behavioral deficits of hemispatial neglect. Both Heilman and Mesulam proposed that neglect is mediated by a distributed cortical/subcortical network for spatial behavior in which different parts of the network are specialized for different forms of neglect. The distinction between perceptual/attention and motor/intentional aspects of neglect was mapped onto the parietal or prefrontal nodes of a fronto-parietal network for spatial behavior and awareness, modulated in their tone by the ascending reticular activating system (ARAS). Mesulam also argued for the presence of a motivational component in neglect localized to the anterior cingulate [32] that affected parietal regions through connections with posterior cingulate. While Heilman emphasized right hemisphere dominance of arousal/vigilance functions to partly explain the lateralization of neglect [6], both authors also proposed that the predominance of left neglect reflected an asymmetric representation of space in posterior parietal and frontal cortex (Figure 13.3, left panels).

Functional mapping studies of attention and spatial neglect

Functional neuroimaging methods have shown that regions involved in directing attention to spatial locations are localized in dorsal frontal and posterior parietal cortex [33,34] and overlap regions involved in eye movement planning/execution (frontal and parietal eye regions) [35,36]. Dorsal fronto-parietal regions contain topographic maps of contralateral space [37–39], their activity is modulated by manipulation of egocentric, but not object-centered, reference frames [40], and they generate top-down signals that bias sensory processing in visual regions [41,42]. These regions form a "dorsal attention network" that controls stimulus–response selection both under goal-driven and stimulus-driven conditions [43].

In the healthy brain, orienting to novel or behaviorally relevant stimuli presented outside the focus of attention involves a second system whose core regions include TPJ cortex and ventral frontal cortex (VFC). This ventral network is "non-spatial" in the sense that it responds equally well to stimuli presented on both sides of space and signals the presence of novel salient stimuli even when they do not

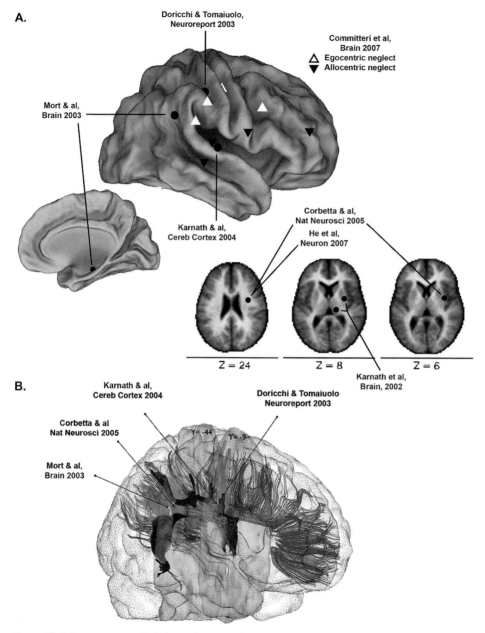

Figure 13.2 Numerous sites of right hemisphere injury have been associated with spatial neglect. (A) Summarizes cortical and subcortical gray matter lesions associated with spatial neglect from studies where Talairach coordinates could be obtained. Coordinates from Committeri *et al.* [21] were converted from MNI to Talairach coordinates using the Nonlinear Yale MNI to Talairach Conversion Algorithm available at http://www. bioimagesuite.org/Mni2Tal/index.html. (B) Recent lesion studies implicating white matter tracts involved in hemispatial neglect. Some results stem from the re-examination of previous studies of cortical damage that revealed concurrent damage to the underlying white matter as well, and hence the contribution of this mechanism to the genesis of spatial neglect could not be completely ruled out. (B) is adapted from Bartolomeo *et al.* [30] and reprinted here with permission from the authors and Oxford Journals.

require a shift of attention. The physiological response of the ventral network may be related to the activity of locus coeruleus (LC) neurons, with the hemispheric asymmetry of the ventral network reflecting a right>left projections from the LC to the cortex [12,44]. During normal perception, the dorsal and ventral attention networks interact, with the ventral network acting as a "sentinel" to detect important events, which are selected by the dorsal network [43,44].

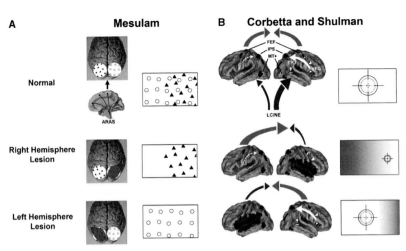

Figure 13.3 Mesulam (left panels) and Corbetta and Shulman (right panels) models that propose different mechanisms to account for the non-lateralized and lateralized aspects of neglect. In this figure the degree of overall vigilance is represented by the density of visual field coverage in the Mesulam model, and by the size of the crosshairs in the Corbetta Shulman model. Tonic bias is represented by a displacement of the crosshairs to the right as well as a gradient of spatial representation favoring one side. (A) In the Mesulam model, the ascending reticular activating system (ARAS) is crucial to maintaining overall attentional tone. The left parietal cortex houses a representation of the right side of space (black triangles), but the right parietal cortex houses a representation for both left and right space (open circles). Damage to the right parietal cortex (shaded region) results in impaired left representation of space, while left parietal damage can be compensated for by the right parietal representation of both sides of space. (B) In the Corbetta and Shulman model, there is a balanced interaction between the two halves of a dorsal attention network (FEF, IPS, MT+ in black). It is modulated by a right dominant ventral attention network (TPJ, VFC in white) which responds to novel unexpected stimuli and provides a circuit breaker signal (solid white arrow) that redirects the resources of the dorsal attention network. The ventral attention network also appears to promote overall vigilance, possibly via asymmetric input from the locus coeruleus/norepinephrine system. After a right hemisphere neglect-inducing stroke (shaded region), the right ventral network is often damaged and deactivated resulting in decreased vigilance (smaller crosshairs) as well as decreased response to novel stimuli. In addition, this damage has remote effects on the right hemisphere dorsal attention network, which is structurally intact but none the less relatively hypoactivated compared to the left (larger arrow from left hemisphere). This relative hypoactivation along with unopposed orienting from the left hemisphere leads to the commonly observed tonic rightward bias. In left hemispheric lesions there is little or no ventral attention network to disrupt, a weak tonic deviation and only a mild decrease in vigilance attributable to non-specific effects of a brain lesion. (FEF: frontal eye fields; IPS: intraparietal sulcus; MT+: middle temporal complex; TPJ: temporo-parietal junction; VFC: ventro-frontal cortex; LC/NE: locus coeruleus–norepinephrine system.)

The physiological properties of dorsal and ventral networks map onto the two major behavioral clusters in neglect, namely *rightward spatial bias* and *non-lateralized deficits* of vigilance/arousal and capacity (Figure 13.3). The locus of attention seems to depend on a competitive interhemispheric mechanism that calculates the position of attention in space from the relative gradient of activity between contralateral and ipsilateral maps in dorsal fronto-parietal regions. These physiological properties make the dorsal network a prime candidate for mediating lateralized spatial biases in neglect. Similarly, the properties of the ventral network, i.e. absence of spatial topography, modulation by behaviorally relevant and unexpected targets, and by arousal/vigilance, map onto the non-lateralized deficits of spatial neglect.

However, lesions causing neglect tend to occur ventrally in temporo-parietal and frontal cortex (see previous section), and typically spare dorsal fronto-parietal regions involved in spatial attention and visuomotor behavior. This sparing is problematic for the Heilman/

Mesulam model, in which structural damage to dorsal spatial representations causes neglect. Furthermore, lesions in dorsal parietal cortex cause visuomotor problems but do not cause neglect. We proposed the following solution to this puzzle: structural lesions causing neglect damage predominantly the ventral network, but in addition produce physiological abnormalities in the dorsal network due to faulty interactions with the damaged ventral network (Figure 13.3B).

This hypothesis was tested in a longitudinal study of neglect patients ($n=11$) with a first right hemisphere stroke, tested at 2–4 weeks and again at 39 weeks post-stroke [45]. Patients received fMRI scans while performing the Posner spatial orienting task, which yields separate behavior measures of rightward bias and non-lateralized attention. As expected, structural lesions occurred in perisylvian regions, with maximal damage in the superior temporal gyrus, frontal operculum, insula, and putamen. The TPJ, supramarginal gyrus, and underlying white matter were also often involved. This area of damage closely overlapped the ventral

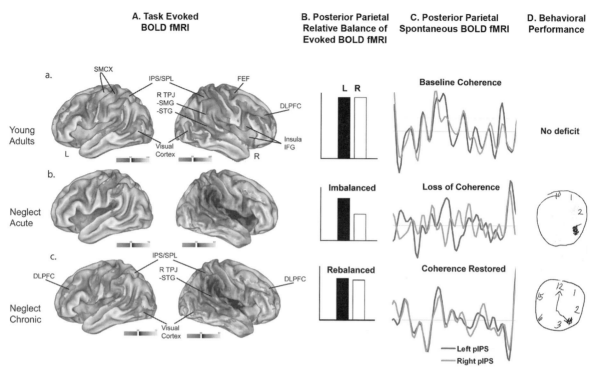

Figure 13.4 For the color version of this figure, see the Plate section. Acutely after stroke there is (A) a reduction of evoked BOLD activity in both hemispheres as compared to young adult controls, (B) a marked imbalance of evoked BOLD activity between the two hemispheres, (C) a loss of interhemispheric coherence of spontaneous BOLD activity between core regions of the attention network, and (D) impaired spatial performance. In the chronic state, there is a reactivation of evoked BOLD activity, rebalancing of relative activity between left and right posterior parietal cortex, return of spontaneous BOLD coherence, and behavioral improvement. A striking finding was that activity of the left dorso-parietal cortex was relatively stronger at the acute stage, but this imbalance decreased at the chronic stage when the right dorso-parietal cortex had reactivated. This "push–pull" pattern was detected in the IPS-SPL and visual cortex, but not in the FEF or TPJ. The relative contributions of interhemispheric imbalance versus loss of spontaneous BOLD coherence to behavioral deficits remain to be determined. Whether a similar pattern of recovery might apply to other bihemispherically represented systems is still unknown. (SMCX: somatomotor cortex; DLFPC: dorsolateral prefrontal cortex; IPS/SPL: intraparietal sulcus/superior parietal lobule; TPJ: temporo-parietal junction; SMG: supramarginal gyrus; STG: superior temporal gyrus; FEF: frontal eye fields; IFG: inferior frontal gyrus.)

attention network but spared the dorsal network (Figure 13.4, column A, note that the areas of right hemisphere activation present in young adult controls overlap with the right hemisphere lesion distribution apparent in both the acute and the chronic stroke neglect patients). Even though the dorsal network was spared, there was a physiological imbalance of task-evoked activity in dorsal parietal cortex acutely, with stronger responses in left than right parietal cortex (Figure 13.4, column B). Finally, the degree of left dorsal parietal activation correlated with the severity of spatial neglect as assessed by the number of missed targets and response speed to targets in the left visual field. These results suggest that acutely, left-field neglect was caused by an imbalance in task-driven responses in posterior parietal cortex that resulted in a decreased and less specific response to stimuli in right visual cortex, presumably because of decreased top-down drive from parietal to occipital areas.

The demonstration that physiological abnormalities in task-evoked activity in the structurally undamaged dorsal attention network are partly responsible for mediating lateralized biases of attention was further supported by the observation that recovery of spatial neglect at 39 weeks paralleled the rebalancing of left and right parietal responses (Figure 13.4, Column B). Consistent with the prediction that ventral network damage correlates with non-lateralized deficits of neglect, activation of the ventral network was correlated with the speed of detection irrespective of visual field.

In summary, this experiment supports the hypothesis that acutely, spatial neglect is caused by structural damage to the ventral network and the parallel physiological dysfunction of the structurally intact dorsal attention network, and that the mechanism responsible for the lateralized spatial bias is an interhemispheric imbalance of activity in cortical regions involved in spatial orienting.

Biases in spatial orienting are also tonically present at rest, as evidenced by tonic attentional and oculomotor biases to the right visual field [46,47]. Interestingly, tonic biases are also observed in the resting-state correlation of the BOLD signal between brain regions. Studies in normal subjects have shown that spontaneous fluctuations of the BOLD signal, measured at rest, are more highly correlated between brain regions that belong to the same functional network [48]. Resting-state interregional correlations may indicate the functional "health" of different anatomical networks without the confounds introduced by differences in task performance between individuals. He *et al.* [27] studied the same neglect subjects as Corbetta *et al.* [45], but removed the mean task-evoked response, and analyzed the residuals containing the intrinsic (not task-driven) signals from different regions of the brain. At 2 weeks, the normally high correlation between left and right dorsal parietal cortex was disrupted and the degree of incoherence correlated with the severity of left spatial neglect (Figure 13.4C). In parallel, incoherence between temporal and prefrontal regions in the ventral network correlated with poor performance in both visual fields. As subjects improved, at 39 weeks, the coherence in the dorsal network but not the damaged ventral network increased toward normal levels. Importantly, the degree of incoherence between ventral prefrontal and dorsal parietal network regions correlated with the degree of neglect, and this physiological imbalance in turn depended on the presence of white matter damage in the superior longitudinal and arcuate fascicles connecting anterior to posterior brain regions. Recently, these results have been confirmed and generalized under resting-state conditions for the entire attention network, and a similar resting-state relationship has been observed between interhemispheric coherence of a motor network and motor impairments [49].

These findings show that focal lesions can result in dysfunction at remote sites through interference with the normal physiological baseline of the brain. Neurological syndromes observed at the bedside do not just reflect the functions of local, structurally damaged regions, but also the effects of this damage on the physiology of distributed brain networks.

Recovery from neglect after stroke

Left hemispatial neglect is a common result of right hemispheric stroke, although right neglect from left hemispheric stroke has also been reported. Spontaneous recovery from neglect after stroke does occur, but time courses for recovery vary by patient age, affected modality and diagnostic test [8,50–52]. Many studies have clearly shown that hemispatial neglect is a poor prognostic factor for overall improvement during acute rehabilitation, maximum level of recovery, and return to independence [53].

Only a handful of experiments have examined the neural correlates of neglect recovery, probably due to the challenges inherent to longitudinal studies. Deuel [54] induced neglect in monkeys with frontal or parietal lesions and found remote hypometabolism in structurally undamaged areas. Reduction of hypometabolism was correlated with behavioral improvement. The earliest human brain mapping studies of spontaneous recovery from neglect confirmed the importance of reactivation of previously damaged areas in the right hemisphere [55]. For example, in a SPECT study of cerebral blood flow in two neglect patients studied within one month and then again after one month, Vallar *et al.* [56] found that recovery from neglect after a subcortical lesion was associated with a reduction in cortical hypoperfusion in the damaged hemisphere. Hillis [57] recently showed that in an individual subject, fluctuations in performance on a task of visuospatial attention are correlated with levels of cerebral perfusion in acute stroke, but large-scale longitudinal studies of cortical perfusion and neglect at the acute and chronic stages have not been performed.

Corbetta *et al.* studied neglect subjects (*N*=11) with fMRI scanned at 2–4 weeks and then again at 39 weeks with a Posner spatial orienting task [45] and reported bilateral depression at the acute stage in both hemispheres that improved over time. Similar observations were reported in fewer patients by Pizzamiglio *et al.* [58] and Thimm *et al.* [59]. The bilateral depression observed in neglect may reflect an overall loss of cortical responsiveness possibly associated with decrements in arousal/vigilance, and lack of cortical modulation by noradrenaline/dopamine. So far this bilateral reactivation has not been correlated with specific improvement in behavioral measures. One prediction is that this bilateral reactivation may correlate with measures of non-lateralized attention.

Corbetta and colleagues have also reported that interhemispheric normalization of task-driven responses and resting-state coherence in parietal regions of the dorsal attention network occurs from acute to chronic stage. In patients with anatomical sparing, task-driven response can also recover in the TPJ, the core region of the ventral attention network, and relate specifically to the recovery of reorienting to visual targets [45,27].

In summary, the best available evidence indicates that spatial neglect recovery depends both on an overall reactivation of task-driven activity in both hemispheres, as well as on a rebalancing of activity across the two hemispheres in regions involved in controlling attention. Whether these changes are predictive or correlate with functional recovery remains to be seen.

Treatment of neglect and neuroimaging

Some studies have investigated the effects of various therapeutic manipulations on both behavioral performance and brain activation in neglect patients. Luaute et al. [60] and Barrett et al. [61] recently reviewed the most promising therapeutic interventions, including top-down approaches such as visual scanning therapy and the use of mental imagery, feedback training to reduce anosognosia, sensory stimulations that recalibrate spatial coordinate frames, and bypass language-mediated attentive learning such as vestibular stimulation, neck muscle vibration and optokinetic (OPK) stimulation, limb activation in the left hemispace, and prism visuomotor adaptation. Few brain mapping studies have correlated changes in patterns of activity with any of these interventions [52].

Thimm et al. [62] studied behavioral and neuroimaging changes in seven chronic neglect patients with right hemisphere lesions and stable deficits in response to computerized alertness training. Training was performed using the AIXTENT program in which the subject drives a car that is heading from the left side to the right side of the computer screen. Using just two buttons (one to accelerate and one to stop), subjects were instructed to drive as rapidly as possible while avoiding collisions. After training, increased evoked activity was observed in the right superior and middle frontal gyrus, medial frontal and anterior cingulate cortex, angular gyrus, and precuneus, consistent with reactivation within the right-hemisphere attentional network. A similar pattern was reported for the left hemisphere, but only increased left middle frontal gyrus activity was associated with improved spatial attention. Four weeks after completion of training, spatial attention behavior returned to pretraining baseline and only increased activations of left temporal and parietal areas and lingual gyrus remained.

Luaute et al. [63] performed a behavioral and PET study of five subjects with chronic left neglect to study the effect of prism adaptation, a promising method for the treatment of neglect based on the occurrence of a leftward subjective shift of the midline following rightward prism adaptation. Subjects performed a line bisection judgment task in the scanner, underwent prism treatment with repeated rapid pointing responses, then repeated the line bisection task in the scanner. The authors found that improvement of left neglect after prism adaptation was correlated with modulation of neuronal activity in the right cerebellum, left thalamus, left temporo-occipital cortex, right posterior parietal cortex, and left medial temporal lobe.

Optokinetic stimulation (OKS) is another visuo-sensory-motor intervention whose imaging correlates have been investigated. Subjects view a stimulus pattern of 30–70 random dots moving coherently from right to left and are encouraged to repeatedly track the dots with smooth pursuit movements and then saccade back to the right side of the screen [64]. In an fMRI study of seven patients with chronic neglect who received this therapy, Sturm et al. found that transient behavioral improvements were associated with bilaterally increased activations in posterior cingulate gyrus and precuneus as well as left hemisphere activations in angular gyrus and temporo-occipital areas (BA 22) [65]. The authors noted that these regions were more posteriorly located than areas implicated in the alertness training paradigm discussed above.

Future directions

The debate over the neuroanatomical basis of visuospatial neglect continues. Progress may come from more consistent definitions of the different subtypes of neglect, normalization of diagnostic tests for neglect, and restriction of study populations to specific types of neglect. However, defining neglect subtypes solely on behavior may overlook common underlying mechanisms, such as the destruction of internal representations, impaired read-out of specific representations, or impairment of a specific sensorimotor transformation. The studies reviewed above clearly show that future studies must not be confined to conventional structural imaging techniques, given the growing evidence for physiologic dysfunction remote from the site of structural damage and the importance of white matter connections between distant cortical areas. Different patterns of structural damage may lead to similar patterns of network dysfunction, just as seemingly unrelated enzymatic deficits along the same metabolic pathway can lead to the same syndrome.

To fully chart the course of brain reorganization of attention systems after injury, well-controlled longitudinal studies are needed, as it is likely that different processes take place at the acute, subacute, and chronic stages. However, because neuroimaging is a correlational technique, imaging alone cannot answer such questions about whether newly recruited regions contribute to recovery or are maladaptive and contribute to further deficits. Interventional techniques such as transcranial magnetic stimulation (TMS) may significantly constrain conclusions drawn from brain mapping studies, allowing us to distinguish between these two possibilities for specific brain regions.

Clinically, research that maps the effects of different interventions on the recovery from neglect is highly important. Unfortunately, rehabilitation science historically has been plagued with difficulties in developing hypothesis-driven interventions, as well as showing that interventions have effects beyond those attributable to spontaneous recovery. Moreover, the majority of the behavioral improvements reported to date have been transient. Neuroimaging of the overlap between areas implicated in attention processes and other sensorimotor networks, such as those responsible for visuomotor adaptation or vestibular function, may reveal networks that can be used as a "back door" mechanism for modulating the damaged attention network (i.e. via prism adaptation, optokinetic stimulation, or vestibular stimulation). The interpretation of neuroimaging changes during recovery is complicated by significant performance confounds, although this problem can be mitigated using approaches such as resting-state functional connectivity MRI. It seems unlikely that any one brain mapping technique used in isolation will provide a conclusive picture of attention network reorganization after stroke. Rather, the convergence of multiple approaches including structural MRI, fMRI, PET, and TMS is necessary for a more complete understanding of the determinants of overall network health and integrity after brain damage.

Acknowledgments

We thank Oxford University Press and Dr Bartolomeo for permission to adapt a figure from their study published in *Cerebral Cortex* 2007 **17**:2479–90.

References

1. Posner MI, Cohen Y. Components of attention. In: Bouman H, Bowhuis D, editors. *Attention and performance X*. Hillsdale, NJ: Erlbaum; 1984: pp. 55–66.

2. Koch C, Ullman S. Shifts in visual attention: Towards the underlying circuitry. *Human Neurobiol.* 1985;**4**:219–27.

3. Desimone R, Duncan J. Neural mechanisms of selective visual attention. *Ann Rev Neurosci.* 1995;**18**:193–222.

4. Jeannerod M, Arbib MA, Rizzolatti G, *et al.* Grasping objects: The cortical mechanisms of visuomotor transformation. *Trends Neurosci.* 1995;**18**:314–20.

5. Mesulam M-M. A cortical network for directed attention and unilateral neglect. *Ann Neurol.* 1981;**10**:309–25.

6. Heilman KM, Bowers D, Valenstein E, *et al.* Hemispace and hemispatial neglect. In: Jeannerod M, editor. *Neurophysiological and neuropsychological aspects of spatial neglect.* Amsterdam: Elsevier; 1987: pp. 115–50.

7. Sapir A, Kaplan JB, He BJ, *et al.* Anatomical correlates of directional hypokinesia in patients with hemispatial neglect. *J Neurosci.* 2007;**27**:4045–51.

8. Rengachary J, d'Avossa G, Sapir A, *et al.* Is the Posner reaction time test more accurate than clinical tests in detecting left neglect in acute and chronic stroke? *Arch Phys Med Rehabil.* 2009;**90**:2081–8.

9. Hillis AE, Newhart M, Heidler J, *et al.* Anatomy of spatial attention: Insights from perfusion imaging and hemispatial neglect in acute stroke. *J Neurosci.* 2005;**25**:3161–7.

10. Hillis AE. Neurobiology of unilateral spatial neglect. *Neuroscientist.* 2006;**12**:153–63.

11. Robertson IH. Do we need the "lateral" in unilateral neglect? Spatially nonselective attention deficits in unilateral neglect and their implications for rehabilitation. *Neuroimage.* 2001;**14**:S85–90.

12. Posner MI, Petersen SE. The attention system of the human brain. *Ann Rev Neurosci.* 1990;**13**:25–42.

13. Heilman KM, Van Den Abell T. Right hemisphere dominance for attention: The mechanism underlying hemispheric asymmetries of inattention (neglect). *Neurology.* 1980;**30**:327–30.

14. Robertson IH, Mattingley JB, Rorden C, *et al.* Phasic alerting of neglect patients overcomes their spatial deficit in visual awareness. *Nature.* 1998;**395**:169–72.

15. Friedrich FJ, Egly R, Rafal RD, *et al.* Spatial attention deficits in humans: A comparison of superior parietal and temporal–parietal junction lesions. *Neuropsychology.* 1998;**12**:193–207.

16. Husain M, Kennard C. Visual neglect associated with frontal lobe infarction. *J Neurol.* 1996;**243**:652–7.

17. Samuelsson H, Jensen C, Ekholm S, *et al.* Anatomical and neurological correlates of acute and chronic visuospatial neglect following right hemisphere stroke. *Cortex.* 1997;**33**:271–85.

18. Leibovitch FS, Black SE, Caldwell CB, *et al.* Brain–behavior correlations in hemispatial neglect using CT

and SPECT: The Sunnybrook Stroke Study. *Neurology.* 1998;**50**:901–08.

19. Karnath HO, Fruhmann Berger M, Kuker W, *et al.* The anatomy of spatial neglect based on voxelwise statistical analysis: A study of 140 patients. *Cereb Cortex.* 2004;**14**:1164–72.

20. Karnath HO, Himmelbach M, Rorden C. The subcortical anatomy of human spatial neglect: Putamen, caudate nucleus and pulvinar. *Brain.* 2002;**125**:350–60.

21. Committeri G, Pitzalis S, Galati G, *et al.* Neural bases of personal and extrapersonal neglect in humans. *Brain.* 2007;**130**:431–41.

22. Grimsen C, Hildebrandt H, Fahle M. Dissociation of egocentric and allocentric coding of space in visual search after right middle cerebral artery stroke. *Neuropsychologia.* 2008;**46**:902–14.

23. Coslett HB, Bowers D, Fitzpatrick E, *et al.* Directional hypokinesia and hemispatial inattention in neglect. *Brain.* 1990;**113**:475–86.

24. Bisiach E, Geminiani G, Berti A, *et al.* Perceptual and premotor factors of unilateral neglect. *Neurology.* 1990;**40**:1278–81.

25. Tegner R, Levander M. Through a looking glass. A new technique to demonstrate directional hypokinesia in unilateral neglect. *Brain.* 1991;**114**:1943–51.

26. Doricchi F, Tomaiuolo F. The anatomy of neglect without hemianopia: A key role for parietal–frontal disconnection? *Neuroreport.* 2003;**14**:2239–43.

27. He BJ, Snyder AZ, Vincent JL, *et al.* Breakdown of functional connectivity in frontoparietal networks underlies behavioral deficits in spatial neglect. *Neuron.* 2007;**53**:905–18.

28. Thiebaut de Schotten M, Urbanski M, Duffau H, *et al.* Direct evidence for a parietal–frontal pathway subserving spatial awareness in humans. *Science.* 2005;**309**:2226–8.

29. Doricchi F, Thiebaut de Schotten M, Tomaiuolo F, *et al.* White matter (dis)connections and gray matter (dys) functions in visual neglect: Gaining insights into the brain networks of spatial awareness. *Cortex.* 2008;**44**:983–95.

30. Bartolomeo P, Thiebaut de Schotten M, Doricchi F. Left unilateral neglect as a disconnection syndrome. *Cereb Cortex.* 2007;**17**:2479–90.

31. Urbanski M, Thiebaut de Schotten M, Rodrigo S, *et al.* Brain networks of spatial awareness: Evidence from diffusion tensor imaging tractography. *J Neurol Neurosurg Psychiatry.* 2008;**79**:598–601.

32. Mesulam MM. Spatial attention and neglect: Parietal, frontal and cingulate contributions to the mental representation and attentional targeting of salient extrapersonal events. *Phil Trans R Soc Lond B Biol Sci.* 1999;**354**:1325–46.

33. Corbetta M, Miezin FM, Shulman GL, *et al.* A PET study of visuospatial attention. *J Neurosci.* 1993;**13**:1202–26.

34. Nobre AC, Sebestyen GN, Gitelman DR, *et al.* Functional localization of the system for visuospatial attention using positron emission tomography. *Brain.* 1997;**120**:515–33.

35. Corbetta M, Akbudak E, Conturo TE, *et al.* A common network of functional areas for attention and eye movements. *Neuron.* 1998;**21**:761–73.

36. Luna B, Thulborn KR, Strojwas MH, *et al.* Dorsal cortical regions subserving visually-guided saccades in humans: An fMRI study. *Cerebral Cortex.* 1998;**8**:40–7.

37. Sereno MI, Pitzalis S, Martinez A. Mapping of contralateral space in retinotopic coordinates by a parietal cortical area in humans. *Science.* 2001;**294**:1350–4.

38. Silver MA, Ress D, Heeger DJ. Topographic maps of visual spatial attention in human parietal cortex. *J Neurophysiol.* 2005;**94**:1358–71.

39. Jack AI, Patel GH, Astafiev SV, *et al.* Changing human visual field organization from early visual to extra-occipital cortex. *PLoS ONE.* 2007;**2**:e452.

40. Galati G, Lobel E, Vallar G, *et al.* The neural basis of egocentric and allocentric coding of space in humans: A functional magnetic resonance study. *Exp Brain Res.* 2000;**133**:156–64.

41. Ruff CC, Blankenburg F, Bjoertomt O, *et al.* Concurrent TMS-fMRI and psychophysics reveal frontal influences on human retinotopic visual cortex. *Curr Biol.* 2006;**16**:1479–88.

42. Bressler SL, Tang W, Sylvester CM, *et al.* Top-down control of human visual cortex by frontal and parietal cortex in anticipatory visual spatial attention. *J Neurosci.* 2008;**28**:10 056–61.

43. Corbetta M, Shulman GL. Control of goal-directed and stimulus-driven attention in the brain. *Nat Rev Neurosci.* 2002;**3**:201–15.

44. Corbetta M, Patel G, Shulman GL. The reorienting system of the human brain: From environment to theory of mind. *Neuron.* 2008;**58**:306–24.

45. Corbetta M, Kincade MJ, Lewis C, *et al.* Neural basis and recovery of spatial attention deficits in spatial neglect. *Nat Neurosci.* 2005;**8**:1603–10.

46. Hornak J. Ocular exploration in the dark by patients with visual neglect. *Neuropsychologia.* 1992;**30**:547–52.

47. Karnath HO. Optokinetic stimulation influences the disturbed perception of body orientation in spatial neglect. *J Neurol Neurosurg Psychiatry.* 1996;**60**:217–20.

48. Biswal B, Yetkin F, Haughton V, *et al.* Functional connectivity in the motor cortex of resting human brain using echo-planar MRI. *Magn Res Med.* 1995;**34**:537–41.

49. Carter AR, Astafiev SV, Lang CE, *et al.* Resting interhemispheric functional magnetic resonance imaging connectivity predicts performance after stroke. *Ann Neurol.* 2010;**67**:365–75.

50. Hier DB, Mondlock J, Caplan LR. Recovery of behavioral abnormalities after right hemisphere stroke. *Neurology.* 1983;**33**:345–50.

51. Stone SP, Patel P, Greenwood RJ, *et al.* Measuring visual neglect in acute stroke and predicting its recovery: The visual neglect recovery index. *J Neurol Neurosurg Psychiatry.* 1992;**55**:431–6.

52. Arene NU, Hillis AE. Rehabilitation of unilateral spatial neglect and neuroimaging. *Eura Medicophys.* 2007;**43**:255–69.

53. Buxbaum LJ, Ferraro MK, Veramonti T, *et al.* Hemispatial neglect: Subtypes, neuroanatomy, and disability. *Neurology.* 2004;**62**:749–56.

54. Deuel RK. Neural dysfunction during hemineglect after cortical damage in two monkey models. In: Jeannerod M, editor. *Neurophysiological and neuropsychological aspects of spatial neglect.* Amsterdam: Elsevier; 1987: pp. 315–34.

55. Perani D, Vallar G, Paulesu E, *et al.* Left and right hemisphere contribution to recovery from neglect after right hemisphere damage – An [18F]FDG study of two cases. *Neuropsychologia.* 1993;**31**:115–25.

56. Vallar G, Perani D, Cappa SF, *et al.* Recovery from aphasia and neglect after subcortical stroke: Neuropsychological and cerebral perfusion study. *J Neurol Neurosurg Psychiatry.* 1988;**51**:1269–76.

57. Hillis AE. Rehabilitation of unilateral spatial neglect: New insights from magnetic resonance perfusion imaging. *Arch Phys Med Rehabil.* 2006;**87**(12 Suppl 2): S43–9.

58. Pizzamiglio L, Perani D, Cappa SF, *et al.* Recovery of neglect after right hemispheric damage: H$_2$(15)O positron emission tomographic activation study. *Arch Neurol.* 1998;**55**:561–8.

59. Thimm M, Fink GR, Kust J, *et al.* Recovery from hemineglect: Differential neurobiological effects of optokinetic stimulation and alertness training. *Cortex.* 2009;**45**:850–62.

60. Luaute J, Halligan P, Rode G, *et al.* Visuo-spatial neglect: A systematic review of current interventions and their effectiveness. *Neurosci Biobehav Rev.* 2006;**30**:961–82.

61. Barrett AM, Buxbaum LJ, Coslett HB, *et al.* Cognitive rehabilitation interventions for neglect and related disorders: Moving from bench to bedside in stroke patients. *J Cogn Neurosci.* 2006;**18**:1223–36.

62. Thimm M, Fink GR, Kust J, *et al.* Impact of alertness training on spatial neglect: A behavioural and fMRI study. *Neuropsychologia.* 2006;**44**:1230–46.

63. Luaute J, Michel C, Rode G, *et al.* Functional anatomy of the therapeutic effects of prism adaptation on left neglect. *Neurology.* 2006;**66**:1859–67.

64. Kerkhoff G, Keller I, Ritter V, *et al.* Repetitive optokinetic stimulation induces lasting recovery from visual neglect. *Restor Neurol Neurosci.* 2006;**24**:357–69.

65. Sturm W, Thimm M, Kust J, *et al.* Alertness-training in neglect: Behavioral and imaging results. *Restor Neurol Neurosci.* 2006;**24**:371–84.

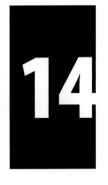

14 Depression and its effects after stroke

Thomas Platz

Description

Emotional symptoms are probably among the most ignored impairments in stroke patients. Depressive symptoms, anxiety, anger and inadequate anger control, fatigue, alexithymia or unawareness of emotions, emotionalism, and pathological crying or laughter are signs and symptoms that can frequently be encountered in stroke victims. Reported changes in personality after stroke include reduced patience and increased frustration, reduced confidence, more dissatisfaction, and a less easy-going nature. The descriptive picture would not be complete if one did not consider the impact of the disease, stroke, on family caregivers of stroke patients. Anxiety, depression, and poor physical health are common sequelae among family caregivers of stroke survivors. Emotional symptoms impact many aspects of stroke recovery in humans, as described below, and so represent a dimension of post-stroke life that is incompletely captured in animal models.

While this chapter will primarily focus on depression and its effects after stroke, the broader perspective of post-stroke emotional disorders is kept in mind; comments on other emotional disorders will amend and contribute to the picture of cause and effects of depression after stroke.

Diagnosis

One important challenge in neuropsychiatry is how to diagnose depression in patients with acute brain lesions, since there may be an overlap between symptoms of depression and signs associated with the neurological disease. The diagnosis of a depressive syndrome should be made using standardized diagnostic criteria for mood disorders due to neurological disease such as in the DSM-IV or the ICD-10. The best approach is to assess the presence of depressive symptoms using semi-structured or structured psychiatric interviews such as the Present State Exam, the Structured Clinical Interview for DSM-IV (SCID), or the Schedules for Clinical Assessment in Neuropsychiatry.

Most studies in acute and chronic neurological disorders demonstrated the specificity of both autonomic and psychological symptoms for the syndrome of depression.

Symptom profiles and thereby the validity of clinically rated DSM-IV depressive symptoms were investigated in stroke patients suffering from (1) major depressive disorder, (2) minor depressive disorder, and (3) those free of any neuropsychiatric disorders [1]. First-ever stroke patients (N=200) were approached within 3 months of the acute stroke and were interviewed with the SCID-P and administered the Hamilton Depression Rating Scale (HDRS) and the Beck Depression Inventory (BDI) among others. The only symptom that did not differ among patient groups (1–3) was Feelings of Guilt; all the other eight DSM-IV symptoms were significantly different. In particular, the frequency of Depressed Mood, Diminished Interest or Pleasure, Fatigue or Loss of Energy, Insomnia, and Psychomotor Agitation/Retardation was higher in minor depressive disorder patients than in those free of any neuropsychiatric disorders.

Depression rating scales may be used to rate the severity of depression and to monitor its changes over time, e.g. with antidepressant treatment. Several diagnostic instruments are in use to identify emotional symptoms in patients who suffer from stroke. Of these, clinician-administered are the Hamilton Depression Rating Scale (HDRS) and the Montgomery–Asberg Depression Rating Scale (MADRS); self-rating scales are the Beck Depression Inventory (BDI), the Center for Epidemiological Studies – Depression Scale (CES-D), the Zung Self-Rating Depression Scale, the Geriatric Depression Scale (GDS), and the Hospital Anxiety and Depression Scale (HADS).

Brain Repair After Stroke, ed. S. C. Cramer and R. J. Nudo. Published by Cambridge University Press.
© Cambridge University Press 2010.

Aphasia and other cognitive impairments may sometimes make these instruments difficult to use. Nevertheless, depression diagnosis (DSM-IV) and severity rating (MADRS) can reliably be made in the acute phase in at least two-thirds of aphasic patients, and feasibility increases over time [2]. Otherwise, the Stroke Aphasic Depression Questionnaire (SADQ) (completed by a spouse or a caregiver; also validated for aphasic patients in the hospital, completed by the nurse) [3] or the Aphasic Depression Rating Scale (ADRS) (validated for the evaluation of depression by the rehabilitation team) [4] can be recommended for screening purposes.

Frequency and evolution

Incidence and prevalence of post-stroke depression

Depression occurs in 20–40% of stroke patients. Other emotional symptoms commonly described include anxiety (20–30%), emotional instability (10–25%), crisis reaction (20%), and reduced initiative and fatigue (50–70%) [5].

An Australian cohort study assessed the frequency and correlates of depression at 3 and 15 months after stroke. A total of 164 consecutive eligible stroke patients and 100 comparison subjects received extensive medical, psychiatric, and neuropsychological assessments. Comprehensive assessments included ratings for DSM-IV major or minor depression at 3–6 months (index assessment) and 15 months (follow-up assessment) after stroke. Major or minor depression was present in 12.0% of stroke patients at index assessment and in 20.7% at follow-up, which included 18 new cases (13.4%) [6].

The Italian multicenter observational DESTRO study included from a total of 53 centers 1064 consecutively admitted patients with ischemic or hemorrhagic stroke who were then periodically assessed in the first 9 months after the event. Patients with depression were followed for two years [7]. Post-stroke depression was detected in 383 patients (36%), most of whom had minor depression (80.17%), with dysthymia, rather than major depression and adaptation disorder. About 80% of these developed their depression within three months of the stroke. Cases with later onset tended to have less severe symptoms.

A Swedish study investigated the risk of depression in elderly patients one and a half years after stroke, and compared it to the risk in a population-based control sample [8]. One hundred and forty-nine elderly stroke survivors and 745 age- and sex-matched controls from the general population were examined with semi-structured psychiatric examinations and cognitive assessments. Diagnoses were made according to DSM-III-R. The frequency of depression was 34% in stroke patients and 13% in population controls (odds ratio, 3.4; 95% CI, 2.3–5.0). The risk of depression was increased in both men and women and in all age groups, but was not related to the predominant side of stroke symptoms.

When patients with post-stroke depression were assessed 1 month and 6 months after stroke, communication impairment was found to be a strong predictor of depression severity and prognosis [9].

In a cohort study with 145 patients, self-rated health was rated as very good or rather good by 62% at 3 months after stroke, and by 78% at 12 months after stroke. Nevertheless, more than half of the patients suffered from symptoms of depression, with no significant improvement at 12 months. The most common general symptoms at 3 months after stroke were fatigue, sadness, pain in the legs, dizziness, and irritability. Fatigue and sadness were still common at 12 months [10].

Frequency of other post-stroke emotional symptoms

Anxiety symptoms had been found to be more frequent than depressive symptoms in the acute stage of ischemic stroke using the Hospital Anxiety and Depression Scale (HADS) between days 3 and 7 after admission to the stroke unit: 26.4% of 178 patients suffered from anxiety symptoms, 14.0% from depressive symptoms, and 7.9% from both during this early stage [11]. Similarly, in another study both patients and caregivers were found to be more anxious than depressed at one year post-stroke [12]. Anxiety symptoms were associated with single marital state and a low Mini Mental State Examination (MMSE) score, whereas depressive symptoms were related to a low Barthel Activities of Daily Living index (BI). In a further cohort study, anxiety remained stable over 3 years post-stroke and was best predicted by prior, early, anxiety, and female gender [13].

The incidence of anger had prospectively been screened in 202 consecutive acute stroke patients (< or = 4 days) using 8 items from 3 psychiatric scales (Catastrophic Reaction Scale, Mania Rating Scale, and Comprehensive Psychopathological Rating Scale) [14]. Anger was considered present if the patient scored in at least one item. Anger was detected in 71 (35%) patients, and 26 of these were severely angry (> or = 4 points). There was no association between anger and the considered variables. Analysis of the items extracted two factors: (i) the emotional-cognitive and (ii) the behavioural components of anger. Using the 10-item Spielberger Trait Anger Scale, another study interviewed 145 patients with stroke regarding inability to control anger or aggression (ICAA) [15]. ICAA was present in 47 patients (32%) and was closely related to motor dysfunction, dysarthria, emotional incontinence, and lesions affecting frontal–lenticulocapsular–pontine base areas.

Post-stroke fatigue is distinct from depression in many instances. It is especially disabling and frustrating in that it typically involves patients with total or near-total neurological recovery, who should have been able to go back to their previous activities but who become severely disabled because of early and persisting exhaustion [16]. A related symptom complex revolves around unawareness. Unawareness may have different forms, such as anosognosia, neglect, and alexithymia or unawareness of emotions. Despite the strong comorbidity rate among the different forms of unawareness, there are patients who suffer from pure forms of these types of lack of awareness [17].

Post-stroke personality changes as reported by the patients' main carer at 9 months after the stroke were reduced patience and increased frustration, reduced confidence, more dissatisfaction, and a less easy-going nature [18].

Cause and effect

The interaction between depression and stroke is complex and the pathophysiological mechanisms have not as yet been fully elucidated, although an interaction between genetic, biochemical, anatomical, and especially psychosocial factors may be important in post-stroke depression development.

Epidemiological reasoning

Depression as a risk factor for stroke

Presence of depressive symptoms has been shown to be a strong risk factor for stroke in men [19,20]; greater depressive symptoms are associated with an increase in the risk of all-cause and, more specifically, cerebrovascular disease mortality in men [21].

A prospective cohort study was conducted on 4120 Framingham Heart Study participants aged 29–100

years with up to 8 years of follow-up and sought to examine whether depressive symptoms are associated with an increased risk of cerebrovascular events in a community-based sample [22]. In participants < 65 years, the risk of developing stroke/transient ischemic attack (TIA) was 4.21 times greater in those with symptoms of depression. After adjusting for components of the Framingham Stroke Risk Profile (hazard ratio = 3.43, 95% CI = 1.60–7.36) and education (hazard ratio = 4.89, 95% CI = 2.19–10.95), similar results were obtained. In subjects aged 65 and older, depressive symptoms were not associated with an increased risk of stroke/TIA. Taking antidepressant medications did not alter the risk associated with depressive symptoms. Depressive symptoms were thus an independent risk factor for incident stroke/TIA in individuals < 65 years.

However, in very elderly persons residing in a continuing-care retirement community ($N = 181$), controlling for demographic factors, both depression and the number of cardiovascular risk factors (CVRFs) at baseline were strongly predictive of stroke [23]. Depression accounted for 12% of the variance in stroke incidence, beyond the contribution of CVRFs.

Thus, pre-existing depression increases the risk for stroke.

Causes of post-stroke depression (and fatigue)

As mentioned above, in the Italian multicenter observational DESTRO study, a total of 53 centers consecutively admitted 1064 patients with ischemic or hemorrhagic stroke and assessed them periodically in the first 9 months after the event [7]. Risk factors for post-stroke depression were a history of depression, severe disability, previous stroke, and female gender, but not the type or site of the vascular lesion.

The relevance of established risk factors for depression in the community (such as female gender, prior personal history of depression, positive family history of depression, and somatic comorbidity other than stroke) and five potential disease-related risk factors (disability, cognitive deterioration, inter- and intra-hemispheric lesion location, and generalized vascular damage on computed tomography (CT) scan) were assessed in a multivariate prediction model for depression in the first year after stroke. The four general risk factors for depression in the community constituted a valid model to predict depression in stroke patients. Of the disease-specific factors, only incorporation of "disability" in this model improved its significance [24]. In the subacute to chronic phase, the causal contribution of stroke-specific factors may therefore be less than might be assumed.

Significantly higher correlations between self-esteem and mood ratings were noted in stroke patients as compared to healthy controls. Thus, lower self-esteem ratings do not appear to be a byproduct of depressive mood. Self-esteem is negatively impacted by stroke and is strongly, but independently, associated with depressive mood [25].

Genetic aspects seem to play a role in modifying the association between incident stroke and depression, as has been shown for the brain-derived neurotrophic factor (BDNF) gene val[66]met polymorphism. Five hundred community residents aged > 65 years without stroke or depression at baseline were re-evaluated after 2 years [26]. The association between incident stroke and depression was strengthened progressively with increasing numbers of met alleles, and was only significant in subjects with the met/met genotype after adjustment for disability and cognitive function.

In conclusion, genetic aspects, post-stroke disability, self-esteem, and certain established risk factors for depression in the community such as female gender and prior personal history of depression each increase the risk for post-stroke depression.

What increases the risk for post-stroke fatigue? A cross-sectional study with 220 consecutive outpatients at an average of 15 months after the onset of stroke assessed the presence of pre- and post-stroke fatigue, post-stroke depression, as well as various other factors [27]. One hundred and twenty-five patients (57%) had post-stroke fatigue, 83 (38%) had pre-stroke fatigue, and 53 (24%) had post-stroke depression. The impact of post-stroke fatigue on patients' daily activities was more severe in the physical domain as compared with the psychological or cognitive domains. Multivariate analyses showed that the presence of pre-stroke fatigue (OR 33.5), a high modified Rankin scale (OR 3.3), and post-stroke depression (OR 2.7) were independently associated with post-stroke fatigue. Thus, pre-stroke fatigue was the most important factor related to post-stroke fatigue in this study.

Associations with post-stroke depression

Early after stroke (within 3 weeks after a first-ever symptomatic stroke), moderate or severe symptoms of depression had been shown to be associated with a specific pattern of cognitive impairment (memory, visual perception, and language), lesion size (but not lesion location), and functional status (Barthel Index, Rankin scale) [28].

A cohort study examined prevalence of depression and anxiety as well as the relationships of age, gender, hemisphere of lesion, functional independence, and cognitive functioning (i.e. memory, attention/impulsivity, cognitive speed) to depression and anxiety at 3 months post-stroke in 73 individuals [29]. Prevalence of moderate to severe depression and anxiety in the sample were high (22.8 and 21.1%, respectively), with comorbidity in 12.3% of cases. In the regression analysis, 74.6% of the variance in depression was explained, with significant relationships between increased depression and younger age, reduced cognitive speed, poorer verbal memory, left hemisphere lesion, and increased impact of interference (Stroop ratio). Having a left-sided hemispheric lesion also contributed to the statistical prediction of anxiety, as did cognitive speed, explaining 50.7% of the variance. While age and side of hemispheric lesion contributed, cognitive performance explained the greatest proportion of variance in both depression and anxiety (51.3 and 38.5%, respectively).

These findings suggest that in the subacute phase of stroke cognition and mood are linked over and above physical independence.

Causes for the evolution of depression after stroke

In the Swedish national quality assessment register (Riks-Stroke), 15 747 stroke survivors were recorded. They were asked about depressive mood and antidepressant treatment 3 months after stroke. At 3 months after stroke, 12.4% of male and 16.4% of female stroke survivors reported that they always or often felt depressed. In a multiple logistic regression model, female gender, age younger than 65 years, living alone, having had a recurrent stroke, being dependent on others, and institutional living 3 months after stroke were independent predictors of self-reported depression [30].

The strength of religious beliefs has also been shown to influence the ability to cope after a stroke event, with stronger religious beliefs acting as a possible protective factor against emotional distress [31].

The aim of another cohort study of stroke patients admitted for rehabilitation was to identify factors that are significantly related to depression in chronic stroke patients, years after stroke onset [32]. A total of 165 first-ever stroke patients over 18 years of age were assessed at 1 and 3 years post-stroke. At 3 years post-stroke, 19% of the patients were depressed. Multivariate logistic regression analysis showed that depression at 3 years post-stroke was predicted by 1-year instrumental activities of daily living (ADL) and fatigue. Sensitivity of the model was 63%, while specificity was 85%.

A further cohort study assessed the correlates of depression at 3 and 15 months after stroke with a focus on dementia and vascular brain pathology. In a total of 164 consecutive eligible stroke patients, depression was not associated with age, intellectual decline prior to stroke, or side or severity of stroke [6]. Patients who experienced a TIA or stroke during the follow-up, who had developed dementia by 3 months, or who were not living with a relative or partner were more likely to be depressed at follow-up. Dementia at 3 months predicted depression, but the reverse did not hold. Depression therefore seemed related to cumulative vascular brain pathology rather than side and severity of single strokes. Fatigue, development of dementia, being dependent on others, living alone, institutional living, as well as recurrent stroke (or TIA) had a negative influence on the evolution of depression after stroke.

Effects of post-stroke depression

In a 6-month prospective cohort study of 141 post-acute stroke patients, demographic and clinical data on admission, and neurological, cognitive, depressive symptoms, and functional variables on admission and at 6 months after stroke were measured. Multivariate analysis indicated that greater magnitudes of functional recovery (Barthel Index change score) were achieved by patients with better baseline depressive symptoms and improvement over time. Functional recovery was not related to baseline cognitive status or its improvement, however [33]. These data suggested that depressive symptoms early after stroke are inversely related to functional recovery that again is improved when depressive symptoms improve, suggesting an independent causal role for depression in limiting functional recovery.

Previous mood disorder, an independent predictor of post-stroke depression [34], also reduces the odds of favorable outcome: among stroke patients who survived hospitalization, those with pre-existing depression had significantly higher odds of being discharged to an institution instead of their home than did patients without any pre-existing mental health condition [35].

Neuroscience reasoning

Neuroimaging evidence

To investigate age-related white matter changes on magnetic resonance imaging (MRI) as an independent predictor of depressive symptoms at 1 year, after controlling for known confounders, a pan-European multicenter study followed 639 older adults without significant disability and assessed MRI white matter changes as well as demographic and clinical variables that included cognitive scores, quality of life, disability, and depressive symptoms. Clinical assessments were repeated at 1 year. Using logistic regression analysis, severity of white matter changes at baseline was shown to independently and significantly predict depressive symptoms at 1 year after controlling for baseline depressive symptoms, quality of life, and worsening disability [36]. Thus, white matter changes (independent of stroke) pre-dated and were related to the development of depressive symptoms, suggesting the possibility of an organic cause.

Some studies have suggested that post-stroke depression and anxiety are specifically related to organic lesions in the anterior parts of the left hemisphere.

To test the independent effects of lesion location (left hemisphere, anterior region) and of co-occurring generalized vascular damage on the development of depression in the first year after ischemic stroke, while other risk factors for depression were controlled for, 190 patients with a first-ever, supratentorial infarct were followed up for 1 year [37]. CT was performed in the acute phase of stroke, while in 75 patients an additional MRI scan was also available. Negative results appeared from one overall, multivariate analysis including variables of both focal and generalized vascular brain damage, as well as other non-cerebral risk factors. In addition, level of handicap and neuroticism were independent predictors of depression in this cohort. A biopsychosocial model including both premorbid (prior to stroke) vulnerability factors, such as neuroticism and (family) history of depression, as well as post-stroke stressors, such as level of handicap, could be substantiated as risk factors in this predictive model while lesion location (left hemisphere, anterior region) or co-occurring generalized vascular damage could not.

However, other studies support a possible contribution of lesion site to depression onset. When 70 patients with a single brain infarct on MRI were studied 3 months after ischemic stroke by a standardized protocol that detailed side, site, type, and extent of the brain infarct, as well as severity of white matter lesions and brain atrophy, it could be shown that affected structures of the frontal–subcortical circuits, i.e. the pallidum and caudate, especially on the left side, predisposed stroke patients to depression (diagnosed by DSM-III-R and DSM-IV criteria) [38]. Note too that the size of the infarcts at these sites was larger among depressed patients. Using a logistic regression analysis, the authors found that a brain infarct that affected the pallidum was a strong independent MRI predictor for post-stroke depression (odds ratio = 7.2).

Further, a meta-analysis of the correlation between severity of depression following stroke and proximity of the lesion to the frontal pole showed that there was a significant inverse correlation between severity of depression and distance of the lesion from the frontal pole among 163 patients with left hemisphere stroke, but not among 106 patients with right hemisphere stroke [39].

Any role of specific sites of brain lesion in the development of post-stroke depression might be further modified by the specific constellation of the individual neuropsychiatric post-stroke disorder.

In a study with 243 stroke patients the severity of *affective depression* (Zung Self-rating Depression Scale scores) was associated with left frontal lobe (but not basal ganglia) damage, while that of *apathetic depression* (Apathy Scale scores) was related to damage to the bilateral basal ganglia (but not to the frontal lobe) [40].

In a separate study, stroke patients who had both post-stroke depression and an executive dysfunction, i.e. a depression–dysexecutive syndrome, were studied. Examination included neurological, psychiatric, and neuropsychological examination carried out 3 months after ischemic stroke, and included an MRI to evaluate brain infarcts, white-matter changes, and brain atrophy. These 21 patients with depression–dysexecutive syndrome had significantly more brain infarcts affecting their frontal–subcortical circuit structures than the 137 patients without depression–dysexecutive syndrome, or the 41 patients with depression but without executive dysfunction [41]. Patients with depression–dysexecutive syndrome also had more severe depressive symptoms and worse psychosocial functioning, and they coped less well in complex activities of daily living.

In addition, right hemisphere damage can influence the presentation of depressive disorders ensuing after stroke by disrupting emotion processing mechanisms. Compared to dysphoric depression, nondysphoric

depression (i.e. depressive ideation without endorsement of sad emotions) in acute stroke patients showed more frequent right anterior hemisphere lesions. The location of damage suggested that nondysphoric depression may be a special presentation of depressive disorder following stroke in which right hemisphere damage limits the apprehension of personal emotional changes [42].

The frontal midline structures have been demonstrated by functional neuroimaging to be involved in the affective control of human behavior. A case study documented a patient with a right anterior cingulate infarct who presented with an alexithymia-like disorder [43].

Inability to control anger or aggression (ICAA) had been shown to be associated with lesions affecting frontal–lenticulocapsular–pontine base areas [15].

Thus, there might be reason to assume that studies that failed to demonstrate an association between lesion side and site and post-stroke depression might have reached their conclusions in some instances because the anatomical correlates of post-stroke depression differ depending on the specific presentation of post-stroke depression (e.g. affective, nondysphoric, or apathetic). As a notion of caution it must, however, be stated that the above-mentioned evidence assessed only a subset of aspects and that this hypothesis requires validation in a pooled multivariate analysis.

The serotonergic system

There is some evidence that points to a role of the serotonergic system in post-stroke depression.

Variations of serotonin transporter-linked promoter region (5-HTTLPR) functional polymorphism were assessed in 26 stroke patients with major depression and in 25 unrelated nondepressed stroke subjects. The findings indicated a significant association between 5-HTTLPR short variant genotype and post-stroke major depression [44].

The intensity dependence of the auditory-evoked potentials (IDAP) is inversely related to serotonergic tone. The linear amplitude/stimulus intensity function (ASF) slope, by measuring the peak-to-peak amplitude of Nl-P2, was found to be markedly increased in stroke patients compared with controls; while stroke patients with depressive symptoms had a significantly steeper ASF slope than controls, there was no statistical difference in ASF slope between stroke patients without depressive symptoms and controls [45]. Together, these findings suggest that the serotonergic system might be involved in post-stroke depression.

For both post-stroke depression and pathological crying, an imbalance of serotonergic neurotransmission has been postulated. To test this hypothesis, patients with acute stroke and pathological crying underwent PET scanning, with results compared to age-matched healthy control subjects [46]. Maps of 5-HT(1A) receptor availability were generated from the images of eight cortical regions and raphe nuclei. The maps showed highest binding in limbic areas and raphe nuclei, while binding in basal ganglia and cerebellum was negligible. Baseline binding potentials of patients were lower than those of control subjects. Treatment with selective serotonin reuptake inhibitor (SSRI) markedly reduced extent of free receptor sites, whereas placebo administration led to a global increase. The study results thus described changes in serotonergic neurotransmission in the early phase of stroke and their modulation with SSRI treatment, and suggested a possible relationship to pathological crying.

Metabolic changes

Metabolic changes might also be associated with post-stroke depression and might be modified by time, i.e. might differ in depression early and late after stroke as a hint to different involved mechanisms. In groups of first-ever stroke patients, the relationship between post-stroke depression and the metabolic/biochemical milieu, as assessed by proton magnetic resonance spectroscopy (1)H-MRS measurements in unaffected frontal lobes, was assessed. Single-voxel proton magnetic resonance spectroscopy ((1)H-MRS) was performed in these lobes to assess N-acetylaspartate/ creatine (NAA)/Cr, glutamate+glutamine (Glx)/Cr, choline (Cho)/Cr and *myo*-inositol (mI)/Cr ratios. Twenty-six patients with a first ischemic stroke located outside the frontal lobes were studied [47]. Patients were assessed within the first 10 days after stroke and again 4 months later. In the group of 26 patients, 8 (31%) met criteria for depression at the first assessment, and 9 (35%) met criteria for depression at follow-up. Patients with depression in the immediate post-stroke phase had significantly higher Glx/Cr ratios in the contralesional hemisphere than non-depressive patients. No biochemical differences were found between the groups at 4-month follow-up. These findings suggested that post-stroke depression is accompanied by changes in frontal lobe glutamate/ glutamine levels, perhaps reflecting abnormalities in

glutamatergic transmission in the immediate post-stroke period. Further, 13 out of a sample of 31 stroke patients (42%) demonstrated apathy. Of these subjects, significantly lowered NAA/Cr ratios were found in the right hemispheres of apathetic patients in the subgroup with left-sided brain lesions. These findings point to the association between apathy and frontal lobe integrity, suggest different reactions of the hemispheres, and indicate that changes in the NAA/Cr ratio could be related to the apathy [48]. Whether these metabolic changes are a contributor to, or a mere reflection of, these emotional states requires further study.

Implications for recovery

Post-stroke depression has been shown to impede the rehabilitation progress following stroke and to be associated with impaired functional outcome, cognitive decline, and increased mortality [49]. Similarly, depression has been linked to increased risk of stroke occurrence.

Post-stroke depression and its impact on activities of daily living functions

A cohort study examined the relationship between depressive symptoms and time courses in achieving independence in basic activities of daily living (bADL) and instrumental activities of daily living (iADL) [50]. At baseline, 1, 3, and 6 months after stroke, 459 stroke patients were prospectively assessed with the Geriatric Depression Scale (GDS) to determine depressive status, outcomes were achieved independence in bADL (Barthel Index scores > 95) and independence in at least three iADL during follow-up. Depressed patients were 0.3 times less likely than nondepressed patients to achieve bADL score of > 95 and 0.4-times less likely to be independent in three or more iADL. The cumulative percentages to achieve a bADL score of > 95 are shown in Figure 14.1. Similarly, the cumulative percentages for nondepressed patients to achieve complete independence in three or more iADL at 1, 3, and 6 months after stroke were 56%, 72%, and 85%, and for the depressed patients, they were 32%, 47%, and 72%, respectively. Thus, depressed patients had significantly poorer functional recovery patterns and took longer to achieve independence with activities of daily living.

Another cohort study investigated the association between stroke and depression, the co-occurrence of

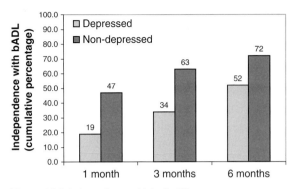

Figure 14.1 Independence with basic ADLs.
The cumulative percentage of non-depressed and depressed stroke patients who are independent with basic activities of daily living (bADL) indicates that stroke patients with depressive symptoms progressed significantly more slowly in achieving independence during the first 6 months after stroke [50].

stroke and depression, and functional health outcomes among adults in the US population using a nationally representative sample of adults aged 25–74. Multiple logistic regression analyses were used to determine the association between stroke (past 12-month prevalence), depression (past 12-month prevalence), and functional health outcomes (past 12 months), and to determine whether there is an interaction between depression and stroke in predicting impairment in functioning. Almost one-third (29.2%) of adults with stroke in the past year also had depression in the past year. The co-occurrence of stroke and depression was associated with significantly greater limitations in walking and climbing stairs and poorer general physical functioning as compared to either stroke or depression alone [51].

Similarly, a further cohort study assessed the frequency and correlates of depression at 3 and 15 months after stroke in a total of 164 consecutive eligible stroke patients [52]. Major or minor depression was present in 20.7% at follow-up. By follow-up, stroke patients with depression had significantly greater impairment of functional ability and global cognition than nondepressed stroke patients or comparison subjects.

While post-stroke depression seems to have a negative impact on ADL activities and quality of life after stroke, there is some evidence to suggest that motor recovery (sensu stricto), i.e. regarding selective innervation and active movement capacity as assessed with the Fugl-Meyer scale, is not affected by post-stroke depression [53].

The picture that emerges from these studies is that post-stroke depression might not impede motor recovery per se in the more restricted sense of regaining selective innervation when paresis followed stroke. However, it seems to affect the ability to use elementary motor behaviors to perform ADL negatively, and to have the effect of retarding the re-acquisition of these functional skills. These effects are not contradictory, since the ability to perform activities of daily living is more complex, i.e. determined by both perceptive and motor recovery, as well as the ability to compensate for any remaining neuro-impairments.

Post-stroke depression and its impact on participation and quality of life

The determinants of "restricted participation", i.e. the degree of inability to perform social roles, had also been investigated among long-term stroke survivors [54]. Self-competence with basic activities of daily living (Functional Independence Measure, FIM) and emotional status (HADS) are the independent determinants of restricted participation for the London Handicap Scale (LHS) domains most related to body function (mobility, physical independence, occupation). Depression was the determinant factor for orientation and social integration. Thus, both functional disability and mood disorders may independently contribute to the restricted participation of post-stroke patients.

In another population-based investigation of 266 patients with incident stroke, among those who were alive at 2 years ($N = 226$; 85%), handicap was also assessed with the LHS [55]. Disability, physical impairment, depression, anxiety, living arrangements, and recurrent stroke at 2 years were also documented; if necessary, proxy assessments were obtained, except for mood. The independent determinants of handicap (LHS) were age and 2-year physical impairment and disability. In the analysis restricted to nonproxy data, depression and anxiety were also independently associated with handicap.

Further, fewer depressive symptoms after stroke – together with walking and acceptance of the stroke – have been documented as the best predictors for participation at 3 months in older adults who had a stroke [56]. Similarly, depression was also most significantly and independently associated with post-stroke handicap at 12 months post-stroke among elderly stroke victims [57].

In a group of stroke patients with a first unilateral, middle cerebral artery (MCA) territory stroke, no significant neurological improvement could be documented between 3 and 12 months after the stroke [58]. The patients as a group were depressed and remained so over the period of the study. The resulting quality of life scores were abnormal at 3 months and improved only slightly. Stepwise regression analysis revealed that depression and degree of paresis were the most important variables for the quality of life outcome (Sickness Impact Profile, SIP).

In another study, post-stroke depression seemed to exert a generalized negative influence on health-related quality of life (at 1 year post-stroke), while dependence on caregivers for ADL affected only some dimensions of health-related quality of life [59].

In summary, post-stroke depression seems to exert a profound negative effect on health-related quality of life and participation including social integration. These detrimental effects seem to be caused by post-stroke depression beyond and above what is attributable to physical impairment and disability.

Can treatment of post-stroke depression ameliorate its negative effects on ADL functions?

Given these suggested profound effects of post-stroke depression, it would be important to know whether intervention for post-stroke depression, to be described in a later section, can effectively treat the disorder and thereby influence functional recovery, participation, and quality of life. This type of knowledge would be important for clinical therapeutic purposes as well as in relationship to above negative associations.

One study examined the differences in functional recovery among post-stroke depressed patients compared to post-stroke nondepressed patients over the course of 6 months after stroke. Patients had suffered from first-time stroke, and did not have a history of premorbid depression. During follow-up, treatment with 20 mg/day citalopram was initiated whenever a diagnosis of depression was established. Functional recovery was assessed using the Scandinavian Stroke Scale, the modified Rankin Scale, and the Barthel Index during acute hospitalization, at the time of depression diagnosis and at the third and sixth month follow-up visits. All stroke patients with post-stroke depression whose mood improved after administration

of citalopram showed also improved ADL functions during the follow-up, suggesting that remission of post-stroke depression was associated with improvement in functional recovery [60].

Another study examined the effect of early versus late treatment with antidepressants on recovery in ADL [61]. Among 62 patients after stroke, the therapeutic effect of a 3-month course of antidepressants begun during the first month after stroke was compared with the effect of treatment begun after 1 month. ADL functions were assessed with the Functional Independence Measure (FIM); post-treatment outcome was assessed over the following 21 months. Although both the early and late treatment groups showed improvements in FIM scores during the 3 months of treatment, the early treatment group improved significantly more than did the late treatment group, consistent with the time course of recovery-related cellular events that take place in the brain after stroke (see also Chapters 1–3 and 6–7). After the treatment, the early treatment group maintained this improvement over 2 years while the late treatment group deteriorated over time. There were no significant differences in the two groups that would explain the findings. Therefore, recovery in ADL functions after stroke appeared to be enhanced by the use of antidepressant medication if treatment was started within the first month after stroke. One might speculate that this earlier antidepressant intervention enables maximum expression of post-stroke cellular repair processes.

These observations strengthen the view that post-stroke depression exerts a negative effect on the recovery in ADL functions and that its negative effects can be ameliorated by antidepressant medication. Early initiation of antidepressant treatment might meet a specific therapeutic window.

It had further been assessed whether antidepressant treatment would even reduce post-stroke mortality (over 9 years of follow-up) [62]. A total of 104 patients had randomly been assigned to receive a 12-week double-blind course of nortriptyline, fluoxetine, or placebo early in the recovery period after a stroke. Mortality data were obtained for all 104 patients 9 years after initiation of the study. Of the 104 patients, 50 (48.1%) had died by the time of the 9-year follow-up. Of 53 patients who were given full-dose antidepressants, 36 (67.9%) were alive at follow-up, compared with only 10 (35.7%) of 28 placebo-treated patients, a significant difference. Logistic regression analysis showed that the beneficial effect of antidepressants remained significant both in patients who were depressed and in those who were nondepressed at enrollment, after the effects of other factors associated with mortality (i.e. age, co-existing diabetes mellitus, and chronic relapsing depression) were controlled. There were no intergroup differences in severity of stroke, impairment in cognitive functioning and ADL, and other medications received. Treatment with fluoxetine or nortriptyline for 12 weeks during the first 6 months post-stroke therefore seemed to have increased the survival of both depressed and nondepressed patients.

It is also of interest to note that veterans who received antidepressant prescription after acute stroke showed a lower 1 year all-cause mortality rate (4.8%) as compared to those who did not (8.0%) [63].

Further implications

Family life

Perception of deficits is a prerequisite for post-stroke management. Goal setting, adjustments, and action plans might best be facilitated, and thereby stress reduced, when they can be agreed on by the patient, his or her family, and healthcare professionals. Anosognosia, the reduced ability to perceive deficits such as neuro-impairments including cognitive and emotional post-stroke disorders, is more frequently and typically seen after right brain damage and poses problems in that respect.

The presence and severity of changes in emotion and cognition as experienced by left- and right-sided stroke patients at 3 months post-stroke has been compared with those observed by their partners [64]. It appeared that while left hemisphere stroke patients agreed with their partners on the number and severity of most changes, partners of right hemisphere patients reported more frequent and more severe changes than did the patients themselves.

Aside from differences in perceiving deficits, family members can be profoundly affected by disability caused by stroke: Both stroke patients' degree of disability and post-stroke depression affect emotional stress and marital dissatisfaction of caregivers and spouses. A consistent association between patients' levels of disability and emotional state and the emotional distress of their caregivers has been documented [65]. Patient depression in particular constitutes a risk factor for marital dissatisfaction in the first few months following stroke [66].

Given that spousal partners provide a large portion of informal support to stroke patients, successful treatment of patient depression may therefore have benefits at the level of the individual and the family.

In a study of sexual dysfunction among 100 patients (75 men and 25 women) following stroke and its relationship to neuropsychiatric impairments or stroke characteristics, 44 men (58.6%) and 11 women (44.0%) reported dissatisfaction with their sexual functioning after stroke, as compared with only 16 men (21.3%) and 5 women (20.0%) before stroke [67]. Based on logistic regression, post-stroke depression (OR, 8.09; 95% CI, 1.28–51.38) was a strong independent predictor of sexual dysfunction.

Healthcare utilization

Post-stroke depression might be one cause of increased healthcare utilization. After adjusting for patient demographic and clinical factors, a study among veterans found that patients with stroke and post-stroke depression had significantly more hospitalizations, outpatient visits, and longer length of stays 12 months post-stroke compared with stroke patients without post-stroke depression [68]. Thus, patients with post-stroke depression had greater 12-month post-stroke healthcare use even when controlling for other demographic and clinical variables.

Therefore, appropriate diagnosis and treatment of post-stroke depression might have the potential not only to benefit the patient, but also to influence healthcare utilization.

Therapeutic options

Treatment of post-stroke depression with antidepressants

At present, pharmacological treatment of post-stroke depression consists mainly of selective serotonin reuptake inhibitors and serotonin noradrenaline reuptake inhibitors [69]. Tricyclic antidepressive therapy is also effective, but often unsuitable due to side effects.

A meta-analysis of randomized placebo-controlled trials (RCTs) of antidepressants in post-stroke patients with depression was conducted using published studies from 1984 to 2006 [70]. Outcome measures of antidepressant treatment included response rate, depression rating scale scores, recovery of neurologic impairments, and improvements in ADLs after stroke. The effect size was presented as rate difference (RD)

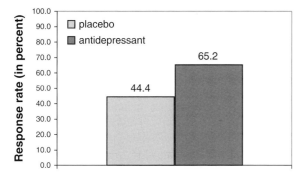

Figure 14.2 Response rate to antidepressants.
The response rate (in percent) to either placebo or antidepressants as indicated by a meta-analysis of a total of 1320 patients with post-stroke depression from 16 RCTs [70].

and weighted mean difference for dichotomous outcomes and continuous outcomes, respectively. A total of 1320 patients who met inclusion criteria were identified from 16 RCTs. The pooled response rates in the active and placebo groups were 65.18% (234/359) and 44.37% (138/311), respectively (see Figure 14.2). The pooled RD was 0.23 (95% CI 0.03–0.43), indicating a significantly higher response rate in the active group compared with the placebo group. From baseline to endpoint, patients in the active group had significantly greater improvement in depressive symptoms compared with patients in the placebo group. Longer duration of treatment was positively correlated with the degree of improvement in depressive symptoms (Spearman's correlation, rho = 0.93). However, no consistent evidence was found for positive antidepressant effects on the recovery of neurological impairments or improvements in ADLs.

A double-blinded, placebo-controlled study evaluated the efficacy and tolerability of the noradrenaline reuptake inhibitor (NARI) reboxetine in a subset of post-stroke patients classified as affected by retarded depression [71], defined by the authors as "a state of clinical depression in which the individual is lethargic and slow to initiate action." Reboxetine (4 mg, twice daily, for 16 weeks) was administered to patients who developed depression after a single ischemic or hemorrhagic stroke. Reboxetine showed good efficacy, safety, and tolerability in post-stroke depression patients affected by retarded depression; at week 16, HDRS and BDI mean scores were, respectively, 22.73 and 18.4 in the placebo group, and 9.26 and 8.06 in the reboxetine group.

Similarly, the efficacy and safety of the selective serotonin reuptake inhibitor (SSRI) citalopram, and the NARI reboxetine, were investigated in post-stroke patients affected by either anxious depression or retarded depression with a randomized double-blind study [72]. Seventy-four post-stroke depressed patients were diagnosed as affected by anxious or retarded depression. Randomization was planned so that 50% of the patients in each subgroup were assigned for 16 weeks to treatment with citalopram and the remaining 50% were assigned to treatment with reboxetine. Both citalopram and reboxetine showed good safety and tolerability. Citalopram exhibited greater efficacy in anxious depressed patients, while reboxetine was more effective in retarded depressed patients.

Effects of antidepressants on other post-stroke emotional disorders

Antidepressants can reduce the frequency and severity of pathological crying or laughing episodes after stroke [73]. The effect was not specific to one drug or class of drugs.

Fluoxetine seems not to be effective in the treatment of post-stroke fatigue (PoSF): a double-blind, placebo-controlled study showed no differences in the number of patients with PoSF between the fluoxetine group and the placebo group at 3 and 6 months after the treatment [74]. However, fluoxetine significantly improved post-stroke emotional incontinence and post-stroke depression in the patients with PoSF.

In another double-blind, placebo-controlled study, fluoxetine significantly improved emotional incontinence, and anger proneness, whereas no definitive improvement of post-stroke depression was found [75]. Improvement of post-stroke depression and anger proneness was noted even at 3 months after the discontinuation of the treatment.

A post-hoc analysis of an antidepressant treatment trial assessed correlates of irritability and aggression after stroke and changes in irritability scores associated with antidepressant treatment [76]. Aggressive patients were compared with nonaggressive patients. All patients were randomized to receive nortriptyline, fluoxetine, or placebo using a double-blind methodology. Among irritable and aggressive patients with depression who responded to antidepressants, there was a significantly greater reduction in irritability after treatment, compared with patients whose depression did not lessen with treatment. The results of this small study suggest that successful treatment of depression may reduce aggressive behavior.

Non-pharmacological treatment of post-stroke depression

Nonmedication treatment options might include repetitive transcranial magnetic stimulation (rTMS). A randomized, parallel, double-blind study of active versus sham rTMS assessed the effects of left prefrontal rTMS in patients with medication-refractory post-stroke depression. After discontinuing antidepressants, patients were randomly assigned to receive 10 sessions of active (10 Hz, 110% of the motor threshold, 20 trains of 5 s duration) or sham left prefrontal rTMS [77]. When compared with sham stimulation, 10 sessions of active rTMS of the left dorsolateral prefrontal cortex were associated with a significant reduction of depressive symptoms. This reduction was not influenced by patient's age, type or location of stroke, volume of left frontal leukoaraiosis, or by the distance of the stimulating coil to the prefrontal cortex. In addition, there were few and mild adverse effects that were equally distributed among groups. Taken together, these preliminary findings suggest that rTMS may be an effective and safe treatment alternative for patients with refractory depression after stroke.

The effect of an adjunct light therapy in stroke victims with major depression receiving citalopram was examined by use of two different intensities of light therapy under double-blind conditions. Altogether, 63 patients were included in the study. After 4 weeks of therapy, the 6-item subscale of the HADRS showed a larger improvement in patients receiving high-intensity light treatment compared to those treated with medium-intensity light [78].

Healthcare management with post-stroke depression

While efficacy of drug therapy is one issue, another issue in treatment of relatively neglected medical conditions such as post-stroke depression is whether and how management of care improves outcome.

When 5-year survivors from a prospective community-based stroke incidence study were assessed for depression, 17% of those assessed were depressed [79]. However, only 22% of these patients with depression were taking an antidepressant medication. Of those taking an antidepressant, 72% were not depressed. Thus, although nearly one-fifth of survivors were depressed, few were taking antidepressants although the treatment is likely to be effective.

A randomized, outcome-blinded multisite trial in 188 ischemic stroke survivors with post-stroke depression investigated the efficacy of a care management program; it performed depression screening and enrollment between 1 and 2 months post-stroke [80]. The Activate–Initiate–Monitor intervention was a care management program that included activation of the patient to recognize depression symptoms and accept treatment, initiation of an antidepressant medication, and monitoring and adjusting treatment. Usual care subjects received nondepression-related education and were prescribed antidepressants at the discretion of their provider. The primary outcome measure was depression response, defined as a Hamilton Depression Inventory score < 8 (remission) or a decrease from baseline of at least 50% at 12 weeks. Both depression response (51% versus 30%) and remission (39% versus 23%) were more likely in the Activate–Initiate–Monitor intervention than in the usual care group. This difference in depression scores was present by 6 weeks and persisted through the 12-week assessment. The Activate–Initiate–Monitor care management model was thus more efficacious than usual care in improving depression outcomes in patients with post-stroke depression.

Are there reasons to promote prevention of post-stroke depression?

Information provision, physical exercise programs, and listening to music

A recent meta-analysis assessed the effectiveness of information provision strategies in improving the outcome for stroke patients and/or their identified caregivers; there is evidence that information improves patient and caregiver knowledge of stroke, aspects of patient satisfaction, and reduces patient depression scores [81].

Physical exercise programs might also help to prevent post-stroke depression and improve physical and emotional outcome. When 100 stroke survivors who had completed acute rehabilitation were randomly assigned to either a progressive, structured, 3-month physical exercise program, or usual care only, significant differences were found: 6 (14%) of the exercise group and 16 (35.6%) of the usual-care group had depressive symptoms at 3 months (93 assessed) (see Figure 14.3) [82]. At 9 months (80 assessed), 3 (7.5%) of the exercisers had significant depressive symptoms compared with 10 (25%) who received usual care.

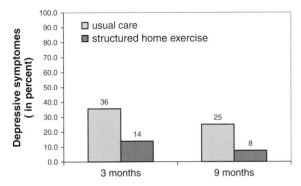

Figure 14.3 Prevalence of depressive symptoms among stroke survivors following a structured, 3-month physical exercise program at home or usual care only.

The prevalence of depressive symptoms (in percent) among stroke survivors was significantly lower among stroke victims who received a structured, 3-month physical exercise program at home as compared to those who received usual care only. Data from a randomized controlled trial [82].

Participants with and without baseline depressive symptoms had equivalent treatment-related gains in impairments and functional limitations, but only participants with depressive symptoms had improved quality of life. It might be concluded that exercise may help to reduce post-stroke depressive symptoms. In this study, depressive symptoms did not limit gains in physical function due to exercise. Further, exercise may contribute to improved quality of life in those with post-stroke depressive symptoms.

Similarly, for bedridden stroke survivors in residential care, it could be demonstrated by a randomized controlled trial that among other effects a simple nurse-led range-of-motion exercise program can generate positive effects on depressive symptoms among bedridden older people with stroke [83].

Further, listening to music could be a preventive measure for negative mood after stroke. In an RCT, MCA stroke patients who listened daily to self-selected music for 2 months showed lower depression scores after 3 months post-stroke as compared to two control groups who either listened to audio books or received usual treatment only [84].

Prophylactic antidepressant treatment

Other studies have examined whether prophylactic antidepressant treatment can prevent depression and improve functional outcome (ADL functions, participation, quality of life), with good tolerability and safety in nondepressed patients with recent stroke.

To test whether prophylactic treatment with the antidepressant mirtazapine (30 mg/day) in patients with acute stroke starting one day after stroke onset prevents post-stroke depression, 70 patients were enrolled in an open randomized controlled study and were re-examined up to day 380 post-stroke [85]. Those post-stroke patients who developed depression (DSM-IV criteria) but had been randomly assigned to the non-treatment group were given the antidepressant mirtazapine after the diagnosis of depression had been established. Forty percent (14/35) of the non-treated patients and only 5.7% (2/35) of the patients who were treated with mirtazapine developed post-stroke depression. Altogether, 16 patients developed post-stroke depression, 15 of whom remitted after initiation of treatment with mirtazapine.

Sertraline (50 mg/day), however, was not effective to prevent post-stroke depression in a double-blind, placebo-controlled 24-week clinical trial [86].

A multisite RCT for prevention of depression among 176 nondepressed patients was conducted within 3 months following acute stroke with a double-blind placebo-controlled comparison of escitalopram with placebo, and a nonblinded problem-solving therapy group [87]. The use of either escitalopram or problem-solving therapy resulted in a significantly lower incidence of depression over 12 months of treatment as compared with placebo. However, only escitalopram, but not the problem-solving therapy, achieved significant results over placebo using an intention-to-treat conservative method of analysis.

A meta-analysis of randomized placebo-controlled trials also provided support for a prophylactic effect of antidepressants in nondepressed patients with stroke [88]. The search included trials from 1950 to August 2006. From 10 RCTs, a total of 703 non-depressed patients after stroke were identified. The pooled occurrence rate of newly developed post-stroke depression cases in the intervention and control groups differed significantly, being 12.54% (41/327) and 29.17% (91/312), respectively (pooled rate difference = −0.17, 95% confidence interval = −0.26 to −0.08). Prophylactic effects of antidepressants were not related to duration of use.

In conclusion, antidepressant prophylaxis is associated with a significant reduction in the occurrence rate of newly developed post-stroke depression, suggesting antidepressants may be considered along with other preventive strategies in the management of stroke patients.

Table 14.1 Risk factors, consequences, and treatment options for post-stroke depression

Risk factors for post-stroke depression	
Pre-existing	Genetic factors, female gender, history of depression, history of stroke, living alone
Current	Severe disability, reduced self-esteem, fatigue, dementia, communication deficits, further TIA or stroke damage to the pallidum and caudate (esp. on the left), left frontal lobe (affective depression), basal ganglia (aphathetic d.), right anterior lobe (nondysphoric d.), frontal midline (alexithymia)
Consequences of post-stroke depression	
Recovery	Reduced ADL function recovery, reduced participation, reduced quality of life
Family life	Emotional distress and marital dissatisfaction of spouse, sexual dysfunction
Mortality	Increased mortality
Health care	Increased utilization
Therapeutic and preventive remedies for post-stroke depression	
Therapy	Antidepressants, e.g. SSRI, NARI, managed health care/clinical pathways, rTMS, high-intensity light therapy
Prevention	Stroke-specific information provision, physical exercise program, antidepressants, listening to music program

Summary and implications for future research

Cause and effects of post-stroke recovery and its treatment

Risk factors for, and consequences of, post-stroke depression, as well as therapeutic and potentially preventive measures, have been summarized in Table 14.1. Pre-existing and current biological, psychological, and social factors all contribute to the risk to develop post-stroke depression. Most importantly, post-stroke depression seems to exert a profound and independent negative effect on ADL functions, participation, and quality of life of stroke victims, has a considerable negative impact on other family members, and is yet a relatively neglected entity. Managed care programs (clinical pathways) might help to improve healthcare for post-stroke depression and thereby foster outcome. Surprisingly little is known, however, about the potential treatment and prevention impact on participation and quality of life after stroke.

Further, our knowledge about complex, e.g. combined non-pharmacological and pharmacological, intervention schemes that could likely treat and prevent post-stroke depression is scarce.

Cortical reorganization of emotion processing

While the above-mentioned evidence sheds light on the association between post-stroke emotional disorders and lesion size and location, functional neuroimaging could also contribute to our understanding of cortical reorganization of emotional experiences and reactions after stroke, providing insights as described with motor, language, and attentional deficits after stroke (see Chapters 9–13).

One behavioral and functional imaging study demonstrates the feasibility of such an approach. In this study, patients with stroke affecting cerebellum reported an unpleasant experience to frightening stimuli similar to healthy controls, yet showed significantly lower activity in the right ventral lateral and left dorsolateral prefrontal cortex, amygdala, thalamus, and retrosplenial cingulate gyrus. However, frightening stimuli led to increased activity in the ventral medial prefrontal, anterior cingulate, pulvinar, and insular cortex [89]. This suggests that focal injury produced a change in the neural circuitry underlying emotional processing, a finding of the sort that could set the stage for gaining greater insights into post-stroke depression and its therapy via functional neuroimaging.

Summary

This chapter has described the scope of post-stroke depression. Contributing factors were summarized, from genetics to anatomical site of injury. The wide-reaching consequences of this condition were described, and include substantial effects at all levels of function. Therapeutic options, from prevention to therapy, were summarized. Post-stroke depression is common and has major effects. Further research can aim to better understand this disorder, individualize its therapy, and increase the fraction of patients for whom post-stroke depression is successfully treated.

References

1. Spalletta G, Ripa A, Caltagirone C. Symptom profile of DSM-IV major and minor depressive disorders in first-ever stroke patients. *Am J Geriatr Psychiatry.* 2005;**13**:108–15.

2. Laska AC, Martensson B, Kahan T, *et al.* Recognition of depression in aphasic stroke patients. *Cerebrovasc Dis.* 2007;**24**:74–9.

3. Bennett HE, Thomas SA, Austen R, *et al.* Validation of screening measures for assessing mood in stroke patients. *Br J Clin Psychol.* 2006;**45**:367–76.

4. Benaim C, Cailly B, Perennou D, *et al.* Validation of the aphasic depression rating scale. *Stroke.* 2004;**35**:1692–6.

5. Fure B. [Depression, anxiety and other emotional symptoms after cerebral stroke.] *Tidsskr Nor Laegeforen.* 2007;**127**:1387–9.

6. Brodaty H, Withall A, Altendorf A, *et al.* Rates of depression at 3 and 15 months post-stroke and their relationship with cognitive decline: The Sydney Stroke Study. *Am J Geriatr Psychiatry.* 2007;**15**:477–86.

7. Paolucci S, Gandolfo C, Provinciali L, *et al.* The Italian multicenter observational study on post-stroke depression (DESTRO). *J Neurol.* 2006;**253**:556–62.

8. Linden T, Blomstrand C, Skoog I. Depressive disorders after 20 months in elderly stroke patients: A case-control study. *Stroke.* 2007;**38**:1860–3.

9. Thomas SA, Lincoln NB. Factors relating to depression after stroke. *Br J Clin Psychol.* 2006;**45**:49–61.

10. Skaner Y, Nilsson GH, Sundquist K, *et al.* Self-rated health, symptoms of depression and general symptoms at 3 and 12 months after a first-ever stroke: A municipality-based study in Sweden. *BMC Fam Pract.* 2007;**8**:61.

11. Fure B, Wyller TB, Engedal K, *et al.* Emotional symptoms in acute ischemic stroke. *Int J Geriatr Psychiatry.* 2006;**21**:382–7.

12. Smith LN, Norrie J, Kerr SM, *et al.* Impact and influences on caregiver outcomes at one year post-stroke. *Cerebrovasc Dis.* 2004;**18**:145–53.

13. Morrison V, Pollard B, Johnston M, *et al.* Anxiety and depression 3 years following stroke: Demographic, clinical, and psychological predictors. *J Psychosom Res.* 2005;**59**:209–13.

14. Santos CO, Caeiro L, Ferro JM, *et al.* Anger, hostility and aggression in the first days of acute stroke. *Eur J Neurol.* 2006;**13**:351–8.

15. Kim JS, Choi S, Kwon SU, *et al.* Inability to control anger or aggression after stroke. *Neurology.* 2002;**58**:1106–08.

16. Bogousslavsky J. William Feinberg lecture 2002: Emotions, mood, and behavior after stroke. *Stroke.* 2003;**34**:1046–50.

17. Spalletta G, Serra L, Fadda L, *et al.* Unawareness of motor impairment and emotions in right hemispheric stroke: A preliminary investigation. *Int J Geriatr Psychiatry.* 2007;**22**:1241–6.

18. Stone J, Townend E, Kwan J, *et al.* Personality change after stroke: Some preliminary observations. *J Neurol Neurosurg Psychiatry.* 2004;**75**:1708–13.

19. Bos MJ, Linden T, Koudstaal PJ, *et al.* Depressive symptoms and risk of stroke: The Rotterdam Study. *J Neurol Neurosurg Psychiatry.* 2008;**79**:997–1001.

20. Gromova HA, Gafarov VV, Gagulin IV. Depression and risk of cardiovascular diseases among males aged 25–64 (WHO MONICA–psychosocial). *Alaska Med.* 2007;**49**:255–8.

21. Gump BB, Matthews KA, Eberly LE, *et al.* Depressive symptoms and mortality in men: Results from the Multiple Risk Factor Intervention Trial. *Stroke.* 2005;**36**:98–102.

22. Salaycik KJ, Kelly-Hayes M, Beiser A, *et al.* Depressive symptoms and risk of stroke: The Framingham Study. *Stroke.* 2007;**38**:16–21.

23. Krishnan M, Mast BT, Ficker LJ, *et al.* The effects of preexisting depression on cerebrovascular health outcomes in geriatric continuing care. *J Gerontol A Biol Sci Med Sci.* 2005;**60**:915–9.

24. Leentjens AF, Aben I, Lodder J, *et al.* General and disease-specific risk factors for depression after ischemic stroke: A two-step Cox regression analysis. *Int Psychogeriatr.* 2006;**18**:739–48.

25. Vickery CD, Sepehri A, Evans CC. Self-esteem in an acute stroke rehabilitation sample: A control group comparison. *Clin Rehabil.* 2008;**22**:179–87.

26. Kim JM, Stewart R, Kim SW, *et al.* BDNF genotype potentially modifying the association between incident stroke and depression. *Neurobiol Aging.* 2008;**29**:789–92.

27. Choi-Kwon S, Han SW, Kwon SU, *et al.* Post-stroke fatigue: Characteristics and related factors. *Cerebrovasc Dis.* 2005;**19**:84–90.

28. Nys GM, van Zandvoort MJ, van der Worp HB, *et al.* Early depressive symptoms after stroke: Neuropsychological correlates and lesion characteristics. *J Neurol Sci.* 2005;**228**:27–33.

29. Barker-Collo SL. Depression and anxiety 3 months post-stroke: Prevalence and correlates. *Arch Clin Neuropsychol.* 2007;**22**:519–31.

30. Eriksson M, Asplund K, Glader EL, *et al*. Self-reported depression and use of antidepressants after stroke: A national survey. *Stroke*. 2004;**35**:936–41.

31. Giaquinto S, Spiridigliozzi C, Caracciolo B. Can faith protect from emotional distress after stroke? *Stroke*. 2007;**38**:993–7.

32. van de Port, I, Kwakkel G, Bruin M, *et al*. Determinants of depression in chronic stroke: A prospective cohort study. *Disabil Rehabil*. 2007;**29**:353–8.

33. Saxena SK, Ng TP, Koh G, *et al*. Is improvement in impaired cognition and depressive symptoms in post-stroke patients associated with recovery in activities of daily living? *Acta Neurol Scand*. 2007;**115**:339–46.

34. Caeiro L, Ferro JM, Santos CO, *et al*. Depression in acute stroke. *J Psychiatry Neurosci*. 2006;**31**:377–83.

35. Nuyen J, Spreeuwenberg PM, Groenewegen PP, *et al*. Impact of preexisting depression on length of stay and discharge destination among patients hospitalized for acute stroke: Linked register-based study. *Stroke*. 2008;**39**:132–8.

36. Teodorczuk A, O'Brien JT, Firbank MJ, *et al*. White matter changes and late-life depressive symptoms: Longitudinal study. *Br J Psychiatry*. 2007;**191**:212–7.

37. Aben I, Lodder J, Honig A, *et al*. Focal or generalized vascular brain damage and vulnerability to depression after stroke: A 1-year prospective follow-up study. *Int Psychogeriatr*. 2006;**18**:19–35.

38. Vataja R, Leppavuori A, Pohjasvaara T, *et al*. Post-stroke depression and lesion location revisited. *J Neuropsychiatry Clin Neurosci*. 2004;**16**:156–62.

39. Narushima K, Kosier JT, Robinson RG. A reappraisal of post-stroke depression, intra- and inter-hemispheric lesion location using meta-analysis. *J Neuropsychiatry Clin Neurosci*. 2003;**15**:422–30.

40. Hama S, Yamashita H, Shigenobu M, *et al*. Post-stroke affective or apathetic depression and lesion location: Left frontal lobe and bilateral basal ganglia. *Eur Arch Psychiatry Clin Neurosci*. 2007;**257**:149–52.

41. Vataja R, Pohjasvaara T, Mantyla R, *et al*. Depression–executive dysfunction syndrome in stroke patients. *Am J Geriatr Psychiatry*. 2005;**13**:99–107.

42. Paradiso S, Vaidya J, Tranel D, *et al*. Nondysphoric depression following stroke. *J Neuropsychiatry Clin Neurosci*. 2008;**20**:52–61.

43. Schafer R, Popp K, Jorgens S, *et al*. Alexithymia-like disorder in right anterior cingulate infarction. *Neurocase*. 2007;**13**:201–08.

44. Ramasubbu R, Tobias R, Buchan AM, *et al*. Serotonin transporter gene promoter region polymorphism associated with post-stroke major depression. *J Neuropsychiatry Clin Neurosci*. 2006;**18**:96–9.

45. Rocco A, Afra J, Toscano M, *et al*. Acute subcortical stroke and early serotonergic modification: An IDAP study. *Eur J Neurol*. 2007;**14**:1378–82.

46. Moller M, Andersen G, Gjedde A. Serotonin 5HT1A receptor availability and pathological crying after stroke. *Acta Neurol Scand*. 2007;**116**:83–90.

47. Glodzik-Sobanska L, Slowik A, McHugh P, *et al*. Single voxel proton magnetic resonance spectroscopy in post-stroke depression. *Psychiatry Res*. 2006;**148**:111–20.

48. Glodzik-Sobanska L, Slowik A, Kieltyka A, *et al*. Reduced prefrontal *N*-acetylaspartate in stroke patients with apathy. *J Neurol Sci*. 2005;**238**:19–24.

49. Dafer RM, Rao M, Shareef A, *et al*. Post-stroke depression. *Top Stroke Rehabil*. 2008;**15**:13–21.

50. Lai SM, Duncan PW, Keighley J, *et al*. Depressive symptoms and independence in BADL and IADL. *J Rehabil Res Dev*. 2002;**39**:589–96.

51. Goodwin RD, Devanand DP. Stroke, depression, and functional health outcomes among adults in the community. *J Geriatr Psychiatry Neurol*. 2008;**21**:41–6.

52. He J, Shen PF. [Clinical study on the therapeutic effect of acupuncture in the treatment of post-stroke depression.] *Zhen Ci Yan Jiu*. 2007;**32**:58–61.

53. Nannetti L, Paci M, Pasquini J, *et al*. Motor and functional recovery in patients with post-stroke depression. *Disabil Rehabil*. 2005;**27**:170–5.

54. D'Alisa S, Baudo S, Mauro A, *et al*. How does stroke restrict participation in long-term post-stroke survivors? *Acta Neurol Scand*. 2005;**112**:157–62.

55. Sturm JW, Donnan GA, Dewey HM, *et al*. Determinants of handicap after stroke: The North East Melbourne Stroke Incidence Study (NEMESIS). *Stroke*. 2004;**35**:715–20.

56. Desrosiers J, Demers L, Robichaud L, *et al*. Short-term changes in and predictors of participation of older adults after stroke following acute care or rehabilitation. *Neurorehabil Neural Repair*. 2008;**22**:288–97.

57. Lo RS, Cheng JO, Wong EM, *et al*. Handicap and its determinants of change in stroke survivors: One-year follow-up study. *Stroke*. 2008;**39**:148–53.

58. Jonkman EJ, de Weerd AW, Vrijens NL. Quality of life after a first ischemic stroke. Long-term developments and correlations with changes in neurological deficit, mood and cognitive impairment. *Acta Neurol Scand*. 1998;**98**:169–75.

59. Kwok T, Lo RS, Wong E, *et al*. Quality of life of stroke survivors: A 1-year follow-up study. *Arch Phys Med Rehabil*. 2006;**87**:1177–82.

60. Bilge C, Kocer E, Kocer A, *et al*. Depression and functional outcome after stroke: The effect of antidepressant therapy on functional recovery. *Eur J Phys Rehabil Med*. 2008;**44**:13–8.

61. Narushima K, Robinson RG. The effect of early versus late antidepressant treatment on physical impairment

associated with post-stroke depression: Is there a time-related therapeutic window? *J Nerv Ment Dis.* 2003;**191**:645–52.

62. Jorge RE, Robinson RG, Arndt S, *et al.* Mortality and post-stroke depression: A placebo-controlled trial of antidepressants. *Am J Psychiatry.* 2003;**160**:1823–9.

63. Ried LD, Tueth MJ, Jia H. A pilot study to describe antidepressant prescriptions dispensed to veterans after stroke. *Res Social Adm Pharm.* 2006;**2**:96–109.

64. Visser-Keizer AC, Meyboom-de JB, Deelman BG, *et al.* Subjective changes in emotion, cognition and behaviour after stroke: Factors affecting the perception of patients and partners. *J Clin Exp Neuropsychol.* 2002;**24**:1032–45.

65. Chow SK, Wong FK, Poon CY. Coping and caring: Support for family caregivers of stroke survivors. *J Clin Nurs.* 2007;**16**:133–43.

66. Blonder LX, Langer SL, Pettigrew LC, *et al.* The effects of stroke disability on spousal caregivers. *NeuroRehabilitation.* 2007;**22**:85–92.

67. Kimura M, Murata Y, Shimoda K, *et al.* Sexual dysfunction following stroke. *Compr Psychiatry.* 2001;**42**:217–22.

68. Jia H, Damush TM, Qin H, *et al.* The impact of post-stroke depression on healthcare use by veterans with acute stroke. *Stroke.* 2006;**37**:2796–801.

69. Starkstein SE, Mizrahi R, Power BD. Antidepressant therapy in post-stroke depression. *Expert Opin Pharmacother.* 2008;**9**:1291–8.

70. Chen Y, Guo JJ, Zhan S, *et al.* Treatment effects of antidepressants in patients with post-stroke depression: A meta-analysis. *Ann Pharmacother.* 2006;**40**:2115–22.

71. Rampello L, Alvano A, Chiechio S, *et al.* An evaluation of efficacy and safety of reboxetine in elderly patients affected by "retarded" post-stroke depression. A random, placebo-controlled study. *Arch Gerontol Geriatr.* 2005;**40**:275–85.

72. Rampello L, Chiechio S, Nicoletti G, *et al.* Prediction of the response to citalopram and reboxetine in post-stroke depressed patients. *Psychopharmacology (Berl).* 2004;**173**:73–8.

73. House AO, Hackett ML, Anderson CS, *et al.* Pharmaceutical interventions for emotionalism after stroke. *Cochrane Database Syst Rev.* 2004; CD003690.

74. Choi-Kwon S, Choi J, Kwon SU, *et al.* Fluoxetine is not effective in the treatment of post-stroke fatigue: A double-blind, placebo-controlled study. *Cerebrovasc Dis.* 2007;**23**:103–08.

75. Choi-Kwon S, Han SW, Kwon SU, *et al.* Fluoxetine treatment in post-stroke depression, emotional

incontinence, and anger proneness: A double-blind, placebo-controlled study. *Stroke.* 2006;**37**:156–61.

76. Chan KL, Campayo A, Moser DJ, *et al.* Aggressive behavior in patients with stroke: Association with psychopathology and results of antidepressant treatment on aggression. *Arch Phys Med Rehabil.* 2006;**87**:793–8.

77. Jorge RE, Robinson RG, Tateno A, *et al.* Repetitive transcranial magnetic stimulation as treatment of post-stroke depression: A preliminary study. *Biol Psychiatry.* 2004;**55**:398–405.

78. Sondergaard MP, Jarden JO, Martiny K, *et al.* Dose response to adjunctive light therapy in citalopram-treated patients with post-stroke depression. A randomised, double-blind pilot study. *Psychother Psychosom.* 2006;**75**:244–8.

79. Paul SL, Dewey HM, Sturm JW, *et al.* Prevalence of depression and use of antidepressant medication at 5 years post-stroke in the North East Melbourne Stroke Incidence Study. *Stroke.* 2006;**37**:2854–5.

80. Williams LS, Kroenke K, Bakas T, *et al.* Care management of post-stroke depression: A randomized, controlled trial. *Stroke.* 2007;**38**:998–1003.

81. Smith J, Forster A, House A, *et al.* Information provision for stroke patients and their caregivers. *Cochrane Database Syst Rev.* 2008;CD001919.

82. Lai SM, Studenski S, Richards L, *et al.* Therapeutic exercise and depressive symptoms after stroke. *J Am Geriatr Soc.* 2006;**54**:240–7.

83. Tseng CN, Chen CC, Wu SC, *et al.* Effects of a range-of-motion exercise programme. *J Adv Nurs.* 2007;**57**:181–91.

84. Sarkamo T, Tervaniemi M, Laitinen S, *et al.* Music listening enhances cognitive recovery and mood after middle cerebral artery stroke. *Brain.* 2008;**131**:866–76.

85. Niedermaier N, Bohrer E, Schulte K, *et al.* Prevention and treatment of post-stroke depression with mirtazapine in patients with acute stroke. *J Clin Psychiatry.* 2004;**65**:1619–23.

86. Almeida OP, Waterreus A, Hankey GJ. Preventing depression after stroke: Results from a randomized placebo-controlled trial. *J Clin Psychiatry.* 2006; **67**:1104–09.

87. Robinson RG, Jorge RE, Moser DJ, *et al.* Escitalopram and problem-solving therapy for prevention of post-stroke depression: A randomized controlled trial. *JAMA.* 2008;**299**:2391–400.

88. Chen Y, Patel NC, Guo JJ, *et al.* Antidepressant prophylaxis for post-stroke depression: A meta-analysis. *Int Clin Psychopharmacol* 2007;**22**:159–66.

89. Turner BM, Paradiso S, Marvel CL, *et al.* The cerebellum and emotional experience. *Neuropsychologia.* 2007;**45**:1331–41.

Epidemiology of stroke recovery

Samir Belagaje & Brett Kissela

Epidemiology is defined as the study of factors influencing health and disease in populations. When applied to stroke recovery, it refers to the natural history of stroke recovery and defining factors that affect recovery derived from post-stroke populations. This is a pillar of stroke recovery knowledge that is important and practical when caring for stroke patients, and that also requires further research attention. One of the most common questions a stroke victim or their family members will ask the physician is to what degree their loved one will recover from their stroke, and over what time frame that recovery can be expected. This question currently poses a huge challenge because of the complex and multifactorial processes involved in recovery, so at present one can only provide best estimates based on epidemiological, natural history knowledge combined with other aspects of the patient's condition that may influence the predicted outcome.

This chapter consists of four sections. The first part of this chapter will provide an overview of the different types of epidemiological studies, highlighting their respective strengths and weaknesses. The second will focus on the current state of knowledge regarding general epidemiological patterns seen in stroke recovery, as well as the gaps in our knowledge. The next portion will discuss the epidemiological data surrounding factors that can affect an individual's recovery from a stroke as well as how those factors interact with each other. In the final section, the application of epidemiology will be discussed with regard to clinical care and planning of future clinical research.

Overview of types of epidemiological studies in stroke

Epidemiological studies primarily are observational in nature but experimental designs also contribute epidemiological information.

Registry

Stroke registries are databases of information collected about patients with stroke. The databases typically collect all details about the patient such as age, sex, comorbidities, and treatments and are primarily descriptive in nature. Analysis of the data then allows one to make inferences about incidence and prevalence. Depending on what data are collected about the patients, these types of studies may be helpful to first generate relationships between diseases and associated factors. By nature of their design, however, these studies by themselves cannot be used to prove those exact relationships, and require further studies. A recent example of a stroke registry is the Paul Coverdell National Acute Stroke Registry [1].

Case control

Case control studies are another type of epidemiological study that attempts to determine factors that influence a disease or condition. In such a study for stroke, a population with stroke ("cases") is compared to a similar population without stroke ("controls"). In the comparison, the investigator looks for differences in the characteristics or factors in cases vs. controls that might have caused the cases to develop stroke. These types of studies are relatively inexpensive compared to other types and are useful in investigating uncommon conditions (such as subarachnoid hemorrhage or intracerebral hemorrhage). Their disadvantages include the inability to make a direct cause and effect relationship because of potentially confounding variables. Furthermore, because of their retrospective nature, the information gained may be subjected to recall bias and investigator bias. A recent example of a case control study in stroke is the Genetics and Environmental Risk Factors for Hemorrhagic Stroke [2,3].

Brain Repair After Stroke, ed. S. C. Cramer and R. J. Nudo. Published by Cambridge University Press.
© Cambridge University Press 2010.

Cohort

A longitudinal cohort is a type of study that takes a group of people with similar characteristics or exposure or experience (cohort) and follows them over a defined period of time. These studies can be prospective or retrospective. The main purpose of these types of studies is to determine an association/causality between an exposure, experience, or some other characteristic, and an outcome (e.g. disease). The advantages of such a study are that it allows for longitudinal observations and more accurate data collection in that they are collected at certain time intervals. However, individuals in cohorts can be lost over time through death and other factors. These studies are also expensive, and time-consuming, and can take years to collect meaningful data. An example in stroke is the Copenhagen Stroke Study, which followed stroke patients over time to determine the time course of recovery [4,5].

Cross-sectional study

These types of studies collect data on the variable(s) of interest at one period of time in a population. To understand these studies, it is often useful to contrast cross-sectional studies with cohorts. While cohorts provide data on relatively small groups over an extended period of time with data collection at several time periods, cross-sectional studies provide data on larger populations at just one time ("snapshot"). These types of studies provide information, such as prevalence data, on the variable of interest and are less expensive to perform than cohorts. An example of a cross-sectional stroke study is the REasons for Geographic And Racial Differences in Stroke (REGARDS) study [6].

Epidemiological data are also gained through experimental studies. The main difference between experimental studies and observational studies is that the investigator will "intervene" with their study population or a portion of the population. The randomized clinical trial is generally considered to provide the highest level of evidence regarding an experimental question. The validity of these trials is highest when they include a valid randomization process that reduces the potential for confounding by randomly distributing potential confounders between placebo and control groups, blinding of both the investigators and participants (to reduce bias in determining outcomes), and a sufficiently large study population that provides adequate power to answer the study question.

While such studies provide most information about the intervention, they may also provide epidemiologic information of use. For example, the EXCITE trial determined that constraint-induced therapy improved post-stroke outcomes vs. traditional therapy, although the therapy-only arm provided useful information on the "natural history" of recovery due to traditional therapy in the 3–9 month time frame of that trial [7].

General patterns of recovery

In 1950, Thomas Twitchell observed the patterns of recovery in a cohort of 121 patients who had hemiplegia in the arm, leg, or both. He examined various factors including onset of spasticity, hyperreflexia, and nature of volitional movements to develop prognostic factors of recovery [8]. Since his published observations, multiple studies have been published subsequently examining populations for their stroke recovery patterns. In these studies, in spite of variations in stroke location and advances in stroke recovery, one can infer several generalizations about the natural history and time course of stroke recovery.

The first observation is that the majority of stroke patients have the ability to recover from their stroke, although the degree of recovery can vary. Statistics show that 50–70% of stroke survivors regain functional independence [9]. However, for the majority of patients, the recovery is incomplete and they do not return to pre-stroke levels of activity [10]. One corollary to these facts is that the severity of deficits is inversely related to the proportion of recovery [11,12]. The biological mechanisms underlying the recovery process and the degree of recovery are incompletely understood in humans and under investigation (see Chapters 9–13).

Another factor related to recovery relates to the rehabilitation therapy provided in various forms after the stroke. In a seminal meta-analysis of 36 clinical trials examining the effectiveness of stroke rehabilitation, people receiving post-stroke rehabilitation had higher levels of function than those stroke survivors who do not receive rehabilitation [12]. This important finding was seen across several measures including ambulation, self-care ability, communication, and independence. Due to such findings, the American Stroke Association recommends that therapy should be considered for all qualifying patients and that rehabilitation access and venues be incorporated in stroke systems of care [13].

With regard to time after stroke, another common finding is that earlier onset of spontaneous recovery from time of stroke onset is associated with a better final outcome than those whose recovery is first observed at later time points after stroke onset. Researchers and clinicians generally believe that the first few weeks post-stroke is the time frame for the greatest rate of spontaneous recovery. By following a cohort of 102 patients with ischemic MCA territory strokes, Kwakkel *et al.* proposed that the amount of recovery of upper extremity function in the first 4 weeks could predict amount of disability in 6 months [14]. In fact, even observations during the first week post-stroke can be used to predict long-term outcome in arm function [14]. Recognizing that earlier recovery offers a better prognosis and rehabilitation also improves outcomes, further epidemiological data are needed to learn more about the optimal timing and dose of rehabilitation. Paolucci *et al.* examined differences in outcomes for patients for whom therapy was initiated 20 days apart and found a strong inverse relationship between the start date and functional outcome, albeit with wide confidence intervals [15]. In other words, the earliest starters had significantly higher effectiveness of treatment than did the medium or latest groups. Treatment initiated within the first 20 days was associated with a significantly higher probability of excellent therapeutic response (OR=6.11; 95% CI, 2.03–18.36), and beginning later was associated with a poorer response (OR=5.18; 95% CI, 1.07–25.00) [15].

There remains conflicting evidence about the dose of therapy. For example, the EXCITE trial, a randomized multicenter trial of constraint-induced movement therapy (CIMT) involving 222 patients 3–9 months post-stroke was successful in the chronic time frame [7], whereas other studies show similar benefit with lower dose of this intervention, referred to as modified constraint-induced therapy [16]. The VECTORS trial, a randomized controlled trial (RCT) of 52 patients, showed that in the acute–subacute time post-stroke, higher intensity (dose) of therapy had an inverse relationship with functional levels at 90 days [17]. Duration of therapy is also important to consider in a discussion of factors determining recovery, although the optimal duration of therapy is not known. In the meta-analysis described above, Ottenbacher and Jannell argued that earlier timing of intervention played a bigger role than the duration of the therapy itself [12]. Studies have also examined the impact that choice of content of therapy might play in maximizing gains.

General patterns of recovery have also been described with respect to the type of deficit after stroke. Proximal recovery usually occurs before distal recovery [8], and lower extremity deficits recover in terms of disability measures faster than upper extremity [18]. Several mechanisms have been proposed for the latter finding, including bihemispheric localization of lower extremity functions such as walking, as well as the presence of a spinal cord nucleus serving as a generator of walking patterns. Bihemispheric functional localization may also play a role in the improvement of deficits seen in swallowing and facial movements [19,20].

The final generalization is that although great strides in recovery are seen initially, most patients who do not achieve early and complete spontaneous recovery reach a plateau phase where further significant spontaneous improvements are not made. In the Copenhagen Stroke Study, a cohort of over 1100 acute stroke patients admitted to the stroke unit in a Copenhagen hospital, maximum arm motor function was seen within 9 weeks post-stroke in 95% of patients [4]. Researchers also looked at 804 patients in the same cohort with lower-extremity paresis and found recovery of walking function occurs in 95% of the patients within the first 11 weeks after stroke. The time and the degree of recovery are related to both the degree of initial impairment of walking function and to the severity of lower-extremity paresis [21]. Similar findings have been observed in patients with aphasia and patients with neglect, with the plateaus occurring approximately at 6 weeks and 3 months, respectively [22,23].

This plateau effect led many to believe that further recovery was not possible and that remaining disabilities were permanent. This belief was propagated amongst healthcare professionals involved in rehabilitation and subsequently hampered the field for many decades. In the past decade, the concept of the plateau has been challenged with new clinical studies and advances in functional neuroimaging. For instance, in the EXCITE trial, traditional therapy was shown to be beneficial in regaining upper-extremity function between 3 and 9 months after stroke [7]; it is important to note that these patients would have plateaued with regard to spontaneous recovery. Furthermore, Page *et al.* showed the CIMT provided significant benefit in patients who were at least 1 year out from their stroke, well past the typical plateau [16]. These findings suggest that the plateau described with spontaneous recovery is not fixed; rather, with newer interventions (see Chapters 16–24), additional recovery might be possible. However, after introducing a new mode of therapy, a typical pattern is to see some improvement initially, after which a new plateau is reached, as reported in studies such as the EXCITE trial [7].

Specific factors in stroke recovery

When examining stroke recovery via epidemiological studies, factors associated with an individual's clinical improvement can be determined. The next section will discuss those factors, both modifiable and non-modifiable, that are generally accepted as important factors in stroke recovery.

Age

Several studies examining stroke outcomes continuously show that age is a factor in determining outcomes. The relationship between age and recovery is an inverse correlation as seen in the Copenhagen Stroke Study cohort and in the EXCITE trial population [5,7]. That is, the older someone is, the less likelihood of recovery they have. Said another way, younger stroke victims have a better prognosis for recovery. Older age is associated with less recovery in virtually all epidemiology studies of stroke outcome. One may argue that older age is associated with other factors that have been associated with lesser recovery, including a larger number of medical comorbidities, higher amount of periventricular white matter disease, a lesser reserve of neurons to assume lost functions, and a greater risk for cognitive dysfunction. And yet, age remains an independent risk factor for less recovery after controlling for all of these other factors in most studies [5,24], suggesting that factors directly related to aging effects influence outcome.

Race/genetics

Certain groups may recover better from their strokes than others. Several studies show that African-American patients have more severe strokes than Caucasians, and that furthermore they do not recover as well. In the Greater Cincinnati Northern Kentucky Stroke Study, a population-based cohort of people living in the Cincinnati area, it was shown that African-American patients have a higher incidence of stroke than Caucasian populations [25]. In general, non-Caucasian races score worse on quality-of-life measures during the recovery process than Caucasian races [24]. There may be some controversy as to whether race actually is a factor, or whether it is mainly a surrogate for other factors such as socio-economic status and access to care. One study examined 1073 African-American and Caucasian stroke patients and showed that rates of utilization and time to referral for inpatient rehabilitation were equal, but that low-income African-American patients had worse functional recovery in 12 months [26]. While these non-biologic factors need further investigation, the disparities in recovery between race/ethnic groups naturally lead to an interest in underlying genetic differences that may be related to the biological processes underlying recovery. For example, it has been shown that the presence of a polymorphism in the gene for brain-derived neurotrophic factor (BDNF) impairs motor cortex plasticity in human subjects [27]. This leads to the suggestion that patients who possess this polymorphism might not recover as well as the general population, and this (or other genotypes associated with poor recovery) may be more prevalent in some race/ethnic groups than others. Such hypotheses require direct study, and if supported, might provide new insights to maximize recovery across the spectrum of human genetics.

Gender

The role of gender in influencing recovery generates some controversy. Earlier studies did not show a difference in recovery by gender [28]. However, other studies from both Europe and North America have consistently shown that women have less favorable outcomes after stroke. In terms of physical outcomes, data from the Riks-Stroke Registry, a national stroke quality registry in Sweden consisting of 9666 women and 9881 men, 54% of women compared to 67% of men were independent in primary ADL within 3 months of stroke onset [29]. Similarly, in the Canadian Stroke Registry covering 21 tertiary hospitals, outcomes of 1527 females were compared against 1796 males as measured by the SIS-16 scale. Women did worse than men, although quality of life (QOL) measures at 6 months were not different [30]. In other studies using stroke-specific QOL measures, such as the Michigan Stroke Registry, women scored significantly lower after stroke [1].

In trying to explain the conflicting data regarding gender and outcomes, some researchers have generally attributed differences to poorer pre-stroke functioning and higher prevalence of depression in the female group. Compared to men, women live slightly longer and might have strokes at older ages. However, even when these factors are accounted for, women still had poorer outcomes [1,31,32]. Post-stroke, women are less likely to be discharged home and tend to be placed in nursing homes and long-term care facilities [29,30,32]. Even though several studies have shown that women have equal access to rehabilitation services, they do not experience the same level of recovery [30,32]. In the only study comparing gender responsiveness to rehabilitation, men were about 3 times more likely than women to be independent as defined by a Barthel index greater than or equal to 95; in this study, the genders were matched in terms of stroke severity, age, and time since stroke onset [32]. As it has been the only study of its kind to date, some of the differences have been argued that the men had more muscular strength at baseline compared to their female counterparts. Further research is needed to clarify whether it is gender that may influence outcome, or whether it serves as a surrogate marker for other factors such as social isolation, baseline premorbid functioning levels, depression, or others.

Nature of stroke and acute treatment

It is intuitive that the size of stroke is correlated with outcomes. Larger strokes in terms of brain volume and clinical severity (measured by scales such as the NIH Stroke Scale) are associated with poorer outcomes. Hemorrhagic strokes typically present with larger deficits than ischemic strokes, and are typically associated with worse outcome. Location of the stroke in terms of involvement of specific tracts and tissue is also important (see below). For instance, a stroke that injures the inferior parietal lobule or causes hemineglect will generally lead to worse outcomes compared to strokes of similar size that do not injure this region or cause hemineglect. The NINDS tPA study group found in their post-hoc subanalysis of their original RCT population that a person receiving tPA for acute stroke treatment, regardless of age or stroke severity, will have better chances for recovery [33].

Medical comorbidities

It is not surprising to imagine that one's comorbidities would affect the ability to recover from a stroke. In addition to limiting the body's ability to repair the brain, medical comorbidities could also affect someone's ability to participate fully in therapy, and influence many other psychosocial functions.

There have been specific comorbidities which have been implicated in the recovery process. For instance, high blood glucose levels have been independently associated with worse outcomes as seen in the populations

of the TOAST study, which was a randomized clinical trial of 1259 stroke patients whose admission blood glucose level was compared to 3-month outcomes, and in the Greater Cincinnati/Northern Kentucky epidemiological cohort [34,35]. Along similar lines, depression has been associated with poorer outcomes (see also Chapter 14). This was seen in the Sunnybrook Stroke Study involving approximately 150 patients who completed the study where depressive symptoms were correlated with functional outcome ($r = -.31$) and handicap ($r = .41$) at 3 months and 1 year [36].

Stroke patients are at a high risk for developing infections such as aspiration pneumonia or urinary tract infections. Such complications may affect their outcomes through multiple mechanisms. For example, as these stroke-related infections occur, they can produce fevers. In a meta-analysis involving 3790 patients, Hajat et al. showed that fever after stroke onset is associated with a marked increase in morbidity and mortality (odds ratio for mortality was 1.19) [37]. In addition to causing pyrexia, one can hypothesize that post-stroke infections prolong hospitalizations and increase the time until rehabilitation referral. Yet, the relationship is not quite clear. In the single randomized, double-blinded clinical trial to date examining prophylactic antibiotic use in stroke patients, patients who received prophylactic levofloxacin did not have significantly better outcomes than patients who received standard preventive care [38]. In another cohort of 229 patients, Vargas et al. showed that stroke-related infections were a marker of stroke severity, and when treated appropriately were not associated with poor outcomes [39]. However, other cohorts such as the Greater Cincinnati Northern Kentucky Epidemiological Cohort have shown that infections such as urinary tract infections are associated with worse outcomes [40].

Not only do comorbidities have the potential to affect stroke outcomes, but the medications used to treat and manage them also have the potential to affect outcomes. For example, Naidech et al. showed in a study of 527 patients that phenytoin adversely affects outcomes in strokes and subarachnoid hemorrhages [41]. Indeed, a range of other drugs has also been suggested as important in this regard [42].

However, some drugs may actually play a role in enhancing recovery. For instance, bromocriptine is used as an adjunct to speech therapy in the subacute phase to help aphasic patients recover their speech [43]. Other dopaminergic medications have also been postulated to help, but research is still in progress. Other medications such as amphetamines have also been proposed to enhance motor recovery, but the largest randomized clinical trial failed to show a positive result [44]. The effect of medications on recovery needs to be investigated further.

While some medical comorbidities can be medically addressed, there are others that cannot. For instance, periventricular white matter disease, or leukoaraiosis, is an independent predictor of poorer outcomes [45,46]. The amount of leukoariosis does not appear to have a dose–effect relationship in terms of outcomes, but rather there appears to be a threshold before the effect is realized [47].

Increasing white matter disease burden is highly associated with cognitive impairment and dementia. Dementia is associated with unfavorable outcomes in stroke recovery. Tatemichi *et al.* followed a cohort of 251 patients and found the mortality rate was 19.8 per 100 person-years among stroke patients with dementia compared to 6.1 deaths per 100 person-years in those stroke patients without dementia [48].

Socio-economic factors

In addition to medical and genetic factors, socio-economic factors also play a role in recovery from stroke. In general, those at a lower socio-economic status do worse than those at higher levels [26]. The level likely acts as a surrogate marker for factors such as access to rehabilitation, the amount of rehabilitation one receives, and access to medical care for management of comorbidities. It may also reflect the amount of social support a person has; for example, the presence of a spouse has been shown to be a beneficial factor in stroke recovery [5].

Preservation of white matter tracts and specific brain tissue

The ability for brain repair post-stroke is dependent on preserved brain tissue to assume lost functions as well as complete repair. While this concept may seem intuitive, it is only in recent years that some of the details have been elicited. For example, Stinear *et al.*, studying 21 patients with chronic stroke, showed that integrity of the corticospinal tracts as measured by fractional anisotropy (FA) with diffusion tensor imaging could be used to predict response to therapy for people who have motor deficits [49]. Furthermore, the same study also showed that the presence of motor-evoked potentials

(MEPs) in the ipsilesional primary motor cortex is also an important predictor of recovery in therapy; this finding has been supported in a subset analysis from the EVEREST study [49,50]. In another clinical trial, decreased motor cortex activation at baseline predicted better outcomes suggesting that underused but intact cortical neurons are recruited for recovery purposes [51]. Along similar lines, mirror neuron preservation may play a role in the rehabilitation of aphasia [52].

Integration of various factors

Multiple prognostic factors have been discussed above. There are certainly others that have yet to be identified. The interaction of the various factors is not yet clear and the clinician will likely have difficulty in determining how to integrate the effects of various stroke recovery factors. As all factors are not weighted equally, the exact contribution of each factor, in each patient, is unclear. This can become even more complicated when the factors interact with each other; for example, while some factors can have additive effects, other factors may offset each other. Models can be used to determine which factors may play the biggest role in determining outcomes as well as demonstrating how factors interact with each other. One proposed theoretical model is provided in Figure 15.1, although the authors recognize that this model does not account for several relevant factors such as medications used.

Importance of epidemiology research in stroke recovery

The final section in this chapter examines the importance of epidemiological research in stroke recovery. First, epidemiological data can be used to help predict the amount of recovery and time during which the recovery process will occur. As mentioned earlier, patients and their families are often very interested in learning about the recovery process, and so such data will be helpful in providing realistic expectations. As seen in the previous section, there are many factors which can play a role in stroke recovery. Understanding these factors will allow one to improve accuracy and tailor expectations for recovery to the specific individual. In turn, providing more realistic expectations can allow for better utilization of the healthcare system through appropriate disposition following hospitalizations.

Such knowledge may also be helpful in developing the rehabilitation plan and maximizing functional outcomes, across the spectrum of patients. For instance, a

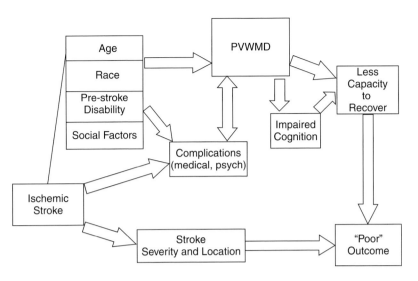

Figure 15.1 A theoretical model ilustrating how various factors interact to determine stroke outcome.
 The figure provides a theoretical model illustrating how various factors interact to determine stroke outcome. Depending on the weighting of each factor in an individual patient, a poor outcome might or might not be likely. (PVWMD, periventricular white matter disease.)

patient whose prognostic factors do not suggest further useful spontaneous recovery is likely to benefit from therapies focused on behavioral compensatory strategies and assistive devices. On the other hand, a stroke survivor with a better prognosis may be better suited for interventions to enhance neuroplasticity with more intense therapy.

Secondly, the factors in stroke recovery outcomes are complex and not well characterized. Although many of these factors such as age or race are fixed, other factors such as depression can be addressed with medications, patient education, and other interventions. Systematic care processes, such as standardized order sets during inpatient stays, are useful for getting therapy started immediately and for preventing complications such as infection. In this way, an epidemiological understanding of factors that affect recovery will allow proper management and treatment of these patients and thereby provide patients with the best chance for recovery. As epidemiological studies continue to progress with further insights into factors of interest, additional interventions will likely be utilized to address modifiable factors.

Any new intervention or treatment for stroke recovery will require careful clinical trials to prove efficacy. Epidemiology can help in developing sharply focused experimental questions and improve experimental design in subsequent clinical trials. In designing a trial, understanding the factors that affect stroke recovery will help achieve better balance between control and intervention populations. An imbalance in a factor relevant to recovery between intervention and control arms in a

recovery trial could lead to a Type II error, where investigators could miss a true difference in the recovery of the two groups. Large clinical trials are time-consuming, challenging to enroll into, expensive, and difficult to conduct. However, such trials are needed to further the field of stroke recovery, and we must maximize what we can learn from each trial that is completed.

Epidemiological data can also be used to create and modify public policy. Stroke is one of the leading causes of disability in the United States and the second leading cause of death worldwide. The economic burden is tremendous and will represent an estimated cost of $2 trillion to the United States healthcare system over the next 50 years [53]. With the population aging, the impact will only continue to grow. Policy decisions impacted by recovery epidemiology should include appropriate reimbursement for effective stroke therapies, provision of effective equipment to help patients recover, and allocation of money for further research in this area.

References

1. Gargano JW, Reeves MJ. Sex differences in stroke recovery and stroke-specific quality of life: Results from a statewide stroke registry. *Stroke*. 2007;**38**:2541–8.

2. Woo D, Sauerback LR, Kissela BK, *et al.* Genetic and environmental risk factors for intracerebral hemorrhage: Preliminary results of a population-based study. *Stroke*. 2002;**33**:1190–5.

3. Flaherty ML, Haverbusch M, Sekar P, *et al.* Long-term mortality after intracerebral hemorrhage. *Neurology*. 2006;**66**:1182–6.

4. Nakayama H, Jorgensen H, Raaschou H, *et al.* Recovery of upper extremity function in stroke patients: The Copenhagen Stroke Study. *Arch Phys Med Rehab.* 1994;**75**:394–8.

5. Jørgensen HS, Reith J, Nakayama H, *et al.* What determines good recovery in patients with the most severe strokes? The Copenhagen Stroke Study. *Stroke.* 1999;**30**:2008–12.

6. Howard VJ, Cushman M, Pulley L, *et al.* The reasons for geographic and racial differences in stroke study: Objectives and design. *Neuroepidemiology.* 2005;**25**:135–43.

7. Wolf S, Winstein CJ, Miller JP, *et al.* Effect of constraint-induced movement therapy on upper extremity function 3 to 9 months after stroke: The EXCITE randomized clinical trial. *JAMA.* 2006;**296**:2095–3015.

8. Twitchell TE. The restoration of motor function following hemiplegia in man. *Brain.* 1951;**74**:443–80.

9. American Heart Association. *Heart Disease and Stroke Statistics – 2004 Update.* Dallas, TX: American Heart Association; 2003.

10. Dobkin B. Principles and practices of neurological rehabilitation. In: Bradley WG, Daroff RB, Fenichel GM, *et al.*, editors. *Neurology in clinical practice.* 4th ed. Philadelphia, PA: Butterworth Heineman; 2004: pp. 1027–70.

11. Shelton FD, Volpe BT, Reding M. Motor impairment as a predictor of functional recovery and guide to rehabilitation treatment after stroke. *Neurorehab Neural Repair.* 2001;**15**:229–37.

12. Ottenbacher KJ, Jannell S. The results of clinical trials in stroke rehabilitation research. *Arch Neurol.* 1993;**50**:37–44.

13. Task Force Members. Recommendations for the establishment of stroke systems of care: Recommendations from the American Stroke Association's task force on the development of stroke systems. *Stroke.* 2005;**36**:690–703.

14. Kwakkel G, Kollen BJ, van der Grond J, *et al.* Probability of regaining dexterity in the flaccid upper limb: The impact of severity of paresis and time since onset in acute stroke. *Stroke.* 2003;**34**:2181–6.

15. Paolucci S, Antonucci G, Grasso MG, *et al.* Early versus delayed inpatient stroke rehabilitation: A matched comparison conducted in Italy. *Arch Phys Med Rehab.* 2000;**81**:695–700.

16. Page SJ, Levine P, Leonard A, *et al.* Modified constraint-induced therapy in chronic stroke: Results of a single-blinded randomized controlled trial. *Phys Ther.* 2008;**88**:333–40.

17. Dromerick AW, Lang CE, Birkenmeier RL, *et al.* Very Early Constraint-Induced Movement (VECTORS). A single-center RCT. *Neurology.* 2009;**73**:195–201.

18. Desrosiers J, Malouin F, Richards C, *et al.* Comparison of changes in upper and lower extremity impairments and disabilities after stroke. *Int J Rehab Res.* 2003;**26**:109–16.

19. Cramer SC, Crafton KR. Somatotopy and movement representation sites following cortical stroke. *Exp Brain Res.* 2006;**168**:25–32.

20. Hamdy S, Aziz Q, Rothwell JC, *et al.* Recovery of swallowing after dysphagic stroke relates to functional reorganization in the intact motor cortex. *Gastro.* 1998;**115**:1104–12.

21. Jongbloed L. Prediction of function after stroke: A critical review. *Stroke.* 1986;**17**:765–76.

22. Pedersen P, Jorgensen H, Nakayama H, *et al.* Aphasia in acute stroke: Incidence, determinants, and recovery. *Ann Neurol.* 1995;**38**:659–66.

23. Hier D, Mondlock J, Caplan L. Recovery of behavioral abnormalities after right hemisphere stroke. *Neuro.* 1983;**33**:345–50.

24. Nichols-Larsen DS, Clark PC, Zeringue A, Greenspan A, Blanton S. Factors influencing stroke survivors' quality of life during subacute recovery. *Stroke.* 2005;**36**:1480–4.

25. Kissela B, Schneider A, Kleindorfer D, *et al.* Stroke in a biracial population: The excess burden of stroke among blacks. *Stroke.* 2004;**35**:426–31.

26. Horner RD, Swanson JW, Bosworth HB, *et al.* Effects of race and poverty on the process and outcome of inpatient rehabilitation services among stroke patients. *Stroke.* 2003;**34**:1027–31.

27. Kleim JA, Chan S, Pringle E, *et al.* BDNF val66met polymorphism is associated with modified experience-dependent plasticity in human motor cortex. *Nat Neurosci.* 2006;**9**:735–7.

28. Wade DT, Hewer RL, Wood VA. Stroke: Influence of patient's sex and side of weakness on outcome. *Arch Phys Med Rehab.* 1984;**65**:513–6.

29. Glader EL, Stegmayr B, Norrving B, *et al.* Sex differences in management and outcome after stroke: A Swedish national perspective. *Stroke.* 2003;**34**:1970–5.

30. Kapral MK, Fang J, Hill MD, *et al.* Sex differences in stroke care and outcomes: Results from the registry of the Canadian Stroke Network. *Stroke.* 2005;**36**:809–14.

31. Lai SM, Duncan PW, Dew P, *et al.* Sex differences in stroke recovery. *Prev Chronic Dis.* 2005;**3**:A13.

32. Fusco R, Morelli D, Venturiero V, *et al.* Is sex a prognostic factor in stroke rehabilitation? A matched comparison. *Stroke.* 2006;**37**:2989–94.

33. The NINDS t-PA Stroke Study Group. Generalized efficacy of t-PA for acute stroke: Subgroup analysis of the NINDS t-PA stroke trial. *Stroke.* 1997;**28**:2119–25.

34. Bruno A, Biller J, Adams HP, *et al.* Acute blood glucose level and outcome from ischemic stroke: Trial of ORG

10172 in Acute Stroke Treatment (TOAST) Investigators. *Neuro.* 1999;**52**:280–4.

35. Kissela BM, Khoury J, Alwell K, *et al.* Long term mortality after ischemic stroke: The effect of diabetes in the greater Cincinnati/Northern Kentucky stroke study [abstract from 2004 International Stroke Conference]. *Stroke.* 2004;**35**:315.

36. Herrmann N, Black SE, Lawrence J, *et al.* The Sunnybrook Stroke Study: A prospective study of depressive symptoms and functional outcome. *Stroke.* 1998;**29**:618–24.

37. Hajat C, Hajat S, Sharma P. Effects of poststroke pyrexia on stroke outcome: A meta-analysis of studies in patients. *Stroke.* 2000;**31**:410–4.

38. Chamorro A, Horcajada JP, Obach V, *et al.* The early systemic prophylaxis of infection after stroke study: A randomized clinical trial. *Stroke.* 2005;**36**:1495–500.

39. Vargas M, Horcajada JP, Obach V, *et al.* Clinical consequences of infection in patients with acute stroke: Is it prime time for further antibiotic trials? *Stroke.* 2006;**37**:461–5.

40. Kissela B, Lindsell CJ, Kleindorfer D, *et al.* Clinical prediction of functional outcome after ischemic stroke: The surprising importance of periventricular white matter disease and race. *Stroke.* 2009;**41**:530–6.

41. Naidech AM, Kreiter KT, Janjua N, *et al.* Phenytoin exposure is associated with functional and cognitive disability after subarachnoid hemorrhage. *Stroke.* 2005;**36**:583–7.

42. Goldstein L, Sygenin Acute Stroke Study Investigators. Common drugs may influence motor recovery after stroke. *Neurology.* 1995;**45**:865–71.

43. Bragoni M, Altieri M, Di Piero V, *et al.* Bromocriptine and speech therapy in non-fluent chronic aphasia after stroke. *Neurol Sci.* 2000;**21**:19–22.

44. Martinsson L, Hårdemark HG, Wahlgren NG. Amphetamines for improving recovery after stroke

(Cochrane systematic review). In: *The Cochrane Library*, 2003. Oxford: Update Software; 2003.

45. Miyao S, Takano A, Teramoto J, *et al.* Leukoaraiosis in relation to prognosis for patients with lacunar infarction. *Stroke.* 1992;**23**:1434–8.

46. Samuelsson M, Soderfeldt B, Olsson GB. Functional outcome in patients with lacunar infarction. *Stroke.* 1996;**27**:842–86.

47. Belagaje SR, Lindsell C, Alwell K, *et al.* The effect of white matter disease (WMD) on post-stroke outcomes: Dose–effect vs. threshold? [Abstract]. Accepted for presentation at the 34th International Conference on Stroke and Cerebral Circulation (February 2009).

48. Tatemichi TK, Desmond DW, Mayeux R, *et al.* Dementia after stroke: Baseline frequency, risks, and clinical features in a hospitalized cohort. *Neuro.* 1992;**42**:1185–93.

49. Stinear CM, Barber PA, Smale PR, *et al.* Functional potential in chronic stroke patients depends on corticospinal tract integrity. *Brain.* 2007;**130**:170–80.

50. Levy RM, Benson RR, Winstein CJ for the Everest Study Investigators. Cortical stimulation for upper-extremity hemiparesis from ischemic stroke: Everest Study primary endpoint results [Abstract]. In: *International Stroke Conference*: 2008, New Orleans.

51. Cramer SC, Parrish TB, Levy RM, *et al.* Predicting functional gains in a stroke trial. *Stroke.* 2007;**38**:2108–14.

52. Buccino G, Solodkin A, Small SL. Functions of the mirror neuron system: Implications for neurorehabilitation. *Cognit Behav Neurol.* 2006;**19**:55–63.

53. Brown DL, Boden-Albala B, Langa KM, *et al.* Projected costs of ischemic stroke in the United States. *Neuro.* 2006;**67**:1390–5.

Issues in clinical trial methodology for brain repair after stroke

Steven C. Cramer

Brain repair after stroke and potential clinical applications

Stroke remains a leading cause of adult disability, the third greatest cause of death in the US (the second greatest cause in the world), and the most common neurologic reason for hospital admission. The annual cost exceeds 68 billion dollars in the US. Approximately 795 000 new symptomatic strokes are diagnosed each year in the US. Note that asymptomatic strokes, which are likely a further source of disability [1], occur with a prevalence that is several-fold higher, for example, being present in 22% of adults 65–69 years of age [2].

Currently approved stroke therapies are limited to the early hours after stroke. As a result, only 2–3% of patients with stroke receive such an intervention [3,4], although this is improving with time, and rates are higher in selected centers. Nonetheless, many patients who do receive thrombolytic therapy in the acute stage of stroke demonstrate significant disability months later [5,6]. Currently approved acute stroke therapies target the vasculature rather than the neural substance of the brain. New therapies are needed that target the brain itself, reduce disability, and can be accessed by a majority of patients with stroke. Repair-based therapies have many candidates that might meet these criteria.

Brain repair after stroke can be defined as a therapeutic strategy whose goal is not to salvage acutely threatened tissue, but instead is to promote the repair and restoration of function in surviving tissue. Repair-based strategies can thus be pursued across a wide range of post-stroke time epochs, from the hours following infarct stabilization to years after stroke onset. Divergent biological targets and therapeutic modalities have been advanced in this regard (see Chapters 17–24). Some focus on specific cellular and molecular events, such as catecholaminergic drugs, while others such as brain stimulation aim to improve brain function through more global means. Clinical trials are underway to evaluate therapies across several post-stroke temporal epochs, ranging from days to weeks to years after stroke onset.

Clinical application of brain repair after stroke is, in general, at an early phase: in most cases, clinical investigations are either preclinical or at phase I or II, although positive phase III data have been published for methods such as intensive physiotherapy [7,8]. As a result, fundamental questions remain to optimize clinical trial methodology for brain repair after stroke, some of which are considered below.

Issues from acute stroke trials inform repair-based stroke trials

To date, the vast majority of acute stroke trials have not shown benefit over placebo. A number of lessons have been gleaned from this acute stroke experience that might be useful to design of clinical trials in the emerging field of brain repair. Issues range from clinical development [9] to entry criteria [10] to outcome measures [11] and beyond.

Methods to identify, then measure, the target tissue or target brain system, are important, and need to be validated [12,13]. Incomplete addressing of this issue might have contributed to the outcome of some previously negative stroke trials [14]. In the setting of brain repair, this might consist of measuring the activity or integrity of a target cortical area [15,16], neurochemical system [17], or white matter tract [18] that is a core component of the therapeutic target. Such methods might be important in relation to improved patient selection, which is likely to be just as important for repair as it is in acute stroke, and in relation to biomarkers (see below). Examples might include measures of brain function via functional MRI, measures of tissue physiology such as transcranial magnetic stimulation, or measures of regional brain injury such as diffusion tensor imaging [16,18].

Dose–response relationships, important in so many other areas of clinical medicine, are likely to be just as important with brain repair [14]. The results of the VECTORS trial, where a higher dose of physiotherapy was associated with poorer behavioral outcome, underscores this point [19]. These relationships might change during the different temporal epochs that follow a stroke [20]. For example, effects of a GABA agonist or NMDA receptor blocker vary depending on whether they are given early [21,22] or late [23–25] after stroke.

When translating the results of animal studies into human clinical trial protocols, many of the lessons from acute stroke trials [26–30] might prove useful for repair-based trials. Issues include matching variables such as treatment time window, route of administration, or dosing schedule. Review of methodological quality of animal studies is an increasing consideration [30]. Use in animal studies of human clinical trial level randomization, concealment of treatment allocation, and blinded outcome assessment might be a key determinant of how well animal studies translate to human trials [31]. Animal models can be of limited relevance to human patients, with animals often being relatively younger [9] and without medical complications or stroke risk factors – for example, in most human but few animal stroke studies, the majority of subjects have hypertension or diabetes mellitus or both (see Chapters 8 and 15). Measures related to executive function, affect, hand dominance, and bipedal gait are generally not considered in animal studies, but can dominate the recovery of a human patient. The organization of rodent brains shows vast differences as compared to humans; for example, white matter constitutes 14% of the rodent brain volume vs. 50% in humans [32,33]. Reorganization after stroke might show differences of a similar magnitude. The experimental infarct in preclinical models tends to be homogeneous, in sharp contrast with humans [34]. Complicating this is that the choice of animal infarct model influences subsequent repair-related molecular events [35–37], and thus might also influence the likelihood of successful translation to humans in the restorative therapy setting.

Repair-based therapies interact with experience, training, and environment

One major difference between acute and repair-based stroke clinical trials is that acute stroke therapies exert

their effect rapidly, around the time of therapy, whereas for a repair-based trial, many of the biological events that improve final behavioral outcome will occur days to weeks after therapy initiation. A subject's experiences, concomitant training, and environment can each interact with a repair-based therapy in defining the final therapy effects. Evidence suggests that both the quantity and the quality of influences can affect brain repair and behavioral outcome [38–45].

One implication of these influences is that for a repair-based trial, many variables that would be considered of limited significance to an acute stroke trial attain increased importance as potential covariates of interest. The details of human experience are complex but become relevant. Furthermore, some of these details are unique to humans, challenging translational efforts from preclinical studies to human trials. Thus, influences that arise between the time that a repair-based therapy is initiated (e.g. time of discharge from the hospital) and the time of final clinical trial outcome assessment (e.g. 90 days after stroke onset) require substantial consideration because they can interact with repair-based therapy and modify its effects.

There are multiple ways that study design might, at least in part, attempt to control these issues. In addition in some cases, these influences can be precisely controlled. In some studies, entry criteria exclude subjects whose post-stroke experience is likely to be highly unusual – for example, subjects who will not be able to receive standard of care physiotherapy. Another way for study design to address this issue relates to the timing of certain study components. For example, in studies of amphetamine that aimed to improve arm motor function early after stroke [46,47], a predefined physiotherapy protocol was initiated at a set number of minutes after medication ingestion, timed to coincide with peak drug levels. In many cases, however, such control would be more difficult. For example, controlling and even monitoring patient experience would be challenging for a growth factor that is thought to exert its effects over days to weeks following its ingestion. Even in the amphetamine examples, enrollees might have had varied experiences and physiotherapy regimens outside of the study – for example, between days of drug provision and the day of final outcome measurements.

When external influences cannot be controlled, study design can insure that they are at least measured. Thus, prospective plans to measure those components of human experience that are most relevant to drug effects or outcome measures can be incorporated into a study's data collection plan. Such an approach provided useful insights in one recent repair-based stroke clinical trial, where the amount of "outside" physiotherapy (i.e. physiotherapy occurring in parallel with trial participation, but prescribed by private physicians, outside of trial jurisdiction), was found to differ significantly between active and placebo treatment arms [20]. Such measures can then be treated as planned covariates of interest in statistical analyses. Note too that such influences might be relatively domain-specific. For example, a study that aims to study how a repair-based therapy affects gait velocity would likely prioritize measurement of non-study therapy focused on gait training over measurement of non-study therapy focused on swallowing. Measurement tools might include questionnaires or selected devices such as pedometers [48] or actigraphy [49].

Other covariates relevant to repair-based trials

Other factors might also influence the likelihood that a repair-based therapy will be found to be effective in human subjects (see Chapters 14 and 15). A number of such factors that influence brain repair, and are thus of potential interest to clinical trials of repair-based therapies, have been described [50]. These include socio-economic factors [51], caregiver status [52,53], and depression/affective state [54–56]. In addition, many of the covariates relevant to acute stroke trials are likely to remain important when trials enroll these patients in repair-based trials. For example, in a study of cognitive recovery after a first stroke, diabetes mellitus was found to be associated with poorer outcome [57].

Genetic factors might also be important to recovery after stroke, and thus therapeutic attempts to improve it [58–61].

An important point is that certain medications can adversely influence brain repair, recovery, and outcome after stroke [62–67]. Thus, medications not only can promote brain repair, evidence suggests they can also impede it (see Chapter 17).

For many of these covariates, a great need exists to standardize methods of measurement. Improved methods and tools are needed to consistently and accurately measure experience-related covariates of interest. Medical comorbidities and complications are common in the early days to weeks after a stroke [68–70], and can influence final outcome [71]. Harmonization is needed for defining, recording, and assigning significance to

such events in the context of a clinical trial. The overall effectiveness of a therapy active during the weeks following a stroke might hinge as much on the accurate assessment of these details as on therapeutic benefits.

Issues of study design for repair-based trials

A number of issues of study design arise when targeting brain repair after stroke. Some are not unique to brain repair; for example, a cross-over study design might not be feasible in many cases [72], as in some cases, e.g. during the first month post-stroke, one can only try one intervention without changing the target neural system forever.

One approach worthy of consideration for repair-based therapies is to focus on within-subject change as the primary means of assessing the endpoint. Many acute stroke trials have been limited in this regard, as measurement of global outcome scales or disability scales can be difficult in the early hours after stroke, when baseline measurements are recorded. However, the trial design of most repair-based trials likely will allow for recording of most endpoints at baseline, prior to initiation of therapy, due to the relatively wide treatment time window typically suggested for this category of intervention. Assessing therapy effects using within-subject change over time, as compared to using cross-sectional subject data acquired at a single late time point, can reduce variance and increase statistical power.

As an extension of this issue, study design for repair-based trials initiated in the acute or early sub-acute period after stroke must carefully define when the baseline measures are acquired. In many forms of stroke, substantial fluctuation of symptoms is not uncommon during the first few days [73]. Baseline measures should be acquired as close as possible to the time of therapy initiation.

Blinding might be more difficult with repair-based studies as compared to acute stroke studies, for multiple possible reasons. For example, this might arise due to use of multiple therapy exposures in many repair-based paradigms, such as the many days of therapy employed in constraint-induced or robot-based therapy, in contrast to briefer therapy exposures for many acute stroke interventions. Also, patients are often more alert during the period of repair-based interventions as versus the early hours [26] post-stroke. Patients in a repair-based trial might be more likely to notice therapy side effects, which could lead to unblinding and thus, to expectation bias [20].

Endpoints and repair-based trials

Brain repair pertains to a broad range of potential target patient populations. However, to date, many of the repair-based stroke clinical trials that have found favorable behavioral effects have emphasized use of domain-specific endpoints [7,47,74,75].

There are several reasons why a repair-based trial might benefit from inclusion of endpoints that measure specific behavioral domains, in addition to endpoints that provide a global view of patient status. First, stroke affects multiple neurological and behavioral domains, and each of these domains can recover to differing extents [76,77]. The time course of recovery in one neurological domain can be independent of recovery in a second domain of neurological function [78–80]. Such differential gains might be best noted with domain-specific endpoints. Also, experience can modulate effects of repair-based therapies, as described above. Indeed, many of the standard therapies provided to patients after stroke are domain-specific, such as hand therapy by an occupational therapist, gait training by a physical therapist, or language therapy by a speech therapist. Domain-specific endpoints might be useful, therefore, to understand the domain-specific effects of standard post-stroke therapy, even if only to measure these effects as covariates in a trial.

A number of domain-specific endpoints have been successfully incorporated into clinical studies in stroke [81,82]. We have been able to effectively incorporate a number of brief, domain-specific measures into recent clinical trials (listed in Table 16.1), such as clinicaltrials. gov NCT00221390, NCT00362414, and NCT00715364. Many reasonable alternatives exist and have been compiled [76,83,84].

Also, the relationship that measures reported in preclinical studies have with the endpoints recorded in clinical trials is unclear [9]. Further studies are needed to clarify these relationships. One potentially fruitful avenue for insight in this regard is to use MRI measures to derive insight, as similar MRI endpoints can be measured in humans and rodents, and might assist in comparing behavioral data across species. Examples include diffusion/perfusion MRI, functional MRI, and diffusion tensor imaging. Such direct comparisons represent a potentially important opportunity in this regard.

Biomarkers and repair-based trials

Direct measurement of the molecular events underlying repair-based therapies would be useful to maximize

Table 16.1 Domain-specific endpoints of potential value to repair-based stroke trials

Test	Domain assessed
Folstein Mini-Mental Status Exam [126]	Global cognitive function
Line cancellation test [127]	Spatial neglect
Boston Naming Test [128]	Aphasia
Alexander's Apraxia Test [129]	Apraxia
Nine Hole Pegboard Test [130]	Manual dexterity
Action Research Arm Test [131], or Arm Motor Fugl–Meyer Score [132]	Arm motor function
Gait velocity [133], or Leg Motor Fugl–Meyer Score [132]	Leg motor function
Nottingham Sensory Assessment [134]	Sensory function
Geriatric Depression Scale [135], or Beck Depression Inventory [136]	Depression

treatment effects. Such data, however, are generally inaccessible in human subjects. Substitute measures, or biomarkers, that can be measured might be valuable towards this goal.

A biomarker can inform clinical trials in many different ways. Such a measure might help define a patient subgroup of interest in a manner not available from bedside exam [62,85]; for example, by measuring the activity or integrity of the CNS treatment target [15–18,62]. By enrolling only those patients in whom the stroke spared a prespecified amount of a target brain region, a trial is likely to reduce variance. Biomarkers such as anatomical scanning or functional neuroimaging might identify survival of such target brain regions better than does a behavioral exam. A biomarker might also provide insight into a treatment's mechanism of action [86–88], which can provide useful insights at the stage of protocol development.

Another major way in which a biomarker might support development of a repair-based therapy is to serve as a surrogate marker, which has been defined as "a laboratory measurement ... used as a substitute for a clinically meaningful endpoint ..." [89]. In general, surrogate markers are particularly useful in phase II trials [90,91]. Examples of successful surrogate markers include blood pressure as a surrogate marker for vascular death, tumor size as a surrogate marker of survival, and HIV RNA level as a surrogate marker of progression to AIDS. Biomarker data can at times be a unique source of information for guiding therapeutic decision-making. This approach has been suggested in the acute stroke setting, where diffusion–perfusion mismatch has been proposed as a surrogate marker of salvable ischemic penumbra [92–94].

A number of caveats exist when considering using a surrogate marker [95]. A good surrogate marker is generally easier to measure than are behavioral end-points, easier to standardize, and saves time and money [90,96]. However, for many of the measures suggested as surrogate markers for brain repair, such as TMS, fMRI, or PET, these features are not clearly established. Nevertheless, a proof of concept study in a carefully defined patient subgroup can be informative and of high guidance, and so investigations into the utility of such measures in this context continue.

Another caveat is that a surrogate marker serves best when its relationships with the disease process and with the therapy are well understood. For example, a surrogate measure has reduced utility when it is not in the causal pathway of the disease process, when the therapy selectively affects physiology of the surrogate, or when the surrogate measure does not fully capture the net effect of therapy on the clinical outcome [90,97]. The usual clinometric properties by which other outcome measures are evaluated, such as validity, reliability, sensitivity, and specificity, remain important to surrogate markers, but limited study of such measures has been performed in the context of brain repair [98–101]. The many covariates influencing brain repair (above) likely also color the utility of surrogate markers in this context.

A number of measures of potential interest are available to serve as biomarkers in this context, some of which are relatively simple to measure. For example, certain blood tests might provide a measure of repair-related biological events that influence subsequent clinical outcome [102,103]. Direct anatomical measures, such as infarct volume [104–106] or regional cortical thickness [107], might have predictive value for response to a repair-based therapy, and so have potential as biomarkers. Measures of injury to a predefined functional brain region, such as the extent of insult to the hand region of primary motor cortex [108], white matter cholinergic projections [109], or left temporal language areas [110], might provide substantial insight into the likelihood that a particular therapy will be able to promote repair in a given patient.

More complex measures are also of potential value as biomarkers of repair-based therapy effects. A number of MRI-based measures have been examined. Diffusion tensor imaging (DTI) provides insight into integrity of white matter tracts and can provide insight into post-stroke brain repair [18,111]. One potential biomarker using this method is the mean value for fractional anisometry within a prespecified region of interest, such as the posterior limb of the internal capsule for a motor-related study [18]. Blood oxygenation level-dependent (BOLD) fMRI provides insights into brain repair [112,113] and can predict treatment response in a clinical stroke trial [16,114]. The impact of cerebrovascular disease on the use of this method, which relies on neuronovascular coupling, remains uncertain, but the convergence of fMRI data findings with results from numerous other human and animal investigations supports its validity [50]. Potential biomarkers using fMRI include the laterality index, a measure of the balance of interhemispheric control [115,116]; task-related signal change, which reflects the magnitude of neuronal activity in relation to task performance [16]; and regional activation volume [20], which describes the spatial extent of task-related activation within a region of interest. Connectivity-based [117], spectroscopic [118,119], and multimodal approaches have also been advanced [120,121].

Other methods might also provide useful biomarkers for trials of repair-based therapies. Physiological measures such as TMS can provide insight into tissue function and its changes with therapy [88,122], especially in the motor system (see Chapter 10). Potential biomarkers with this method include the motor threshold, which describes the amount of energy required to elicit a criterion motor system response; motor-evoked potential (MEP), which describes the skeletal muscle response to motor cortex stimulation; and the latency, which reflects the time between cortical stimulation and the MEP. Brain function can also be measured with PET, as well as with electroencephalography or magnetoencephalography. PET is also able to measure many other brain processes, such as receptor occupation, oxygen extraction, protein synthesis, and metabolism [123–125].

The choice of biomarker might also be driven by pragmatic issues. Many patients with stroke are often frail or unwell, with limited capacity to undergo extended testing. Many stroke patients have disability in a number of neurological domains [77] that might limit testing. For example, a patient with aphasia, hemi-inattention, depression, or dementia might not be able to properly undergo surrogate marker testing when testing requires a high level of cooperation or participation.

Much work remains to bring biomarkers of stroke recovery to the point of utility. The degree of variance in behavioral outcome after therapy explained by biomarkers remains limited. For example, a measure of CNS injury based on DTI accounted for only 38% of the variance in clinical gains in one study [18]; an fMRI-based measure of CNS function, only 20% [16]. Much study is needed for all repair-based candidates as biomarkers to understand their value to clinical trials.

Conclusions

A number of classes of therapy are under evaluation to promote brain repair after stroke. Clinical trials of these agents are emerging. In some regards, the design of these trials is directly informed by experience with acute stroke trials. In other regards, there are unique features to repair-based trials. Issues related to covariates of interest, endpoints, and biomarkers in this context have been considered above. Improvements in the design of repair-based trials will help translate preclinical findings, and maximize the application of this class of therapy to the large population of patients living with stroke.

Measures of global outcome such as the NIH Stroke Scale, the Barthel Index, and the modified Rankin Scale are of potential value to measuring effects of repair-based therapies. In addition, measuring therapy effects in specific domains might have value. Table 16.1 lists selected domain-specific endpoints of potential interest.

References

1. Yue NC, Longstreth WT Jr., Elster AD, *et al.* Clinically serious abnormalities found incidentally at MR imaging of the brain: Data from the Cardiovascular Health Study. *Radiology.* 1997;**202**:41–6.

2. Lloyd-Jones D, Adams R, Carnethon M, *et al.* Heart disease and stroke statistics – 2009 update: A report from the American Heart Association Statistics Committee and Stroke Statistics Subcommittee. *Circulation.* 2009; **119**:480–6.

3. Reed S, Cramer S, Blough D, *et al.* Treatment with tissue plasminogen activator and inpatient mortality rates for patients with ischemic stroke treated in community hospitals. *Stroke.* 2001;**32**:1832–40.

4. Katzan I, Furlan A, Lloyd L, *et al.* Use of tissue-type plasminogen activator for acute ischemic stroke: The Cleveland area experience. *JAMA.* 2000;**283**:1151–8.

5. The National Institute of Neurological Disorders and Stroke rt-PA Stroke Study Group. Tissue plasminogen activator for acute ischemic stroke. *N Engl J Med.* 1995;**333**:1581–7.

6. Furlan A, Higashida R, Wechsler L, *et al.* Intra-arterial prourokinase for acute ischemic stroke. The PROACT II study: A randomized controlled trial. Prolyse in Acute Cerebral Thromboembolism. *JAMA.* 1999;**282**:2003–11.

7. Wolf SL, Winstein CJ, Miller JP, *et al.* Effect of constraint-induced movement therapy on upper extremity function 3 to 9 months after stroke: The EXCITE randomized clinical trial. *JAMA.* 2006;**296**:2095–104.

8. Wolf SL, Winstein CJ, Miller JP, *et al.* Retention of upper limb function in stroke survivors who have received constraint-induced movement therapy: The EXCITE randomised trial. *Lancet Neurol.* 2008;**7**:33–40.

9. Savitz SI, Fisher M. Future of neuroprotection for acute stroke: In the aftermath of the SAINT trials. *Ann Neurol.* 2007;**61**:396–402.

10. Uchino K, Billheimer D, Cramer S. Entry criteria and baseline characteristics predict outcome in acute stroke trials. *Stroke.* 2001;**32**:909–16.

11. Duncan P, Jorgensen H, Wade D. Outcome measures in acute stroke trials: A systematic review and some recommendations to improve practice. *Stroke.* 2000;**31**:1429–38.

12. Toth G, Albers GW. Use of MRI to estimate the therapeutic window in acute stroke: Is perfusion-weighted imaging/diffusion-weighted imaging mismatch an EPITHET for salvageable ischemic brain tissue? *Stroke.* 2009;**40**:333–5.

13. Donnan GA, Baron JC, Ma H, *et al.* Penumbral selection of patients for trials of acute stroke therapy. *Lancet Neurol.* 2009;**8**:261–9.

14. Feuerstein GZ, Zaleska MM, Krams M, *et al.* Missing steps in the STAIR case: A Translational Medicine perspective on the development of NXY-059 for treatment of acute ischemic stroke. *J Cereb Blood Flow Metab.* 2008;**28**:217–9.

15. Cramer S, Benson R, Burra V, *et al.* Mapping individual brains to guide restorative therapy after stroke: Rationale and pilot studies. *Neurol Res.* 2003;**25**:811–4.

16. Cramer SC, Parrish TB, Levy RM, *et al.* Predicting functional gains in a stroke trial. *Stroke.* 2007;**38**:2108–14.

17. Tardy J, Pariente J, Leger A, *et al.* Methylphenidate modulates cerebral post-stroke reorganization. *NeuroImage.* 2006;**33**:913–22.

18. Stinear CM, Barber PA, Smale PR, *et al.* Functional potential in chronic stroke patients depends on corticospinal tract integrity. *Brain.* 2007;**130**:170–80.

19. Dromerick A, Lang C, Powers W, *et al.* Very Early Constraint-Induced Movement Therapy (VECTORS): Phase II trial results. *Stroke.* 2007;**38**:465.

20. Cramer S, Dobkin B, Noser E, *et al.* A randomized, placebo-controlled, double-blind study of ropinirole in chronic stroke. *Stroke.* 2009;**40**:3034–8.

21. Green AR, Hainsworth AH, Jackson DM. GABA potentiation: A logical pharmacological approach for the treatment of acute ischaemic stroke. *Neuropharmacology.* 2000;**39**:1483–94.

22. Ovbiagele B, Kidwell CS, Starkman S, *et al.* Neuroprotective agents for the treatment of acute ischemic stroke. *Curr Neurol Neurosci Rep.* 2003;**3**:9–20.

23. Kozlowski D, Jones T, Schallert T. Pruning of dendrites and restoration of function after brain damage: Role of the NMDA receptor. *Restor Neurol Neurosci.* 1994;**7**:119–26.

24. Wahlgren N, Martinsson L. New concepts for drug therapy after stroke. Can we enhance recovery? *Cerebrovasc Dis.* 1998;**8**(Suppl 5): 33–8.

25. Barth T, Hoane M, Barbay S, *et al.* Effects of glutamate antagonists on the recovery and maintenance of behavioral function after brain injury. In: Goldstein L, editor. *Restorative neurology: Advances in pharmacotherapy for recovery after stroke.* Armonk, NY: Futura Publishing Co., Inc.; 1998.

26. Grotta J, Bratina P. Subjective experiences of 24 patients dramatically recovering from stroke. *Stroke.* 1995;**26**:1285–8.

27. Fisher M, Ratan R. New perspectives on developing acute stroke therapy. *Ann Neurol.* 2003;**53**:10–20.

28. Gladstone D, Black S, Hakim A. Toward wisdom from failure: lessons from neuroprotective stroke trials and new therapeutic directions. *Stroke.* 2002;**33**:2123–36.

29. Fisher M, Feuerstein G, Howells DW, *et al.* Update of the Stroke Therapy Academic Industry Roundtable Preclinical Recommendations. *Stroke.* 2009;**40**:2244–50.

30. Philip M, Benatar M, Fisher M, *et al.* Methodological quality of animal studies of neuroprotective agents currently in phase II/III acute ischemic stroke trials. *Stroke.* 2009;**40**:577–81.

31. Macleod MR, van der Worp HB, Sena ES, *et al.* Evidence for the efficacy of NXY-059 in experimental focal cerebral ischaemia is confounded by study quality. *Stroke.* 2008;**39**:2824–9.

32. Goldberg MP, Ransom BR. New light on white matter. *Stroke.* 2003;**34**:330–2.

33. Cramer S. Clinical issues in animal models of stroke and rehabilitation. *ILAR J.* 2003;**44**:83–4.

34. Endres M, Engelhardt B, Koistinaho J, *et al.* Improving outcome after stroke: Overcoming the translational roadblock. *Cerebrovasc Dis.* 2008;**25**:268–78.

35. Napieralski JA, Butler AK, Chesselet MF. Anatomical and functional evidence for lesion-specific sprouting of corticostriatal input in the adult rat. *J Comp Neurol.* 1996;**373**:484–97.

36. Voorhies A, Jones T. The behavioral and dendritic growth effects of focal sensorimotor cortical damage depend on the method of lesion induction. *Behav Brain Res.* 2002;**133**:237–46.

37. Windle V, Szymanska A, Granter-Button S, *et al.* An analysis of four different methods of producing focal cerebral ischemia with endothelin-1 in the rat. *Exp Neurol.* 2006;**201**:324–34.

38. Kwakkel G. Impact of intensity of practice after stroke: Issues for consideration. *Disabil Rehabil.* 2006;**28**:823–30.

39. Kwakkel G, Wagenaar R, Twisk J, *et al.* Intensity of leg and arm training after primary middle-cerebral-artery stroke: A randomised trial. *Lancet.* 1999;**354**:191–6.

40. Dobkin B. *The clinical science of neurologic rehabilitation.* New York, NY: Oxford University Press; 2003.

41. Van Peppen RP, Kwakkel G, Wood-Dauphinee S, *et al.* The impact of physical therapy on functional outcomes after stroke: What's the evidence? *Clin Rehabil.* 2004;**18**:833–62.

42. Cicerone KD, Dahlberg C, Malec JF, *et al.* Evidence-based cognitive rehabilitation: Updated review of the literature from 1998 through 2002. *Arch Phys Med Rehabil.* 2005;**86**:1681–92.

43. Bhogal S, Teasell R, Speechley M. Intensity of aphasia therapy, impact on recovery. *Stroke.* 2003;**34**:987–93.

44. Jones T, Chu C, Grande L, *et al.* Motor skills training enhances lesion-induced structural plasticity in the motor cortex of adult rats. *J Neurosci.* 1999;**19**:10 153–63.

45. Johansson B. Brain plasticity and stroke rehabilitation. The Willis lecture. *Stroke.* 2000;**31**:223–30.

46. Gladstone DJ, Danells CJ, Armesto A, *et al.* Physiotherapy coupled with dextroamphetamine for rehabilitation after hemiparetic stroke: A randomized, double-blind, placebo-controlled trial. *Stroke.* 2006;**37**:179–85.

47. Walker-Batson D, Smith P, Curtis S, *et al.* Amphetamine paired with physical therapy accelerates motor recovery after stroke. Further evidence. *Stroke.* 1995;**26**:2254–9.

48. Macko RF, Haeuber E, Shaughnessy M, *et al.* Microprocessor-based ambulatory activity monitoring in stroke patients. *Med Sci Sports Exerc.* 2002;**34**:394–9.

49. Reiterer V, Sauter C, Klosch G, *et al.* Actigraphy – A useful tool for motor activity monitoring in stroke patients. *Eur Neurol.* 2008;**60**:285–91.

50. Cramer SC. Repairing the human brain after stroke: I. Mechanisms of spontaneous recovery. *Ann Neurol.* 2008;**63**:272–87.

179

51. McFadden E, Luben R, Wareham N, *et al*. Social class, risk factors, and stroke incidence in men and women: A prospective study in the European prospective investigation into cancer in Norfolk cohort. *Stroke*. 2009;**40**:1070–7.

52. Smith J, Forster A, Young J. Cochrane review: Information provision for stroke patients and their caregivers. *Clin Rehabil*. 2009;**23**:195–206.

53. Glass TA, Matchar DB, Belyea M, *et al*. Impact of social support on outcome in first stroke. *Stroke*. 1993;**24**:64–70.

54. Lai SM, Duncan PW, Keighley J, *et al*. Depressive symptoms and independence in BADL and IADL. *J Rehabil Res Dev*. 2002;**39**:589–96.

55. Jonsson AC, Lindgren I, Hallstrom B, *et al*. Determinants of quality of life in stroke survivors and their informal caregivers. *Stroke*. 2005;**36**:803–8.

56. Mukherjee D, Levin RL, Heller W. The cognitive, emotional, and social sequelae of stroke: Psychological and ethical concerns in post-stroke adaptation. *Topics Stroke Rehabil*. 2006;**13**:26–35.

57. Nys GM, Van Zandvoort MJ, De Kort PL, *et al*. Domain-specific cognitive recovery after first-ever stroke: A follow-up study of 111 cases. *J Int Neuropsychol Soc*. 2005;**11**:795–806.

58. Kleim JA, Chan S, Pringle E, *et al*. BDNF val66met polymorphism is associated with modified experience-dependent plasticity in human motor cortex. *Nat Neurosci*. 2006;**9**:735–7.

59. Siironen J, Juvela S, Kanarek K, *et al*. The Met allele of the BDNF Val66Met polymorphism predicts poor outcome among survivors of aneurysmal subarachnoid hemorrhage. *Stroke*. 2007;**38**:2858–60.

60. Alberts MJ, Graffagnino C, McClenny C, *et al*. ApoE genotype and survival from intracerebral haemorrhage. *Lancet*. 1995;**346**:575.

61. Pearson-Fuhrhop KM, Kleim JA, Cramer SC. Brain plasticity and genetic factors. *Top Stroke Rehabil*. 2009;**16**:282–99.

62. Butefisch C, Davis B, Wise S, *et al*. Mechanisms of use-dependent plasticity in the human motor cortex. *Proc Natl Acad Sci USA*. 2000;**97**:3661–5.

63. Feeney D, Gonzalez A, Law W. Amphetamine, haloperidol, and experience interact to affect the rate of recovery after motor cortex injury. *Science*. 1982;**217**:855–7.

64. Goldstein L, Sygen in Acute Stroke Study Investigators. Common drugs may influence motor recovery after stroke. *Neurology*. 1995;**45**:865–71.

65. Troisi E, Paolucci S, Silvestrini M, *et al*. Prognostic factors in stroke rehabilitation: The possible role of pharmacological treatment. *Acta Neurol Scand*. 2002;**105**:100–06.

66. Conroy B, Zorowitz R, Horn SD, *et al*. An exploration of central nervous system medication use and outcomes in stroke rehabilitation. *Arch Phys Med Rehabil*. 2005;**86**(12 Suppl 2):S73–S81.

67. Lazar R, Fitzsimmons B, Marshall R, *et al*. Reemergence of stroke deficits with midazolam challenge. *Stroke*. 2002;**33**:283–5.

68. Dromerick AW, Khader SA. Medical complications during stroke rehabilitation. *Adv Neurol*. 2003;**92**:409–13.

69. Kalra L, Yu G, Wilson K, *et al*. Medical complications during stroke rehabilitation. *Stroke*. 1995;**26**:990–4.

70. McLean D. Medical complications experienced by a cohort of stroke survivors during inpatient, tertiary-level stroke rehabilitation. *Arch Phys Med Rehabil*. 2004;**85**:466–9.

71. Berlowitz DR, Hoenig H, Cowper DC, *et al*. Impact of comorbidities on stroke rehabilitation outcomes: Does the method matter? *Arch Phys Med Rehabil*. 2008;**89**:1903–06.

72. Piantadosi S. *Clinical trials. A methodologic perspective*. New York, NY: John Wiley & Sons, Inc.; 1997.

73. Ozdemir O, Beletsky V, Chan R, *et al*. Thrombolysis in patients with marked clinical fluctuations in neurologic status due to cerebral ischemia. *Arch Neurol*. 2008;**65**:1041–3.

74. Volpe BT, Ferraro M, Lynch D, *et al*. Robotics and other devices in the treatment of patients recovering from stroke. *Curr Neurol Neurosci Rep*. 2005;**5**:465–70.

75. Scheidtmann K, Fries W, Muller F, *et al*. Effect of levodopa in combination with physiotherapy on functional motor recovery after stroke: A prospective, randomised, double-blind study. *Lancet*. 2001;**358**:787–90.

76. Gresham G, Duncan P, Stason W, *et al*. *Post-stroke rehabilitation*. Rockville, MD: US Department of Health and Human Services. Public Health Service, Agency for Health Care Policy and Research; 1995.

77. Rathore S, Hinn A, Cooper L, *et al*. Characterization of incident stroke signs and symptoms: Findings from the Atherosclerosis Risk in Communities study. *Stroke*. 2002;**33**:2718–21.

78. Hier D, Mondlock J, Caplan L. Recovery of behavioral abnormalities after right hemisphere stroke. *Neurology*. 1983;**33**:345–50.

79. Marshall R, Perera G, Lazar R, *et al*. Evolution of cortical activation during recovery from corticospinal tract infarction. *Stroke*. 2000;**31**:656–61.

80. Markgraf C, Green E, Hurwitz B, *et al*. Sensorimotor and cognitive consequences of middle cerebral artery occlusion in rats. *Brain Res*. 1992;**575**:238–46.

81. Hillis A, Newhart M, Heidler J, *et al*. Anatomy of spatial attention: Insights from perfusion imaging and

hemispatial neglect in acute stroke. *J Neurosci.* 2005;**25**:3161–7.

82. Hillis A, Wityk R, Barker P, *et al.* Subcortical aphasia and neglect in acute stroke: The role of cortical hypoperfusion. *Brain.* 2002;**125**:1094–104.

83. Duncan PW, Zorowitz R, Bates B, *et al.* Management of adult stroke rehabilitation care: A clinical practice guideline. *Stroke.* 2005;**36**:e100–43.

84. Salter K, Jutai J, Zettler L, *et al.* Outcome measures in stroke rehabilitation. http://wwwebrsrcom/uploads/ Outcome_Measures_SREBR11_finalpdf. 2008.

85. Collins JM. Functional imaging in phase I studies: Decorations or decision making? *J Clin Oncol.* 2003;**21**:2807–09.

86. Carey J, Kimberley T, Lewis S, *et al.* Analysis of fMRI and finger tracking training in subjects with chronic stroke. *Brain.* 2002;**125**:773–88.

87. Johansen-Berg H, Dawes H, Guy C, *et al.* Correlation between motor improvements and altered fMRI activity after rehabilitative therapy. *Brain.* 2002;**125**:2731–42.

88. Koski L, Mernar T, Dobkin B. Immediate and long-term changes in corticomotor output in response to rehabilitation: Correlation with functional improvements in chronic stroke. *Neurorehabil Neural Repair.* 2004;**18**:230–49.

89. Temple R. A regulatory authority's opinion about surrogate endpoints. In: Nimmo W, Tucker G, editors. *Clinical measurement in drug evaluation.* New York, NY: John Wiley and Sons; 1995.

90. Fleming T, DeMets D. Surrogate end points in clinical trials: Are we being misled? *Ann Intern Med.* 1996;**125**:605–13.

91. Stephen RM, Gillies RJ. Promise and progress for functional and molecular imaging of response to targeted therapies. *Pharm Res.* 2007;**24**:1172–85.

92. Lansberg MG, Thijs VN, Hamilton S, *et al.* Evaluation of the clinical-diffusion and perfusion–diffusion mismatch models in DEFUSE. *Stroke.* 2007;**38**:1826–30.

93. Furlan AJ, Eyding D, Albers GW, *et al.* Dose Escalation of Desmoteplase for Acute Ischemic Stroke (DEDAS): Evidence of safety and efficacy 3 to 9 hours after stroke onset. *Stroke.* 2006;**37**:1227–31.

94. Hacke W, Albers G, Al-Rawi Y, *et al.* The Desmoteplase in Acute Ischemic Stroke trial (DIAS): A phase II MRI-based 9-hour window acute stroke thrombolysis trial with intravenous desmoteplase. *Stroke.* 2005;**36**:66–73.

95. Hsia A, Kidwell C. Magnetic resonance imaging for surrogate outcomes and patient selection. In: Woodbury-Harris K, Coull B, editors. *Clinical trials in the neurosciences.* Basel: Karger; 2009: pp. 89–92.

96. Boissel J, Collet J, Moleur P, *et al.* Surrogate endpoints: A basis for a rational approach. *Eur J Clin Pharmacol.* 1992;**43**:235–44.

97. Bucher H, Guyatt G, Cook D, *et al.* Users' guides to the medical literature: XIX. Applying clinical trial results. A. How to use an article measuring the effect of an intervention on surrogate end points. Evidence-Based Medicine Working Group. *JAMA.* 1999;**282**:771–8.

98. Takahashi CD, Der-Yeghiaian L, Le V, *et al.* Robot-based hand motor therapy after stroke. *Brain.* 2008;**131**:425–37.

99. Bosnell R, Wegner C, Kincses ZT, *et al.* Reproducibility of fMRI in the clinical setting: Implications for trial designs. *NeuroImage.* 2008;**42**:603–10.

100. Eaton KP, Szaflarski JP, Altaye M, *et al.* Reliability of fMRI for studies of language in post-stroke aphasia subjects. *NeuroImage.* 2008;**41**:311–22.

101. Kimberley TJ, Khandekar G, Borich M. fMRI reliability in subjects with stroke. *Exp Brain Res/Experimentelle Hirnforschung.* 2008;**186**:183–90.

102. Geiger S, Holdenrieder S, Stieber P, *et al.* Nucleosomes as a new prognostic marker in early cerebral stroke. *J Neurol.* 2007;**254**:617–23.

103. Yip HK, Chang LT, Chang WN, *et al.* Level and value of circulating endothelial progenitor cells in patients after acute ischemic stroke. *Stroke.* 2008;**39**:69–74.

104. Brott T, Marler J, Olinger C, *et al.* Measurements of acute cerebral infarction: Lesion size by computed tomography. *Stroke.* 1989;**20**:871–5.

105. Saver J, Johnston K, Homer D, *et al.* Infarct volume as a surrogate or auxiliary outcome measure in ischemic stroke clinical trials. The RANTTAS Investigators. *Stroke.* 1999;**30**:293–8.

106. Schiemanck SK, Kwakkel G, Post MW, *et al.* Predictive value of ischemic lesion volume assessed with magnetic resonance imaging for neurological deficits and functional outcome poststroke: A critical review of the literature. *Neurorehabil Neural Repair.* 2006;**20**:492–502.

107. Schaechter JD, Moore CI, Connell BD, *et al.* Structural and functional plasticity in the somatosensory cortex of chronic stroke patients. *Brain.* 2006;**129**:2722–33.

108. Crafton K, Mark A, Cramer S. Improved understanding of cortical injury by incorporating measures of functional anatomy. *Brain.* 2003;**126**:1650–9.

109. Bocti C, Swartz RH, Gao FQ, *et al.* A new visual rating scale to assess strategic white matter hyperintensities within cholinergic pathways in dementia. *Stroke.* 2005;**36**:2126–31.

110. Hillis AE, Gold L, Kannan V, *et al.* Site of the ischemic penumbra as a predictor of potential for recovery of functions. *Neurology.* 2008;**71**:184–9.

181

111. Ding G, Jiang Q, Li L, *et al.* Magnetic resonance imaging investigation of axonal remodeling and angiogenesis after embolic stroke in sildenafil-treated rats. *J Cereb Blood Flow Metab.* 2008;**28**:1440–8.

112. Hodics T, Cohen LG, Cramer SC. Functional imaging of intervention effects in stroke motor rehabilitation. *Arch Phys Med Rehabil.* 2006;**87**(12 Suppl):36–42.

113. Richards LG, Stewart KC, Woodbury ML, *et al.* Movement-dependent stroke recovery: A systematic review and meta-analysis of TMS and fMRI evidence. *Neuropsychologia.* 2008;**46**:3–11.

114. Dong Y, Dobkin BH, Cen SY, *et al.* Motor cortex activation during treatment may predict therapeutic gains in paretic hand function after stroke. *Stroke.* 2006;**37**:1552–5.

115. Cramer S, Nelles G, Benson R, *et al.* A functional MRI study of subjects recovered from hemiparetic stroke. *Stroke.* 1997;**28**:2518–27.

116. Naccarato M, Calautti C, Jones PS, *et al.* Does healthy aging affect the hemispheric activation balance during paced index-to-thumb opposition task? An fMRI study. *NeuroImage.* 2006;**32**:1250–6.

117. Grefkes C, Nowak DA, Eickhoff SB, *et al.* Cortical connectivity after subcortical stroke assessed with functional magnetic resonance imaging. *Ann Neurol.* 2008;**63**:236–46.

118. Parsons M, Li T, Barber P, *et al.* Combined (1)H MR spectroscopy and diffusion-weighted MRI improves the prediction of stroke outcome. *Neurology.* 2000;**55**:498–505.

119. Pendlebury S, Blamire A, Lee M, *et al.* Axonal injury in the internal capsule correlates with motor impairment after stroke. *Stroke.* 1999;**30**:956–62.

120. Nair DG, Hutchinson S, Fregni F, *et al.* Imaging correlates of motor recovery from cerebral infarction and their physiological significance in well-recovered patients. *NeuroImage.* 2007;**34**:253–63.

121. Ward NS, Newton JM, Swayne OB, *et al.* Motor system activation after subcortical stroke depends on corticospinal system integrity. *Brain.* 2006;**129**:809–19.

122. Talelli P, Greenwood RJ, Rothwell JC. Arm function after stroke: Neurophysiological correlates and recovery mechanisms assessed by transcranial magnetic stimulation. *Clin Neurophysiol.* 2006;**117**:1641–59.

123. Powers W, Raichle M. Positron emission tomography and its application to the study of cerebrovascular disease in man. *Stroke.* 1985;**16**:361–76.

124. Heiss WD. Imaging the ischemic penumbra and treatment effects by PET. *Keio J Med.* 2001;**50**:249–56.

125. Ward NS. Neural plasticity and recovery of function. *Prog Brain Res.* 2005;**150**:527–35.

126. Folstein MF, Folstein SE, McHugh PR. "Mini-mental state". A practical method for grading the cognitive state of patients for the clinician. *J Psychiatr Res.* 1975;**12**:189–98.

127. Albert ML. A simple test of visual neglect. *Neurology.* 1973;**23**:658–64.

128. Kent PS, Luszcz MA. A review of the Boston Naming Test and multiple-occasion normative data for older adults on 15-item versions. *Clin Neuropsychol.* 2002;**16**:555–74.

129. Alexander MP, Baker E, Naeser MA, *et al.* Neuropsychological and neuroanatomical dimensions of ideomotor apraxia. *Brain.* 1992;**115**: 87–107.

130. Wade DT. Measuring arm impairment and disability after stroke. *Int Disabil Stud.* 1989;**11**:89–92.

131. Yozbatiran N, Der-Yeghiaian L, Cramer SC. A standardized approach to performing the action research arm test. *Neurorehabil Neural Repair.* 2008;**22**:78–90.

132. Fugl-Meyer A, Jaasko L, Leyman I, *et al.* The post-stroke hemiplegic patient: a method for evaluation of physical performance. *Scand J Rehabil Med.* 1975;**7**:13–31.

133. Richards C, Malouin F, Dumas F, *et al.* Gait velocity as an outcome measure of locomotor recovery after stroke. In: Craik R, Oates C, editors. *Gait analysis: Theory and application.* St. Louis: Mosby; 1995: pp. 355–64.

134. Lincoln N, Jackson J, Adams S. Reliability and revision of the Nottingham Sensory Assessment for stroke patients. *Physiotherapy.* 1998;**84**:358–65.

135. Agrell B, Dehlin O. Comparison of six depression rating scales in geriatric stroke patients. *Stroke.* 1989;**20**:1190–4.

136. Beck AT, Beck RW. Screening depressed patients in family practice. A rapid technique. *Postgrad Med.* 1972;**52**:81–5.

17

Neuropharmacology in stroke recovery

Isabelle Loubinoux & François Chollet

Introduction

Clinicians have long recognized that most stroke survivors recover over time, albeit to varying degrees. Until now, rTPA thrombolysis within the first hours of the stroke is recognized as the only validated treatment able to improve the spontaneous – and most of the time incomplete – recovery of neurological functions after stroke. However, we have learnt from research over the last decade, in part based on the considerable improvement of neuroimaging techniques, that spontaneous recovery of neurological functions was associated with a large intracerebral reorganization of the damaged human brain (see Chapters 9–13). Recruitment of remote functional areas, overactivation of primary cortices, and changes in cortical maps are now considered as the physiological substratum of clinical recovery. Moreover, it has now been demonstrated that brain post-stroke plasticity can be modulated in order to reduce the residual neurological deficit and the subsequent disability. Rehabilitation, rTMS, peripheral stimulations, local anesthetic blocks, drugs, and other interventions have demonstrated in certain conditions a capacity to induce an intracerebral reorganization after focal lesion (see also Chapters 18–24). All are potential therapeutic agents for recovery. They rely on induced functional changes in a damaged intracerebral network. Each of these therapeutic interventions requires extensive validation. We review in this chapter the data concerning drug and other neuropharmacological aspects of the issue. We also address the clinical questions concerning the repair of damaged neuronal networks and potential future therapy using external cellular material.

Animal models

Studies in laboratory animals clearly show that the rate and extent of functional recovery after focal brain injury can be modulated by drugs affecting certain neurotransmitters in the central nervous system. Those laboratory experiments indicate that the rate and degree of recovery can be affected by changes in selected neurotransmitters in the central nervous system (CNS).

Norepinephrine and motor recovery

Several lines of evidence suggest that motor recovery after injury to the cerebral cortex can be modulated through the effects of norepinephrine on the CNS. Detailed reviews have been published [1–3]. For example, in rats, central infusion of norepinephrine hastens locomotor recovery after a unilateral sensorimotor cortex lesion. In addition, bilateral or unilateral selective lesions of the locus ceruleus, the major source of noradrenergic projection fibers to the cerebral cortex and cerebellum, also impair motor recovery after a subsequent unilateral cortical lesion. In a provocative initial experiment, Feeney and Sutton [1] found that, when combined with task-relevant experience, a single dose of dextroamphetamine given the day after a unilateral sensorimotor cortex ablation in the rat resulted in an enduring enhancement of motor recovery. The amphetamine effect found by Feeney and Sutton has subsequently been confirmed in relation to functional deficits arising from focal lesions produced through a variety of mechanisms, to lesions affecting other areas of the cortex, and to a range of other behaviors.

Norepinephrine agonists and antagonists

Given the hypothesis that the effect of amphetamine on recovery is exerted through its effect on norepinephrine, other drugs that enhance norepinephrine tone would be expected to have similarly favorable effects on behavioral recovery after stroke. In fact, yohimbine and idazoxan (α2-adrenergic receptor

Brain Repair After Stroke, ed. S. C. Cramer and R. J. Nudo. Published by Cambridge University Press.
© Cambridge University Press 2010.

antagonists that increase the release of norepinephrine in the CNS) facilitate motor recovery when given as a single dose after unilateral sensorimotor cortex injury. Similarly, phentermine, an amphetamine analog with weaker cardiovascular effects, phenylpropanolamine, and methylphenidate hydrochloride also accelerate motor recovery after experimental focal brain injury.

If drugs that enhance norepinephrine release are beneficial, then drugs that decrease norepinephrine release, increase its catabolism, or block its postsynaptic effects would be hypothesized to be harmful to recovery. In experiments designed to test this hypothesis, a single dose of the α2-adrenergic receptor agonist clonidine hydrochloride, given the day after cortex injury, was found to have a prolonged detrimental effect on motor recovery in rats and to reinstate the deficit in recovered animals. Prazosin and phenoxybenzamine, α1-adrenergic receptor antagonists that act on the CNS, also interfere with recovery.

Other drugs

Antidepressants

Depression is common after stroke (see Chapter 14) and often prompts the use of antidepressant medications. The administration of a single dose of trazodone, a 5HT reuptake blocker, transiently slows motor recovery in rats with sensorimotor cortex injury and reinstates the hemiparesis in recovered animals. A single dose of desipramine, a NE reuptake blocker, facilitates motor recovery.

GABA

Intracortical infusion of gamma-aminobutyric acid (GABA) was found to increase the hemiparesis produced by a small motor cortex lesion in rats. The short-term administration of the benzodiazepine diazepam, an indirect GABA agonist, permanently impedes recovery from the sensory asymmetry caused by damage to the anteromedial neocortex in the rat [4]. The deleterious effect of GABA on motor recovery after motor cortex injury is increased by the peripheral administration of phenytoin. Phenobarbital also delays behavioral recovery after injury to the cerebral cortex in laboratory studies. In contrast, neither carbamazepine nor vigabatrin has detrimental effects.

Dopamine and dopaminergic drugs

Dopaminergic agents may influence recovery from neglect caused by prefrontal cortical injury. Apomorphine, a dopamine agonist, reduces the severity of experimentally induced neglect, and spiroperidol, a dopamine receptor antagonist, reinstates neglect in recovered animals. Concurrent administration of dopamine-blocking drugs such as haloperidol also blocks amphetamine-promoted recovery, and haloperidol, as well as other butyrophenones (fluanisone, droperidol), transiently reinstates the deficits in recovered animals.

General trends from experimental studies

From published experimental studies, several main conclusions can be emphasized.

- First, one can be convinced from these studies that there is obviously a large interaction between certain drugs and the recovery process in animal models. Norepinephrine and its agonists and antagonists have probably been the most studied drugs, but others with potentially fewer side effects might also be beneficial. This is undoubtedly sufficient data from animal studies to support the need for further human studies [5].
- Second, it appears that the cellular mechanisms underlying these significant effects of drugs acting on the CNS are still not well understood. Additional basic research is needed to better understand such pharmacological actions in the setting of rewiring and cellular growth in the damaged brain.
- Third, drugs can have varying effects based on the dosage and also the dose regimen. For example, animal studies have found that with increasing dose, amphetamine has increasing then decreasing benefit. We have demonstrated kinetics in human subjects; for example, with increasing dose of paroxetine, primary motor cortex activation increases then decreases.
- Motor deficits have been the most frequently studied domain of recovery after a focal lesion. Other neurological domains require further study.
- Moreover, the timing of drug administration may be crucial. A therapeutic time window probably exists. Some drugs, such as benzodiazepines, that may be neuroprotective when given soon after the stroke, are harmful when given later [6]. Amphetamine may no longer be effective after a therapeutic window of opportunity has passed [7].
- Last, the effects of many drugs, particularly the effects of noradrenergic agents on motor recovery after injury to the cerebral cortex, are highly dependent on experimental details. For example, drug infusion paired with behavioral training does

not have the same behavioral effect as compared to drug infusion without training.

Clinical trials

Trials reported here were considered reliable since they were all randomized, double-blind, and placebo-controlled. In this part of the chapter we will only mention trials where the main evaluation criterion was clinical outcome. Ideally, the optimal pharmacological treatment of an individual patient should be predictable and hypothesis-driven. Hypotheses can in some instances be derived from findings in animal experiments. Other approaches are possible. For example, functional imaging tools such as fMRI, PET, electroencephalography, or TMS allow evaluation of the effects of a drug on brain activity in greater detail. In some cases, they can be considered as surrogate markers for drug activity on the human damaged brain (see Chapter 16). They might represent the initial step of clinical evaluation of the drug, but the final judgment must be clinical. The interest of neuroimaging will be detailed in the next part of the chapter. The below review considers selected trials. More comprehensive reviews regarding clinical trials have been published [8,9].

Amphetamine

Dextroamphetamine enhances the release of noradrenaline and dopamine in the synaptic cleft. Such a mechanism seemed promising because animal experiments have indicated that the two neurotransmitters modulated by this drug support activity and motor functions.

Recovery of motor function

Several studies have tested the effects of D-amphetamine on motor recovery after stroke, including a total of at least 280 patients.

The first study of the effects of amphetamine on recovery after stroke in humans [10] was carefully designed to simulate the paradigm used in the laboratory. Eight patients with stable motor deficits were randomized to receive a single dose of amphetamine or a placebo within 10 days of ischemic stroke, with drug administration tightly coupled with physical therapy. The following day, the amphetamine-treated group had a significant improvement in motor performance ($P < .05$), whereas there was little change in the placebo-treated group. A second double-blind, placebo-controlled trial involving 12 patients [57]

found no treatment effect, but it differed in several ways from the previous study. A different dosing regimen was used, interventions began more than 1 month after the stroke, and the administration of the drug or placebo was not tightly linked with physical therapy. In a third double-blind, placebo controlled trial [11], a short course of treatment began between 15 and 30 days after the stroke, with each dose of amphetamine or placebo given in tight conjunction with physical therapy. Patients treated with amphetamine had significantly greater improvements in motor scores compared with placebo-treated patients ($P < .05$), and that benefit persisted for as long as 10 months after the intervention ceased. In combination with the principles learned from the laboratory, these three clinical studies suggest that drug dosage, timing, and the tight coupling of drug therapy with physical therapy may be critical determinants of whether the treatment is efficacious.

Despite these results, subsequent studies failed to show a superiority of D-amphetamine compared with placebo [12–17], even though some adhered to key principles such as tight coupling of peak drug blood levels with physical therapy. A recent review summarized that it is currently impossible to draw any definite conclusions about the potential role of D-amphetamine in motor rehabilitation [18].

Recovery of aphasia

Two placebo-controlled studies have evaluated changes of aphasic symptoms during treatment with D-amphetamine. Walker-Batson et al. [19] studied 21 stroke patients in the subacute phase. Ten milligrams of D-amphetamine were administered every third or fourth day, combined with a 1-h session of speech therapy. Altogether, 10 sessions were performed. The Porch Index of Communicative Ability was used as a measure of changes. Patients receiving D-amphetamine improved significantly, and 6 months later there was still a trend for greater improvement in the D-amphetamine group.

Whiting et al. [20] published a study, although only two patients were enrolled, making it difficult to draw large conclusions. In this report, one patient showed greater improvement during D-amphetamine treatment, whereas the other did not.

Methylphenidate

Methylphenidate produces an increase in dopamine and noradrenaline signaling through multiple actions.

A prospective, randomized, double-blind, placebo-controlled trial with 21 patients early after stroke indicated that the combination of methylphenidate with physical therapy over a period of 3 weeks improved motor functions (as measured with the Fugl–Meyer Motor Scale and with a modified version of the Functional Independence Measure) and decreased depression [21]. A subsequent neuroimaging study by Tardy et al. confirmed these findings [22].

Levodopa: chronic dose versus single dose

Chronic dose: conflicting results

A randomized study with stroke patients (n=53) 6 weeks after stroke onset demonstrated that 100 mg levodopa given once a day over a period of 3 weeks in combination with carbidopa was significantly better than placebo in reducing motor deficits as measured with the Rivermead Motor Assessment. The improvement persisted over the subsequent 3 weeks [23]. However, the study results have not been replicated by others up to now. Rather, on the contrary, a recent study with subacute stroke patients who received 100 mg levodopa per day for 2 weeks did not find a stronger improvement of motor functions than in the group treated with placebo [24]. Sample sizes were smaller in the latter study, and carbidopa was not concomitantly administered, complicating direct comparison of the two studies.

Single dose: conflicting results again

Three placebo-controlled studies have tested the effect of a single dose of 100 mg levodopa in chronic stroke patients. Floel et al. [25] used a paradigm that is thought to reflect short-term plasticity in motor neuronal circuits. Thumb movements evoked by transcranial magnetic stimulation (TMS) are trained in the opposite direction for 30 min. After the training period, this paradigm generally finds that TMS typically evokes thumb movements in the trained direction. After another 15–20 min, TMS-induced movements return to the original (pretraining) direction. Using this paradigm, Floel et al. demonstrated that, compared with placebo, ingestion of levodopa was associated with more frequent TMS-evoked movements in the trained direction. The authors interpreted their results as an indicator that levodopa is able to enhance the ability to encode a motor memory with training. The design of this study is elegant, but the findings do not necessarily imply that levodopa is also effective in improving activities of daily living.

Restemeyer et al. [26] used other parameters to test the effects of levodopa in 10 chronic stroke patients who participated in a double-blind, placebo-controlled crossover trial. The authors employed the nine-hole peg test as a measure of dexterity, a dynamometer to measure grip strength, and the Action Research Arm Test, which allows evaluation of proximal and distal arm functions. In addition, motor excitability was measured by a variety of TMS techniques. There was no difference between levodopa and placebo – neither in the clinical tests nor in the TMS results. A third study [27] found that levodopa was superior to placebo for improving reaction time in 18 patients with chronic stroke undergoing procedural motor learning. Each study applied the same dose of levodopa, suggesting that other factors might be important to effectiveness of this intervention.

Selective serotonin reuptake inhibitors

The effectiveness of the selective serotonin reuptake blocker fluoxetine on recovery of motor functions has been tested in two main studies.

Single-dose study

In a double-blind, placebo-controlled crossover trial, a recent study with eight chronic stroke patients investigated the effects of a single dose of 40 mg citalopram [28]. Grip strength was measured with a mechanical dynamometer, and dexterity was evaluated with the nine-hole peg test. After citalopram intake, dexterity (but not grip strength) was significantly more improved than after placebo. The drug effect was present only in the affected, and not the unaffected, hand.

Chronic-dose study

In an early study, Dam et al. [29] applied 20 mg fluoxetine per day in severely disabled stroke patients and compared the effects with those in the control groups receiving either 150 mg maprotiline per day or placebo. They found the greatest improvements regarding walking and activities of daily living in the fluoxetine-treated patient group. Other effects of selective serotonin reuptake inhibitors on activities of daily living, mood, and cognitive status are reviewed in Chapter 14.

Pending study

The FLAME trial is a double-blinded randomized trial that is comparing placebo with 3 months of 20 mg fluoxetine in 110 patients presenting with an ischemic stroke with motor deficit. The results should be available within the following year. Effects of selective serotonin reuptake inhibitor therapy on depression following stroke are considered in Chapter 14.

Piracetam

Very little is known about the mechanism of action, but there is some evidence that piracetam enhances glucose utilization and cellular metabolism in the brain. Placebo-controlled trials in subacute stroke patients ($n=203$) indicated that application of 4.800 mg piracetam daily reduced aphasic symptoms as evaluated by the Aachener Aphasie Test [30,31]. The drug was given for either 12 weeks [30] or 6 weeks [31]. In the study by Huber et al. [31], piracetam-associated improvements were detected in the patients' "written language" and "profile level." Kessler et al. [32] performed a positive prospective, double-blind, placebo-controlled PET study in 24 stroke patients with aphasia, included in the study within 14 days after stroke. A Cochrane Review concluded that "treatment with piracetam may be effective in the treatment of aphasia after stroke" [33].

Others

Reboxetine

Reboxetine inhibits the reuptake of noradrenaline. Ten chronic stroke patients receiving a single dose of 6 mg reboxetine were studied in a double-blind, placebo-controlled crossover design [34] by Zittel et al. Grip strength, dexterity and hand tapping speed were evaluated before drug ingestion, 3 h after drug intake, and after a single session of physiotherapy aimed at improvement of hand function. In addition, motor excitability changes were investigated with TMS. Reboxetine induced a significant improvement of tapping speed and grip strength. Dexterity and TMS results remained unchanged.

Moclobemide

Moclobemide is an inhibitor of monoamine oxidase A. Compared to placebo, treatment with moclobemide (600 mg per day) for 6 months did not enhance the regression of aphasia following an acute stroke [35].

Donepezil

Donepezil inhibits the acetylcholine esterase. Donepezil has been tested in 26 patients with post-stroke aphasia [36]. The patients received donepezil (10 mg per day) or placebo for 16 weeks. The Aphasia Quotient of the Aphasia Test Battery showed a drug-associated improvement, indicating less severity. However, the Communicative Ability Log, a scale that assesses the patient's communicative behavior in everyday life, remained unchanged.

Summary of clinical trials

Currently, there is only limited evidence for supporting or refuting the use of centrally acting drugs to enhance effects of neurorehabilitation. Many reasons can be underlined to explain the difficulties encountered by the investigators: recruitment of patients (25–40 screened for 1 enrolled), heterogeneity in stroke types, size, location of lesion, concomitant neurological symptoms (within-subject variability in recovery), standardization of rehabilitation programs, dose of the drug, specific chemical formulation of the drug under study (D or DL amphetamines), time of prescription, duration of the treatment, and more. Most studies were performed in well-selected small patient groups and rather serve as a proof-of-principle investigation. The interpretation is further complicated by conflicting results, for example, with D-amphetamine and levodopa. One could interpret the current limited data as suggesting that the most promising post-stroke pharmacological strategies might be piracetam for aphasia, and levodopa for improvement of motor functions. These drugs have only minor side effects and might prove to be reasonably well tolerated. No regulatory agency will grant approval for use of such drugs until evidence is also provided by properly powered, formal, phase 3 clinical trials. Such trials would likely have to evaluate effects in the long term, and consider effects on function and disability.

Neuroimaging and pharmacotherapy

Neuroimaging can provide useful insights for optimal use of pharmacotherapy towards stroke recovery. A number of such applications are considered below, as well as in Chapter 16.

Neuroimaging trials in aphasia

For aphasia, as mentioned above, there may be mild positive effect of piracetam on behavioral status [9,33]. The only neuroimaging trial in aphasia was performed by Kessler et al. [32] in a study combining serial language assessment with serial positron emission tomography (PET) measurements using O^{15}-labeled water in an activation experiment (word repetition against resting state). Twenty-four patients were included after 2 weeks post-stroke, and randomized to either a placebo or a piracetam group (2.4 g/twice day) for a 6-week session. No significant difference existed between the two groups for language deficits at enrollment. Improvements of language functions were assessed using subscores from the Aachen aphasia test. Over the course of treatment, the placebo group showed improvements in three subscores, while the piracetam group improved on seven of them. More left hemisphere areas showed an increase in activation across the period of therapy in the piracetam group as compared to the placebo group. rCBF was increased in the left inferior precentral gyrus (BA 6) for the placebo group and in preserved left areas (Broca, Wernicke's areas, Helsch's gyrus) for the piracetam group. A reduction of rCBF was observed in the right hemisphere. This study supports the idea that recovery is better when occurring in the hemisphere to which language is normally localized. However, although activation correlated with performance in the first PET scan, no such correlation was present at the post-therapy PET scan, raising questions as to whether the observed PET changes were indeed responsible for the observed drug-related behavioral recovery.

Neuroimaging trials in hemiparesis

Depletion in norepinephrine (NE) and dopamine (DA) has been demonstrated after the acute phase following cortical infarction [37]. In light of this, pharmacological strategies have been based on monoaminergic supplementation, although other excitatory neurotransmitters such as acetylcholine might also prove to be good candidates. Below, neuroimaging findings relevant to pharmacological studies of stroke recovery are considered.

Functional MRI

Our group in Toulouse have investigated monoaminergic drugs (noradrenergic-, dopamine-, and serotonine enhancers) on motor deficits. Only single-dose studies have been conducted in patients, whereas single- and multiple-dose treatments have been tested in healthy subjects [38–42]. In the scanner, task parameters were controlled so that placebo or drug intake was the only parameter that changed between both evaluations. Briefly, first, it was demonstrated that a single dose of monoaminergic enhancer increases sensorimotor activity and motor performance, which cannot be attributed to an antidepressant effect that

requires weeks to occur, that was not a placebo effect, a dose effect could be evidenced, and cortical motor excitability was modified. Second, chronic treatments disclosed an increase in motor performance, decrease in sensorimotor activation, and an increased facilitation explained by excitatory interneurons projecting on motorneurons [38]. Moreover, as a general arousing system, the serotoninergic system may modulate and facilitate other functions such as language [43].

In patients, the serotoninergic pathway was first explored by Pariente et al. [44] with a crossover design in eight stroke patients with subcortical lesion on the pyramidal tract and pure motor deficit. They demonstrated that a single dose of fluoxetine, a selective serotoninergic reuptake inhibitor, was able to enhance BOLD signal in the ipsilesional sensorimotor cortex compared to placebo (parameters of the task being similar), and that this enhancement was correlated with better performances on grip force and tapping speed. Significant improvements were observed only on the paretic side, and furthermore, no imaging effect was seen when they moved the "healthy" side. This study demonstrated that drug can target a preserved sensorimotor network. Slight displacements in the z-direction of the ipsilesional sensorimotor area were evidenced [45], demonstrating a very localized reorganization. Those displacements have been demonstrated functionally relevant [46].

Similar results were found by Tardy et al. [22] with methylphenidate (a noradrenergic and dopaminergic enhancer). A passive training (electrical stimulation) was applied twice during 10 min. The finger tapping speed was improved by 9% on average 2 h after intake at peak plasma concentration. The main difference relied on the brain region whose activation was recruited by drug, which was demonstrated to be towards the ipsilesional face sensorimotor area. Activity in this region demonstrated a correlation with motor performance (finger tapping speed), demonstrating that a drug is able to target efficiently areas that are recruited. The anterior cingulum was hypoactivated after drug intake, suggesting an effect on attention expected with this type of drug. This second study highlighted the pharmacological targeting of a compensatory reorganized network.

Transcranial magnetic stimulation

A number of studies have also examined pharmacological effects using TMS. The preserved primary motor cortex was explored on the ipsilesional side in the study conducted by Zittel et al. [47]. A single dose

(6 mg) of reboxetine, a noradrenaline reuptake inhibitor, was tested at peak plasma concentration before and after a 1-h physiotherapy session. TMS investigation disclosed no effect on motor-evoked potential (MEP) amplitude. Compared with placebo, reboxetine ingestion was followed by an increase of tapping speed and grip strength in the paretic but not in the unaffected hand. No further improvement was noticed after physiotherapy. Restemeyer et al. [26] also found no TMS changes in their study of levodopa, although this negative TMS result was in association with absence of behavioral effects of the drug. Although these two trials do not provide support for TMS as a means to examine pharmacological effects in stroke recovery, TMS has performed well in many non-pharmacological studies, such as constraint-induced therapy [48].

Lessons regarding pharmacotherapy mechanisms

The effects of a single dose can be explained by short-term plasticity. Mechanisms might include alleviation of metabolic depression, stimulation of sensorimotor pathways, increase in cortical excitability [38,22], and partial re-establishment of interhemispheric inhibition between both M1. In analogy with amphetamine, monoaminergic drugs can increase the signal/noise ratio, i.e. the ratio between task-dependent activity and tonic activity [22]. Applying this to post-stroke recovery, drugs could increase adaptive brain activity in a compensatory network.

More specifically, DA through attention and reward may reinforce associative learning, and the effects of dopamine drugs might be mediated through dopamine projections to cerebral areas related to these functions. Noradrenaline (NA) modulates saliency of sensory inputs, attention, and memory. One additional hypothesis is that a primary function of the brain serotoninergic system would be to facilitate motor output [49], which underlines the fact that drug intake would be more efficient when paired with training. Further, 5HT enhances arousal and vigilance [40] and enhances energetic supply by stimulating glycogenolysis. 5HT is also involved in spatial memory acquisition, learning, consolidation, short-term facilitation (enhancement of transmitter release), storage of long-term memory in aplysia sensorimotor synapses, and long-term facilitation (growth of new synaptic contacts between sensory and motor neuron and facilitation of synaptic strength), growth factor gene expression, declarative memory, and the associated hippocampal neurogenesis in animals and humans [41].

All monoamines (NE, DA, 5HT), and Ach, may drive long-term potentiation (LTP), optimize activity-dependent learning in humans and possibly relearning after stroke. Finally, amphetamine takes part in post-lesional remodeling of motor areas through NA modulation in ref. [22].

Conclusion

In studies of pharmacotherapy for stroke recovery, consideration must be given to a broad range of issues including choice of drug, the dose, the treatment window, and the treatment duration. In many cases, single-dose studies will be of less value than chronic, recurrent strategies. Attention must be given to cortical vs. white matter injury, as biological targets might vary across such groups. Individual levels of monoamines, genetic profile, dose, and location of stroke injury might each contribute to variability in subject response, and so might be important to measure as covariates.

In conclusion, neuroimaging and single-dose studies may identify therapeutic targets, and lead to larger clinical trials. Studies will likely eventually involve multiple treatment modalities, such as pharmacotherapy combined with direct cortical stimulation, repetitive TMS, transcranial direct cortical stimulation, or paired stimulation (coupled cortical and sensory stimulation) to improve post-lesional plasticity.

Stem cells in relation to pharmacotherapy

The biology of stem cells and their effects in animal models of stroke are reviewed in Chapter 24. There have been very few human clinical trials of stem cell therapies published to date. Stem cell applications in humans with other conditions, such as acute myocardial infarction, suggest safety and possible clinical benefit.

Four stem cell trials have been published to date in human subjects. One study [50] examined intravenous injection of 1×10^8 autologous mesenchymal stem cells 1–2 months after a severe hemispheric stroke ($n = 5$ transplanted, $n = 25$ controls), and reported that, up to 1 year post-therapy, cell therapy was safe and improved outcome on measures such as the Barthel Index. A second study examined neural stem cells derived from embryonic porcine striatum, implanted into the striatum of five patients who were 1.5–10 years after a basal ganglia strokes (no control group). The trial was terminated by the US FDA after the occurrence of two adverse events, including one patient with cortical vein occlusion possibly related to surgery [51].

Two stem cell trials examined intracerebral implantation of differentiated hNT cells, also known as NT2N cells or LBS neurons (Layton Bioscience, Inc.), which are postmitotic human neuronal cells generated from an immortalized NT2 (ntera-2) cell line derived from a human teratocarcinoma upon exposure to retinoic acid. In contrast to the above two studies, administration of these cells required concomitant immunosuppression. The first study [52] examined a dose of 2–6 million cells 7–55 months post-stroke. No safety concerns were raised after one year of follow-up. At 24 weeks, 6 patients showed neurological improvement; 3, decline. Positron emission tomography scanning 6 months after implantation showed increased glucose consumption at the implant site, possibly reflecting cell survival or effects on host cells. Autopsy examination of one patient who did not show clinical improvement and died of myocardial infarction found no signs of inflammation, neoplasia, or infectious disease 27 months after implantation [53]. Fluorescent in-situ hybridization detected NT2N DNA in this patient, suggesting long-term stem cell survival. A second trial [54] in 14 subjects examined 5–10 million cells or control ($n = 4$, no surgery), with implantation 1–6 years post-stroke. Cell therapy was safe. However, no statistically significant gains were seen in any of several stroke scales.

Debate continues as to the extent to which some stem cell therapies might replace, or regenerate, actual neural circuitry after brain injury such as stroke. Evidence suggests, however, that some stem cells are preferentially attracted to sites of brain injury, where they are transformed by local factors and begin releasing a range of neurotrophic factors [55]. In this regard, some stem cells, such as mesenchymal stromal cells, represent a mobile, inducible source of local pharmacological therapies (see Chapter 24). Favorable effects of such cells combined with measurement of the local factors released by such cells when introduced after stroke might provide insights useful for planning pharmacological interventions.

The optimal conditions for cell transplant therapy after stroke are not known [56,57]. Future stem cell trials must be designed in accordance with the Consolidated Standards of Reporting Trials (CONSORT) guidelines.

Also, guidelines for stem cells clinical trials were developed by a group of basic scientists and research clinicians actively involved with CNS transplantation and published as the recommendation of the American Association of Neural Transplantation and Repair [53].

An exciting future direction for research pertains to monitoring stem cells introduced therapeutically. Tagging cells with nanoparticles such as superparamagnetic iron oxide particles (SPIO) or gadonanotubes (carbon nanotubes complexed with a paramagnetic contrast agent such as gadolinium) allows them to be monitored with the use of MRI [56]. SPIO labeling allows in-vivo cell tracking over several weeks. Data to date suggest that this method of tagging does not have obvious effects on cell migration, integration, or differentiation. The complete safety profile of this approach in humans remains under investigation. If feasible, in-vivo MRI of labeled transplanted stem cells might be helpful in detecting whether sufficient cells enter and remain viable in the injured brain area. However, this technique will not differentiate whether labeled cells have been trapped by macrophages or not.

To bring such innovative cell-based therapies to the clinic, many questions have to be solved. Do the cells survive in a sufficient number; how do they act on neural tissue; how do they impact impairment and disabilities? The robustness of their effects on neuromodulation, reorganization, regeneration, and behavioral recovery is a work in progress [57,58–60].

Summary

Neuropharmacological intervention, directly via pharmacological therapies and perhaps indirectly via factors elaborated by stem cells, has the potential to improve recovery from stroke. Many studies have focused on the chronic phase of stroke, but likely biological targets of interest exist in early phases too. Many possible therapeutic strategies have been suggested, and require further study. Functional neuroimaging has the potential to be of guiding value to many of these studies.

References

1. Feeney DM, Sutton RL. Pharmacotherapy for recovery of function after brain injury. *Crit Rev Neurobiol.* 1987;3:135–97.

2. Feeney DM, Weisend MP, Kline AE. Noradrenergic pharmacotherapy, intracerebral infusion and adrenal transplantation promote functional recovery after cortical damage. *J Neural Transplant Plast.* 1993;4:199–213.

3. Goldstein LB. Basic and clinical studies of pharmacologic effects on recovery from brain injury. *J Neural Transplant Plast.* 1993;**4**:175–92.

4. Schallert T, Jones TA, Weaver MS, *et al.* Pharmacologic and anatomic considerations in recovery of function. *Phys Med Rehabil.* 1992;**6**:375–93.

5. Goldstein LB. Influence of common drugs and related factors on stroke outcome. *Curr Opin Neurol.* 1997;**10**:52–7.

6. Jones TA, Schallert T. Subcortical deterioration after cortical damage: effects of diazepam and relation to recovery of function. *Behav Brain Res.* 1992; **51**: 1–13.

7. Reding M, Solomon B, Borucki S. The effect of dextroamphetamine on motor recovery after stroke. *Neurology.* 1995;**45**(Suppl 4):A222.

8. Liepert J. Pharmacotherapy in restorative neurology. *Current Opin Neurol.* 2008; **21**: 639–43.

9. de Boissezon X, Peran P, de Boysson C, *et al.* Pharmacotherapy of aphasia: Myth or reality? *Brain Lang.* 2007;**102**:114–25.

10. Crisostomo EA, Duncan PW, Propst M, *et al.* Evidence that amphetamine with physical therapy promotes recovery of motor function in stroke patients. *Ann Neurol.* 1988;**23**:94–7.

11. Walker-Batson D, Smith P, Curtis S, *et al.* Amphetamine paired with physical therapy accelerates motor recovery after stroke. Further evidence. *Stroke.* 1995;**26**:2254–9.

12. Sonde L, Lökk J. Effects of amphetamine and/or L-dopa and physiotherapy after stroke: A blinded randomized study. *Acta Neurol Scand.* 2007;**115**:55–9.

13. Sonde L, Nordstrom M, Nilsson CG, *et al.* A double-blind placebo-controlled study of the effects of amphetamine and physiotherapy after stroke. *Cerebrovasc Dis.* 2001;**12**:253–7.

14. Martinsson L, Eksborg S, Wahlgren NG. Intensive early physiotherapy combined with dexamphetamine treatment in severe stroke: A randomized, controlled pilot study. *Cerebrovasc Dis.* 2003;**16**:338–45.

15. Treig T, Werner C, Sachse M, *et al.* No benefit from D-amphetamine when added to physiotherapy after stroke: A randomized, placebo-controlled study. *Clin Rehabil.* 2003;**17**:590–9.

16. Platz T, Kim IH, Engel U, *et al.* Amphetamine fails to facilitate motor performance and to enhance motor recovery among stroke patients with mild arm paresis: Interim analysis and termination of a double blind, randomised, placebo-controlled trial. *Restor Neurol Neurosci.* 2005;**23**:271–80.

17. Gladstone DJ, Danells CJ, Armesto A, *et al.* Subacute therapy with amphetamine and rehabilitation for stroke study investigators. Physiotherapy coupled with dextroamphetamine for rehabilitation after hemiparetic stroke: A randomized, double-blind, placebo-controlled trial. *Stroke.* 2006;**37**:179–85.

18. Martinsson L, Hårdemark H, Eksborg S. Amphetamines for improving recovery after stroke. *Cochrane Database Syst Rev* 2007:CD002090. A comprehensive review of published and unpublished studies.

19. Walker-Batson D, Curtis S, Natarajan R, *et al.* A double-blind, placebo-controlled study of the use of amphetamine in the treatment of aphasia. *Stroke.* 2001;**32**:2093–8.

20. Whiting E, Chenery HJ, Chalk J, *et al.* Dexamphetamine boosts naming treatment effects in chronic aphasia. *J Int Neuropsychol Soc.* 2007;**13**:972–9.

21. Grade C, Redford B, Chrostowski J, *et al.* Methylphenidate in early poststroke recovery: a double-blind, placebo-controlled study. *Arch Phys Med Rehabil.* 1998;**79**:1047–50.

22. Tardy J, Pariente J, Leger A, *et al.* Methylphenidate modulates cerebral post-stroke reorganization. *Neuroimage.* 2006;**33**:913–22.

23. Scheidtmann K, Fries W, Muller F, *et al.* Effect of levodopa in combination with physiotherapy on functional motor recovery after stroke: A prospective, randomized, double-blind study. *Lancet.* 2001;**358**:787–90.

24. Sonde L, Lökk J. Effects of amphetamine and/or L-dopa and physiotherapy after stroke: a blinded randomized study. *Acta Neurol Scand.* 2007;**115**:55–9.

25. Floel A, Hummel F, Breitenstein C, *et al.* Dopaminergic effects on encoding of a motor memory in chronic stroke. *Neurology.* 2005;**65**:472–4.

26. Restemeyer C, Weiller C, Liepert J. No effect of a levodopa single dose on motor performance and motor excitability in chronic stroke. A double-blind placebo-controlled cross-over pilot study. *Restor Neurol Neurosci.* 2007;**25**:143–50.

27. Rosser N, Heuschmann P, Wersching H, *et al.* Levodopa improves procedural motor learning in chronic stroke patients. *Arch Phys Med Rehabil.* 2008;**89**:1633–41.

28. Zittel S, Weiller C, Liepert J. Citalopram improves dexterity in chronic stroke patients. *Neurorehabil Neural Repair.* 2008;**22**:311–4.

29. Dam M, Tonin P, De Boni A, *et al.* Effects of fluoxetine and maprotiline on functional recovery in poststroke hemiplegic patients undergoing rehabilitation therapy. *Stroke.* 1996;**27**:1211–4.

30. Enderby P, Broeckx J, Hospers W, *et al.* Effect of piracetam on recovery and rehabilitation after stroke: A double-blind, placebo-controlled study. *Clin Neuropharmacol.* 1994;**17**:320–31.

31. Huber W, Willmes K, Poeck K, et al. Piracetam as an adjuvant to language therapy for aphasia: A randomized double-blind placebo-controlled pilot study. Arch Phys Med Rehabil. 1997;78:245–50.

32. Kessler J, Thiel A, Karbe H, et al. Piracetam improves activated blood flow and facilitates rehabilitation of poststroke aphasic patients. Stroke. 2000;31:2112–6.

33. Greener J, Enderby P, Whurr R. Pharmacological treatment for aphasia following stroke. Cochrane Database Syst Rev. 2001:CD000424.

34. Zittel S, Weiller C, Liepert J. Reboxetine improves motor function in chronic stroke: A pilot study. J Neurol. 2007;254:197–201.

35. Laska AC, von Arbin M, Kahan T, et al. Long-term antidepressant treatment with moclobemide for aphasia in acute stroke patients: A randomised, double-blind, placebo-controlled study. Cerebrovasc Dis. 2005;19:125–32.

36. Berthier ML, Green C, Higueras C, et al. A randomized, placebo-controlled study of donepezil in poststroke aphasia. Neurology. 2006;67:1687–9.

37. Robinson RG, Shoemaker WJ, Schlumpf M, et al. Effect of experimental cerebral infarction in rat brain on catecholamines and behaviour. Nature. 1975;255:332–4.

38. Gerdelat-Mas A, Loubinoux I, Tombari D, et al. Chronic administration of selective serotonin reuptake inhibitor (SSRI) paroxetine modulates human motor cortex excitability in healthy subjects. Neuroimage. 2005;27:314–22.

39. Loubinoux I, Boulanouar K, Ranjeva JP, et al. Cerebral functional magnetic resonance imaging activation modulated by a single dose of the monoamine neurotransmission enhancers fluoxetine and fenozolone during hand sensorimotor tasks. J Cereb Blood Flow Metab. 1999;19:1365–75.

40. Loubinoux I, Pariente J, Boulanouar K, et al. A single dose of serotonin neurotransmission agonist paroxetine enhances motor output. A double-blind, placebo-controlled, fMRI study in healthy subjects. NeuroImage. 2002;15:26–36.

41. Loubinoux I, Pariente J, Rascol O, et al. Selective serotonin reuptake inhibitor paroxetine modulates motor behavior through practice. A double-blind, placebo-controlled, multi-dose study in healthy subjects. Neuropsychologia. 2002;40:1815–21.

42. Loubinoux I, Tombari D, Pariente J, et al. Modulation of behavior and cortical motor activity in healthy subjects by a chronic administration of a serotonin enhancer. Neuroimage. 2005;27:299–313.

43. Peran P, Demonet JF, Cardebat D. Paroxetine-induced modulation of cortical activity supporting language representations of action. Psychopharmacology (Berl). 2008;195:487–96.

44. Pariente J, Loubinoux I, Carel C, et al. Fluoxetine modulates motor performance and cerebral activation of patients recovering from stroke. Ann Neurol. 2001;50:718–29.

45. Tombari D, Loubinoux I, Pariente J, et al. A longitudinal fMRI study: in recovering and then in clinically stable sub-cortical stroke patients. Neuroimage. 2004;23:827–39.

46. Thickbroom GW, Byrnes ML, Archer SA, et al. Motor outcome after subcortical stroke correlates with the degree of cortical reorganization. Clin Neurophysiol. 2004;115:2144–50.

47. Zittel S, Baumer T, Liepert J. Modulation of intracortical facilitatory circuits of the human primary motor cortex by digital nerve stimulation. Exp Brain Res. 2007;176:425–31.

48. Sawaki L, Butler AJ, Xiaoyan L, et al. Constraint-induced movement therapy results in increased motor map area in subjects 3 to 9 months after stroke. Neurorehabil Neural Repair. 2008;22:505–13.

49. Jacobs BL, Fornal CA. Serotonin and motor activity. Curr Opin Neurobiol. 1997;7:820–5.

50. Bang OY, Lee JS, Lee PH, et al. Autologous mesenchymal stem cell transplantation in stroke patients. Ann Neurol. 2005;57:874–82.

51. Meltzer CC, Kondziolka D, Villemagne VL, et al. Serial [18F] fluorodeoxyglucose positron emission tomography after human neuronal implantation for stroke. Neurosurgery. 2001;49:586–91; discussion 91–2.

52. Kondziolka D, Steinberg GK, Wechsler L, et al. Neurotransplantation for patients with subcortical motor stroke: a phase 2 randomized trial. J Neurosurg. 2005;103:38–45.

53. Nelson PT, Kondziolka D, Wechsler L, et al. Clonal human (hNT) neuron grafts for stroke therapy: Neuropathology in a patient 27 months after implantation. Am J Pathol. 2002;160:1201–06.

54. Kondziolka D, Wechsler L, Goldstein S, et al. Transplantation of cultured human neuronal cells for patients with stroke. Neurology. 2000;55:565–9.

55. Kornblum HI. Introduction to neural stem cells. Stroke. 2007;38(2 Suppl):810–6.

56. Bliss T, Guzman R, Daadi M, et al. Cell transplantation therapy for stroke. Stroke. 2007;38(2 Suppl):817–26.

57. Dobkin BH. Behavioral, temporal, and spatial targets for cellular transplants as adjuncts to rehabilitation for stroke. Stroke. 2007;38(2 Suppl):832–9.

58. Savitz SI, Dinsmore J, Wu J, *et al.* Neurotransplantation of fetal porcine cells in patients with basal ganglia infarcts: A preliminary safety and feasibility study. *Cerebrovasc Dis.* 2005;**20**:101–07.

59. Bakay RA. Neural transplantation. *J Neurosurg.* 2005;**103**:6–8; discussion.

60. Redmond DE, Jr, Freeman T. The American Society for Neural Transplantation and Repair Considerations and guidelines for studies of human subjects. The practice committee of the society. Approved by council. *Cell Transplant.* 2001;**10**:661–4.

18 Robotic approaches to stroke recovery

David J. Reinkensmeyer

Introduction

Research on robot-assisted movement therapy is increasing exponentially, as measured by estimates of the number of publications in the field (Figure 18.1). Most of this work has focused on rehabilitation of movement after stroke, because stroke is a leading cause of adult disability in industrialized nations, and therefore survivors of stroke are a large target population, although there is also some work on robotic movement training after spinal cord injury, cerebral palsy, and multiple sclerosis.

The most commonly explored paradigm is to use a robotic device to physically assist in completing desired motions of the arms, hands, or legs as the patient plays computer games presented on a screen (Figure 18.2). A wide variety of assistive control strategies have been designed (see [1] for review), ranging from robots that rigidly move limbs along fixed paths, to robots that assist only if patient performance fails to stay within some spatial or temporal bound, to soft robots that form a model of the patient's weakness. There is also some preliminary work on devices that perturb patient movements ("error-amplification strategies" [2]), or that act as non-contacting coaches [3]. Most robotic therapy devices are currently used as stationary exercise machines in clinics, although there is substantial interest in making devices that are portable, wearable, and usable at home (e.g. [4–7]).

There is now substantial clinical evidence that exercise with robotic therapy devices can benefit stroke patients (see [13–15] for reviews). As reviewed below, improvements in movement ability following robot-assisted training in acute, subacute, or chronic stroke are statistically significant, but modest. Less clear is the specific role that robotic actuation itself plays in these findings [16]. A robot is commonly defined as a device that can apply forces (and therefore move itself and

other things) in response to computerized commands. Adopting this focused definition of robotic therapy – i.e. that robot therapy is the application of computer-controlled forces to limbs – clearly distinguishes robotic therapy and non-robotic approaches, such as sensor-based computer games and passive exercise machines, which also show promise for stroke rehabilitation [17–22]. Under what conditions should one expect that applying forces to a limb will enhance motor recovery?

The purpose of this chapter is to critically review existing clinical evidence for efficacy of robotic movement training, with a view toward identifying the mechanisms of neuroplasticity that are stimulated by robot-assisted movement training. This chapter focuses on upper extremity training because of space limitations, although results are similar for robotic gait training after stroke. Evidence for sufficiency of robotic assistance in providing therapeutic benefit during movement training is extensive, but evidence for necessity of robotic actuation in providing therapeutic benefit is limited. From a mechanistic perspective, the evidence is consistent with the following working hypothesis: movement practice, consisting of the repetitive execution of descending commands to try to achieve a presented motor goal, is the key stimulus for motor recovery, independently of whether this movement practice is accompanied by robotic assistance. The benefits of robotic therapy devices may therefore be more related to providing motivating, quantifiable, and economic delivery of training, rather than a specific enhancement of plasticity attributable to robotic forces, although it is still a possibility that some motor benefits might be derived from the somatosensory signals generated when robotic therapy moves a limb. A practical implication then is that non-robotic technology that improves the motivating, quantifying, or economic qualities

---

Brain Repair After Stroke, ed. S. C. Cramer and R. J. Nudo. Published by Cambridge University Press.
© Cambridge University Press 2010.

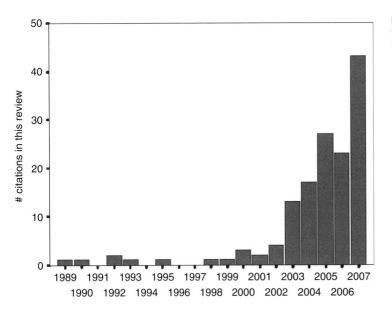

Figure 18.1 Number of publications on robotic therapy devices, plotted as a function of publication year. From [1].

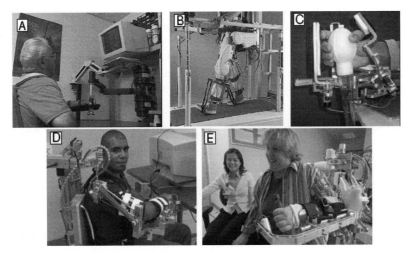

Figure 18.2 Examples of robotic and non-robotic movement training devices. A: The first device to undergo extensive clinical testing was MIT-MANUS [8], which assists in movement of the supported arm in the horizontal plane. B. The Lokomat is a motorized orthosis that can assist in hip flexion/extension and knee flexion/extension [9]. C. The hand robot HWARD [10] uses triggered assistance, which means that it allows free movement for a fixed time for each desired task, and then responds by moving the hand if the patient does not achieve the task. D. T-WREX [11] is a non-robotic device that uses passive gravity balancing to provide assistance; the number of elastic bands determines the amount of assistance. E. Pneu-WREX [12] builds a real-time computer model of the patient's weakness, and uses it to provide feedforward assistance with a compliant position controller for 3D movement. From [1].

associated with robots may ultimately be a more viable solution for clinical implementation.

Clinical studies analyzing the effect of additional therapy provided by a robotic device

An important question for acute stroke rehabilitation is whether therapy provided by a robotic device beyond standard amounts of therapy can improve recovery. Likewise, for chronic stroke patients with a stable motor function baseline, does additional therapy, in the form of robotic therapy, produce a benefit? If so, then at the least it would seem justifiable to use robotic devices as adjuncts to traditional therapy inasmuch as they allow additional therapy and thus additional recovery to be obtained at a reduced cost.

In discussing the answer to this question, we will refer to the upper extremity Fugl-Meyer (FM) score [23] as an outcome measure, because it has been frequently used and provides a basis for comparing studies. The upper extremity Fugl-Meyer score is an impairment-based scale that measures movement ability on a scale from 0 (complete paralysis) to 66 (normal movement). It is calculated by asking patients to make 33 test movements, scoring them 0 (unable to perform), 1 (performed imperfectly), or 2 (performed perfectly). Most studies have included groups of patients with an average beginning FM score in the range of 10–30 points (pts), although a few have included higher-level patients (e.g. [10]). A patient with an FM score of 10–30 is severely to moderately impaired, and thus a logical candidate for robotic assistance, since unassisted movements are severely disrupted. An additional factor to keep in mind when reading the following summary is that most studies to date have used exercise protocols lasting from 3 to 8 weeks, with the patients receiving 3–5 h of robotic therapy per week.

Arm exercise

The first randomized clinical tests of a robotic therapy device measured the effect of additional therapy delivered to subacute stroke patients with MIT-MANUS [8,24,25]. This device (Figure 18.2A), now sold as the InMotion2, sits across from the patient on a tabletop, attaches to the patient's hand/forearm, and compliantly assists the patient in moving the supported arm in a horizontal workspace, requiring shoulder and elbow motion as the patient plays simple video games. About 1h per day of extra therapy delivered with MIT-MANUS resulted in a significantly greater improvement in the FM score (2 points on the 66-point scale) [8,25]. Additional therapy with MIT-MANUS also improved motor function of chronic stroke patients (3.2 FM pts) (n=20) [26], and was maintained at 4 month follow-up (3.4 FM pts) (n=42) [27]. Chronic, severely impaired stroke subjects (initial mean FM=10 pts) who received a shorter duration of training with MIT-MANUS improved by 1.2 FM pts [28].

Robot therapy has also been applied to acute stroke survivors, beginning during the first week after stroke, using the cable-based NeReBot to mobilize the arm [29]. This robot can be rolled up to the patient's bed, and uses a motorized, overhead suspended sling to move the shoulder and elbow in 3D space along a therapist-demonstrated path. Acute stroke survivors (n=17) who received active-assist arm mobilization, compared to a control group that did not receive additional therapy (n=18), improved 5 pts more in FM, as well as on a functional measure (the Functional Independence Measure, or "FIM"). These incremental gains were sustained at 8-month follow-up (10 pt additional FM gain).

A simple design for a robot that assists in reaching is to use a linear bearing to guide the hand, since for many reaching movements, the hand moves along an approximately straight-line path. A study with one of the first robots of this design, the ARM Guide, found a benefit of robotic therapy in chronic stroke subjects (n=3), in terms of range and speed of reaching motion [30]. Chronic stroke subjects (n=20) who practiced with a bilateral robotic arm trainer consisting of two linear slides improved by 2.8 pts on the FM scale [31]. Therapy with a robotic arm trainer (MEMOS) that assisted in horizontal plane arm motion of chronic stroke subjects (n=9) with two perpendicular linear slides found a significant gain in FM score by 6.7 points [32]. In a second study of the same device, there was a 10 pt FM gain in subacute stroke patients (n=9) and a 5 pt gain in chronic stroke subjects (n=13) [33].

A recently developed control approach is to use EMG measurements from elbow muscles to help drive the assisting robot. A robot that assisted in elbow extension by measuring triceps EMG activity and providing proportional robot assistance helped chronic stroke patients (n=8) to improve their movement ability by 4.1 points on the FM score [34]. EMG-triggered assistance for another elbow-assisting robot improved FM score by 3.5 points in chronic stroke subjects (n=6) [35].

Hand/wrist/forearm exercise

Most initial robot therapy devices focused on arm movement, but there are now several studies of hand/wrist/forearm robots, as reviewed in this section and the following sections. One of the first devices, the Rutgers Glove, uses small, frictionless pneumatic cylinders mounted in the palm of the hand to help move the fingers [36]. Additional exercise with this haptic glove in a virtual reality (VR) environment resulted in measurable benefits by quantitative and clinical measures [36]. Exercise with a device that assisted solely in wrist flexion/extension resulted in a significant 5.7 pt FM gain after 3 weeks of therapy for chronic stroke subjects (n=7) [32]. This is comparable to the 7.6 pt FM gain seen with HWARD (Hand Wrist Assistive Rehabilitation Device) [10], which is a pneumatically actuated robotic device that helps move the wrist and fingers after the patient initiates movement.

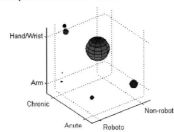

Figure 18.3 Summary of gains in upper extremity Fugl-Meyer (FM) score, as a function of robotic or non-robotic therapy, chronic versus acute training, or hand/wrist versus arm therapy. The FM score varies from 0 (complete paralysis) to 66 (normal movement). Most of the studies reported here included subjects with an initial FM score between 10 and 30. The size of the sphere is the size of the FM gain for a study. A sphere with a diameter corresponding to 7 FM points is labeled. Red spheres denote hand/wrist studies; blue, arm studies. A: FM Gains reported from studies reviewed here that examined the effect of an additional dose of movement therapy delivered with a robotic or non-robotic device. For studies on acute and subacute patients, only studies that controlled for intrinsic recovery by including a control group that did not receive additional therapy are included, and only the change on top of that due to intrinsic recovery is plotted. FM gains are modest but consistently positive. B: Differential FM gains due to robotic therapy, when the control therapy was duration matched. Only one study [46] with a distal robot and subacute stroke patients showed a substantial differential benefit. For both A and B, there is no obvious advantage to the distal versus proximal, chronic versus acute, or arm versus hand/wrist parameters.

A recent study examined the effect of a combination of robot assistance of the wrist and fingers through a cyclic motion, while vibrating the tendons of the lengthening muscles for chronic stroke subjects ($n=11$) [4]. The goal of this "AMES" (Assisted Movement with Enhanced Sensation) technique was to enhance the sensory input associated with movement, and thus to strengthen functional connections between somatosensory neurons and motor output neurons in the cortex. Notably, subjects treated themselves at home with this technique, 30 minutes per day for 6 months, complying to complete an average of 70% of the recommended treatments. Subjects significantly improved their strength and range of motion, as well as a functional outcome score.

Another recent study combined training with the BiManuTrac device with a brief period of transcranial direct current stimulation (tDCS, see Chapter 19) over the motor cortex at the beginning of each training session [37]. The BiManuTrac device allows bilateral forearm supination/pronation or wrist flexion/extension movements, after a quick configuration change. For subacute stroke patients, the combined robotic/brain stimulation approach resulted in large improvements in FM score (+33 pts) in 3 patients, 2 of which had subcortical lesions, and smaller improvements (5 pts) in 7 patients, all with cortical lesions.

Summary

Additional motor training provided with a robotic device can significantly improve movement ability following acute, subacute, or chronic stroke, but the reduction is modest – typically on the order of 2–6 additional FM points, leaving patients well short of the peak possible score of 66 (Figure 18.3). A plausible use-dependent plasticity mechanism that robotic training stimulates to achieve these gains is simply the mechanism (or mechanisms) by which all forms of repetitive practice improve movement ability.

Clinical studies comparing a matched amount of two therapy types, at least one of them being robotic, and finding benefits, but no difference between groups

Given that additional therapy delivered with a robotic device is beneficial, it is logical to ask whether robot-assisted therapy is more effective than other types of therapy a patient could undertake. Several studies that have tried to address this question have produced inconclusive results. We review these studies in this section.

Arm exercise

The first study to compare robot therapy with another dose-matched therapy compared a matched amount of robot-assisted therapy using the MIME device with therapist-provided neurodevelopmental therapy with chronic stroke subjects [38]. The MIME device uses an industrial robot to assist the arm in moving in three-dimensional space, and can be used in a mirror-image mode in which movements of the less-impaired arm are used to specify movements of the paretic arm. The robot-trained group (n=13) had larger improvements in FM score compared to the control group (n=14) after 2 months of treatment (by 4.7 compared to 3.1 points), but not at 6-month follow-up. A follow-up study [39] compared different forms of robot-assisted treatment (unilateral n=9, bilateral n=5, combined bilateral and unilateral n=10) to conventional therapy (n=6) for subacute stroke patients (about 10 weeks post-stroke). The FM point gains after 2 months were 7.9 for unilateral, 3.8 for bilateral, 7.6 for combined, and 5.8 for conventional, with the only significant difference being the one between combined and conventional groups. Gains in all treatment groups were not significantly different at the 6-month follow-up.

A study with the ARM Guide compared robot-assisted reaching (n=10) with a repetition-matched amount of unassisted exercise (n=9) in chronic stroke patients and found that both groups improved significantly in quantitative measures of reaching (range of motion and speed of reach), but comparably, so that there were no significant differences between groups [40]. A follow-up study examined training with the ARM Guide in a mode in which it resisted movements when the patient pushed abnormally against the device, requiring the patient to generate forces in the correct direction, as shown using visual feedback of forces, before allowing reaching along the linear guide [41]. Comparison groups received a matched amount of conventional therapy, and free reaching therapy, in which the patients simply practiced reaching a matched amount of time. Chronic stroke patients improved their FM score by similar amounts: 5.0, 4.4, and 4.1 pts for the robot (n=7), conventional (n=7), and free reaching (n=7) training groups, respectively.

Another MIT-MANUS study compared a matched amount of robot (n=11) or therapist-delivered (n=10) movement training with chronic stroke patients and found significant gains in impairment measures in each group (3 pt FM gain in robot group, 3.5 pt FM gain in therapist-delivered training group) that were not different from each other, but were sustained at 3-month follow-up [42].

Perhaps the only study that has directly compared two different types of *robotic* therapy compared assistive (n=14) robotic therapy versus resistive robotic

therapy (n=14) for chronic stroke subjects using the MIT-MANUS device [43]. Training produced a significant increase by 4.4 FM points and 4.0 FM points in each group. The gains for the two training techniques did not differ from each other.

Hand/wrist/forearm exercise

Stroke patients often have difficulty opening the hand. A recent study compared motor gains for chronic stroke subjects who exercised with a cable-driven orthosis that helped extend the fingers (n=5), a pneumatic glove that helped extend the fingers (n=5), or no assistance, in a VR environment [5]. All groups improved in the outcome measures, including time to complete functional tasks, but there were no differences between groups. The change in FM score was 4 pts (cable-driven), −1 pt (pneumatic), and 3 pts (no assistance).

Summary

The lack of difference in outcomes between robotic therapy and other therapy types would be expected if: (1) practice is the primary stimulus for improvement; and (2) the comparison therapy includes comparable amounts of practice. A confounding factor in interpreting these inconclusive studies, however, is their limited statistical power due to relatively small sample sizes.

Clinical studies comparing a matched amount of two therapy types, at least one of them being robotic, and finding a benefit of robotic therapy

Other studies have found a difference between robotic therapy and another type of therapy.

Arm exercise

The ARMOR robot can move all the joints of the arm, as well as supinate/pronate the forearm, and flex/extend the wrist and hand [44]. It was used in a crossover design with 8 stroke patients, 2.4 months following stroke on average, to compare robotic training with EMG-triggered functional electrical stimulation (EMG-FES). ARMOR training resulted in a greater improvement of muscle tone, range of movement and dexterity, but less improvement of strength, than EMG-FES.

The Gentle-S robot uses a force-feedback controlled 3D commercial robot to assist in moving the arm [45]. A study of Gentle-S compared robot-assisted 3D movements to sling-suspension based exercises in a crossover design, and found a nearly significant (p=0.06) greater rate of improvement during the robot therapy.

Hand/wrist/forearm exercise

Robotic training of the forearm and wrist using the BiManuTrac device produced greater improvements than EMG-triggered FES of the wrist in subacute stroke patients (n=44) [46]. The FM score was 15 points higher at study end and 13 points higher at 3-month follow-up than the FES group. It is important to note that the intensity of the exercise achieved with the two modalities was quantified and found to be different: the robot group performed about 800 repetitions per session, whereas the FES group performed about 80 repetitions per session.

Perhaps the only study to show a direct benefit of robotic forces per se during robotic training examined hand training [10]. Chronic stroke patients who received robot assistance using the HWARD device (Figure 18.2C), which assists in hand opening and closing and wrist flexion/extension, for all of their training movements (n=7) recovered significantly more hand function than patients who received robot assistance for only half of their training movements (i.e. for only the last 7.5 sessions of a 15 session protocol, n=6). The increase in FM score was 9.1 versus 5.8 points, for the two groups. Caveats include a small sample size that was slightly mismatched in impairment level at baseline, and uncertainty in whether the group that received half the amount of assistance completed as many training movements when assistance was absent. This study is also different from most others in that the patients had a higher beginning FM score (mean score of 45 out of 66).

A recent study with MIT-MANUS compared training with three forms of assistance for combined arm and hand movements for chronic stroke subjects (n=47) [13]. All groups received active-assistance for reaching to targets. One group did not use the hand during training; another group interacted with objects at the target; and another group grasped, transported, and released virtual objects between targets by controlling isometric grip force against a sensor. The no-hand group improved the most in FM score (3 FM pts), followed by the group that gripped actual objects (2.7 FM pts), followed by the group gripping virtual objects (0.8 FM pts). Note that the virtual grip group trained at a different hospital and was evaluated by a different therapist. The improvement in the group that trained without using the hand was significantly greater than the groups that incorporated hand training.

It is possible that robot therapy could be less effective than other therapy types. We mention one recent gait training study in this regard. This study compared a matched amount of gait training with the Lokomat robot (Figure 18.2B) in chronic stroke subjects (n=48) to gait training with a physical therapist [9]. The subjects randomized to receive gait training with a physical therapist exhibited greater improvements in self-selected and maximum gait speed (~2× greater gain). In a separate study, this same group quantified patient energy expenditure in the Lokomat compared to during therapist-assisted gait training, and found it to be about 50% less, as gauged by oxygen uptake, unless the patient is instructed to work against the machine [54]. These studies suggest that some forms of assistance provided by robotic therapy devices might encourage slacking by patients, reducing the recovery possible with a fixed amount of training. For the upper extremity, a tendency for patients to reduce effort in response to robotic assistance provided with a compliant device Pneu-WREX (Figure 18.2E) has also been observed [12], but no relative reduction in training effects with robotic therapy has been reported to our knowledge. A partial exception is that training with the ARMOR robot resulted in less improvement of strength than EMG-FES, although it also resulted in greater improvements in muscle tone, range of movement, and dexterity [44].

Summary

A few studies have demonstrated that robot-assisted therapy is modestly more effective than another type of therapy, with the largest difference coming for a distal robot (BiManuTrac) compared to EMG-FES (13 FM pt advantage at study follow-up) [46] (Figure 18.3). However, a confounding factor for this study, as well as several others showing a difference, is that patients received more repetitions in, and thus a higher dose of, the robot-assisted therapy compared to the comparison therapy. Thus, the working hypothesis that practice is the key mechanistic stimulus to practice rather than robotic assistance could still explain these studies.

Clinical studies with non-robotic technology showing a comparable benefit to robotic technology

Several non-robotic devices are being developed to assist patients in practicing upper extremity movements and have produced comparable results to robotic devices. We briefly review several of these studies.

Arm exercise

The NudelHoltz device provides mechanically assisted exercise using a rolling-pin like mechanism that requires patients to use two hands to slide up and down a ramp [19]. This non-robotic exercise modality was compared with EMG-triggered FES of the wrist extensors for 54 subacute patients with severe impairment (FM score ~ 8 out of 66), 20–30 min per day, 5 days per week, for 6 weeks [19]. Both groups improved significantly (10 and 5 pts on FM score), but there were no significant differences between the two groups. More NudelHolz patients became able to move blocks (5 responders versus 0 at end of 6 weeks). Note that the number of movements performed by the mechanically assisted group was larger (18 000 movements versus ~2000 movements), included more degrees of freedom (DOF) of the upper extremity, and incorporated a bilateral approach.

The BATRAC device incorporates two low-friction linear tracks on which the patient slides handles, and provides auditory cueing for movement [47]. Training bilateral push–pull movements with BATRAC improved arm function in 14 chronic stroke subjects by 3 pts after 6 weeks of training, and by 10 pts at 2-month follow-up [47]. When BATRAC training was compared to standard, dose-matched exercises in chronic stroke patients ($n=21$), patients in the BATRAC group increased brain activation during a distal motor task, but there was no difference in functional outcome between groups, unless only considering patients with fMRI response ($n=6$), in which case BATRAC improved arm function more than the standard exercises did [18]. However, a subsequent study found no benefit of training with a modified form of BATRAC in chronic stroke ($n=14$), as evidenced by no significant change in FM or Wolf Motor Function Test scores [17].

The Sensorimotor Active Rehabilitation Training (SMART) Arm is comprised of a sensorized, low-friction linear track [21]. Training with the SMART Arm alone ($n=13$) was compared with SMART ARM training plus EMG-triggered FES ($n=10$), and no intervention ($n=13$) in chronic stroke patients [21]. Both SMART Arm groups demonstrated significant improvements in all impairment and activity measures after training and at follow-up. There was no significant difference between these two SMART Arm groups. There was no change in the control group.

The T-WREX (Figure 18.2D) is an elastic-band driven, passive, arm-supporting orthosis that is connected to simple VR games [11]. Training with T-WREX produced greater benefits than conventional table-top exercises for chronic stroke subjects ($n=28$), resulting in a 3.8 FM increase at 6-month follow-up compared to a 1.5 pt FM increase [11]. T-WREX is now sold as ARMEO by Hocoma, A. G., the maker of the Lokomat.

A very simple non-robotic technology is the rocking chair. When acute stroke patients ($n=100$) rocked in a chair by pushing with their air-splinted paretic arm, they improved by 7 more FM points at 1-year follow-up compared to a group that did not receive the extrasensory motor stimulation [48]. The FM difference was 17 pts at 5-year follow-up ($n=64$) [49].

Hand/wrist/forearm exercise

For the hand, an example of a non-robotic therapeutic approach is to measure finger movements and provide computer feedback in the form of movement tracking games [50]. Practice with the system at home improved scores of hand movement ability in chronic stroke subjects ($n=20$) [50]. Another device, the Auto-Cite, consists of a motorized table that automatically presents trays of sensor-based hand exercise activities [22]. In three groups of chronic stroke patients ($n=9$ in each group) with varying levels of therapist supervision (25, 50, and 100%), there were significant motor gains after training with Auto-Cite and no differences between groups.

Summary

Non-robotic training devices that facilitate autonomous practice also produce significant reductions in impairment that are comparable with results from robotic devices (Figure 18.3).

Discussion

In its current state, robot-assisted therapy produces modest but consistent benefits that appear attributable to the practice undertaken, rather than a specific drive of plasticity attributable to the robotic forces applied. Non-robotic technology shows comparable therapeutic promise at this stage, as well, and may thus be a more clinically viable approach as it is potentially less expensive and safer.

What can be done to optimize robotic therapy? An important direction is to challenge the assumptions on which robotic therapy is based. For example, several design goals that are often stated for robotic therapy devices need to be rigorously evaluated, including the goals of:

(1) Physically assisting the patient in completing desired motions normally. Rationales given for this goal include providing enhanced somatosensory stimulation, stretching limbs to maintain their soft tissue compliance and reduce spasticity, and encouraging patient practice by allowing patients to accomplish meaningful tasks. However, providing assistance may reduce motor learning by changing the nature of the task to be learned or by encouraging slacking. Assistance has been found to enhance learning by unimpaired subjects only slightly in specific tasks [51–53]. In contrast, increasing performance errors may better provoke plasticity from some motor tasks, since performance errors drive adaptation [2,52]. The relationship between patient effort during training and therapeutic outcome is actually not established – is it a strong relationship?

(2) Allowing motions to be as naturalistic as possible. Although many devices assist in single degree of freedom (DOF) or two DOF movements because such movements require less complex devices, an often-stated goal is to allow more naturalistic movement. The rationale is that motor learning is task-specific, and therefore it would be desirable for patients to train the movements that they seek to perform in activities of daily living. This rationale needs to be rigorously tested. There is a possibility that the greater amount of repetitions possible in a fixed amount of time with simpler movements may ultimately be more effective. In addition, even simple movements require complex multiple muscle coordination as well, to stabilize the non-moving joints. The robotic therapy device that produced the largest differential therapeutic gain compared to a time-matched therapy focused on single joint distal movement [46].

(3) Providing bilateral training. Some devices use a bilateral training approach [19,38,46,47], using neural science on bilateral movements to infer that bilateral movements may produce brain activation patterns beneficial for plasticity. One study that addressed this hypothesis in a controlled therapeutic context failed to verify it [39]. Again, this approach requires rigorous evaluation.

(4) Providing intense but relatively brief therapy. Most robotic therapy studies have used therapeutic protocols lasting from 3 to 8 weeks, with the patients receiving 3–5 h of robotic therapy per week. Is residual capacity exhausted by this dosage? Constraint-induced therapy protocols often provide therapy for 6 or more hours per day. These trials tend to be in more mildly affected patients, and so the answer to the question of therapy intensity and duration might vary in relation to individual patient features. The issue of therapy intensity is also considered in Chapter 20.

Another direction for optimizing robotic therapy is to couple it with other techniques to stimulate plasticity, with the hopes of synergy – the combination of the parts greater that their simple sum. As reviewed above, there are at least two studies along these lines so far, one using tendon vibration to enhance somatosensory input during robotic therapy [4], and the other using tDCS to prime the motor cortex during robotic therapy [37]. Neither study was controlled with a matched-dose comparison group, so conclusions are not possible at this point.

Ultimately, optimizing robotic therapy will require a much more detailed understanding of how practice provokes plasticity. We have suggested the working hypothesis that movement practice, consisting of the repetitive execution of descending commands to try to achieve a presented motor goal, is the key stimulus for motor recovery, independently of whether this movement practice is accompanied by robotic assistance. This is a general statement that provides little insight into how practice actually improves performance. Measures of stroke-induced injury and brain function in individual patients might provide insights useful for optimizing an individual patient's robotic therapy protocol (see also Chapter 16). Another key direction for future research is to identify the behavioral/biomechanical signals that trigger the neurochemical signals that result in implementation of neuroplasticity mechanisms during movement practice. Defining these signals would allow exercise protocols and devices to then be designed that optimize them.

Acknowledgments

This work was supported in part by NIH N01-HD-3-3352 from NCMRR and NIBIB, and by the NIDRR RERC on Robotics and Telerehabilitation

References

1. Marchal-Crespo L, Reinkensmeyer DJ. Review of control strategies for robotic movement training after neurologic injury. *J Neur Eng Rehab*. 2009;**6**:20.

2. Patton J, Kovic M, Mussa-Ivaldi F. Custom-designed haptic training for restoring reaching ability to individuals with poststroke hemiparesis. *J Rehabil Res Dev*. 2006;**43**:643–56.

3. Eriksson J, Mataric M, Winstein C. Hands-off assistive robotics for post-stroke arm rehabilitation. *Proceedings of the 2005 IEEE International Conference on Rehabilitation Robotics*, 28 June –1 July, Chicago, Illinois 2005: 21–4.

4. Cordo P, Lutsep H, Cordo L, *et al.* Assisted Movement With Enhanced Sensation (AMES): Coupling motor and sensory to remediate motor deficits in chronic stroke patients. *Neurorehabil Neural Repair*. 2010;**23**:67–77.

5. Fischer HC, Stubblefield K, Kline T, *et al.* Hand rehabilitation following stroke: A pilot study of assisted finger extension training in a virtual environment. *Top Stroke Rehabil*. 2007;**14**:1–12.

6. Sugar TG, He J, Koeneman EJ, *et al.* Design and control of RUPERT: A device for robotic upper extremity repetitive therapy. *IEEE Trans Neural Syst Rehabil Engng*. 2007;**15**:336–46.

7. Ferris D. Powered lower limb orthoses for gait rehabilitation. *Top Spinal Cord Injury Rehab*. 2005;**11**(2):34–49.

8. Aisen ML, Krebs HI, Hogan N, *et al.* The effect of robot-assisted therapy and rehabilitative training on motor recovery following stroke. *Arch Neurol*. 1997;**54**:443–6.

9. Hornby TG, Campbell DD, Kahn JH, *et al.* Enhanced gait-related improvements after therapist- versus robotic-assisted locomotor training in subjects with chronic stroke: A randomized controlled study. *Stroke*. 2008;**39**:1786–92.

10. Takahashi CD, Der-Yeghiaian L, Le V, *et al.* Robot-based hand motor therapy after stroke. *Brain*. 2008;**131**:425–37.

11. Housman SJ, Scott KM, Reinkensmeyer DJ. A randomized controlled trial of gravity-supported, computer-enhanced arm exercise for individuals with severe hemiparesis. *Neurorehab Neural Repair*. 2009;**23**:505–14.

12. Wolbrecht ET, Reinkensmeyer DJ, Bobrow JE. Optimizing compliant, model-based robotic assistance to promote neurorehabilitation. *IEEE Trans Neural Syst Rehab Engng*. 2008;**16**:286–97.

13. Krebs HI, Mcrnoff S, Fasoli SE, *et al.* A comparison of functional and impairment-based robotic training in severe to moderate chronic stroke: A pilot study. *NeuroRehabilitation*. 2008;**23**:81–7.

14. Brewer BR, McDowell SK, Worthen-Chaudhari LC. Poststroke upper extremity rehabilitation: A review of robotic systems and clinical results. *Top Stroke Rehabil*. 2007;**14**(6):22–44.

15. Mehrholz J, Platz T, Kugler J, *et al.* Electromechanical and robot-assisted arm training for improving arm function and activities of daily living after stroke. *Cochrane Database Syst Rev*. 2008;**4**(4):CD006876.

16. Kahn L, Lum P, Rymer W, *et al.* Robot-assisted movement training for the stroke-impaired arm: Does it matter what the robot does? *J Rehab Res Dev*. 2006;**43**:619–30.

17. Richards LG, Senesac CR, Davis SB, *et al.* Bilateral arm training with rhythmic auditory cueing in chronic stroke: Not always efficacious. *Neurorehabil Neural Repair*. 2008;**22**:180–4.

18. Luft AR, McCombe-Waller S, Whitall J, *et al.* Repetitive bilateral arm training and motor cortex activation in chronic stroke: A randomized controlled trial. *JAMA*. 2004;**292**:1853–61.

19. Hesse S, Werner C, Pohl M, *et al.* Mechanical arm trainer for the treatment of the severely affected arm after a stroke: A single-blinded randomized trial in two centers. *Am J Phys Med Rehabil*. 2008;**87**:779–88.

20. Sanchez R, Liu J, Rao S, *et al.* Automating arm movement training following severe stroke: Functional exercises with quantitative feedback in a gravity-reduced environment. *IEEE Trans Neural RehabEngng*. 2006;**14**:378–89.

21. Barker RN, Brauer SG, Carson RG. Training of reaching in stroke survivors with severe and chronic upper limb paresis using a novel nonrobotic device: A randomized clinical trial. *Stroke*. 2008;**39**:1800–07.

22. Taub E, Lum PS, Hardin P, *et al.* AutoCITE: Automated delivery of CI therapy with reduced effort by therapists. *Stroke*. 2005;**36**:1301–04.

23. Fugl-Meyer AR, Jaasko L, Leyman I, *et al.* The post-stroke hemiplegic patient. 1. A method for evaluation of physical performance. *Scand J Rehabil Med*. 1975;**7**:13–31.

24. Krebs HI, Hogan N, Aisen ML, *et al.* Robot-aided neurorehabilitation. *IEEE Trans Rehabil Engng*. 1998;**6**:75–87.

25. Volpe B, Krebs H, Hogan N, *et al.* Robot training enhanced motor outcome in patients with stroke maintained over 3 years. *Neurology*. 1999;**53**:1874–6.

203

26. Fasoli S, Krebs H, Stein J, *et al*. Effects of robotic therapy on motor impairment and recovery in chronic stroke. *Arch Phys Med Rehabil*. 2003;**84**:477–82.

27. Fasoli SE, Krebs HI, Stein J, *et al*. Robotic therapy for chronic motor impairments after stroke: Follow-up results. *Arch Phys Med Rehabil*. 2004;**85**:1106–11.

28. Finley MA, Fasoli SE, Dipietro L, *et al*. Short-duration robotic therapy in stroke patients with severe upper-limb motor impairment. *J Rehabil Res Dev*. 2005;**42**:683–92.

29. Masiero S, Celia A, Rosati G, *et al*. Robotic-assisted rehabilitation of the upper limb after acute stroke. *Arch Phys Med Rehabil*. 2007;**88**:142–9.

30. Reinkensmeyer DJ, Kahn LE, Averbuch M, *et al*. Understanding and treating arm movement impairment after chronic brain injury: Progress with the ARM Guide. *J Rehab Res Dev*. 2000;**37**:653–62.

31. Chang JJ, Tung WL, Wu WL, *et al*. Effects of robot-aided bilateral force-induced isokinetic arm training combined with conventional rehabilitation on arm motor function in patients with chronic stroke. *Arch Phys Med Rehabil*. 2007;**88**:1332–8.

32. Colombo R, Pisano F, Micera S, *et al*. Robotic techniques for upper limb evaluation and rehabilitation of stroke patients. *IEEE Trans Neural Syst Rehabil Engng*. 2005;**13**:311–24.

33. Colombo R, Pisano F, Micera S, *et al*. Assessing mechanisms of recovery during robot-aided neurorehabilitation of the upper limb. *Neurorehabil Neural Repair*. 2008;**22**:50–63.

34. Song R, Tong KY, Hu X, *et al*. Assistive control system using continuous myoelectric signal in robot-aided arm training for patients after stroke. *IEEE Trans Neural Syst Rehabil Engng*. 2008;**16**:371–9.

35. Stein J, Narendran K, McBean J, *et al*. Electromyography-controlled exoskeletal upper-limb-powered orthosis for exercise training after stroke. *Am J Phys Med Rehabil*. 2007;**86**:255–61.

36. Adamovich SV, Merians AS, Boian R, *et al*. A virtual reality based exercise system for hand rehabilitation post-stroke: Transfer to function. *Conf Proc IEEE Engng Med Biol Soc*. 2004;**7**:4936–9.

37. Hesse S, Werner C, Schonhardt EM, *et al*. Combined transcranial direct current stimulation and robot-assisted arm training in subacute stroke patients: A pilot study. *Restor Neurol Neurosci*. 2007;**25**:9–15.

38. Lum PS, Burgar CG, Majmundar M, *et al*. Robot-assisted movement training compared with conventional therapy techniques for the rehabilitation of upper limb motor function following stroke. *Arch Phys Med Rehabil*. 2002;**83**:952–9.

39. Lum P, Burgar C, Van der Loos M, *et al*. MIME robotic device for upper-limb neurorehabilitation in subacute stroke subjects: A follow-up study. *J Rehabil Res Dev*. 2006;**43**:631–42.

40. Kahn LE, Zygman ML, Rymer WZ, *et al*. Robot-assisted reaching exercise promotes arm movement recovery in chronic hemiparetic stroke: A randomized controlled pilot study. *J Neuroengng Neurorehabil*. 2006;**3**:12.

41. Fischer H, Kahn L, Pelosin E, *et al*. Can robot-assisted therapy promote generalization of motor learning following stroke? Preliminary results. *Proceedings of the First IEEE/RAS-EMBS International Conference on Biomedical Robotics and Biomechatronics 2006 (BioRob 2006), 20–22 February 2006, Pisa, Italy*. IEEE Press: 865–8.

42. Volpe BT, Lynch D, Rykman-Berland A, *et al*. Intensive sensorimotor arm training mediated by therapist or robot improves hemiparesis in patients with chronic stroke. *Neurorehabil Neural Repair*. 2008;**22**:305–10.

43. Stein J, Krebs HI, Frontera WR, *et al*. Comparison of two techniques of robot-aided upper limb exercise training after stroke. *Am J Phys Med Rehabil*. 2004;**83**:720–8.

44. Mayr A, Kofler M, Saltuari L. ARMOR: An electromechanical robot for upper limb training following stroke. A prospective randomised controlled pilot study. *Handchir Mikrochir Plast Chir*. 2008;**40**:66–73.

45. Coote S, Murphy B, Harwin W, *et al*. The effect of the GENTLE/s robot-mediated therapy system on arm function after stroke. *Clin Rehabil*. 2008;**22**:395–405.

46. Hesse S, Werner C, Pohl M, *et al*. Computerized arm training improves the motor control of the severely affected arm after stroke: A single-blinded randomized trial in two centers. *Stroke*. 2005;**36**:1960–6. Epub 2005 Aug 18.

47. Whitall J, McCombe Waller S, Silver KH, *et al*. Repetitive bilateral arm training with rhythmic auditory cueing improves motor function in chronic hemiparetic stroke. *Stroke*. 2000;**31**:2390–5.

48. Feys H, De Weerdt W, Selz B, *et al*. Effect of a therapeutic intervention for the hemiplegic upper limb in the acute phase after stroke: A single-blind, randomized, controlled multicenter trial. *Stroke*. 1998;**29**:785–92.

49. Feys H, De Weerdt W, Verbeke G, *et al*. Early and repetitive stimulation of the arm can substantially improve the long-term outcome after stroke: A 5-year follow-up study of a randomized trial. *Stroke*. 2004;**35**:924–9.

50. Carey JR, Durfee WK, Bhatt E, *et al*. Comparison of finger tracking versus simple movement training via telerehabilitation to alter hand function and cortical reorganization after stroke. *Neurorehabil Neural Repair*. 2007;**21**:216–32.

51. Marchal-Crespo L, McHughen S, Cramer SC, *et al.* The effect of haptic guidance, aging, and initial skill level on motor learning of a steering task. *Exp Brain Res*, 2009;**201**:209–20.

52. Reinkensmeyer DJ, Patton JL. Can robots help the learning of skilled actions? *Exp Sports Sci Rev.* 2009;**37**:43–51.

53. Milot MH, Marchal-Crespo L, Green CS, *et al.* Comparison of error amplification and haptic guidance training techniques for learning of a timing-based motor task by healthy individuals. *Exp Brain Res.* 2009 Sep 29 [Epub ahead of print].

54. Israel JF, Campbell DD, Kahn JH, *et al.* Metabolic costs and muscle activity patterns during robotic- and therapist-assisted treadmill walking in individuals with incomplete spinal cord injury. *Phys Ther.* 2006;**86**:1466–78.

19 Electromagnetic approaches to stroke recovery

Gottfried Schlaug & Leonardo G. Cohen

Neurophysiological studies in chronic stroke patients have demonstrated that *disinhibition* of *contralesional* motor regions co-exists with *increased inhibition* of *ipsilesional* motor regions that results in an imbalance of interhemispheric interactions [1–3]. The indirect effect of this imbalance on the lesioned hemisphere combined with the stroke's direct effect on the unimpaired parts of the lesioned motor cortex and its efferent motor system appears to interfere with the recovery process under some circumstances. Similarly, imaging studies in well-recovered patients have shown that brain reorganization during the recovery phase is associated with reactivation or overactivation of unimpaired sensorimotor and premotor networks in the lesional hemisphere [4–7], while the significance of activation in the contralesional motor regions when the affected arm/hand performs a motor task remains under study [8,9]. One explanation is that this activation is a sign of *disinhibition* (the lesional hemisphere's lack of inhibitory effect on the contralesional hemisphere's motor region) that could potentially impede recovery. Although this model of interhemispheric imbalance may appear to be a simplified representation of the many underlying pathophysiological processes involved in recovery from stroke, it provides a framework for hypotheses focused on two facets: (1) downregulating activity in the contralesional motor region to check its unbalanced influence on the lesional motor region, and/or (2) facilitating activity in the ipsilesional motor region [10–15]. Support for these approaches can be found in pilot and proof-of-principle studies that have shown temporary beneficial effects in motoric measures, primarily in single session experiments using either transcranial magnetic stimulation (TMS), or, more recently, transcranial direct current stimulation (tDCS) [11,12,15–17]. TMS used as a diagnostic tool (see Chapter 10) has

also revealed that the re-emergence of motor-evoked potentials (MEPs) recorded from muscles in the paretic extremity after stimulation of the ipsilesional M1 in some cases indicates good motor recovery after stroke [18,19], although some patients with undetectable MEPs have shown good motor recovery [18]. TMS studies also have suggested that increased cortical excitability in contralesional M1 is not associated with good recovery [20,21].

The concept of therapeutic electricity on excitable tissues such as the brain is not new considering the attempts to cure epileptic disorders using electric catfish as early as the eleventh century (for a historic perspective, see [22]). The initial experiments of Eduard Hitzig (1870; cited in [23]) on dog cortex subsequent to a serendipitous discovery of abnormal involuntary movements in patients treated with high-voltage transcranial electric currents led to an interest in using electric currents to identify the cortical representations of limb movements (for more historic details see [23]). Electro-sleep therapy, which later came to be known as cranial electrical stimulation (CES), was used to treat sleep disorders and depression since 1902.

In the 1960s, the experiments of Bindman [24], suggesting long-lasting polarization effects following electric stimulation of the exposed motor cortex of animals, led to a resurgence of studies focusing on its clinical applications, including the use of brain polarization in depressed patients. Although these studies showed some benefits, replicating these beneficial effects in controlled settings yielded mixed results which subsequently led to a diminished interest in transcranial electrical treatments [25].

Several forms of electromagnetic stimulation are under evaluation to improve behavioral status after stroke. This stimulation is targeted towards a particular brain region, such as the motor cortex. This

---

Brain Repair After Stroke, ed. S. C. Cramer and R. J. Nudo. Published by Cambridge University Press.

chapter focuses on three of these: repetitive transcranial magnetic stimulation (rTMS), epidural cortical stimulation, and transcranial direct current stimulation (tDCS), which all lead to changes in polarity, but differ among others with regard to how focal and specific the stimulation is being applied and whether or not the intervention leads to neuronal discharges.

Several means for defining the stimulation target have been used. In some studies, landmarks on the scalp are used to direct stimulation to the underlying brain structures. Other studies use neurophysiological methods such as TMS to identify a specific neural target. Yet others have used functional magnetic resonance imaging (fMRI) activation sites to focus the stimulation. The relative strengths of each approach is a topic that requires further study.

Repetitive transcranial magnetic stimulation

One stimulation approach that has been examined in patients with stroke is rTMS. Depending on the stimulation frequency, rTMS has inhibitory or excitatory effects on cortical excitability [26]. As such, goals can include increasing excitation in ipsilesional cortical regions [27–30], or decreasing excitation in contralesional cortical regions that are uninhibitied and show increased cortical excitability [31–33].

Several studies have examined high frequency ($\geq$ 3–20 Hz) rTMS in patients with stroke applied to the ipsilesional hemisphere. Khedr et al. [27] found that 10 sessions of 3 Hz rTMS to the motor cortex improved disability and overall neurological status to a greater extent than sham rTMS did in patients with subacute stroke, all of whom received standard of care physiotherapy. No effect was seen in the patients with the largest stroke. Also, no correlation was found between behavioral gains and changes in cortical excitability, a finding that suggests that electrostimulation effects on behavior are not mediated by simply changing motor cortex excitability. Kim et al. [28], in a cohort of patients with chronic hemiparetic stroke, found that a single session of 10 Hz rTMS applied to the ipsilesional motor cortex as subjects practiced a complex finger-sequencing motor task improved motor learning more than did sham rTMS. Application of rTMS induced a significantly larger increase in the MEP amplitude than did sham rTMS. In this case, a change in motor cortex excitability was associated with greater motor behavioral gains. In a small sample, Talelli et al. [34] found that a single

session of excitatory theta burst stimulation, consisting of 3 pulses at 50 Hz repeated 5 times/s, increased MEP amplitude from the affected hemisphere and also improved reaction time. Yozbatiran et al. [30], in a study of patients with chronic hemiparetic stroke, found small increases in blood pressure when applying a single session of 20 Hz rTMS.

Application of low-frequency rTMS to the contralesional hemisphere is intended to reduce its excitability and activity, and thereby reduce its unbalanced inhibitory effects on the ipsilesional hemisphere, resulting in improvements in motor control of the ipsilesional motor cortex upon the affected hand [2,35–37]. Even a single session of such stimulation can improve motor function in the affected hand after stroke, at least transiently [38]. This suppressive approach was effective in modifying cortical silent periods [39], and increasing excitability of the ipsilesional motor cortex [31]. A single session of low-frequency (1 Hz) rTMS to the affected hemisphere in subacute stroke patients, followed by motor training, tended to increase cortical excitability, but without an effect on motor behavior [40].

Many questions remain with using TMS for a noninvasive brain stimulation. Furthermore, the mechanisms underlying spontaneous functional recovery after stroke are likely to differ depending on a variety of factors that may include magnitude of impairment, lesion site and size, affected hemisphere, and hemispheric dominance among others. Such factors likely also have an influence regarding the extent of effects from electromagnetic stimulation. Similarly, the optimal approach to pairing with behavioral experience [41], the role that adjuvant cellular or pharmacological therapy might play [42,43], the proper dose of rTMS [44], the preferred stimulation site(s), safety, and other issues require clarification, possibly with prescription being individualized according to features of individual stroke.

Epidural cortical stimulation

An alternative approach to non-invasive cortical stimulation involves surgical placement of electrodes in the epidural space above targeted brain regions. This approach was supported by a series of studies in rodents [45–47] and primates [48], where animals receiving epidural stimulation during rehab training showed greater stroke recovery than did animals receiving sham stimulation during rehab training. A small phase II study [49] evaluated 3 weeks of therapy in 8 patients, 4 of whom were randomized to epidural motor cortex stimulation, and 4 of whom were randomized to no stimulation. Both groups received concurrent arm physiotherapy. Results were suggestive of but did not substantiate significantly greater motor gains in the stimulation-treated group. A follow-up study [50] evaluated 6 weeks of therapy in 24 patients with chronic hemiparetic stroke. Patients were randomized to either epidural motor cortex stimulation concomitant with physiotherapy or to physiotherapy alone. Patients receiving stimulation appear to experience greater, albeit non-significantly larger, arm motor gains on several scales over 6 months of follow-up, and the intervention failed to evidence significant complications. However, a phase III study [51] of 164 patients found that epidural motor cortex stimulation combined with physiotherapy was not superior to physiotherapy alone. Different reasons could have contributed to this negative outcome, including different patient selection across trials (the ability to evoke a motor-evoked response was much less common in the phase III trial), choice of parameters of stimulation or choice of relatively focal stimulation site versus stimulation a large area of premotor/motor cortex.

Transcranial direct current stimulation

tDCS is a safe, portable, non-invasive brain polarization technique and its property of modulating cortical excitability in a polarity-specific manner is destined to be applied in the context of a model that assumes that the imbalance of interhemispheric inhibition and local excitation is an important pathophysiological barrier in the recovery process. Although the efficacy of tDCS has not been formally compared against TMS, there are advantages for using tDCS to induce polarity-specific excitability changes in stroke patients. First, tDCS does not directly lead to neuronal discharges and may be safer than TMS with a lower incidence of adverse effects [52]. Second, the current is usually transmitted through large electrodes, possibly modulating a larger neural network [53] that might include multiple brain regions shown to play a role in the recovery process (e.g. premotor, somatosensory, primary motor cortex). Third, tDCS has a sham mode, making it possible to be used in controlled experiments and randomized controlled clinical trials [54]. Lastly, a key advantage of tDCS over TMS is that tDCS

can be combined in real-time with motor training protocols or cognitive training (e.g. simultaneous occupational therapy or aphasia therapy), thus optimizing the brain's plasticity by inducing Hebbian or long-term potentiation-like mechanisms [55]. Furthermore, tDCS can be used in a dual mode applying anodal stimulation to one hemisphere and cathodal stimulation to a homolog region on the other hemisphere. This dual hemispheric stimulation has been shown to lead to stronger behavioral effects in normal subjects than a uni-hemispheric montage [56].

Studies on the effects of anodal direct currents on brain tissue in rats [57], such as increased accumulation of calcium ions leading to increased cortical excitability, as well as evidence for intracerebral currents during electro-sleep therapy studies in humans, prompted Priori and colleagues to develop a novel approach of non-invasive brain stimulation with weak direct currents which came to be known as tDCS [58,59]. Subsequent experiments by Nitsche and Paulus demonstrated modulatory effects of anodal (increasing cortical excitability) and cathodal (decreasing cortical excitability) tDCS on brain tissue whose effects surprisingly outlasted the duration of stimulation [60,61]. Residual electrophysiological effects were detectable up to 90 min and sensorimotor/cognitive effects up to 30 min after a 20–30-min stimulation period [60]. These early reports and others over the last 8–10 years have renewed the interest in the use of non-invasive regional brain polarization for various neurological disorders. Current research studies make use of the excitability-depressing effects of cathodal tDCS to create temporary cortical dysfunctions ("virtual lesions") that allow investigators to establish cause–effect links between activation in specific brain regions (as shown in fMRI, for example) and the behavioral consequences of its disruption. Similarly, several studies have examined whether anodal tDCS can be used to facilitate performance of certain sensorimotor or cognitive tasks if these tasks draw on the region that receives anodal stimulation (as an example of these two approaches, see [62,63]).

The components required for tDCS include a constant current stimulator and surface electrodes. A constant current stimulator can be either battery operated or connected to a power source (Figure 19.1). It should provide an uninterrupted direct current supply through the anodal and cathodal ends while monitoring the system for any change in resistance resulting from dryness of the electrodes, loss of contact, or other

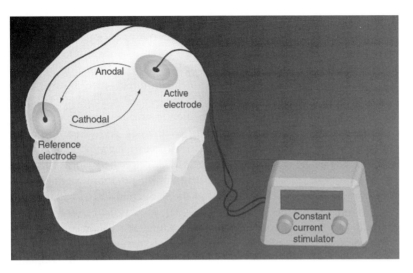

Figure 19.1 tDCS setup.

This figure shows a mobile, battery-operated direct current stimulator connected with two electrodes. One electrode (active) is positioned over C3 (corresponding to the precentral gyrus) and the reference electrode is positioned over the contralateral supra-orbital region. If current flows from C3 to the supra-orbital region, then the tissue underlying C3 is subjected to anodal (increase in excitability) stimulation. If current is reversed, then the tissue underlying C3 is subjected to cathodal (decrease in excitability) stimulation. (This figure is reprinted from [73] with permission from Future Science Group.)

causes. Available current stimulators have current settings from 0–4 mA and can supply up to 80 mA/min for a session. Saline soaked electrodes with variable surface areas (areas between 5 and 50 cm^2 have been reported) are placed on the desired region of interest (e.g. C3 or C4 for left or right primary motor cortex). The direction of the current flow determines the effect on the underlying tissue. If the positive electrode is placed over C3 or C4 and a reference electrode for example over a supra-orbital region, which acts as a terminal to complete the circuitry, then the brain tissue underlying the C3 or C4 region receives anodal polarization. If the negative electrode is placed over the motor cortex, then it is subject to cathodal inhibition (see [55] for more details on technical components).

Location of the reference electrode is important in both situations as it can influence the underlying tissue as well. In order to reduce any unwanted effects on brain tissue by the reference electrode, this electrode is frequently chosen to be in the supra-orbital region or outside the skull, over the collarbone or the chest. However, one has to be careful with regard to the location of the reference electrode, since at least one report showed that placing an electrode at a position which involves passage of current through the brain-stem might influence respiratory function [24]. Once the constant current stimulator is switched on, subjects usually have a tingling, itching, or a warming sensation under and around the electrodes as the current ramps up which usually fades away in 30 s to 1 min due to tolerance. Current density might also have an effect on the perceived intensity and how quickly this tingling/itching/warming sensation

might fade away. However, this transient sensation enables tDCS to have a sham mode which entails turning off the current stimulator unnoticed by the subject after letting it ramp up and giving the subject this initial experience of a tingling sensation, which has been shown to be undistinguishable from the initial sensory experience of real stimulation by research subjects [54].

tDCS has been shown to be a relatively safe intervention. Nitsche and colleagues described general safety limits for tDCS [64]. They identified "current density" and "total charge" as the most important parameters for judging the safety of tDCS studies. McCreery and colleagues found that current densities below 25 mA/cm^2 do not cause brain tissue damage [65]. The current density in protocols that apply 1 mA through an electrode with a size of 15–25 cm^2 is approximately 0.1 mA/cm^2, about 4/1000ths of the magnitude at which stimulation begins to be potentially dangerous for tissue. Yuen and colleagues found that no brain tissue damage occurs for a total charge less than 216 C/cm^2 [66]. Our own protocols typically involve a maximum total charge of 2.4 C/cm^2, about 1/100th of the minimum magnitude at which tissue damage can occur. The stimulation protocols in various laboratories around the world use 1–2 mA current strength applied for 20–40 min which is well within the safety limits reported above.

How does tDCS exert its effect on brain tissue? tDCS provides a subthreshold stimulus that modulates the likelihood that neurons will fire by hyperpolarizing or depolarizing the brain tissue, without direct neuronal depolarization [24,60]. The prolonged sensory, motor, and cognitive effects of tDCS have been attributed to a persistent bidirectional modification of post-synaptic connections similar to long-term potentiation (LTP) and long-term depression (LTD) effects [57,67,68]. Dextromethorphan, an *N*-methyl-D-aspartate (NMDA) antagonist, suppressed both anodal and cathodal tDCS effects, strongly suggesting the involvement of NMDA receptors in both types of DC-induced neuroplasticity. In contrast, carbamazepine selectively eliminated anodal effects. Since carbamazepine stabilizes the membrane potential through voltage-gated sodium channels (stabilizing the inactivated state of sodium channels), the results were interpreted as indicative that aftereffects of anodal tDCS require a depolarization of membrane potentials [69]. Ardolino and colleagues also proposed a non-synaptic mechanism involving changes in membrane excitability and ionic shifts [70]. Nevertheless, more studies are needed, in humans as well as in animal models, to verify the effects of tDCS on brain tissue, to better understand the underlying mechanisms of action, its sustained effects, and to determine relations between current strength/duration and neural tissue/behavioral effects interactions. Recent studies on brain modeling and current density distribution have suggested that in spite of a large fraction of the direct current being shunted through the scalp, tDCS carries adequate currents to the underlying cortex to be able to modulate neuronal excitability [71,72] and corresponding regional blood flow changes have been seen using non-invasive arterial spin labeling techniques [55].

Targeting the affected, unaffected, or both hemispheres

The model of an imbalance in the interhemispheric inhibitory interactions after a stroke led to the formulation of hypotheses focused on downregulating activity in the contralesional M1, facilitating it in the ipsilesional M1 or applying both at the same time resulting in three modes (Figure 19.2) of interventions [10,11,13,55,56,73–75]. The first set of studies that reported a significant improvement in motor function after stroke [12,14] applied anodal tDCS to the stroke-affected hemisphere. Later the same year, Fregni *et al.* found similar effects applying cathodal tDCS to the contralesional hemisphere [11]. However, these studies only used a single session of tDCS (1 mA for 20 min) in a pre–post assessment design and showed short-lasting effects. In a double-blind, sham-controlled, crossover study, Hummel *et al.*

reported an improvement in reaction time and pinch force in chronic stroke patients following anodal tDCS of the lesional hemisphere [76]. A more recent study in healthy subjects indicated that daily applications of anodal tDCS over M1 for 5 days in association with motor training led to a substantial improvement in skill acquisition through facilitation of off-line learning that remained present 3 months after the end of the training-stimulation period relative to controls [77], an effect possibly present also in elderly healthy human subjects [78]. Ongoing studies in chronic stroke patients are assessing longer-lasting effects using multiple daily sessions, often in combination with peripheral sensorimotor activities such as occupational therapies [16].

Anodal or cathodal stimulation have both led to relatively consistent effects across various laboratories around the world, suggesting that some aspects of the model of an imbalance in interhemispheric inhibition may be correct. Further support for this model comes also from the facilitatory influence of somatosensory stimulation of the paretic hand or anesthesia or disuse of the healthy hand in patients with stroke [79–82]. It is quite obvious that a technique that would allow the stimulation of ipsilesional M1, invasive or non-invasive, in addition to modulating interhemispheric interactions, might take advantage of facilitating perilesional cortical activity in the case of small cortical strokes [83]. There have also been attempts to apply cathodal and anodal stimulation to the motor regions of both hemispheres simultaneously in normal subjects in order to increase motor skill acquisition in the hand that is controlled by the hemisphere receiving anodal polarization. The interhemispheric inhibitory effect on this hemisphere was dampened by applying cathodal stimulation to the opposite hemisphere. Results showed significant differences in a motor skill acquisition between this "dual" stimulation approach compared to the unihemispheric stimulation [56].

Nevertheless, despite similarities with other cognitive models of interhemispheric inhibitory interactions [84], it remains to be investigated whether this mechanism operates in regions other than M1 after stroke. It is also important to keep in mind that cortical reorganization is likely to operate at a network level and approaches that focus on only one brain region at a time, while a reasonable start, are likely to represent only a partial aspect of a more complex full picture of recovery of function.

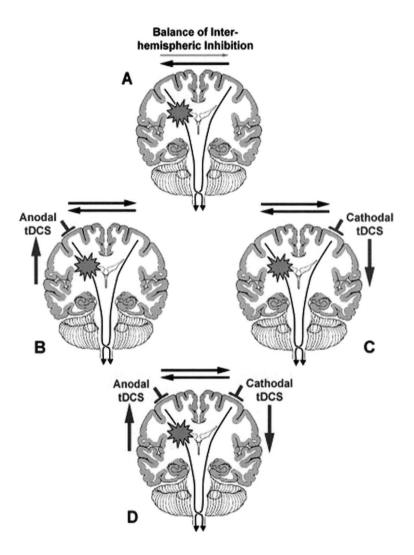

Balance of Inter-hemispheric Inhibition

A

Anodal tDCS   B

Cathodal tDCS   C

Anodal tDCS   Cathodal tDCS

D

Figure 19.2 Brain model of altered interhemispheric inhibition in patients with a unihemispheric stroke and the therapeutic options to ameliorate this imbalance.

The balance of interhemispheric inhibition becomes disrupted after a stroke (A). This leaves the healthy hemisphere in a position that it could exert too much of an unopposed influence onto the lesional hemisphere and possibly interfere in the recovery process. There are three possible ways to ameliorate this process: either the excitability in the affected (lesional) hemisphere (B) is upregulated, the excitability in the unaffected (normal) hemisphere (C) is downregulated, or a combination of both approaches (D).

Combining non-invasive brain stimulation with peripheral sensorimotor activities and neuromodulatory agents

Several recent studies [7,15] combined tDCS with rehabilitative therapy to further enhance the facilitating effect of non-invasive brain stimulation that had some effect already by itself. The idea behind this simultaneous approach is that combined peripheral sensorimotor activities (which also provide increased sensory feedback) and central brain stimulation (which has the ability to increase or decrease regional excitability) can enhance synaptic plasticity and motor skill acquisition/consolidation by increasing or modulating afferent inputs to the cortex at a time when it is receiving central stimulation. Cortical stimulation studies in experimental stroke models have shown stronger effects when peripheral sensorimotor activities were combined with central stimulation [85]. It has also been shown that paired associative brain stimulation and repetitive median nerve stimulation raised motor cortical excitability to a level higher than that produced by cortical stimulation alone [86]. This increase was not seen when the same procedure was performed under the influence of dextromethorphan, which is known to block LTP [87]. Motor skill learning has shown to produce LTP and LTD changes in the primary motor cortex in animal studies [88]. It seems possible that combined repetitive peripheral stimulation or rehabilitative therapy with non-invasive brain

Pre TDCS   Post TDCS

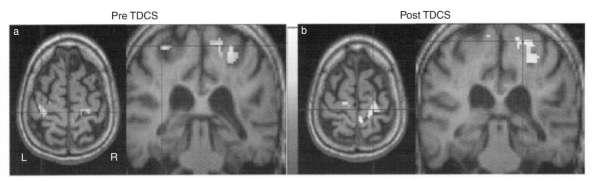

Figure 19.3 For the color version of this figure, see the Plate section. fMRI activation pattern in a stroke patient before and after tDCS fMRI studies in patients recovering from a stroke have shown that the ipsilateral (to the moving hand) sensorimotor cortex can become active when a patient performs a movement with their recovering hand. Applying cathodal stimulation to the non-lesional motor cortex (the motor cortex that activated when the recovering wrist was moving) significantly decreased the activation on the ipsilateral site and was associated with an improvement in this patient's functional motor status. (This figure is reprinted from [73] with permission from Future Science Group.)

stimulation can potentiate relearning and consolidation of motor skills to a level unattainable by any of these interventions alone in subacute or chronic stroke patients [89]. One of the first studies to test the efficacy of this approach was by Hesse *et al.*, who used multiple sessions of anodal tDCS (1.5 mA for 7 min) in an open-label pilot study without sham control and combined brain stimulation with a robot-assisted arm training protocol in severely affected subacute stroke patients (UE-FM scores were less than 18 [15]). Although the authors failed to find significant improvements in motor function in all patients, some of their subacute patients showed a pronounced effect. A second study was recently done by our group in which we applied cathodal tDCS (1 mA for 30 min) to the contralesional, unaffected hemisphere while chronic patients (at least 6 months after their first stroke; mean UE-FM was 28) received simultaneous occupational therapy for 60 min per day for 5 days in a row [16]. Preliminary analyses of this randomized, double-blind, sham-controlled study showed a significant improvement in motor outcomes that lasted for at least 1 week [16]. The improvement in motor outcomes correlated with a decrease in the contralesional excitability using TMS-induced MEPs and determining the slope of the input–output curve of the contralesional hemisphere. Furthermore, in some subjects following cathodal tDCS of the contralesional (unaffected) hemisphere there was a decrease in the ipsilateral activation when the recovered hand was moving as determined by functional magnetic resonance imaging (Figure 19.3).

Besides combining physical/occupational therapy or peripheral nerve stimulation with tDCS, combining tDCS with neuromodulatory substances might also enhance the tissue and behavioral effects. Kuo *et al.* recently showed that administering L-dopa to normal healthy subjects prolonged the cathodal tDCS-induced reduction in excitability and it prolonged all of the aftereffects typically seen after a 20–30-min stimulation session by a factor of about 20 [90]. The explanation for this effect might be that dopamine affects synaptic plasticity in cortical networks affected by the regional brain cathodal stimulation.

So far, most of the applications that we have mentioned have used a direct current. However, other forms of current are also under investigation such as alternating currents and random noise. Recently, Terney *et al.* used a novel method of electrical stimulation, transcranial random noise stimulation (tRNS), whereby a random electrical oscillation spectrum is applied to a particular region of the brain [91]. tRNS induced consistent excitability increases lasting 60 min after stimulation, possibly due to repeated opening of sodium channels. Although the associated behavioral effects of this type of intervention would still have to be shown, tRNS avoids the constraint of current flow direction sensitivity that is characteristic of tDCS.

Conclusions

The efficacy, safety, and full potential of non-invasive brain stimulation in stroke rehabilitation continue to be explored. Additional physiological and brain imaging studies as well as bench work will be necessary to understand the neural changes that are associated with the various forms of non-invasive brain stimulation and to elucidate the neural correlates of the therapeutic effects that such interventions may induce. There is preliminary evidence that different forms of cortical stimulation lead to clear modulation of measures of cortical excitability and interhemispheric interactions when functional motor activation is compared between pre- and post-stimulation (Figure 19.3). Second, patient selection may have to be improved to better determine which patients might benefit from this approach considering the variability in post-stroke recovery and which physiological, structural, and/or functional imaging parameters can be used to determine which form of brain stimulation will maximize gains. For example, different patients might show differential benefits from anodal, cathodal, or dual hemispheric tDCS. Factors that might contribute to the variance in outcome data include the anatomical and functional integrity of the descending pyramidal tract as well as other descending motor tracts [17], lesion load affecting descending motor fibers, hemisphere affected (dominant versus nondominant), age, gender, handedness, and presence or absence of electrophysiological markers of excitability or inhibition. Third, it will need to be explored whether there is an optimal therapeutic window during which the application of electromagnetic brain stimulation leads to beneficial effects and what stimulation parameters and application modes are optimal to make the effects last as long as possible. Last but not least, the combination of brain stimulation with peripheral stimulation techniques and pharmacological therapies, in order to optimally modulate neural plasticity, similar to paired associative stimulation protocols, needs to be further explored [86,92].

References

1. Shimizu T, Hosaki A, Hino T, *et al.* Motor cortical disinhibition in the unaffected hemisphere after unilateral cortical stroke. *Brain.* 2002;**125**:1896–907.

2. Murase N, Duque J, Mazzocchio R *et al.* Influence of interhemispheric interactions on motor function in chronic stroke. *Ann Neurol.* 2004;**55**:400–09.

3. Duque J, Mazzocchio R, Dambrosia J, *et al.* Kinematically specific interhemispheric inhibition operating in the process of generation of a voluntary movement. *Cereb Cortex.* 2005;**15**:588–93.

4. Cramer SC, Mark A, Barquist K, *et al.* Motor cortex activation is preserved in patients with chronic hemiplegic stroke. *Ann Neurol.* 2002; **52**:607–16.

5. Calautti C, Baron JC. Functional neuroimaging studies of motor recovery after stroke in adults: A review. *Stroke.* 2003;**34**:1553–66.

6. Loubinoux I, Carel C, Pariente J, *et al.* Correlation between cerebral reorganization and motor recovery after subcortical infarcts. *Neuroimage.* 2003;**20**:2166–80.

7. Nair DG, Hutchinson S, Fregni F, *et al.* Imaging correlates of motor recovery from cerebral infarction and their physiological significance in well-recovered patients. *Neuroimage.* 2007;**34**:253–63.

8. Johansen-Berg H, Rushworth MF, Bogdanovic MD, *et al.* The role of ipsilateral premotor cortex in hand movement after stroke. *Proc Natl Acad Sci USA.* 2002;**99**:14 518–23.

9. Lotze M, Markert J, Sauseng P, *et al.* The role of multiple contralesional motor areas for complex hand movements after internal capsular lesion. *J Neurosci.* 2006;**26**:6096–102.

10. Mansur CG, Fregni F, Boggio PS, *et al.* A sham stimulation-controlled trial of rTMS of the unaffected hemisphere in stroke patients. *Neurology.* 2005;**64**:1802–04.

11. Fregni F, Boggio PS, Mansur CG, *et al.* Transcranial direct current stimulation of the unaffected hemisphere in stroke patients. *Neuroreport.* 2005;**16**:1551–5.

12. Hummel F, Celnik P, Giraux P, *et al.* Effects of noninvasive cortical stimulation on skilled motor function in chronic stroke. *Brain.* 2005;**128**:490–9.

13. Ward NS, Cohen LG. Mechanisms underlying recovery of motor function after stroke. *Arch Neurol.* 2004; **61**:1844–8.

14. Hummel F, Cohen LG. Improvement of motor function with noninvasive cortical stimulation in a patient with chronic stroke. *Neurorehabil Neural Repair.* 2005;**19**:14–9.

15. Hesse S, Werner C, Schonhardt EM, *et al.* Combined transcranial direct current stimulation and robot-assisted arm training in subacute stroke patients: A pilot study. *Restor Neurol Neurosci.* 2007;**25**:9–15.

16. Nair D, Renga V, Hamelin S, *et al.* Improving motor function in chronic stroke patients using simultaneous occupational therapy and tDCS. *Restor Neurol Neurosci.* 2010; in press.

17. Lindenberg R, Renga V, Zhu LL, *et al.* Bihemispheric brain stimulation facilitates motor recovery in chronic stroke. *Neurology.* 2010; in press.

18. Escudero JV, Sancho J, Bautista D, *et al.* Prognostic value of motor evoked potential obtained by transcranial magnetic brain stimulation in motor function recovery in patients with acute ischemic stroke. *Stroke.* 1998;**29**:1854–9.

19. Heald A, Bates D, Cartlidge NE, *et al.* Longitudinal study of central motor conduction time following stroke. 2. Central motor conduction measured within

72 h after stroke as a predictor of functional outcome at 12 months. *Brain*. 1993;**116**:1371–85.

20. Caramia MD, Iani C, Bernardi, G. Cerebral plasticity after stroke as revealed by ipsilateral responses to magnetic stimulation. *Neuroreport*. 1996;**7**:1756–60.

21. Turton A, Wroe S, Trepte N, *et al*. Contralateral and ipsilateral EMG responses to transcranial magnetic stimulation during recovery of arm and hand function after stroke. *Electroencephalogr Clin Neurophysiol*. 1996;**101**:316–28.

22. Priori A. Brain polarization in humans: A reappraisal of an old tool for prolonged non-invasive modulation of brain excitability. *Clin Neurophysiol*. 2003;**114**:589–95.

23. Gross CG. The discovery of motor cortex and its background. *J Hist Neurosci*. 2007;**16**:320–31.

24. Bindman LJ, Lippold OC, Redfearn JW. The action of brief polarizing currents on the cerebral cortex of the rat (1) during current flow and (2) in the production of long-lasting after-effects. *J Physiol*. 1964;**172**:369–82.

25. Arfai E, Theano G, Montagu JD, *et al*. A controlled study of polarization in depression. *Br J Psychiatry*. 1970;**116**:433–4.

26. Valero-Cabre A, Payne BR, Pascual-Leone A. Opposite impact on (14)C-2-deoxyglucose brain metabolism following patterns of high and low frequency repetitive transcranial magnetic stimulation in the posterior parietal cortex. *Exp Brain Res*. 2007;**176**:603–15.

27. Khedr EM, Ahmed MA, Fathy N, *et al*., Therapeutic trial of repetitive transcranial magnetic stimulation after acute ischemic stroke. *Neurology*. 2005;**65**:466–8.

28. Kim YH, You SH, Ko MH, *et al*. Repetitive transcranial magnetic stimulation-induced corticomotor excitability and associated motor skill acquisition in chronic stroke. *Stroke*. 2006;**37**:1471–6.

29. Malcolm MP, Triggs WJ, Light KE, *et al*. Repetitive transcranial magnetic stimulation as an adjunct to constraint-induced therapy: An exploratory randomized controlled trial. *Am J Phys Med Rehabil*. 2007;**86**:707–15.

30. Yozbatiran N, Alonso-Alonso M, See J, *et al*. Safety and behavioral effects of high-frequency repetitive transcranial magnetic stimulation in stroke. *Stroke*. 2009;**40**:309–12.

31. Fregni F, Boggio PS, Valle AC, *et al*. A sham-controlled trial of a 5-day course of repetitive transcranial magnetic stimulation of the unaffected hemisphere in stroke patients. *Stroke*. 2006;**37**:2115–22.

32. Martin P, Naeser M, Theoret H, *et al*. Transcranial magnetic stimulation as a complementary treatment for aphasia. *Semin Speech Lang*. 2004;**25**:181–91.

33. Takeuchi N, Tada T, Toshima M, *et al*. Inhibition of the unaffected motor cortex by 1 Hz repetitive transcranical magnetic stimulation enhances motor performance and training effect of the paretic hand in patients with chronic stroke. *J Rehabil Med*. 2008;**40**:298–303.

34. Talelli P, Greenwood RJ, Rothwell JC. Exploring theta burst stimulation as an intervention to improve motor recovery in chronic stroke. *Clin Neurophysiol*. 2007;**118**:333–42.

35. Webster BR, Celnik PA, Cohen LG. Noninvasive brain stimulation in stroke rehabilitation. *NeuroRx*. 2006;**3**:474–81.

36. Butefisch CM, Wessling M, Netz J, *et al*. Relationship between interhemispheric inhibition and motor cortex excitability in subacute stroke patients. *Neurorehabil Neural Repair*. 2008;**22**:4–21.

37. Nowak DA, Grefkes C, Dafotakis M, *et al*. Effects of low-frequency repetitive transcranial magnetic stimulation of the contralesional primary motor cortex on movement kinematics and neural activity in subcortical stroke. *Arch Neurol*. 2008;**65**:741–7.

38. Liepert J, Zittel S, Weiller C. Improvement of dexterity by single session low-frequency repetitive transcranial magnetic stimulation over the contralesional motor cortex in acute stroke: A double-blind placebo-controlled crossover trial. *Restor Neurol Neurosci*. 2007;**25**:461–5.

39. Takeuchi N, Chuma T, Matsuo Y, *et al*. Repetitive transcranial magnetic stimulation of contralesional primary motor cortex improves hand function after stroke. *Stroke*. 2005;**36**:2681–6.

40. Pomeroy VM, Cloud G, Tallis RC, *et al*. Transcranial magnetic stimulation and muscle contraction to enhance stroke recovery: A randomized proof-of-principle and feasibility investigation. *Neurorehabil Neural Repair*. 2007;**21**:509–17.

41. Stefan K, Classen J, Celnik P, *et al*. Concurrent action observation modulates practice-induced motor memory formation. *Eur J Neurosci*. 2008;**27**:730–8.

42. Kirschner J, Moll GH, Fietzek UM, *et al*. Methylphenidate enhances both intracortical inhibition and facilitation in healthy adults. *Pharmacopsychiatry*. 2003;**36**:79–82.

43. Lang N, Speck S, Harms J, *et al*. Dopaminergic potentiation of rTMS-induced motor cortex inhibition. *Biol Psychiatry*. 2008;**63**:231–3.

44. Hiscock A, Miller S, Rothwell J, *et al*. Informing dose-finding studies of repetitive transcranial magnetic stimulation to enhance motor function: A qualitative systematic review. *Neurorehabil Neural Repair*. 2007;**22**:228–49.

45. Adkins-Muir D, Jones T. Cortical electrical stimulation combined with rehabilitative training: Enhanced functional recovery and dendritic plasticity following focal cortical ischemia in rats. *Neurol Res*. 2003;**25**:780–8.

46. Kleim J, Bruneau R, VandenBerg P, *et al*. Motor cortex stimulation enhances motor recovery and

reduces peri-infarct dysfunction following ischemic insult. *Neurol Res.* 2003;**25**:789–93.

47. Teskey G, Flynn C, Goertzen C, *et al.* Cortical stimulation improves skilled forelimb use following a focal ischemic infarct in the rat. *Neurol Res.* 2003;**25**:794–800.

48. Plautz E, Barbay S, Frost S, *et al.* Post-infarct cortical plasticity and behavioral recovery using concurrent cortical stimulation and rehabilitative training: A feasibility study in primates. *Neurol Res.* 2003;**25**:801–10.

49. Brown JA, Lutsep HL, Weinand M, *et al.* Motor cortex stimulation for the enhancement of recovery from stroke: A prospective, multicenter safety study. *Neurosurgery.* 2006;**58**:464–73.

50. Huang M, Harvey RL, Stoykov ME, *et al.* Cortical stimulation for upper limb recovery following ischemic stroke: A small phase II pilot study of a fully implanted stimulator. *Top Stroke Rehabil.* 2008;**15**:160–72.

51. Levy R, Benson R, Winstein C, for the Everest Study Investigators. Cortical stimulation for upper-extremity hemiparesis from ischemic stroke: Everest study primary endpoint results. In *International Stroke Conference.* 2008. New Orleans, LA.

52. Poreisz C, Boros K, Antal A, *et al.* Safety aspects of transcranial direct current stimulation concerning healthy subjects and patients. *Brain Res Bull.* 2007;**72**:208–14.

53. Lang N, Siebner HR, Ward NS, *et al.* How does transcranial DC stimulation of the primary motor cortex alter regional neuronal activity in the human brain? *Eur J Neurosci.* 2005;**22**:495–504.

54. Gandiga PC, Hummel FC, Cohen LG. Transcranial DC stimulation (tDCS): A tool for double-blind sham-controlled clinical studies in brain stimulation. *Clin Neurophysiol.* 2006;**117**:845–50.

55. Schlaug G, Renga V, Nair D. Transcranial direct current stimulation in stroke recovery. *Arch Neurol.* 2008;**65**:1571–6.

56. Vines BW, Cerruti C, Schlaug G. Dual-hemisphere tDCS facilitates greater improvements for healthy subjects' non-dominant hand compared to uni-hemisphere stimulation. *BMC Neurosci.* 2008;**9**:103.

57. Islam N, Aftabuddin M, Moriwaki A, *et al.* Increase in the calcium level following anodal polarization in the rat brain. *Brain Res.* 1995;**684**:206–08.

58. Priori A, Berardelli A, Rona S, *et al.* Polarization of the human motor cortex through the scalp. *Neuroreport.* 1998;**9**:2257–60.

59. Priori A, Egidi M, Pesenti A, *et al.* Do intraoperative microrecordings improve subthalamic nucleus targeting in stereotactic neurosurgery for Parkinson's disease? *J Neurosurg Sci.* 2003;**47**:56–60.

60. Nitsche MA, Paulus W. Excitability changes induced in the human motor cortex by weak transcranial direct current stimulation. *J Physiol.* 2000;**527**:633–9.

61. Nitsche MA, Paulus W. Sustained excitability elevations induced by transcranial DC motor cortex stimulation in humans. *Neurology.* 2001;**57**:1899–901.

62. Vines BW, Nair DG, Schlaug G. Contralateral and ipsilateral motor effects after transcranial direct current stimulation. *Neuroreport.* 2006;**17**:671–4.

63. Vines BW, Schnider NM, Schlaug G. Testing for causality with transcranial direct current stimulation: Pitch memory and the left supramarginal gyrus. *Neuroreport.* 2006;**17**:1047–50.

64. Nitsche MA, Liebetanz D, Lang N, *et al.* Safety criteria for transcranial direct current stimulation (tDCS) in humans. *Clin Neurophysiol.* 2003; **114**:2220–2; author reply 2222–3.

65. McCreery DB, Agnew WF, Yuen TG, *et al.* Charge density and charge per phase as cofactors in neural injury induced by electrical stimulation. *IEEE Trans Biomed Engng.* 1990;**37**:996–1001.

66. Yuen TG, Agnew WF, Bullara LA, *et al.* Histological evaluation of neural damage from electrical stimulation: Considerations for the selection of parameters for clinical application. *Neurosurgery.* 1981;**9**:292–9.

67. Hattori Y, Moriwaki A, Hori Y. Biphasic effects of polarizing current on adenosine-sensitive generation of cyclic AMP in rat cerebral cortex. *Neurosci Lett.* 1990;**116**:320–4.

68. Moriwaki A. Polarizing currents increase noradrenaline-elicited accumulation of cyclic AMP in rat cerebral cortex. *Brain Res.* 1991;**544**:248–52.

69. Liebetanz D, Nitsche MA, Paulus W. Pharmacology of transcranial direct current stimulation: Missing effect of riluzole. *Suppl Clin Neurophysiol.* 2003;**56**:282–7.

70. Ardolino G, Bossi B, Barbieri S, *et al.* Non-synaptic mechanisms underlie the after-effects of cathodal transcutaneous direct current stimulation of the human brain. *J Physiol.* 2005;**568**:653–63.

71. Miranda PC, Lomarev M, Hallett M. Modeling the current distribution during transcranial direct current stimulation. *Clin Neurophysiol.* 2006;**117**:1623–9.

72. Wagner T, Fregni F, Fecteau S, *et al.* Transcranial direct current stimulation: A computer-based human model study. *Neuroimage.* 2007;**35**:1113–24.

73. Schlaug G, Renga V. Transcranial direct current stimulation: A noninvasive tool to facilitate stroke recovery. *Expert Rev Med Devices.* 2008;**5**:759–68.

74. Hummel FC, Cohen LG. Non-invasive brain stimulation: A new strategy to improve neurorehabilitation after stroke? *Lancet Neurol.* 2006;**5**:708–12.

75. Vines BW, Nair D, Schlaug G. Modulating activity in the motor cortex affects performance for the two hands differently depending upon which hemisphere is stimulated. *Eur J Neurosci.* 2008;**28**:1667–73.

76. Hummel FC, Voller B, Celnik P, *et al.* Effects of brain polarization on reaction times and pinch force in chronic stroke. *BMC Neurosci.* 2006;**7**:73.

77. Reis J, Schambra HM, Cohen LG, *et al.* Noninvasive cortical stimulation enhances motor skill acquisition over multiple days through an effect on consolidation. *Proc Natl Acad Sci USA.* 2009;**106**:1590–5.

78. Hummel FC, Heise K, Celnik P, *et al.* Facilitating skilled right hand motor function in older subjects by anodal polarization over the left primary motor cortex. *Neurobiol Aging.* 2009.

79. Taub E, Uswatte G, Pidikiti R. Constraint-induced movement therapy: A new family of techniques with broad application to physical rehabilitation – a clinical review. *J Rehabil Res Dev.* 1999;**36**:237–51.

80. Voller B, Floel A, Werhahn KJ, *et al.* Contralateral hand anesthesia transiently improves poststroke sensory deficits. *Ann Neurol.* 2006;**59**:385–8.

81. Floel A, Hummel F, Duque J, *et al.* Influence of somatosensory input on interhemispheric interactions in patients with chronic stroke. *Neurorehabil Neural Repair.* 2008;**22**:477–85.

82. Floel A, Nagorsen U, Werhahn KJ, *et al.* Influence of somatosensory input on motor function in patients with chronic stroke. *Ann Neurol.* 2004;**56**:206–12.

83. Nudo RJ, Wise BM, SiFuentes F, *et al.* Neural substrates for the effects of rehabilitative training on motor recovery after ischemic infarct. *Science.* 1996;**272**:1791–4.

84. Kinsbourne M, Swanson JM, Ledlow A. Measuring interhemispheric transfer time in man. *Trans Am Neurol Assoc.* 1977;**102**:163–7.

85. Adkins-Muir DL, Jones TA. Cortical electrical stimulation combined with rehabilitative training: Enhanced functional recovery and dendritic plasticity following focal cortical ischemia in rats. *Neurol Res.* 2003;**25**:780–8.

86. Stefan K, Kunesch E, Cohen LG, *et al.* Induction of plasticity in the human motor cortex by paired associative stimulation. *Brain.* 2000;**123**:572–84.

87. Stefan K, Kunesch E, Benecke R, *et al.* Mechanisms of enhancement of human motor cortex excitability induced by interventional paired associative stimulation. *J Physiol.* 2002;**543**:699–708.

88. Rioult-Pedotti MS, Friedman D, Donoghue JP. Learning-induced LTP in neocortex. *Science.* 2000;**290**:533–6.

89. Celnik P, Paik NJ, Vandermeeren Y, *et al.* Effects of combined peripheral nerve stimulation and brain polarization on performance of a motor sequence task after chronic stroke. *Stroke.* 2009;**40**:1764–71.

90. Kuo MF, Paulus W, Nitsche MA. Boosting focally-induced brain plasticity by dopamine. *Cereb Cortex.* 2008;**18**:648–51.

91. Terney D, Bergmann I, Poreisz C, *et al.* Pergolide increases the efficacy of cathodal direct current stimulation to reduce the amplitude of laser-evoked potentials in humans. *J Pain Symptom Manage.* 2008;**36**:79–91.

92. Celnik P, Hummel F, Harris-Love M, *et al.* Somatosensory stimulation enhances the effects of training functional hand tasks in patients with chronic stroke. *Arch Phys Med Rehabil.* 2007;**88**:1369–76.

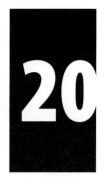

20 Intensive physical therapeutic approaches to stroke recovery

Steven L. Wolf & Carolee J. Winstein

The notion of "intensity"

The Merriam-Webster Dictionary defines "intensity" as the quality or state of being intense; especially: extreme degree of strength, force, energy or feeling (www.merrriam-webster.com/dictionary/intnsity), and the Free Dictionary defines it as exceptionally good concentration, power or force (www.thefreedictionary.com/intensity). While both these definitions share the notion of "force", reality dictates that "intensity" is a concept defined within the unique construct for which it is intended. In physics, for example, intensity means the amount or degree of strength of electricity, light, heat, or sound per unit area or volume, while in the context of sports competition, intensity means showing a great energy of emotion or a component of motivation that relates to the amount of effort an athlete makes in a particular situation. In the context of a jubilant youth, it means excessive and mindless enthusiasm for an activity that might be considered trivial or pointless (www.urbandictionary.com/define.php?term=intensity). Inevitably, what this myriad of definitions shares is a biological or physical sense of concentrated if not confined energy.

Intensity applied to stroke rehabilitation

If one now shifts this definition toward rehabilitation in general and stroke rehabilitation in particular, without wanting to lose a general perspective, indeed, we can readily become lost. As Kwakkel [1] has noted, intensity of practice has defied a clearly accepted definition. Are we referring to the number of repetitions of one or multiple movements (frequency) per unit of time (duration) within one treatment session or over multiple sessions, or the totality of effort exerted during practice, including both mental and physical aspects? Do we measure intensity in terms of energy expenditure or some combination of frequency and duration of effort? Or should any definition of treatment intensity in stroke rehabilitation be referenced primarily to what is being attempted as a function of chronicity, thus unveiling modifiers including age, concordance, or changes in fatigue, pain, and cognitive states as critical factors for consideration? What can be said, at this time, is that the prevailing data suggest earlier is better in terms of potential exploitation of cortical plasticity and that more may be better [2], although with some limits [3]. The extensiveness of such plasticity and how one operationalizes the meaning of "more" remain profoundly open-ended questions. Additionally, our collective failure to control for intensity of practice in many stroke studies, including randomized Phase III clinical trials, may have led to inconsistent results and multiple interpretations, both within and outside the stroke rehabilitation communities [4,5]. In fact, arguments have been made that in the absence of precisely specifying at least frequency and duration of treatment, replication of treatment approaches can be compromised [6].

Perhaps our free-spirited approach to stroke survivor treatment finds its historical roots in the advocacy of our rehabilitation stalwarts, such as Karl and Berta Bobath [7,8], Signe Brunnstrom [9], Maggie Knott or Dorothy Voss [10]. These dedicated individuals were keen on extracting fundamental principles of reflex organization, hierarchies of postural control, including the expression of synergies, and the impact of sensory stimuli on normal and abnormal motor responses. The genesis of their treatment approaches and the emergence of derivations, such as neurodevelopmental treatment (NDT) [11], arose from extricating findings in fundamental scientific studies from such notables as Sherrington, Magnus,

Denny-Brown, and Hughlings Jackson. While dissemination of approaches for the treatment of patients with stroke excited practitioners because, for the first time, efforts had been set in motion to apply sound scientific observations from animal models of movement pathology to the human condition, those advocates were blinded by the collective failure to quantitatively validate the observations from these fundamental studies. In fact, the literature derived from the enthusiasm generated by these clinical approaches was deplete of quantitative data to support the observations, lacked long-term follow-up, and failed to demonstrate relationships between magnitude of impairment, reacquisition of ability, and treatment specificity. Observation without rigorous quantitative analysis is insufficient.

What was generated from such empirical approaches, however, was a sense that prolonged and rigorous treatment, using Bobath or Brunnstrom treatment techniques, for example, could lead to less impairment. The time course over which such treatment would be delivered was not an essential consideration; yet, the intimacy and longevity of exposure to patients quite satisfactorily met the altruistic desire of many physical and occupational therapists to validate their commitment to improve movement capability in catastrophically injured patients. Hence, for over 40 years, health-related professionals within the stroke community were trained with the belief that prolonged treatment, often in the absence of data to support such extended treatment, was the appropriate form of interaction.

When one undertakes a retrospective "look at the data," it becomes apparent that few studies advocating specific "neuromuscular treatment techniques," especially those espoused by many of our neurorehabilitation founders and their disciples, have any substantive data to support the benefits derived from their implementation. In fact, there is uncertainty surrounding the justification of the amount of time in treatment relative to the outcome, and this reality now confronts all of us treating stroke survivors.

Accordingly, this chapter focuses on upper extremity rehabilitation by exploring the fundamental question regarding the relationship between the amount of time spent in treatment (to designate "intensity") and outcome. In the process, a review of some approaches will exemplify the paucity of support for unequivocal blanket treatments, and several limitations that have impeded our comprehension of intensity will be identified. The suggestion will be made that the strongest data to demonstrate enhanced measures of function have been derived from patients who might be classified as having sustained a mild to moderate stroke. Last, a confluence of circumstance and fact will be used to suggest that future applications of upper-extremity stroke rehabilitation must consider elements of patient self-efficacy as a potential cornerstone to promote both treatment effectiveness and retention of functional improvements.

Performing literature searches

These searches were not intended to be all inclusive, but, rather, to provide for a grasp of information relevant to the notion of intensity of practice and outcomes as they relate to reasonably well-recognized forms of treatment. Thus, intensive reviews that characterize the Cochrane Collection or PEDro have been forsaken in favor of simple PubMed searches that cross-reference key terms. This exploratory form also represents what most clinicians would undertake to gain information to address the primary question.

The relationship between treatment and outcome: Brunnstrom

In an effort to appreciate the relationship between treatment and outcome, the current search cross-referenced the terms "Brunnstrom," "stroke," and "outcome." The search yielded 19 eligible studies, 5 of which addressed upper-extremity rehabilitation approaches. They are summarized in Table 20.1. The decision to include them was based solely on reference to the use of Brunnstrom treatment techniques or the Brunnstrom stage of stroke recovery as an outcome measure. While each had appropriately matched control groups (not shown), the approaches varied considerably as did the measure of intensity and relative chronicity of the participants. Moreover, "Brunnstrom" as a term varied between use of the six-level synergy scale and combining Brunnstrom with Fugl-Meyer into what is more contemporarily referred to as the Fugl-Meyer Assessment Scale [12]. Only one study actually made reference to the Brunnstrom approach to treatment. Perhaps most disconcerting is the fact that while several studies reported significant outcomes, only the Feys *et al.* study [13] showed a statistical change that might have implications for clinical importance.

Table 20.1 Stroke outcome and Brunnstrom approach

Study	Intervention	Intensity	Outcome
Werner and Kessler [57]	Neuromuscular facilitation (N=49)	1 h PT/1 h OT 4/wk, 12 wks	FIM motor score improved; Brunnstrom motor score = no change
Feys et al. [13]	Repetitive sensory motor stimulation, air splint/rocking chair (N=62 at 5 years post-Rx)	6 weeks (30 min, 30 sessions)	17 point increase in Brunnstrom/Fugl-Meyer score
Chan et al. [58]	Thermal stimulation and standard therapy (N=29/46)	Standard treatment + 30 min/day, 6 weeks, thermal stim	Brunnstrom stage of recovery improved significantly at each evaluation
Hemmen and Seelen [59]	Imagery and EMG triggered biofeedback (N=27)	3 mo, 5 d/wk, 30 min/d	Brunnstrom/Fugl-Meyer score improved 8.7 points
Yavuzer et al. [60]	Mirror therapy + conventional therapy (N=40)	5 d/wk, 2–5 h/d, 4 wks	Brunnstrom stage of motor recovery improved .83 (units) hand, .89 arm

Table 20.2 Stroke outcome and proprioceptive neuromuscular facilitation approach

Study	Intervention	Intensity	Outcome
Quin [61]	Observational		
Dickstein et al. [15]	Traditional exercise + functional training PNF Bobath (N=131)	Regularly for 6 weeks	Barthel Index Muscle Tone Wrist/ankle ROM and strength No between group differences
Kraft et al. [62]	PNF FES No treatment	3 months	Fugl-Meyer Score PNF=18%↑; FES=42%↑

The relationship between treatment and outcome: proprioceptive neuromuscular facilitation (PNF)

If the same exercise is undertaken just exploring articles on PNF, 99 studies can be identified through a PubMed search, but only 4 of them are applied to patients with stroke, while the remaining appear more relevant to patients with musculoskeletal disorders. One of the four articles [14] was a review of all Bobath-based outcomes and cited only the Dickstein article [15]. These studies, shown in Table 20.2, lacked specificity about treatment elements and intensities. The outcomes are equivocal.

The relationship between treatment and outcome: the Bobath approach

Cross-referencing Bobath with treatment intensity resulted in the identification of three articles, one of which addressed pediatric treatments, one a comparison of measurement techniques, and one considered to be a major paper [16] addressed below. When both "stroke" and "outcomes" were added to the referencing, 33 articles were identified, of which 12 contained data related to upper extremity treatment, 1 was a review article, 8 were brief commentaries, and the remainder addressed lower-extremity treatment. The information from these studies is presented in Table 20.3. One of the lower extremity studies [17] is included because of its relatively good design and the fact that it was the only comparative study demonstrating preferential favorable outcomes using this approach. One publication [14] reviewed 688 papers on this subject and only found 8 that met 4 fundamental criteria for consideration: (1) adults (18 years or older) diagnosed with a stroke; (2) use of the Bobath concept or neurodevelopmental therapy in isolation; that is, outcomes for upper extremity training that used the Bobath concept but without combining other treatments, such as PNF, or motor learning; (3) a control for Bobath training using either a "no intervention" control group or a comparison intervention,

Table 20.3 Stroke outcome and the Bobath approach

Study	Intervention	Intensity	Outcome
Basmajian et al. [63]	Bobath or EMG biofeedback (N=29)	5 weeks	Upper extremity function test; No differences
Partridge et al. [64]	Bobath or cryotherapy (N=65)	4 weeks	Shoulder pain rating; Less pain with NDT
Nakayama et al. [65]	"Bobath" technique with outcomes assessed by Scandinavian Stroke Severity Scale (N=636 acute)	69–74 hospital days with no defined treatment duration or frequency	Discharged: 64/115=no use and subsequently: 26/64=compensate Xlat UE 10/64=full function 28/64=partial
Lincoln et al. [16]	Typical British approach (N=282)	Routine PT (standard Bobath treatment, 5 d/wk, 30–45 min) Qualified PT (standard PT + 2 h/wk senior research PT) Assistant PT (standard treatment given by PTA + 2 h/wk Bobath); each treatment option given for 5 weeks	Barthel Index, Rivermead Motor Assessment; No differences between groups
Van der Lee et al. [66]	Bobath or forced use	2 weeks 5 d/wk	More improved in Action Research Arm Test (forced use); less pain (Bobath)
Langhammer and Stanghelle [67]	Motor relearning program or Bobath (N=61) stratified into equal groups by gender and lesion site	At least 40 min, 5 d/wk throughout hospitalization (21–34 days)	Motor Assessment Scale Barthel Index; Both groups improved but motor relearning group significantly more
Luke [14]	8/688 studies reviewed	30–45 min, 5 d/wk in 7/8 studies; amount of therapist experience varied across studies	Reduce shoulder pain but no difference compared to functional training
Platz et al. [68]	No augmented treatment time; Augmented with Bobath; Augmented with Arm BASIS, systematic repetition training (N=62 severely impaired)	20 additional sessions per group; 45 min over 4 weeks	No overall between-group differences in Fugl-Meyer Assessment scores but BASIS training superior to Bobath in Fugl-Meyer change score
Wang et al. [17]	Bobath program or orthopedic treatment (N=21 stroke with spasticity; N=23 relative recovery stage)	20 treatments, 40 min, 5 d/wk	Motor Assessment Scale and Stroke Impact Scale improved more in both groups with Bobath treatment
Hofsteinsdottir [69]	Bobath versus task-oriented training (N=324), 1 year post-stroke	Not specified	Bobath treatment had no effect upon shoulder pain or health-related quality of life
Van Vliet et al. [70]	Bobath-based vs. movement science-based (N=120) 2 wks post stroke	As long as needed but matched between groups	Motor Assessment Scale; 10-hole peg test; muscle tone; sensation; No difference between groups through 6-month follow-up

or a baseline phase; and (4) an outcome that reflected change in upper limb impairment, activity limitation or participation restriction. Many of these studies can be categorized by provision of treatments that spanned 4–5 weeks, but the actual dosage varied considerably (Table 20.3). Most outcomes described in that publication [14] were either not favorable or equivocal.

A closer examination of intensity: contemporary approaches

A PubMed search that cross-referenced the terms "stroke," "upper extremity," and "intensity of treatment," without specifying the nature of the intervention, yielded 79 articles, 14 of which specifically addressed intensity of training and 10 of which specified constraint-induced movement therapy (CIMT) as the intervention. Inevitably, if more specific or alternative terms had been chosen, undoubtedly many more articles would appear. Of the 14, 2 [5,18] provide critical reviews of published studies to date, and one [19] was a critique of the Kwakkel et al. 1999 study [20]. Two points of view by Dobkin [4] and Wolf et al. [5] discussed recent clinical trials on ambulation in the Spinal Cord Injury Locomotor Trial (SCILT) and in the Extremity Constraint Induced Therapy Evaluation (EXCITE Trial). While not included in Table 20.4, both papers noted a pervasive shortcoming in the rehabilitation literature including clinical trial studies, and poorly defined characterization of intensity of training.

The studies depicted in Table 20.4 are more contemporary than many of the neuromuscular re-education studies that have preceded them, and are characteristically defined by novel treatment techniques, several of which engage new technologies. While the issue of delineating and condensing intensity can still be seen as elusive, several interesting patterns have emerged. The outstanding studies and analyses by the Kwakkel group [5,20,21] have exposed issues related to variability in stroke patient attributes and poorly defined control over blinding. Langhorne [19] noted that differences in outcomes and a failure to observe persistence of improvements in the long term may be attributable to heterogeneity of study groups that are not appropriately counterbalanced, thus permitting improvement in controls over time. Efforts to compare treatments comprised of Bobath techniques with or without additional therapy [22] or by differentiating unimanual from bilateral training [23] still produce equivocal results and, for the first time, suggest that intensity per se may not be a determining factor in outcome, although this might be less true in the very early weeks after a stroke [3]. In fact, the emerging discussions now suggest a need to examine dosing more closely and, indeed, Morris et al. [23] quantified frequency of movements across tasks during training. In this context, the review by Van Peppen et al. [18] draws attention to the fact that focused task training studies yield greater effect sizes than those that are more oriented towards application of a technique.

Yet, beyond the review of traditional "hands on" interventions, introducing novel technologies, such as robotics and virtual environments (see also Chapter 18), offers hope for further improving upper-extremity outcomes in stroke rehabilitation. The numbers of comprehensive studies in these two areas are limited, but they share in common the very unique opportunity for participants to work without detailed instruction and to potentially better impose their own thought processes toward rendering solutions toward further movement control with prospects for functional restitution. Thus, while only representative of the emerging work in mental imagery as a rehabilitation technique, Liu et al. [24] found that their patients showed greater improvements in retention and transfer to relevant tasks than those patients undergoing functional training. They noted that mental imagery subjects were left to their own thoughts with minimal clinician intrusion in efforts to optimize their imaging. This same strategy has been employed by Steve Page and his colleagues in their use of mental imagery as a therapeutic technique [25,26] (see also Chapter 21).

Opportunities to more effectively exploit advances in robotics and virtual environments are plentiful. However, the articles represented herein point to the need for investigators to better stratify patients and more effectively link these interventions to changes in ability as well as impairment. Thus far, few studies have made much headway in this direction. Moreover, the novelty of these approaches creates a potential to thwart systematic examination of dosing in favor of the excitement ensconced in enthusiastic endorsement and engagement without thinking about patient fatigue or motoric capabilities, let alone cognitive acumen. In addition and perhaps more importantly, the field must move past the "feasibility" stage to one where these innovative therapies are shown to bring about better outcomes than those achieved through dose-matched standard methods.

Intensity revisited

In summary, it would appear that newer approaches offer chances for patients to become more directly involved in their upper extremity therapy. Comments within review articles [5,18] indicate that earlier and more intense, goal-directed interventions among less severely impaired stroke survivors produce better changes in impairment and ability. Interestingly, in 2000, the Heart and Stroke Foundation of Ontario supported the work of the Consensus Panel on Hemiplegic Arm and Hand, who undertook the difficult task of assembling and classifying all available literature

Table 20.4 Contemporary approaches addressing intensity

Study	Intervention	Intensity	Outcome
Kwakkel et al. [5]	Meta-analysis, 9 studies (1051 patients)	Small but significant intensity effect	Interpretation confounded by poor contrast to control group descriptions, inadequate blinding, patient heterogeneity
Kwakkel et al. [20]	Arm splint immobilization (N=37); Arm training (N=33); Leg training (N=31); 14 days post-stroke	Immobilization (30 min, 5 d/wk arm or leg (30 min, 5 d/wk, 20 wks)	Leg>Control (ADL ability, walking, dexterity) Arm>Control (dexterity Arm = Leg group; Specificity of training effect
Kwakkel et al. [21]	1 year follow-up to Kwakkel et al. [18]	Not applicable	No difference between treatment groups at one year
Langhorne [19]	Commentary on Kwakkel et al. [18]		Possibly due to continued improvement in control group; therefore earlier recovery that may not persist
Hesse et al. [71]	Robotic bilateral upper extremity training (N=12) > 6 months post-stroke	15 min, 5 d/wk, 3 weeks + 45 min, 5 d/wk NDT training	Short-term improvement in modified Ashworth for 8/12 participants
Rodgers et al. [21]	Stroke unit care + enhanced upper limb rehab (N=62) versus stroke unit care (N=61), 10 d post-stroke	30 min/d, 5 d/wk, 6 wks; enhanced therapy defined as additional home treatment at discharge	All treatment was Bobath-based. No differences in outcomes ARAT, Barthel, Nottingham) at 3 and 6 months. More treatment did not enhance outcomes
Van Peppen et al. [18]	Review 151 studies using PEDro criteria to assess impact of PT; assess effect sizes	Varied, more acute patients with more intense upper-extremity focused training showed greater effect sizes	Largest effect sizes for upper-extremity therapy for focused training including CI movement therapy; poor or no evidence for neuromuscular retraining approaches
Liu et al. [24]	Mental imagery (N=27) or functional retraining (N=22) Acute in-patients	15 sessions; 1 h/d, 3 wks	Fugl-Meyer and Color Trails Test; better retention and transfer to other tasks
MacClellan et al. [72]	Robotic training N=8 (moderate), N=19 (severe). No controls	18 sessions over 3 weeks (2 sessions/d, 1 h each, 3 d/wk)	Greater improvements seen in shoulder and hand motion severe>moderate; no change in disability
Gladstone et al. [73]	Double-blind stratified by severity 10 sessions PT with amphetamine (N=34) or placebo (N=37) administration 5–10 d post-stroke	2 d/wk, 5 wks using NDT principles	Fugl-Meyer and FIM no between-group differences in improvement by severity; trends toward improvement within the moderate group
Merians et al. [74]	Virtual environment training; Chronic stroke (N=8); mild to moderate impairment	13 days, 2–2.5 h/d	Baseline to 1 wk retention; significant changes in Jepsen Test for Hand Function and digit movements
Muller et al. [75]	Mental imagery of sequential hand movements (N=6), repetition of same movement as imaged (N=6), and conventional (Bobath and PNF) PT (N=5) 1 month post-stroke	3 weekly baselines; 4 wks training (5 d/wk, 30 min), 1 wk follow-up	Jepsen Hand Test with both imagery and repetition of movements superior to conventional PT
Morris et al. [23]	Bilateral (N=56) vs. unilateral (N=50) upper extremity retraining, 2–4 wks post-stroke	5 d/wk, 20 min/d, 6 wks ; numbers of tasks and frequency of repetitions specified	ARAT=no change at 6 weeks; but at 18 weeks bilateral group had improved less based upon pinch ARAT and 9 HPT scores; importance of dosing noted
Volpe et al. [76]	Upper extremity intensive robotic training (N=11) vs. intensive therapy (N=10) based on Bobath chronic stroke with moderate to severe (NIHSS)	Dose matched (1 h, 3 d/wk, 6 wks)	Comparable improvement in shoulder and elbow movement but no changes in disability

on upper-extremity rehabilitation of stroke survivors with the intent of developing predictive equations for the expected magnitude of functional restoration [27]. The assembled panel cleverly categorized all the data by intervention type and then applied the evidence to nine case scenarios of decreasing complexity (less impairment). As a result, the panel could produce a quantitative value, based upon the Chedoke–McMaster Stroke Assessment Scale, for expected return of shoulder, elbow, and wrist/hand function.

The results validated the same conclusions reached independently by Kwakkel [20] and later by van Peppen [18]. Fundamentally, the evidence suggested that the best functional restoration would be generated for patients with Chedoke–McMaster Assessment scores of ≥ 4, indicative of isolated movement out of flexion synergy. Moreover for patients who were severely impaired, provision of passive motion, maintaining joint alignment, and preventing shoulder subluxation would be the best use of available time and resources. A summary of these observations was published subsequently [27], and highlighted the fact that one important element, intensity of training, had not been studied sufficiently during the review of studies comprising the consensus report. Recently, The Canadian Stroke Network [28], one of the world's outstanding clinical and research stroke organizations, has provided a summary statement about stroke study priorities, based upon their 2003 consensus conference. Indeed, defining the ideal timing and intensity of rehabilitation after mild to moderate stroke is now one of the Network's top five priorities. Inevitably, the emphasis on mild to moderate stroke may well have been determined by the compilation of data, suggesting that these patients have the greatest potential to overcome impairments and to maximize function.

Yet, the elements that should constitute "intensity of practice" remain elusive. Previously, Wolf [29] discussed factors that can influence outcomes using CIMT and which, to date, had not been investigated. These factors included patient fatigue, family compliance, and socio-economic factors that can increasingly impede cooperation and optimization of treatment results. When one adds to these important considerations the fact that reimbursement for services continues to constrict and the factors contributing to decisions to pay for services are dictated by private and governmental agencies whose policies and procedures vary throughout the world, there is little wonder why defining intensity can be difficult. If, in fact,

non-clinical factors control rehabilitation treatment exposure, reaching any form of consensus on defining intensity becomes a most onerous task. These realities often make the inclusion of more clinically sound contributions to defining intensity, such as location of lesion, severity of impairment, and implementation of supportive evidence, more difficult. Last, clinician treatment biases, often driven by an educational environment that might have been provided by teachers resistant to processing supportive or contrary data, obstruct a desire to achieve rational boundaries to delineate intensity.

Providing a perspective

No matter the preferences for treatment approaches to reduce impairments and improve upper-extremity function among stroke survivors, several clinician behaviors have withstood the test of time. Inevitably, most health professionals, given the remarkable responsibility for improving the status of catastrophically injured individuals, have been motivated to do so because of their remarkable sense of compassion and their desire to work regularly and directly with patients, often independently from other healthcare providers. These individuals are usually physical and occupational therapists, who have enjoyed a tradition of "hands on" approaches to form the core of their treatment repertoires, often perceived as remarkably "unique" and self-defining. Historically, many of the neuromuscular re-education approaches (see above) do indeed require manual guidance with some form of repetition, often dictated and directed by the clinician. The number of trials and their consistency varies considerably across these various approaches, as does the form of feedback provided to patients. Many approaches have lacked true goal direction that includes strategies and decision-making within the context of a function. Rather, treatments have addressed single or multi-joint motions directed toward reducing tone or enhancing volitional movement, but often at the expense of incorporating the movement within a context that has limited function or relevance to the patient. In addition, the construct of the repetition varies, as does the nature of the feedback. Are movements repeated the same way and, if so, how often? Are they repeated within a session or over treatment sessions? When are they modified, and on what basis? Answers to these questions have often been intuitive to clinicians, but made without respect to a vast literature that indicates that varying the train-ing (blocked versus random trials), the nature and timing of the feedback, and the problem-solving based challenge to the patient can all have a profound effect upon learning and retention (see for example, references [30,31]).

We have often become so obsessed with the spe-cifics of treatment delivery that we may lose sight of functional goals. These specifics characterize many of the hands-on approaches inherent in traditional neuromuscular re-education techniques. However, the reality is that we have less time to spend with our stroke survivors and must, from necessity, adhere to findings for which there is definitive evidence for func-tional gains. Thus, at least among patients with mild–moderate (i.e. less than profoundly severe) impair-ments, the emerging evidence suggests earlier interventions that foster more goal-directed and con-centrated training yield more positive results, although this too might have a limit [3]. Such a reality cogni-tively engages patients as proactive participants in the rehabilitation process.

A model to depict this situation is shown in Figure 20.1. While patients with stroke are undeniably participatory during the provision of neuromuscular re-education techniques, such approach-based thera-pies often enlist the therapist as the driver for problem solving, with the patient participating secondarily as a problem solver. The major direction of such approaches has emphasized a reduction in impairment with some evidence for improved outcomes. Often the therapist becomes so immersed in applying techniques using appropriate psychomotor skills that patient responsiveness and appropriate feedback may be either delayed or totally lacking [32]. Clinicians often become very attentive to manual contact and to inter-pretation of tactile input so that integrating informa-tion from other sources as a basis for modifying instruction or patient behavior can be forsaken. For example, efforts to monitor electromyographic responses in the form of visual and auditory cueing (biofeedback signals) often resulted in the therapist actually ignoring this additional information because it compromised internal processing of tactile input [32]. Under such a circumstance, it seems unreasonable to expect that therapists can use these additional resources to foster patient-initiated problem-solving. Thus one must ask whether relying upon traditional

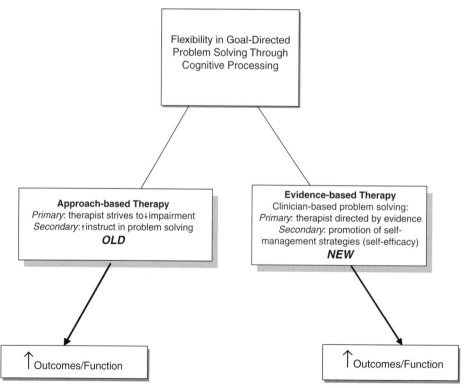

Figure 20.1 Conceptualization of how problem-solving aspects of upper-extremity rehabilitation post-stroke have changed from a more empirical therapist-driven approach toward more evidence-based, patient-driven approach.

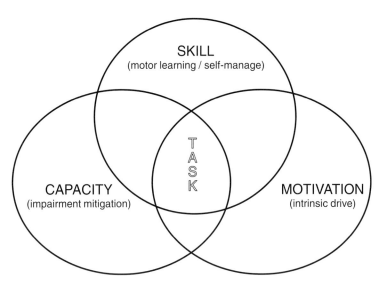

Figure 20.2 Conceptual model for the accelerated skill acquisition program (ASAP). The patient-selected task at the center provides the vehicle for the three elements. See text for details.

intrinsic (tactile) feedback or extrinsic (biofeedback equipment during manual contact) can optimize patient problem-solving. While outcomes might be improved (Figure 20.1, left), the magnitude and sustainability of such improvements can be justifiably questioned. Moreover, such customary approaches have failed to take into account the intensity of treatment as defined by any standard, and, historically, may never have been required to do so.

On the other hand, the newer movement toward incorporating evidence as a basis for treatment selection still requires the clinician to direct efforts toward problem-solving, but now permits the patient to play a more active role (Figure 20.1, right). Evidence-based treatment also bestows upon the stroke survivor the need to entertain not only seeking solutions towards improving function while minimizing compensatory behavior, but affords him/her the chance to initiate problem-solving. The result when this approach is undertaken through, for example, strength training or CIMT has been substantial improvement in functional restoration. Using CIMT as a model, data from the EXCITE Trial suggest that perhaps intensity defined as dosage over time may not be a key element to account for improvement [33], and that use of task-specific training can induce sustainable improvements [34]. Such a possibility raises the intriguing question about whether improvement might be driven more by the nature of the problem-solving as it relates to the defined functional goal, existing impairments, and patient comprehension, rather than the nature of the treatment itself.

Given the continuing reduction in available treatment time, the evidence-based approach noted here seems relevant, if not essential, for optimization of future rehabilitation outcomes. Its very nature requires promoting patient self-efficacy, which, upon contemplation, perhaps places "intensity" on a new plane. Here the patient becomes the problem-solver, and the process engenders a behavior that transcends the formalized treatment time. If, indeed, a patient incorporates elements of self-efficacy into most, if not all activities, then one can ask somewhat rhetorically, where does "intensity" of practice begin and end? This question can be examined in relation to a newly developed task-oriented training model for post-stroke upper extremity rehabilitation, called "Accelerated Skill Acquisition Program" (ASAP) [35]. ASAP may be the quintessential form of intensity training, whose dimensions transcend formalized training, and that embraces three essential ingredients.

The three major components embraced by ASAP are *skill* (motor learning and self-management); *capacity* (impairment mitigation); and *motivation* (intrinsic drive) within the context of task practice (Figure 20.2). Re-learning motor skills can favorably impact neural reorganization [36,37] while also encouraging self-directed post-training activities. Skill reacquisition is facilitated by improving impairments, such as muscle weakness, limitations in active range of motion, or low self-efficacy to enhance capacity. Attention to motor learning, motor control (e.g. goal-directed whole tasks with natural synergies [38]), and exercise physiology (e.g. overload in terms

Accelerated Skill Acquisition Program (ASAP)

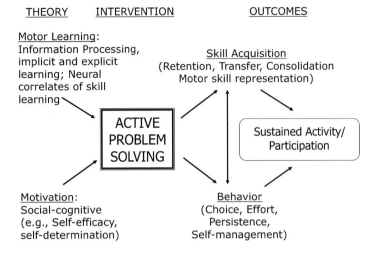

THEORY   INTERVENTION   OUTCOMES

Motor Learning:
Information Processing,
implicit and explicit
learning; Neural
correlates of skill
learning

Skill Acquisition
(Retention, Transfer, Consolidation
Motor skill representation)

ACTIVE PROBLEM SOLVING

Sustained Activity/
Participation

Motivation:
Social-cognitive
(e.g., Self-efficacy,
self-determination)

Behavior
(Choice, Effort,
Persistence,
Self-management)

Figure 20.3 Schematic showing putative elements at the theoretical, intervention, and outcome levels for the accelerated skill acquisition (ASAP) program.

of training load/intensity, speed) principles are also relevant to ASAP.

The scientific rationale and evidence for impairment mitigation (capacity) is derived from studies that have shown the importance of fundamental impairments including strength and control [39–47] to regain upper-extremity function. Moreover, contributions for enhancing motivation stress the importance of self-regulation, self-management, and self-efficacy to induce lasting behavioral changes known to support beneficial outcomes [48–53]. Motivational enhancements strengthen self-confidence and support patient control or autonomy (intrinsic motivation), thus reinforcing the important conceptual linkage between the capacity for intrinsic motivation and the development of self-efficacy. Many of the successes inherent in CIMT may build capacity and promote self-efficacy through repetitive performance or operant conditioning, but provide *extrinsic* rather than *intrinsic* motivation for affected limb use.

ASAP addresses social–cognitive psychological theories of motivation that have been applicable in motor learning/performance and clinical contexts [54–56] and are relevant here as an integrated model for immediate, and particularly longer-term, participant motivation. These theories assume that intrinsic sources of motivation, including perceptions of self-determination (choice, control, collaboration) and self-efficacy (confidence in one's capabilities) are key contributors of continued choice, effort, and persistence to use paretic limbs, which in turn leads to mitigation of disability and of self-imposed

participation restrictions (Figure 20.3). These concepts are reminiscent of the successful strategies used in falls prevention programs that combine balance training with development of self-efficacy for tasks (e.g. stairs, bathtub, curbs) that were initially perceived as unachievable, in large part because of low self-efficacy. Further engaging the patient in this process is the therapist–patient collaboration about the functional tasks that are important to the individual patient. In this context, the functional task (defined with metrics related to patient satisfaction, e.g. "I want to be able to carry a full plate of food using my affected arm and hand across the room approximately 10 meters, to my satisfaction and without spilling it") becomes the vehicle during practice to build capacity and improve capability.

Within a clinical context, ASAP can be thought of as a fully defined, evidence-based, hybrid combination of CIMT and skill-based/impairment-mitigating motor skill training with embedded motivational enhancements. ASAP with its constituent components is currently being tested within a national multisite clinical trial (clinicaltrials.gov ID # NCT00871715) to determine whether the collective ASAP package is superior to usual and customary care. As noted earlier, in the context of "intensity of training," ASAP offers a unique chance to view intensity in the more conventional manner of measuring time over which the training occurs or, alternatively, as a motivational tool that instills in stroke survivors the desire to practice skills well beyond this time domain through self-management and self-discovery as efforts to attempt task execution and solve new motor problems as they present in the absence of an awareness of time. In essence, this new model is designed to sustain the improved skills and capacity and thereby enable participation in meaningful activities (Figure 20.3).

Summary

There is little question that the concept of "intensity" of upper extremity re-training during recovery from stroke has assumed different perspectives among clinicians. Foremost is the fact that historically the relationship between dosing and outcomes has been poorly elucidated in the stroke rehabilitation literature, and often there has been a dependence upon persistent and prolonged delivery of several neuromuscular re-education techniques for which a paucity of evidence exists to support efficacy. As a result, a substantial effort is extended toward teaching stroke survivors compensatory behaviors that forsake the intrinsic possibilities to maximize functional restitution for the more impaired limb.

This situation has now been influenced substantially by cuts in length of hospital stay, outpatient services, and availability of fiscal resources. Accordingly, a more practical approach has emerged that builds upon the specific aspects of task-specific training that can include elements of strengthening, skill reacquisition, and self-efficacy. In fact, evidence is accruing to indicate that such a constellation of elements within the treatment "package" may be efficacious. Inevitably, allocation of time and resources will determine the extent to which a more contemporary approach must be embraced by clinicians and family members.

References

1. Kwakkel G. Impact of intensity of practice after stroke: Issues for consideration. *Disabil Rehabil.* 2006;**28**:823–30.

2. Richards L, Senesac C, McGuirk T, *et al.* Response to intensive upper extremity therapy by individuals with ataxia from stroke. *Top Stroke Rehabil.* 2008;**15**:262–71.

3. Dromerick AW, Lang CE, Birkenmeier RL, *et al.* Very Early Constraint-Induced Movement during Stroke Rehabilitation (VECTORS): A single-center RCT. *Neurology.* 2009;**73**:195–201.

4. Dobkin BH. Confounders in rehabilitation trials of task-oriented training: Lessons from the designs of the EXCITE and SCILT multicenter trials. *Neurorehabil Neural Repair.* 2007;**21**:3–13.

5. Wolf SL, Winstein CJ, Miller JP, *et al.* Looking in the rear view mirror when conversing with back seat

drivers: The EXCITE trial revisited. *Neurorehabil Neural Repair.* 2007;**21**:379–87.

6. Kwakkel G, Wagenaar RC, Koelman TW, *et al.* Effects of intensity of rehabilitation after stroke. A research synthesis. *Stroke.* 1997;**28**:1550–6.

7. Bobath B. *Adult hemiplegia: Evaluation and treatment.* 3rd ed. Oxford: Heinemann; 1990.

8. Bobath B. *Abnormal postural reflex activity caused by brain lesions.* 2nd ed. London: Heinemann; 1971.

9. Brunnstrom S. *Movement therapy in hemiplegia.* 1st ed. New York, NY: Harper & Row; 1970.

10. Voss DE, Ionta MK, Myers B. *Proprioceptive neuromuscular facilitation: Patterns and techniques.* 3rd ed. Philadelphia: Harper & Row; 1985.

11. Howle JM. *Neuro-developmental treatment approach: Theoretical foundations and principles of clinical practice.* 1st ed. Laguna Beach: The North American Neurodevelopmental Tretment Association; 2003.

12. Fugl-Meyer AR, Jaasko L, Leyman I, *et al.* The post-stroke hemiplegic patient. 1. A method for evaluation of physical performance. *Scand J Rehab Med.* 1975;**7**:13–31.

13. Feys H, De Weerdt W, Verbeke G, *et al.* Early and repetitive stimulation of the arm can substantially improve the long-term outcome after stroke: A 5-year follow-up study of a randomized trial. *Stroke.* 2004;**35**:924–9.

14. Luke C, Dodd KJ, Brock K. Outcomes of the Bobath concept on upper limb recovery following stroke. *Clin Rehabil.* 2004;**18**:888–98.

15. Dickstein R, Hocherman S, Pillar T, *et al.* Stroke rehabilitation. Three exercise therapy approaches. *Phys Ther.* 1986;**66**:1233–8.

16. Lincoln NB, Parry RH, Vass CD. Randomized, controlled trial to evaluate increased intensity of physiotherapy treatment of arm function after stroke. *Stroke.* 1999;**30**:573–9.

17. Wang RY, Chen HI, Chen CY, *et al.* Efficacy of Bobath versus orthopaedic approach on impairment and function at different motor recovery stages after stroke: A randomized controlled study. *Clin Rehabil.* 2005;**19**:155–64.

18. Van Peppen RP, Kwakkel G, Wood-Dauphinee S, *et al.* The impact of physical therapy on functional outcomes after stroke: What's the evidence? *Clin Rehabil.* 2004;**18**:833–62.

19. Langhorne P. Intensity of rehabilitation: Some answers and more questions? *J Neurol Neurosurg Psychiatry.* 2002;**72**:430–1.

20. Kwakkel G, Wagenaar RC, Twisk JW, *et al.* Intensity of leg and arm training after primary middle-cerebral-artery stroke: A randomised trial. *Lancet.* 1999;**354**:191–6.

21. Kwakkel G, Kollen BJ, Wagenaar RC. Long term effects of intensity of upper and lower limb training after stroke: A randomised trial. *J Neurol Neurosurg Psychiatry*. 2002;**72**:473–9.

22. Rodgers H, Mackintosh J, Price C, *et al.* Does an early increased-intensity interdisciplinary upper limb therapy programme following acute stroke improve outcome? *Clin Rehabil*. 2003;**17**:579–89.

23. Morris JH, van Wijck F, Joice S, *et al.* A comparison of bilateral and unilateral upper-limb task training in early poststroke rehabilitation: A randomized controlled trial. *Arch Phys Med Rehabil*. 2008;**89**:1237–45.

24. Liu KP, Chan CC, Lee TM, *et al.* Mental imagery for promoting relearning for people after stroke: A randomized controlled trial. *Arch Phys Med Rehabil*. 2004;**85**:1403–08.

25. Page SJ, Levine P, Leonard AC. Effects of mental practice on affected limb use and function in chronic stroke. *Arch Phys Med Rehabil*. 2005;**86**:399–402.

26. Page SJ, Levine P, Leonard A. Mental practice in chronic stroke: Results of a randomized, placebo-controlled trial. *Stroke*. 2007;**38**:1293–7.

27. Barreca S, Wolf SL, Fasoli S, *et al.* Treatment interventions for the paretic upper limb of stroke survivors: A critical review. *Neurorehabil Neural Repair*. 2003;**17**:220–6.

28. Bayley MT, Hurdowar A, Teasell R, *et al.* Priorities for stroke rehabilitation and research: Results of a 2003 Canadian Stroke Network consensus conference. *Arch Phys Med Rehabil*. 2007;**88**:526–8.

29. Wolf SL. Revisiting constraint-induced movement therapy: Are we too smitten with the mitten? Is all nonuse "learned"? and other quandaries. *Phys Ther*. 2007;**87**:1212–23.

30. Lee TD, Swanson LR, Hall AL. What is repeated in a repetition? Effects of practice conditions on motor skill acquisition. *Phys Ther*. 1991;**71**:150–6.

31. Schmidt RA, Lee TD. *Motor control and learning: A behavioral emphasis*. 4th ed. Champaign, IL: Human Kinetics; 2005.

32. Wolf SL, Edwards DI, Shutter LA. Concurrent assessment of muscle activity (CAMA). A procedural approach to assess treatment goals. *Phys Ther*. 1986;**66**:218–24.

33. Wolf SL, Newton H, Maddy D, *et al.* The Excite Trial: Relationship of intensity of constraint induced movement therapy to improvement in the Wolf motor function test. *Restor Neurol Neurosci*. 2007;**25**:549–62.

34. Wolf SL, Winstein CJ, Miller JP, *et al.* Retention of upper limb function in stroke survivors who have received constraint-induced movement therapy: The EXCITE randomised trial. *Lancet Neurol*. 2008;**7**:33–40.

35. Winstein C, Wolf SL. Task-oriented training to promote extremity recovery. In: Stein RLH, Macko RF, Winstein CJ, Zorowitz RD, editors. *Stroke recovery & rehabilitation*. New York, NY: Demos Medical; 2008: pp. 267–390.

36. Dobkin BH. Strategies for stroke rehabilitation. *Lancet Neurol*. 2004;**3**:528–36.

37. Nudo RJ, Plautz EJ, Frost SB. Role of adaptive plasticity in recovery of function after damage to motor cortex. *Muscle Nerve*. 2001;**24**:1000–19.

38. Wu C, Trombly CA, Lin K, *et al.* A kinematic study of contextual effects on reaching performance in persons with and without stroke: Influences of object availability. *Arch Phys Med Rehabil*. 2000;**81**:95–101.

39. Duncan P, Studenski S, Richards L, *et al.* Randomized clinical trial of therapeutic exercise in subacute stroke. *Stroke*. 2003;**34**:2173–80.

40. Platz T. Impairment-oriented training (IOT) – Scientific concept and evidence-based treatment strategies. *Restor Neurol Neurosci*. 2004;**22**:301–15.

41. Platz T, van Kaick S, Moller L, *et al.* Impairment-oriented training and adaptive motor cortex reorganisation after stroke: A fTMS study. *J Neurol*. 2005;**252**:1363–71.

42. Platz T, Winter T, Muller N, *et al.* Arm ability training for stroke and traumatic brain injury patients with mild arm paresis: A single-blind, randomized, controlled trial. *Arch Phys Med Rehabil*. 2001;**82**:961–8.

43. Winstein CJ, Rose DK, Tan SM, *et al.* A randomized controlled comparison of upper-extremity rehabilitation strategies in acute stroke: A pilot study of immediate and long-term outcomes. *Arch Phys Med Rehabil*. 2004;**85**:620–8.

44. Sunderland A, Tuke A. Neuroplasticity, learning and recovery after stroke: A critical evaluation of constraint-induced therapy. *Neuropsychol Rehabil*. 2005;**15**:81–96.

45. Winstein CJ, Wing AM, Whitall J. Motor control and learning principles for rehabilitation of upper limb movements after brain injury. In: Boller F, Grafman J, editors. *Handbook of neuropsychology*. 2nd ed. Amsterdam: Elsevier Science; 2003: pp. 77–137.

46. Patten C, Dozono J, Schmidt SG, *et al.* Combined functional task practice and dynamic high intensity resistance training promotes recovery of upper-extremity motor function in post-stroke hemiparesis: A case study. *J Neurol Phys Ther*. 2006;**30**:99–115.

47. Zackowski KM, Dromerick AW, Sahrmann SA, *et al.* How do strength, sensation, spasticity and joint individuation relate to the reaching deficits of people with chronic hemiparesis? *Brain*. 2004;**127**:1035–46.

48. Bandura A. Self-efficacy: Toward a unifying theory of behavioral change. *Psychol Rev*. 1977;**84**:191–215.

49. Bandura A. *Self-efficacy: The exercise of control*. New York, NY: Freeman; 1997.

50. Jones F. Strategies to enhance chronic disease self-management: How can we apply this to stroke? *Disabil Rehabil*. 2006;**28**:841–7.

51. Kendall E, Catalano T, Kuipers P, *et al.* Recovery following stroke: The role of self-management education. *Soc Sci Med*. 2007;**64**:735–46.

52. Williams GC, McGregor HA, Sharp D, *et al.* Testing a self-determination theory intervention for motivating tobacco cessation: Supporting autonomy and competence in a clinical trial. *Health Psychol*. 2006;**25**:91–101.

53. Williams GC, McGregor HA, Zeldman A, *et al.* Testing a self-determination theory process model for promoting glycemic control through diabetes self-management. *Health Psychol*. 2004;**23**:58–66.

54. Ewart CK, Stewart KJ, Gillilan RE, *et al.* Self-efficacy mediates strength gains during circuit weight training in men with coronary artery disease. *Med Sci Sports Exerc*. 1986;**18**:531–40.

55. Taylor CB, Bandura A, Ewart CK, *et al.* Exercise testing to enhance wives' confidence in their husbands' cardiac capability soon after clinically uncomplicated acute myocardial infarction. *Am J Cardiol*. 1985;**55**:635–8.

56. Sniehotta FF, Scholz U, Schwarzer R, *et al.* Long-term effects of two psychological interventions on physical exercise and self-regulation following coronary rehabilitation. *Int J Behav Med*. 2005;**12**:244–55.

57. Werner RA, Kessler S. Effectiveness of an intensive outpatient rehabilitation program for postacute stroke patients. *Am J Phys Med Rehabil*. 1996;**75**:114–20.

58. Chen G, Patten C, Kothari DH, *et al.* Gait differences between individuals with post-stroke hemiparesis and non-disabled controls at matched speeds. *Gait Posture*. 2005;**22**:51–6.

59. Hemmen B, Seelen HA. Effects of movement imagery and electromyography-triggered feedback on arm hand function in stroke patients in the subacute phase. *Clin Rehabil*. 2007;**21**:587–94.

60. Yavuzer G, Selles R, Sezer N, *et al.* Mirror therapy improves hand function in subacute stroke: A randomized controlled trial. *Arch Phys Med Rehabil*. 2008;**89**:393–8.

61. Quin CE. Observations on the effects of proprioceptive neuromuscular facilitation techniques in the treatment of hemiplegia. *Rheumatol Phys Med*. 1971;**11**:186–92.

62. Kraft GH, Fitts SS, Hammond MC. Techniques to improve function of the arm and hand in chronic hemiplegia. *Arch Phys Med Rehabil*. 1992;**73**:220–7.

63. Basmajian JV, Gowland CA, Finlayson MA, *et al.* Stroke treatment: Comparison of integrated behavioral–physical therapy vs. traditional physical therapy programs. *Arch Phys Med Rehabil*. 1987;**68**:267–72.

64. Partridge C, Edwards S, Mee R, *et al.* Hemiplegic shoulder pain: A study of two methods of physiotherapy treatment. *Clin Rehab*. 1990;**4**:43–9.

65. Nakayama H, Jorgensen HS, Raaschou HO, *et al.* Recovery of upper extremity function in stroke patients: The Copenhagen Stroke Study. *Arch Phys Med Rehabil*. 1994;**75**:394–8.

66. van der Lee JH, Wagenaar RC, Lankhorst GJ, *et al.* Forced use of the upper extremity in chronic stroke patients: Results from a single-blind randomized clinical trial. *Stroke*. 1999;**30**:2369–75.

67. Langhammer B, Stanghelle JK. Bobath or motor relearning programme? A comparison of two different approaches of physiotherapy in stroke rehabilitation: A randomized controlled study. *Clin Rehabil*. 2000;**14**:361–9.

68. Platz T, Eickhof C, van Kaick S, *et al.* Impairment-oriented training or Bobath therapy for severe arm paresis after stroke: A single-blind, multicentre randomized controlled trial. *Clin Rehabil*. 2005;**19**:714–24.

69. Hafsteinsdottir TB, Kappelle J, Grypdonck MH, *et al.* Effects of Bobath-based therapy on depression, shoulder pain and health-related quality of life in patients after stroke. *J Rehabil Med*. 2007;**39**:627–32.

70. van Vliet PM, Lincoln NB, Foxall A. Comparison of Bobath based and movement science based treatment for stroke: A randomised controlled trial. *J Neurol Neurosurg Psychiatry*. 2005;**76**:503–08.

71. Hesse S, Schmidt H, Werner C, *et al.* Upper and lower extremity robotic devices for rehabilitation and for studying motor control. *Curr Opin Neurol*. 2003;**16**:705–10.

72. Macclellan LR, Bradham DD, Whitall J, *et al.* Robotic upper-limb neurorehabilitation in chronic stroke patients. *J Rehabil Res Dev*. 2005;**42**:717–22.

73. Gladstone DJ, Danells CJ, Armesto A, *et al.* Physiotherapy coupled with dextroamphetamine for rehabilitation after hemiparetic stroke: A randomized, double-blind, placebo-controlled trial. *Stroke*. 2006;**37**:179–85.

74. Merians AS, Poizner H, Boian R, *et al.* Sensorimotor training in a virtual reality environment: Does it improve functional recovery poststroke? *Neurorehabil Neural Repair*. 2006;**20**:252–67.

75. Muller K, Butefisch CM, Seitz RJ, *et al.* Mental practice improves hand function after hemiparetic stroke. *Restor Neurol Neurosci*. 2007;**25**:501–11.

76. Volpe BT, Lynch D, Rykman-Berland A, *et al.* Intensive sensorimotor arm training mediated by therapist or robot improves hemiparesis in patients with chronic stroke. *Neurorehabil Neural Repair*. 2008;**22**:305–10.

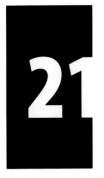

21 Cognitive approaches to stroke recovery

Valerie M. Pomeroy, Stephen J. Page & Megan Farrell

The international incidence of acquired brain injury (ABI) (e.g. stroke; traumatic brain injury) is several million new cases annually, and is not changing over time [1]. The efficacy and speed with which acutely based ABI care is delivered are also each increasing. Given these factors, and an increasingly aged and obese population, the prevalence of ABI survivors is expected to grow exponentially in the next decade.

Most ABI survivors exhibit psychological, social, motor, and/or cognitive sequelae [2,3]. Among these deficits, hemiparesis may be the most disabling, because it diminishes ability to perform valued activities of daily living (ADLs) (e.g. writing, feeding oneself, dressing). For example, following stroke, arm hemiparesis is the primary impairment underlying disability [4], is the most frequent impairment treated by therapists [5], and is a primary reason why stroke is the leading cause of disability. Upper limb hemiparesis in traumatic brain injury (TBI) can be similarly problematic [6].

Despite the increasing prevalence and devastating impact of ABI, conventional rehabilitative techniques targeting hemiparesis are incompletely effective [7] (see also Chapter 20), with several factors believed to be responsible. Most notably, skill is improved as a direct result of practice [8]; yet, most patients are receiving diminished focused practice time with therapists, less task-specific practice, and often spend substantial time doing little to nothing when they could be practicing [9–12]. With significant reduction in rehabilitation length of stay and outpatient services, therapists are also often forced to spend valuable therapy time focusing on compensatory strategies rather than restitution of function [13].

Besides the frequency of motor practice, the nature of motor practice provided during rehabilitation may also be suboptimal. Indeed, it is now believed that repeated, task-specific practice with the more affected limb induces cortical reorganization and correlative functional improvement. Due to the above factors, 30–50% of community-dwelling stroke survivors do not regain the ability to live independently; 10–30% are permanently disabled, and 20% require institutional care at 3 months post-onset [14]. Thus, a fundamental gap exists, centering on growing stroke incidence and prevalence, and the paucity of efficacious, easily implemented, non-invasive rehabilitative approaches.

A new age for ABI rehabilitative therapy?

Over the past 50 years, neurorehabilitative therapies have often focused on compensation using the unaffected arm (e.g. one-handed shoe tying; eating with the unaffected arm), rather than restitution of the affected arm. Studies have also reported learned non-use in humans and reliance on contralesional motor systems in primates [15]. Corresponding changes in brain structure or function resulting from these disuse patterns can sometimes be found. For example, following neurologic insult, individuals with certain symptomatologies (e.g. phantom limb pain, focal hand dystonia in musicians, hemiparesis) exhibit massive cortical reorganizations that largely explain their symptoms [16].

The good news is that the size of cortical representations of the affected limbs depends on the use of those limbs [17]. Consequently, the representations of anatomical regions can be modified through repeated, task-specific practice [18]. Jenkins and colleagues [19] similarly showed that repeated tapping training with the second, third, and fourth fingers caused expansion in the cortical representations corresponding to these areas, and correlative motor improvements. Karni and colleagues [20] similarly

Brain Repair After Stroke, ed. S. C. Cramer and R. J. Nudo. Published by Cambridge University Press.
© Cambridge University Press 2010.

reported enlargement in human primary motor cortices engaging in daily practice of several motor tasks, while Classen and colleagues [21] showed that even simple thumb movements repeated over a short period of time induce lasting cortical representational changes. Others have repeated this finding, using a number of practice scenarios [22–24]. Further summaries of the brain events underlying stroke recovery can be found in many of the other chapters in this book.

Recently, this knowledge has been harnessed to improve rehabilitative care after ABI. Specifically, when repetitive, task-specific, affected arm practice (RTP) is provided to hemiparetic patients, the size of the cortical areas representing that limb increase, and correlative functional changes can be seen [25–27]. A number of programs have taken advantage of this information to produce motor changes after stroke, with the most notable example being constraint-induced movement therapy (CIMT) [28–30]. CIMT emphasizes affected arm RTP by: (1) restricting participants' less-affected upper limbs during 90% of waking hours of a 2-week period; and (2) requiring subjects to engage in 6-h activity sessions using their more affected limbs on the 10 weekdays of the same 2-week period. Shaping (see [31] for a description) is also applied during the 6-h therapy sessions, in which the subject is verbally encouraged to perform progressively more difficult components of the movement.

Although CIMT efficacy was shown in a recently completed multicenter trial [32], the broader impact and feasibility have been questioned by some [33], as for some subjects its intensive parameters may be difficult to clinically implement and/or may encounter resistance or low adherence. Shorter CIMT versions have been developed with comparable efficacy [34–36], yet issues of intensive home and/or clinical practice still linger. To provide RTP, yet assuage CIMT contact time concerns, a variety of researchers have developed robotic (see Volpe and colleagues [37] for a review; also see Chapter 18) or other mechanized approaches to administering affected arm RTP [38–40]. Still others are attempting to facilitate RTP with implanted devices [41–43], or other machinery (see also Chapters 19 and 22).

Despite this explosion in the number and diversity of RTP approaches, some of the above regimens often require particular equipment to administer, can be intensive and/or taxing for the patient and therapist, and/or can be invasive. Many of the strategies and devices inherent in the above approaches are also costly for individual clinics or hospitals, and are not reimbursed by insurance plans, making them also implausible for individual patient purchase. Thus, there remains a need for easily implemented, inexpensive, non-invasive RTP approaches for hemiparesis, which indeed in some cases complement and enhance more invasive approaches.

Towards this goal, and given the difficulties associated with implementing current RTP therapies, this chapter examines the application of cognitively based approaches in ABI. This discussion has been purposefully limited to stroke, primarily because the greatest amount of literature and, thus, evidence, is available in this population. None the less, most of the findings reported herein are also applicable to other types of ABI, such as TBI and cerebral palsy.

Cognitive interventions – techniques and evidence

Active participation in stroke rehabilitation for motor recovery

Changes in connectivity of the central nervous system (CNS) after stroke disrupt the ability to perform motor tasks such as walking or writing. Consequently, many stroke survivors have to learn to perform previously learnt motor tasks or to learn new motor skills such as using an assistive device to enable walking [44]. In this chapter, motor learning is defined as "a change in the capability of a person to perform a skill that must be inferred from a relatively permanent improvement in performance as a result of practice or experience" [45]. The aim of motor learning after stroke therefore is that an improvement in ability to perform a motor task is retained after a period of training of that task [46]. The process of motor learning is generally described in terms of stages of learning. Several models exist, but all have in common the need for cognitive problem-solving ability in the early stages and for the ability to detect error and produce appropriate corrective adjustments in a variety of environment conditions in the later stages [45].

Rehabilitation of motor function is thus an active participatory process that is most effective when stroke survivors are engaged in activities that are functional, challenging, and meaningful. Hence, interventions designed to enhance motor recovery are not, and cannot, be delivered in the absence of consideration of stroke survivors' attention capacity, communication ability, problem-solving ability, and priorities for recovery. Two examples of important cognitive processes are working memory and attention. Working memory within the domain of executive functions is important for modifying a motor plan in response to the specific requirements of subsequent performance of the task in different environmental contexts [47]. Attention is also important, and if this is disrupted then stroke survivors could have difficulty in having conscious awareness of stimuli, selecting relevant stimuli in the environment to direct desired activity, being able to undertake more than one activity at the same time, and/or concentrating on an activity over a period of time [48]. Indeed, in a group of people 3–24 months after stroke, improvements in motor function in response to repetitive upper limb pointing training were associated with cognitive function [49].

Interventions to enhance motor function should not, therefore, ignore cognitive impairments. A therapist is "in essence a designer of the learning situations" [50]. The learning situation which forms the focus of this chapter is that concerned with the restoration of motor control and function after stroke. Hence we will focus on motor learning and outline some cognitive interventions to provide alongside physical interventions for the purpose of enhancing motor learning after stroke.

Motor learning after stroke

Learning a motor task after stroke is influenced by a combination of ability to produce voluntary contraction of paretic muscle; ability to adapt force appropriately in groups of muscles to achieve the intended action; and by cognitive functions such as attention, memory and communication [48]. The process of motor learning after stroke can therefore be disrupted by lesions in several different brain areas and not just in those specifically associated with planning or execution of a motor task.

Many brain regions are often implicated in motor learning, including the prefrontal cortex, premotor cortex, primary motor cortex, parietal regions, occipital regions, basal ganglia, and cerebellum (reviewed by [47,51,52]). Not all of these are activated to the same level, with different neural substrates supporting different forms and stages of learning.

For implicit learning, the medial temporal lobe may be important [53] and discrete lesions in the basal ganglia may not be detrimental [54]. However, the basal ganglia may be involved in explicit learning of a

stimulus–response task [53]. Stages of motor learning may also be associated with different neural substrates. Investigation of healthy adults learning a novel sequence of pressing buttons with digits of the right hand found that during the early stages of learning, activation was mainly in superior parietal lobes bilaterally, ipsilateral middle frontal gyrus, and the left caudate nucleus [51]. In the later stages of learning, activation moved to the contralateral occipito-temporal cortex, contralateral superior frontal cortex, and bilateral parahippocampal region [51]. Within the basal ganglia activation moved from rostrodorsal (associative) regions to caudoventral (sensorimotor) regions of the putamen as healthy adults increased in motor skill [52]. These anatomical findings have implications for stroke, as specific lesion locations might disrupt particular aspects of motor learning.

Some specific experiments have investigated motor learning ability in well-characterized groups of stroke survivors. Findings from these investigations indicate that:

a. People at least 6 months after unilateral stroke with upper-limb hemiparesis ranging from severe to mild (Fugl-Meyer scores 19–66) who were able to understand the instructions and perform the task were able to use correction strategies similar to those used by healthy adults after one trial of perturbation by adding a resistance to movement if their cognitive and sensorimotor impairment was mild. Those with more severe impairments persisted in showing errors after three trials [47,55]. These findings support the clinical practice of considering sensorimotor function together with cognitive processes involved in motor memory and problem-solving ability.

b. Stroke survivors may be able to learn motor tasks implicitly [56], but this ability may not be present in all stroke survivors. After unilateral stroke, individuals with lesions in the sensorimotor area or sensorimotor output area were unable to demonstrate implicit learning of a key pressing sequence even after a period of extra practice [57]. In contrast, stroke survivors with unilateral cerebellar lesions did demonstrate implicit learning of a tracking task although this was only evident for spatial accuracy. Temporal accuracy was not learned [60]. In summary, aspects of implicit learning may be achievable depending on the site of the stroke lesion.

c. Individuals with unilateral stroke lesions in sensorimotor areas or sensorimotor output demonstrated learning of a motor task as assessed by a decrease in reaction time to the go signal when they were informed that there was a sequence to learn and given time to study it visually. This finding suggests that stroke survivors might need to be provided with explicit knowledge about the motor task to be learnt before beginning physical practice [57]. However, provision of explicit knowledge about the task to be learnt might not be beneficial in all situations. For example: explicit information adversely affected learning of a motor sequence task in stroke survivors with lesions in the MCA territory [59] and stroke survivors with basal ganglia lesions were able to decrease tracking error but did not benefit from explicit information [58]. Decisions about whether or not to provide explicit information about the motor task to be learnt therefore need to consider the site of the stroke lesion.

d. Stroke survivors with minimal residual paresis of the paretic upper limb, resulting in the majority of cases from basal ganglia lesions, were able to learn a 3D motor task and two precision tasks, but demonstrated a longer time to complete the tasks, more time to correct errors and higher variability in performance [61]. None of the stroke survivors had "rigidity, bradykinesia, dyskinesia, somatosensory impairment, perceptual, apraxic or other cognitive deficits," and therefore poorer performance than healthy adults probably resulted from motor paresis and/or reduced motor learning ability.

Implications for using motor learning strategies in stroke rehabilitation

The therapist needs to understand the cognitive abilities of an individual stroke survivor and also stage of learning. At the basic level there is a need to differentiate between motor deficits resulting from motor execution deficits and from motor learning deficits. By so doing, the intervention session can be structured around an individual's motor needs and cognitive abilities [48]. For example, a therapist may have to use different communication strategies including chunking information, physical demonstration/guidance, visual feedback and checking for understanding to enable stroke survivors to problem-solve for themselves (reviewed by [62]). Opportunity to practice is also

important; specifically, the opportunity to practice variants of the task in different environmental contexts. There are several distinct strategies to enhance motor learning and thus recovery after stroke. The remainder of this chapter describes some of these strategies. It needs to be appreciated that it is likely that there is not a one-size-fits-all approach and that assessment of what strategies to use will need to be undertaken, which might include site of brain lesion and specific testing of physical and cognitive abilities.

Cognitive strategies to enhance motor learning after stroke

Therapists use physical interventions to enhance motor recovery after stroke, such as muscle strength training and weight transfer training. Delivery of such physical interventions needs to consider not just the ability of individuals to produce appropriate temporal–spatial activation of voluntary muscle contraction for a motor task, but also whether or not cognitive impairments are present that may have a detrimental effect on motor learning. Therapists therefore need to be able to adapt the mode of delivery of physical interventions to maximize stroke survivors' ability for motor learning. There are a variety of cognitive strategies available for use, and for ease of description these can be loosely grouped into those designed to enhance instruction, practice, and feedback. In practice, of course, the strategies outlined below are not used exclusively within these groups.

Providing information and/or instruction

Providing information and or instruction is important especially during the early stages of learning [48]. Information/instruction can be provided verbally, via auditory stimulus (rhythm), and by action observation (demonstration).

Verbal

Verbal information and instructions need to be tailored to stroke survivors' ability to attend to pertinent information, to retain information, and to communicate. This could mean:

- curtailing the number of instructions if attention span and/or working are affected adversely;
- directing verbal instructions towards aspects of the task pertinent for improved performance [45]. For example, attention might be directed to the intended effect of a task such as grasping a cup or

to the performance of the task such as moving smoothly;

- directing verbal instruction towards a feature of the environment with the aim of distracting conscious attention from motor performance. An example of this strategy is asking an individual to bounce a ball whilst standing up when the aim is to enhance balance ability;

- using verbal instruction to focus an individual onto specific aspects of the environment and thus enhance selective attention.

Whatever the focus of verbal instruction, in the presence of cognitive impairment, enhanced communication strategies need to be used. Enhanced communication strategies could include: chunking information into small bits, repeating information, checking for understanding, writing/drawing, facial expression, gesture, and demonstration (see below). Such enhanced communication strategies have been found to be beneficial especially for people with aphasia after stroke. See Cherney *et al.* [63] for a fuller discussion.

Auditory stimulus

When the motor task to be learnt has an inherent rhythmic component, then auditory cues to emphasis the rhythm are beneficial [45]. Several studies have found benefits for using rhythmic auditory stimuli to augment retraining of lower limb motor function after stroke. Benefits have been found for temporal–spatial gait parameters [64,65], walking speed [64,65], and balance during movement.

Benefits have also been found on spatial–temporal control of sequential reaching movements of the paretic upper limb after stroke. Improvements were found for variability of timing, variability of reaching trajectories, increases in elbow range of motion, and increases in smoothness of movement [66]. Lessons from contextual interference apply in this regard, with random practice being more effective than blocked practice for motor learning after stroke [67].

Action observation

A systematic review has concluded that observation of another person's movement produces activation of the observer's neural network responsible for the planning and execution of the observed movement [68]. Even more important clinically is that this activation may also found in the muscles that would be used to produce the observed movement [68]. Essentially,

observation of motor sequences may be encoded in an effector-specific fashion, i.e. motor learning occurs and primes effector muscles for physical action [69]. This so-called mirror neuron system is not exclusive to motor function: "The same neural structures that are involved in processing and controlling executed actions, felt sensations and emotions are also active when the same actions, sensations and emotions are to be detected in others. It therefore appears that a whole range of different 'mirror matching mechanisms' may be present in our brains" [70].

In healthy adults observation enhances learning of what movements to make (reviewed by Mattar and Gribble [71]) and how to make them [71,72]. Furthermore, action observation has been found to encode a motor memory in the primary motor cortex of healthy adults [73] and in some cases actual physical practice may not always be necessary for implicit motor learning [74]. Demonstration of the motor task to be learnt may therefore be a beneficial strategy to include in the treatment of stroke survivors. Perhaps not unexpectedly, in older adults a combination of action observation and motor practice might produce the best effect [75]. Details by which therapy based on action observation is delivered must be carefully considered [76].

The position of the demonstrator may also be an important variable. First-person perspective appears to be superior. This was illustrated by a study which found that the best effect on learning a sequence of postures resulted from a video film showing the model from the rear, rather than from either (a) the front with ipsilateral posture, or (b) the front with contralateral posture (mirror effect) [77]. Other studies support this finding of better motor learning when observation occurs from a first-person perspective [78,79]. Of interest is that a first-person perspective was associated with a higher level of activity in brain sensorimotor areas than viewing from a third-person perspective [79].

Most studies investigating the effects of action observation have used video film or still pictures. However, this type of presentation of the posture or movement to be learnt may be less effective than viewing a live human hand, which has been found to produce higher activity in the primary motor cortex of healthy adults than watching the same action from the same perspective via a video film [78]. Indeed, receiving the stimulus via a human hand produces better effect than when the stimulus is a robotic hand

[80]. This is probably because observation of a movement performed by a robotic form does not activate neural networks that are involved in motor execution to the same extent as observation of a movement performed by another human [81].

There is as yet only a limited evidence base for the use of action observation with stroke survivors. Published preliminary studies provide proof-of-concept for using action observation of daily upper limb actions together with actual physical practice in people at least 6 months after stroke in terms of motor function [82] and encoding a motor memory in the primary motor cortex [83]. Current findings provide important information for the design of subsequent exploratory (Phase II) and definitive (Phase III) clinical trials. Therefore, at present there is insufficient evidence on which to change current clinical practice regarding therapist demonstration of the activity to be learned.

Motor imagery

Motor imagery (MI) has been defined as "a dynamic state during which a subject mentally simulates a given action" [84]. Imaging of a specific movement or functional task is undertaken in the first person, i.e. the individual imagines themselves actually doing the task in terms of how it feels rather than as an observer of themselves (third person or visual imagery). Most importantly, there is no command to perform an actual movement during MI.

There is evidence for common neural mechanisms in MI and planning the execution of the same motor action [84–86]. Brain areas involved include: prefrontal cortex, inferior frontal gyrus, supplementary motor area, premotor area, anterior cingulate cortex, inferior parietal lobule, basal ganglia, caudate nucleus, and the cerebellum. Primary motor cortex is activated but to a lesser extent than during executed action [84,87,88] with the level of activation possibly influenced by characteristics of the motor task being imagined [86]. Lateralization of MI ability after stroke may be important in this context [89], and lesions in the left parietal lobe could affect ability to perform mental imagery [90]. Decety highlights that MI processing is closely related to the network activation during directed attention but does not overlap completely [84]. Moreover, MI has been found to increase EMG activity in target muscles in the absence of actual movement (reviewed by Jeannerod [91]) and increase cardiac and respiratory activity (reviewed by Decety [84] and Jeannerod [91]). The central effects of MI thus prepare for the energy needs to execute the imagined action.

Because the same neural and muscular structures are activated during MI as physical practice, MI may be a useful means of accessing the motor network in the presence of paresis, and improving outcome after stroke [92]. Consistently, there is evidence that MI is beneficial for learning a motor skill and for increasing force production in target muscles [84,91]. Below, we review selected studies showing MI efficacy after ABI. Specifically, we highlight MI efficacy in stroke, as the largest number of studies with MI have been performed in this group. However, MI is also likely to improve performance in other ABI diagnoses.

Motor imagery efficacy for the affected arm in stroke

Motor imagery reduces affected arm impairment: a pilot study [93]

We initially provided 8 chronic stroke patients with right-arm hemiparesis a 4-week program combining MI and RTP (Group 1), while 8 controls received exposure to stroke information + RTP (Group 2). At the pretesting period (PRE), mean scores of Group 1 and Group 2 on the upper extremity section of the Fugl-Meyer Assessment (FM), a stroke-specific impairment measure, were nearly identical. However, after treatment (POST), scores indicated that MI + RTP patients exhibited significantly greater reductions in impairment than patients in Group 2 ($F[1,14]=14.71$; $p<.05$). A case report was concordant with these findings [94].

Motor imagery improves reaching kinematics [95]

We also showed that MI + RTP use improves the kinematics with which the affected arm performs a reaching task. In other words, not only did MI improve function, but the quality and efficiency with which patients performed a functional activity improved.

Before and after MI + RTP, five chronic stroke patients (3 males; mean age= 52.6±15.4 years, age range 38–76 years; mean time since stroke=51.2 months, range 13–126 months) were instrumented with 15 retro reflective markers placed bilaterally. Subjects were seated at an adjustable chair and feet positioned flat. They then randomly performed two different reaching tasks: reach out and reach up. Both tasks consisted of reaching a plastic cylinder (5 cm diameter; 17 cm high) positioned in line with the olecranon and at a height of either the olecranon (reach out) or the acromioclavicular joint (reach up). Before MI + RTP, mean horizontal reaching distance was 8.3±1.7 cm and 10.9±2.2 cm for the reach up and reach out tasks, respectively. After intervention, ability to reach up significantly improved to 9.9±1.6 cm ($P<0.001$); horizontal reach distance improved non-significantly during the reach out task (11.7±2.2 cm, $P=0.366$). Subjects exhibited marked, nonsignificant increases in linear hand velocity (reach out: pre 20.5±3.4 cm/s, post 27.3±4.8 cm/s, $P=0.068$; reach up: pre 19.3±3.9 cm/s, post 26.1±3.8 cm/s, $P=0.072$) by 7 cm/s (approximately 35%).

A randomized, placebo-controlled study of MI in chronic stroke [96]

The above studies culminated in a recently completed clinical trial. Using a multiple baseline design, all subjects ($n=32$) were administered the Fugl-Meyer (FM) and the Action Research Arm Test (ARAT) on two occasions. Patients were then randomly assigned to either (a) MI + RTP or (b) relaxation tape + RTP. No baseline group differences were found on any demographic variable or movement scale. Subjects receiving MI + RTP showed significantly greater reductions in affected arm impairment and functional limitation as compared to subjects randomized to relaxation tape + RTP (both at the $P<0.0001$ level). Functionally, patients receiving MI + RTP were able to perform valued activities that they had not performed in years, such as writing, and using a computer keyboard with the affected hand.

Other research groups have corroborated the finding that MI reduces affected arm impairment and increases movement in stroke patients [97,98].

Motor imagery use for affected leg retraining after stroke

As mentioned above, MI is especially useful in situations where physical practice may be difficult or unsafe. For example, walking is, perhaps, the primary goal after stroke. Indeed, Lord et al. [99] found that the ability to "get out and about" in the community was considered to be either essential or very important by 75% of stroke patients. Yet, practicing walking in one's hospital room or one's home is unwise for most patients, especially if they lack substantive care partner support. In such situations, MI may be a viable, safe method of practicing walking, since skills are cognitively rehearsed without actual, physical practice.

Spurred by the above findings, MI has been tested in small pilot studies targeting the stroke-affected leg. These studies included: (a) a case series [100] in which four chronic stroke subjects were administered MI in combination with exercises addressing gait impairments, and some gait training, all occurring 3 days/week for 6 weeks. Subjects exhibited increased gait velocity, stride length, and cadence, and a decrease in double support time; (b) a single case [101] who also received the above intervention. He also showed a 23% increase in gait velocity, and reduced double support time; (c) finally, a group [85] has suggested that M1 and the orbitofrontal cortex are implicated in motor skill relearning of the affected leg following mental practice. Note that, of relevance, one other study [94] has shown that MI participation increases serial response time to a task performed with the affected leg, while another [102] showed that subjects who incorporated MI with visual feedback exhibited better responses to a symmetrical weight-bearing training program compared to those who used visual feedback only.

Mechanisms during motor imagery

Although individuals do not physically move during MI, decades of research show that widespread muscular activations occur during MI as if the activity is being physically performed. Indeed, in one group's words, MI produces "an identical, minute innervation in localized muscles activated during the same overt movement" [103].

Evidence for this finding first came from Jacobsen [104], who reported activations in the biceps brachii of participants who were asked to visualize bending their right arms. More recent studies have confirmed Jacobsen's findings using electromyography (EMG) [105,106]. Moreover, the EMG force characteristics observed during MI are proportional to the force characteristics of the task imaged, and vegetative responses (e.g. heart rate, oxygen consumption) during MI covary with degrees of imagined effort on a particular task [107]. In other words, an imagined task that is physically more strenuous elicits greater physiologic responses than one that is less strenuous. A number of studies have also reported correlative neural activity during MI. Indeed, motor-evoked potentials, EEG activity, and increased cerebral blood flow to cortical areas that are used during physical performance of a particular task are all observed during MI [108,109].

Not all stroke survivors, or indeed healthy adults, are able to perform MI. It has been postulated that increasing age might be a factor, although the correlation between age and ability to perform MI as assessed by the Vividness of Movement Imagery Questionnaire is rather weak ($r = 0.31$, $p < 0.001$) [110]. Damage to the left parietal lobe might also affect ability to perform MI [90], and so this might constitute an additional factor limiting capacity to derive gains from MI. Whatever the mechanism, after stroke it is possible that a substantial proportion of stroke survivors may be unable to perform MI [86,111,112]. It is important therefore for both clinical practice and research to assess individuals for MI ability.

Time to perform a MI task is considered to be a useful means of assessing MI ability [86]. In healthy adults, MI and execution of the same movement takes essentially the same time [84,113,114]. In people with hemiplegia, this time relationship between imagined and executed movement is probably also present. Interestingly MI of action of the paretic limb has been found to take more time than for the non-paretic limb and to be consistent with Fitts Law of speed/accuracy trade off (reviewed by [84,91]). A specific form of assessment is to measure how long an individual takes to identify whether pictures of hands presented in different orientations are of a left or right hand. Such tasks have been found to be reliable [114] and are now being used in evaluative studies of the effects of MI in stroke survivors [111].

In clinical practice, MI is rarely provided on its own but is used as an adjunct to physical practice. This is reflected in evaluative studies to date, for example, (a) a combination of MI and physical practice and visual feedback of performance [102] and (b) MI, physical practice, a virtual reality system, and audio-visual feedback of performance [116]. Whatever combination of MI and physical practice is used, it is important to know what duration and intensity of MI to provide, and of what imagined motor tasks/movements. Meta-analysis of published reports of evaluative studies of MI is of limited value as there is heterogeneity in interventions [92]. Recently, Simmons and colleagues [111] identified, in consultation with stroke survivors, that the most appropriate daily dose was two 20-min periods separated by a 10-min rest. A standardized list of tasks (treatment schedule) was used for MI training and some benefits were found, although this was only an exploratory trial. This treatment schedule and daily dose required further evaluation.

Feedback

An important role for therapists is to provide feedback to enhance learning [45–62]. Two general types of feedback can be augmented. The first is *intrinsic* feedback, which consists of the sensorimotor information resulting from performing the motor task. The second is *extrinsic* feedback, which consists of *knowledge of the results* of the motor task and *knowledge of performance* of the motor task [45].

Intrinsic feedback

The theoretical rationale for providing intrinsic feedback is that enhancing the learner's conscious knowledge of physiological processes will facilitate ability to manipulate these and thus improve motor function [117]. The most common means to provide intrinsic feedback of physical performance is by using EMG biofeedback [117].

There has been much research interest in the effects of EMG biofeedback to improve motor function after stroke, but the number of high-quality clinical trials is limited. A systematic review of augmented feedback to enhance upper limb motor recovery of rehabilitation patients identified 11 trials of EMG biofeedback in stroke [118]. Only 3 of the 11 primary trials reported a positive result. Findings are limited, however, by poor methodological quality of some of the primary trials; for example, only two used both concealment of the order of random allocation and blinded assessment [118]. A subsequent systematic review, performed within the Cochrane Collaboration, found 13 randomized and quasi-randomized trials. Meta-analysis was limited, however, by the small sample sizes, lack of high methodological quality, and by the differences across the primary trials in outcome measures used [119]. This review concluded that there may be some benefits for:

- muscle strength (one trial, WMD 1.09, 95% CI 0.48–1.70);
- range of movement at the shoulder (one trial, SMD 0.88, 95% CI 0.07–1.70), but not at ankle, knee or wrist; and
- functional ability (two trials, SMD 0.69, 95% CI 0.15–1.23), but not for stride length or walking speed [119].

Overall, the current evidence base neither supports nor rejects the use of EMG biofeedback after stroke, although it is unclear whether published studies considered the important issue as to how "learning is specific to the sources of sensory feedback available during practice" [45]. Thus, future trials need to consider the potential for disruption to intrinsic feedback networks arising from specific stroke lesions which might inhibit response to augmented biofeedback [120].

A further consideration is that the trials included in these systematic reviews were focused on specific impairments. It has been argued that a focus on performance of functional tasks in their entirety would be a more appropriate focus for biofeedback therapy [121]. Such a focus involves mostly the use of extrinsic feedback.

Extrinsic feedback

Extrinsic feedback takes two forms of knowledge, one of results and one of performance. Feedback focused on enhancing knowledge of *results* concentrates on provision of information about how successful a motor action has been in achieving the desired goal. In contrast, feedback focused on enhancing knowledge of *performance* concentrates on provision of information about the quality of the movement used to achieve the goal, such as smoothness of the trajectory, joint range of movement, and whether compensatory movements were present in adjacent body segments. Comparisons of the two types of extrinsic feedback have found that:

- in a study of subjects with stroke, verbal feedback of knowledge of results of upper limb pointing movements to a target in front of the contralateral workspace of subjects improved precision of pointing at movement end, whereas verbal feedback of knowledge of performance improved movement speed and variability [49]; and
- improvement in the kinematics of a pointing movement occurred only in those stroke survivors provided with feedback focused on knowledge of performance [122].

These findings suggest that if the aim of therapy is to enhance recovery of normal movement patterns, then feedback of knowledge of performance may be the preferred strategy. However, if the aim of therapy is to enable stroke survivors to perform a functional task irrespective of the presence of compensatory movement patterns, then feedback to enhance knowledge of results may be the preferred approach. These suggestions have not yet been tested robustly [120].

The evidence for the clinical use of feedback of knowledge of results with stroke survivors is sparse. Indeed, a systematic review of the effects of augmented feedback on motor function of the paretic upper limb in rehabilitation patients found no primary trials [118]. More research is needed to investigate whether stroke survivors benefit from receiving feedback focused on knowledge of results [120].

A larger number of clinical trials have investigated the use of knowledge of performance modalities to enhance motor function after stroke. These have been included in systematic reviews [118,123,124]. However, these systematic reviews have been unable to make unequivocal recommendations as to whether or not providing knowledge of performance has a beneficial effect on motor recovery after stroke. Some primary trials report beneficial effects [118], but a key limitation to interpretation of the collated findings in systematic reviews has been limited methodological quality of these primary clinical trials, for example due to lack of use of concealment of group allocation and/or blinded assessment [118]. Although the results of meta-analyses are mostly equivocal [123,124], there are some small indications of probable benefit in laboratory environments for visual feedback (two trials, SMD −0.68, 95% CI −1.31 to −0.04) and concurrent visual and auditory feedback (two trials, WMD −4.02, 95% CI −5.99 to −2.04) [123]. No benefits on balance were found, however, when moving or walking [123,124]. Furthermore, differences between the experimental and control groups found at outcome were not present at follow-up of one month or more after the intervention [123].

Many questions remain unanswered about the effects of extrinsic feedback on motor recovery after stroke including the following [120].

- Is motor recovery enhanced more by feedback on (a) errors made (see also Chapter 18) or (b) elements of correct performance exhibited?
- Do stroke survivors gain more benefit from feedback after every trial or from a lower frequency of feedback?
- Does most benefit arise from providing feedback immediately after performance of the motor task or from providing feedback after a delay?
- Is there an interaction between type and frequency of feedback and stage of learning a motor task after stroke?

Conclusion

In this chapter, we have discussed evidence and promise of several promising cognitive techniques, including various forms of feedback, and the use of MI. Current evidence suggests that these techniques will one day hold a place in the rehabilitation milieu, given their easy administration, and high efficacy. Yet, there is still much work to do. Studies examining the window during which these techniques are most efficaciously administered, their optimal duration, and their optimal frequency and intensity are but a few of the questions that must be answered to assure their appropriate, cost-effective administration. Future authors must consider these questions, as well as the ways in which cognitive techniques can be co-administered with promising physical techniques, to continue to optimize rehabilitation after ABI.

References

1. Kleindorfer D, Broderick J, Khoury J, *et al*. The unchanging incidence and case-fatality of stroke in the 1990s: A population-based study. *Stroke*. 2006;**37**:2473–8.

2. Centers for Disease Control and Prevention, National Center for Injury Prevention and Control. *Traumatic brain injury in the United States: A report to Congress*. Atlanta: CDC; 1999.

3. American Heart Association. Stroke Statistics. [On-line]. Available from: http://www.americanheart. org/Heart_and_Stroke_A_Z_Guide/strokes.html; 2000.

4. Carr J, Shepherd R. *Neurological rehabilitation: Optimizing motor performance*. Oxford: Butterworth-Heineman; 1998.

5. Ottenbacher K. Cerebral vascular accident: Some characteristics of occupational therapy evaluation forms. *Am J Occ Ther*. 1980;**34**:268–71.

6. Wallen MA, Mackay S, Duff SM, *et al*. Upper-limb function in Australian children with traumatic brain injury: A controlled, prospective study. *Arch Phys Med Rehabil*. 2001;**82**:642–9.

7. Duncan PW. Synthesis of intervention trails to improve motor recovery following stroke. *Top Stroke Rehabil*. 1997;**3**:1–20.

8. Newell A., Rosenbloom PS. Mechanisms of skill acquisition and the law of practice. In Anderson JR, editor. *Cognitive skills and their acquisition*. Hilisdale, NJ: Erlbaum; 1981:1–55.

9. Keith RA, Cowell KS. Time use of stroke patients in three rehabilitation hospitals. *Soc Sci Med*. 1987;**24**:524–33.

10. Lincoln NB, Willis D, Phillips SA, *et al*. Comparison of rehabilitation practice on hospital wards for stroke patients. *Stroke* 1996;**27**:18–23.

11. Mackay F, Ada L, Heard R, *et al*. Stroke rehabilitation: Are highly structured units more conducive to physical activity than less structured units? *Arch Phys Med Rehabil*. 1996;**77**:1066–70.

12. Bernhardt J, Dewey H, Thrift A, *et al*. Inactive and alone: Physical activity within the first 14 days of acute stroke unit care. *Stroke*. 2004;**35**:1005–09.

13. Wolf SL. Approaches to facilitating movement control. *Top Stroke Rehabil*. 1997;**3**:v–vi.

14. Broderick JP. William M. Feinberg lecture: Stroke therapy in the year 2025: Burden, breakthroughs, and barriers to progress. *Stroke*. 2004;**35**:205–11.

15. Nudo R, Milliken GW. Reorganization of movement representations in primary cortex following focal ischemic infarcts in adult squirrel monkeys. *J Neurophysiol*. 1996;**75**:2144–9.

16. Elbert T, Flor H, Birbaumer N, *et al*. Extensive reorganization of the somatosensory cortex in adult humans after nervous system injury. *Neuroreport*. 1994;**5**:2593–7.

17. Nudo RJ, Wise BM, SiFuentes F, *et al*. Neural substrates for the effects of rehabilitative training on motor recovery following ischemic infarct. *Science*. 1996;**272**:1791–4.

18. Butefisch C, Hummeisheim H, Denzler P, *et al*. Repetitive training of isolated movements improves the outcome of motor rehabilitation of the centrally paretic hand. *J Neurol Sci*. 1995;**130**:59–68.

19. Jenkins WM, Merzenich MM, Ochs MT, *et al*. Functional reorganization of primary somatosensory cortex in adult owl squirrel monkeys after behaviorally controlled tactile stimulation. *J Physiol*. 1990;**63**:82–104.

20. Karni A, Meyer G, Jezzard P, *et al*. Functional MRI evidence for adult motor cortex plasticity during motor skill learning. *Nature*. 1995;**377**:155–8.

21. Classen J, Liepert J, Wise SP, *et al*. Rapid plasticity of human cortical movement representation induced by practice. *J Neurophysiol*. 1998;**79**:1117–23.

22. Liepert J, Terborg C, Weiller C. Motor plasticity induced by synchronized thumb and foot movements. *Exp Brain Res*. 1999;**125**:435–9.

23. Elbert T, Pantev C, Wienbruch C, *et al*. Increased cortical representation of the fingers of the left hand in string players. *Science*. 1995;**270**:305–07.

24. Sterr A, Müller MM, Elbert T, *et al*. Changed perceptions in Braille readers. *Nature*. 1998;**391**:134–5.

25. Dean CM, Shepherd RB. Task-related training improves performance of seated reaching tasks after stroke. A randomized controlled trial. *Stroke*. 1997;**28**:722–8.

26. Galea MP, Miller KJ, Kilbreath SL. Early task-related training enhances upper limb function following stroke. *Poster presented at the annual meeting of the Society for Neural Control of Movement*, Sevilla, Spain; 2001.

27. Smith GV, Silver KH, Goldberg AP, *et al*. "Task-oriented" exercise improves hamstring strength and spastic reflexes in chronic stroke patients. *Stroke*. 1999;**30**:2112–8.

28. Taub E, Miller NE, Novack TA, *et al*. Technique to improve chronic motor deficit after stroke. *Arch Phys Med Rehabil*. 1993;74:347–54.

29. Miltner W, Bauder H, Sommer M, *et al*. Effects of constraint-induced movement therapy on patients with chronic motor deficits after stroke: A replication. *Stroke*. 1999;30:586–92.

30. van der Lee JH, Wagenaar RC, Lankhorst GJ, *et al*. Forced use of the upper extremity in chronic stroke patients: Results from a single-blind randomized clinical trial. *Stroke*. 1999; 30:2369–75.

31. Taub E. Movement in nonhuman primates deprived of somatosensory feedback. In *Exercise and sports science reviews*. Santa Barbara, CA: Journal Publishing Affiliates; 1977: pp. 335–74.

32. Wolf SL, Winstein CJ, Miller JP, *et al*. Effect of constraint-induced movement therapy on upper extremity function 3 to 9 months after stroke: the EXCITE randomized clinical trial. *JAMA*. 2006;296:2095–104.

33. Siegert RJ, Lord S, Porter K. Constraint-induced movement therapy: Time for a little restraint? *Clin Rehabil*. 2004;18:110–4.

34. Sterr A, Elbert T, Berthold I, *et al*. Longer versus shorter daily constraint-induced movement therapy of chronic hemiparesis: An exploratory study. *Arch Phys Med Rehabil*. 2002;83:1374–7.

35. Pierce SR, Gallagher KG, Schaumburg SW, *et al*. Home forced use in an outpatient rehabilitation program for adults with hemiplegia: A pilot study. *Neurorehabil Neural Repair*. 2003;17:214–9.

36. Page SJ, Sisto S, Levine P, *et al*. Efficacy of modified constraint-induced therapy in chronic stroke: A single blinded randomized controlled trial. *Arch Phys Med Rehabil*. 2004;85:14–8.

37. Volpe BT, Ferraro M, Lynch D, *et al*. Robotics and other devices in the treatment of patients recovering from stroke. *Curr Neurol Neurosci Rep*. 2005;5:465–70.

38. Whitall J, McCombe Waller S, Silver KH, *et al*. Repetitive bilateral arm training with rhythmic auditory cueing improves motor function in chronic hemiparetic stroke. *Stroke*. 2000;31:2390–5.

39. Merians AS, Poizner H, Boian R, *et al*. Sensorimotor training in a virtual reality environment: Does it improve functional recovery poststroke? *Neurorehabil Neural Repair*. 2006;20:252–67.

40. Taub E, Lum PS, Hardin P, *et al*. AutoCITE: Automated delivery of CI therapy with reduced effort by therapists. *Stroke*. 2005;36:1301–04. Epub 2005 May 5.

41. Northstar Neuroscience, Inc. Safety and effectiveness of cortical stimulation in hemiparetic stroke patients. Northstar study code "Everest"; study # VO267.

42. Baker LL, Eberly V, Rakoski D, *et al*. CSM 2007 Poster Presentations: Preliminary experience with implanted microstimulators for management of post-stroke impairments. *J Neurol Phys Ther*. 2006;30:209–22.

43. Chae J, Hart R. Intramuscular hand neuroprosthesis for chronic stroke survivors. *Neurorehabil Neural Repair*. 2003;17:109–17.

44. Bakkes ES, Groenewald SJ, Hughes JR. The use of functional activities in therapy. *SA J Physiotherapy* 1996;52(2):33–36.

45. Magill RA. *Motor learning and control. Concept and applications*. 8th ed. New York, NY: McGraw-Hill; 2007.

46. Dobkin BH. Strategies for stroke rehabilitation. *Lancet Neurol*. 2004;3:528–36.

47. Dancause N, Ptito A, Levin MF. Error correction strategies for motor behaviour after unilateral brain damage: Short-term motor learning processes. *Neuropsychologia*. 2002;40:1313–23.

48. Hochstenbach J, Mulder T. Neuropsychology and the relearning of motor skills following stroke. *Int J Rehab Res*. 1999;22:11–9.

49. Cirstea VM, Ptito A, Levin MF. Feedback and cognition in arm motor skill reacquisition after stroke. *Stroke*. 2006;37:1237–42.

50. Mulder T. A process-orientated model of human behaviour: Toward a theory-based rehabilitation approach. *Phys Ther*. 1991;71:157–64.

51. Muller R-A, Kleinhans N, Pierce K, *et al*. Functional MRI of motor sequence acquisition: Effects of learning stage and performance. *Cogn Brain Res*. 2002;14:277–93.

52. Lehericy S, Benali H, Van de Moortele P-F, *et al*. Distinct basal ganglia territories are engaged in early and advanced motor sequence learning. *Proc Natl Acad Sci USA*. 2005;102:12 566–71.

53. Rose M, Haider H, Weiller C, *et al*. The role of medial temporal lobe structures in implicit learning: An event-related fMRI study. *Neuron*. 2002;36:1221–31.

54. Vakil E, Kahan S, Huberman M, *et al*. Motor and non-motor sequence learning in patients with basal ganglia lesions: The case of serial reaction time (SRT). *Neuropsychologia*. 2000;38:1–10.

55. Weeks DL, Aubin MP, Feldman AG, *et al*. One-trial adaptation of movement to changes in load. *J Neurophysiol*. 1996;75:60–74.

56. Pohl PS, McDowd JM, Filion DL, *et al*. Implicit learning of a perceptual-motor skill after stroke. *Phys Ther*. 2001;81:1780–90.

57. Boyd LA, Winstein CJ. Implicit motor-sequence learning in humans following unilateral stroke: The impact of practice and explicit knowledge. *Neurosci Lett*. 2001;298:65–9.

58. Boyd LA, Winstein CJ. Providing explicit information disrupts implicit motor learning after basal ganglia stroke. *Learning Memory*. 2004;**11**:388–96.

59. Boyd LA, Winstein CJ. Impact of explicit information on implicit motor-sequence learning following middle cerebral artery stroke. *Phys Ther*. 2003;**83**:976–89.

60. Boyd LA, Winstein CJ. Cerebellar stroke impairs temporal but not spatial accuracy during implicit motor learning. *Neurorehabil Neural Repair*. 2004;**18**:134–43.

61. Platz T, Denzler P, Kaden B, *et al*. Motor learning after recovery from hemipareis. *Neuro Neuropsychologia*. 1994;**32**:1209–23.

62. Gilmore PE, Spaulding SJ. Motor control and motor learning: Implications for treatment of individuals post stroke. *Phys Occup Ther Geriatrics*. 2001;**20**:1–15.

63. Cherney LR, Patterson JP, Raymer A, *et al*. Evidence-based systematic review: Effects of intensity of treatment and constraint-induced language therapy for individuals with stroke-induced aphasia. *J Speech Lang Hear Res*. 2008;**51**:1282–99.

64. Schauer M, Mauritz K-H. Musical motor feedback (MMF) in walking hemiparetic stroke patients: Randomised trials of gait improvement. *Clin Rehabil*. 2003;**17**:713–22.

65. Thaut MH, Leins AK, Rice RR, *et al*. Rhythmic auditory stimulation improves gait more than NDT/Bobath training in near ambulatory patients early poststroke: A single-blind, randomized trial. *Neurorehabil Neural Repair*. 2007;**21**:455–9.

66. Thaut MH, Kenyon GP, Hurt CP, *et al*. Kinematic optimization of spatiotemporal patterns in paretic arm training with stroke patients. *Neuropsychologia*. 2002;**40**:1073–81.

67. Hanlon RE. Motor learning following unilateral stroke. *Arch Phys Med Rehabil*. 1996;**77**:811–5.

68. Pomeroy VM, Clark CA, Miller JSG, *et al*. The potential for utilising the "mirror neurone system" to enhance recovery of the severely affected upper limb early after stroke. A review and hypothesis. *Neurorehabil Neural Repair*. 2005;**19**;4–13.

69. Heyes CM, Foster CL. Motor learning by observation: Evidence from a serial reaction task. *Q J Exp Psychol*. 2002;**55A**:593–607.

70. Gallese V. The roots of empathy: The shared manifold hypothesis and the neural basis of intersubjectivity. *Psychopathology*. 2003;**36**:171–80.

71. Mattar AAG, Gribble PL. Motor learning by observing. *Neuron*. 2005;**46**:153–60.

72. Osman M, Bird G, Heyes C. Action observation supports effector-dependent learning of finger movement sequences. *Exp Brain Res*. 2005;**165**:19–27.

73. Stefan K, Cohen LG, Duque J, *et al*. Formation of a motor memory by action observation. *J Neurosci*. 2005;**25**:9339–46.

74. Vinter A, Perruchet P. Implicit motor learning through observational training in adults and children. *Memory Cognition*. 2002;**30**:256–61.

75. Celnik P, Stefan K, Hummel F, *et al*. Encoding a motor memory in the older adult by action observation. *NeuroImage*. 2006;**29**:677–84.

76. Weeks DL, Anderson LP. The interaction of observational learning with overt practice: Effects on motor skill learning, *Acta Psychol*. 2000;**104**:259–71.

77. Ishikura T, Inomata K. Effects of angle of model-demonstration on learning of motor skill. *Percept Motor Skills*. 1995;**80**:651–8.

78. Jarvelainen J, Schurmann M, Avikainen S, *et al*. Stronger reactivity of the human primary motor cortex during observation of live rather than video motor acts. *NeuroReport*. 2001;**12**:3493–5.

79. Jackson PL, Meltzoff AN, Decety J. Neural circuits involved in imitation and perspective-taking. *NeuroImage*. 2006;**31**:429–39.

80. Press C, Bird G, Flach R, *et al*. Robotic movement elicits automatic imitation. *Cogn Brain Res*. 2005;**25**:632–40.

81. Kilner JM, Paulignan Y, Blakemore SJ. An interference effect of observed biological movement on action. *Curr. Biol*. 2003;**13**:522–5.

82. Ertelt D, Small S, Solodkin A, *et al*. Action observation has a positive impact on rehabilitation of motor deficits after stroke. *Neuroimage*. 2007;**36**:T164–73.

83. Celnik P, Webster B, Glasser DM, *et al*. Effects of action observation on physical training after stroke. *Stroke*. 2008;**39**:1814–20.

84. Decety J. The neurophysiological basis of motor imagery. *Behav Brain Res*. 1996;**77**:45–52.

85. Jackson PL, Lafleur MF, Malouin F, *et al*. Functional cerebral reorganization following motor sequence learning through mental practice with motor imagery. *NeuroImage*. 2003;**20**:1171–80.

86. De Vries S, Mulder T. Motor imagery and stroke rehabilitation: A critical discussion. *J Rehabil Med*. 2007;**39**:5–13.

87. Sharma N, Jones PS, Carpenter TA, *et al*. Mapping the involvement of BA 4a and 4p during motor imagery. *NeuroImage*. 2008;**41**:92–9.

88. Huda S, Rodriguez R, Lastra L, *et al*. Cortical activation during foot movements: II effect of movement rate and side. *NeuroReport*. 2008;**19**:1573–7.

89. Stinear CM, Fleming MK, Barber PA, *et al*. Lateralization of motor imagery following stroke. *Clin Neurophysiol*. 2007;**118**:1794–801.

90. Sirigu A, Duhamel JR, Cohen L, *et al.* The mental representation of hand movements after parietal cortex damage. *Science.* 1996;**273**:1564–8.

91. Jeannerod M. Mental imagery in the motor context. *Neuropsychologia.* 1995;**33**:1419–32.

92. Sharma N, Pomeroy VM, Baron J-C. Motor imagery. A backdoor to the motor system after stroke? *Stroke.* 2006;**37**:1941–52.

93. Page SJ. Imagery improves motor function in chronic stroke patients with hemiplegia: A pilot study. *Occup Ther J Res.* 2000;**20**:200–15.

94. Jackson PL, Doyon J, Richards CL, *et al.* The efficacy of combined physical and mental practice in the learning of a foot-sequence task after stroke: A case report. *Neurorehabil Neural Rep.* 2004;**18**:106–11.

95. Hewitt TE, Ford K, Levine P, *et al.* Reaching kinematics to measure motor changes after motor imagery in stroke. *Top Stroke Rehabil.* 2007;**14**:23–9.

96. Page SJ, Levine P, Leonard A. Motor imagery in chronic stroke: Results of a randomized, placebo controlled trial. *Stroke.* 2007;**38**:1293–7.

97. Crosbie JH, McDonough SM, Gilmore DH, *et al.* The adjunctive role of mental practice in the rehabilitation of the upper limb after hemiplegic stroke: A pilot study. *Clin Rehabil.* 2004;**18**:60–8.

98. Dijkerman HC, Letswaart M, Johnston M, *et al.* Does motor imagery training improve hand function in chronic stroke patients? A pilot study. *Clin Rehabil.* 2004;**18**:538–49.

99. Lord SE, McPherson K, McNaughton HK, *et al.* Community ambulation after stroke: How important and obtainable is it and what measures appear predictive? *Arch Phys Med Rehabil.* 2004;**85**:234–9.

100. Dunsky A, Dickstein R, Ariav C, *et al.* Motor imagery practice in gait rehabilitation of chronic post-stroke hemiparesis: Four case studies. *Int J Rehabil Res.* 2006;**29**:351–6.

101. Dickstein R, Dunsky A, Marcovitz E. Motor imagery for gait rehabilitation in post-stroke hemiparesis. *Phys Ther.* 2004;**84**:1167–77.

102. Yoo EY, Chung BI. The effect of visual feedback plus mental practice on symmetrical weight-bearing training in people with hemiparesis. *Clin Rehabil.* 2006;**20**:388–97.

103. Hale BD. The effects of internal and external imagery on muscular and ocular concomitants. *J Sport Psychol.* 1982;**4**:379–87.

104. Jacobsen E. Electrical measurement of neuromuscular states during mental activities: A note on mental activities concerning an amputated limb. *Am J Physiol.* 1931;**43**:122–5.

105. Bakker FC, Boscher M, Chung J. Changes in muscular activity while imagining weight lifting using stimulus response propositions. *J Sport Exerc Psychol.* 1996;**18**:313–24.

106. Livesay JR, Samras MR. Covert neuromuscular activity of the dominant forearm during visualization of a motor task. *Percept Motor Skills.* 1998;**86**:371–4.

107. Decety J, Jeannerod M, Germain M, *et al.* Vegetative response during imagined movement is proportional to mental effort. *Behav Brain Res.* 1991;**42**:1–5.

108. Izumi S, Findley T, Ikai T, *et al.* Facilitatory effect of thinking about movement on motor evoked potentials to transcranial magnetic stimulation of the brain. *Am J Phys Med Rehabil.* 1995;**74**:207–13.

109. Salford E, Ryding E, Rosen I, *et al.* Motor performance and motor ideation of arm movements after stroke: A SPECT rCBF study. In: *Proceedings of the World Confederation of Physical Therapy Congress:* Washington, DC; 1995: 793.

110. Mulder TH, Hochstenbach JBH, van Heuvelen MJG, *et al.* Motor imagery: The relation between age and imagery capacity. *Human Movt Sci.* 2007;**26**:203–11.

111. Simmons L, Sharma N, Baron J-C, *et al.* Motor imagery to enhance recovery after subcortical stroke: Who might benefit, daily dose and potential effects. *Neurorehabil Neural Repair.* 2008;**22**:458–67.

112. Malouin F, Richards CL, Durand A, *et al.* Clinical assessment of motor imagery ability after stroke. *Neurorehabil Neural Repair.* 2008;**22**:330–40.

113. Papaxanthis C, Schieppati M, Gentili R, *et al.* Imagined and actual arm movements have similar durations when performed under different conditions of direction and mass. *Exp Brain Res.* 2002;**143**:447–52.

114. Gentili R, Cahouet V, Ballay Y. Inertial properties of the arm are accurately predicted during motor imagery. *Behav Brain Res.* 2004;**155**:231–9.

115. Malouin F, Richards CL, Durand A, *et al.* Reliability of mental chronometry for assessing motor imagery ability after stroke. *Arch Phys Med Rehabil.* 2008;**89**:311–9.

116. Gaggioli A, Meneghini A, Morganti F, *et al.* A strategy for computer-assisted mental practice in stroke rehabilitation. *Neurorehabil Neural Repair.* 2006;**20**:503–07.

117. Glanz M, Klawansky S, Chalmers T. Biofeedback therapy in stroke rehabilitation: A review. *J R Soc Med.* 1997;**90**:33–9.

118. Van Dijk H, Jannink MJA, Hermens HJ. Effect of augmented feedback on motor function of the affected upper extremity in rehabilitation patients: A systematic review of randomized controlled trials. *J Rehabil Med.* 2005;**37**:202–11.

119. Woodford H, Price C. EMG biofeedback for the recovery of motor function after stroke. *Cochrane Database of Systematic Reviews* 2007. Issue 2. Art. No.: CD004585. DOI: 10.1002/14651858.CD004585.pub2.

120. van Vliet PM, Wulf G. Extrinsic feedback for motor learning after stroke: What is the evidence? *Disabil Rehabil.* 2006;**28**:831–40.

121. Huang H, Wolf SL, He J. Recent developments in biofeedback for neuromotor rehabilitation. *J NeuroEngng Rehabil.* 2006;**3**:11.

122. Cirstea MC, Levin MF. Improvement of arm movement patterns and endpoint control depends on type of feedback during practice in stroke survivors. *Neurorehabil Neural Repair.* 2007;**21**:398–411.

123. Barclay-Goddard R, Stevenson T, Poluha W, *et al.* Force platform feedback for standing balance training after stroke. *Cochrane Database of Systematic Reviews* 2004, Issue 4. Art. No.: CD004129. DOI: 10.1002/14651858. CD004129.pub2.

124. Van Peppen RPS, Kortsmit M, Lindeman E, *et al.* Effects of visual feedback therapy on postural control in bilateral standing after stroke: a systematic review. *J Rehabil Med.* 2006;**38**:3–9.

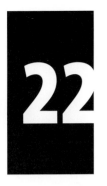

22 Electrical stimulation approaches to stroke recovery

John Chae & Leigh R. Hochberg

Electrical stimulation can modify the function of peripheral or central nervous system elements. Neuromuscular electrical stimulation (NMES) in stroke rehabilitation provides both therapeutic and functional benefits. NMES produces muscle contractions by directly exciting peripheral motor nerves or motor points. Therapeutic applications may lead to a specific effect that enhances, but does not directly provide, function. Specific NMES therapeutic applications reviewed in this chapter include post-stroke motor relearning and reduction of hemiplegic shoulder pain. The term *functional electrical stimulation* or FES refers to the use of NMES to directly accomplish functional tasks. Devices that provide FES are also referred to as *neuroprostheses*, and are also reviewed in this chapter. Specific "functional" or neuroprosthetic applications reviewed in this chapter include upper and lower limb motor movement for activities of daily living (ADL) and mobility, respectively. Finally, the fourth section of this chapter considers a range of emerging electrical stimulation techniques for promoting recovery and repair after stroke, some of which specifically target the central nervous system.

Motor relearning

Basic science and theoretical considerations

Motor relearning is defined as "the recovery of previously learned motor skills that have been lost following localized damage to the central nervous system" [1]. In non-human primate models, goal-oriented, active repetitive movement training of the paretic limb after local damage to the motor cortex shapes subsequent functional reorganization in the adjacent intact cortex, and the undamaged motor cortex plays an important role in motor relearning. Specific types of tasks that appear to induce long-term plasticity entail the development of

motor skills [2] (task features and effects on restoring movement are also considered in Chapters 18, 20, and 21). If goal-oriented repetitive movement therapy facilitates motor relearning via cortical mechanisms, NMES-mediated goal-oriented repetitive movement therapy may also facilitate motor relearning.

Spinal mechanisms may also have a role in motor relearning. Rushton theorized that the corticospinal–anterior horn cell synapse is a Hebb-type, modifiable synapse and that the synapse can be modified by NMES [3]. Under normal circumstances, neural activity in the pyramidal tract easily discharges the anterior horn cells and the strength of the presumed Hebb-type pyramidal tract/anterior horn cell synapse is maintained. However, following brain injury, the failure to restore this traffic leads to "decorrelation" of presynaptic and postsynaptic activity. Rushton suggested that NMES-mediated antidromic impulses provide an artificial means to resynchronize presynaptic and postsynaptic activity. Accordingly, he predicted that combining NMES with simultaneous voluntary effort is an effective means of facilitating motor relearning.

As many stroke survivors lack sufficient motor ability to take part in volitional, active repetitive movement therapy, NMES-mediated motor activation may have an important role in motor restoration following stroke. Regardless of cortical or spinal mechanisms, the experimental and theoretical considerations suggest that the necessary prerequisites for NMES-mediated motor relearning include high repetition, novelty of activity, concurrent volitional effort, and high functional content [2].

Three forms of NMES are available for motor relearning: cyclic NMES, EMG-mediated NMES, and neuroprostheses. Cyclic NMES-mediated activity is novel in that the stroke survivor has difficulty performing the task without the NMES; however, there is no volitional input and the task is not functionally relevant.

Brain Repair After Stroke, ed. S. C. Cramer and R. J. Nudo. Published by Cambridge University Press.

EMG-mediated NMES couples cognitive intent and NMES-mediated muscle contraction. This approach may be applied to patients who can partially activate a paretic muscle but are unable to generate sufficient muscle contraction for adequate exercise or functional purposes. Although this approach utilizes novel tasks and includes cognitive investment, the task itself is not functionally relevant. Neuroprosthetic applications provide FES for completion of ADL and mobility tasks. Because repetitive movement training is performed in the context of meaningful, functional behavioral tasks that are novel, neuroprostheses have a theoretical advantage over both cyclic and EMG-mediated NMES for motor relearning. Neuroprosthesis applications independent of therapeutic benefits are discussed in greater detail below.

Upper limb applications

Numerous randomized clinical trials (RCT) have evaluated the efficacy of cyclic and EMG-mediated NMES for upper limb motor relearning. The initial survey of these studies suggested that NMES is efficacious in reducing motor impairment but not activities limitation [4]. The authors suggested that the effect is more significant for those with milder impairments. A subsequent review by the same group concluded that EMG-mediated NMES may be more effective than cyclic NMES [5]. However, a more recent meta-analysis concluded that EMG-mediated NMES was no more efficacious than "usual care" in facilitating motor relearning [6]. However, they noted that most studies were with chronic stroke survivors and that results might be different among acute stroke survivors. Consistent with this conclusion, two small RCT failed to demonstrate the superiority of EMG-mediated NMES over cyclic NMES [7] or usual care [8] among chronic stroke survivors. While acute studies are ongoing, at present there is no persuasive evidence that cyclic and EMG-mediated NMES are efficacious in facilitating upper limb motor relearning among chronic stroke survivors.

There are considerably fewer data regarding the efficacy of neuroprostheses for motor relearning; nevertheless, emerging experience with acute stroke survivors is encouraging. Two recent RCT using a hybrid brace–NMES device that incorporates surface electrodes into a brace for hand grasp and release (Figure 22.1) demonstrated improvements in motor impairments [9,10]. A third RCT of multichannel NMES also resulted in significant improvement in upper limb motor function [11].

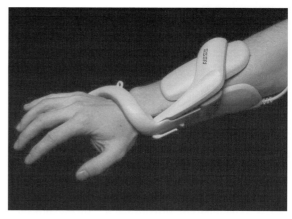

Figure 22.1 A hybrid brace–transcutaneous neuroprosthesis system (NESS H200) that is worn on the hand and forearm. The exoskeleton positions the wrist in a functional position and the five surface electrodes built into the exoskeleton stimulate specific muscles to provide coordinated hand opening and closing. (Courtesy of Bioness Inc., Valencia, CA.)

Several novel neuroprosthesis approaches with encouraging preliminary results are presently under investigation, including injectable microstimulators [12], contralaterally controlled surface FES [13], and the incorporation of work stations [14].

Lower limb applications

Lieberson and associates described the first single-channel surface peroneal nerve stimulator to provide ankle dorsiflexion assist during the swing phase of gait for stroke survivors [15]. However, they also commented, "On several occasions we observed, after training with the electrophysiologic brace [peroneal nerve stimulator] … patients acquire the ability of dorsiflexing the foot by themselves." Since then, numerous studies of single- or dual-channel stimulators have reported similar findings [16]. In a recent double-blinded RCT, Yan and associates reported that cyclic NMES reduces spasticity, strengthens ankle dorsiflexors, improves mobility, and increases home discharge rate after acute inpatient stroke rehabilitation [17]. Given the importance of functional content in motor relearning, gait training with peroneal nerve stimulation may have significant clinical impact [18].

Because gait deviation in hemiplegia is not limited to ankle dysfunction, several studies evaluated multichannel surface neuroprosthesis systems that additionally provide hip and knee control. A controlled trial demonstrated significantly greater improvement in gait performance and motor function among participants treated with the neuroprosthesis compared to those treated with conventional therapy [19]. Similarly, a single-blinded RCT demonstrated that a multichannel percutaneous NMES-mediated ambulation training improves gait components and knee flexion coordination relative to controls [20].

Motor relearning: summary and future directions

Although earlier studies suggested that cyclic and EMG-mediated NMES reduce motor impairment, more recent data, especially among chronic stroke survivors, raise considerable doubts regarding their therapeutic benefits, particularly for the upper extremity. They may be efficacious among acute stroke survivors, but there are insufficient data to confirm this. While the efficacy of cyclic and EMG-mediated NMES in facilitating motor relearning remains uncertain, the implementation of neuroprostheses will likely have significant clinical impact due to the higher functional content.

Future investigations on NMES for motor relearning should demonstrate impact on clinical outcomes at the level of activity limitation and quality of life. These studies should be large, multicenter RCT, which should be at least single-blinded. Studies should carefully define the subject populations, identify potential confounders, and evaluate long-term outcomes using valid and reliable measures of motor impairment, activity limitations, and quality of life. These trials should directly compare the various types of NMES to at least the standard of care to identify the most effective clinical paradigm and the populations that will likely benefit from each approach. Future studies should determine the optimal dose and prescriptive parameters. Systems that harness the natural command signals for limb movement, such as those generated from the primary motor cortex, should also be developed. Neuroprostheses that provide clear functional, cost-effective benefit to a broad range of stroke survivors should be developed to provide goal-oriented, repetitive movement therapy in the context of functional and meaningful tasks. Finally, studies should further investigate mechanisms in order to optimize the treatment paradigm.

Post-stroke shoulder pain

Theoretical considerations

Shoulder pain is a common complication following stroke [21]. The exact cause of shoulder pain remains uncertain. However, spasticity and weakness following stroke, which can lead to mechanical instability and immobility of the glenohumeral joint, may be important contributing factors [22]. These conditions may cause pain directly or place the capsule and extracapsular soft tissue at risk for micro and macro trauma, subsequently leading to inflammation or degenerative changes, immobility, and pain. Numerous treatment approaches have been reported, but with limited success [23]. However, the use of NMES of the muscles surrounding the shoulder to improve biomechanical integrity of the shoulder complex may be an effective strategy for reducing post-stroke shoulder pain.

Surface systems

A number of RCT of surface NMES for the treatment of post-stroke shoulder pain have been reported. Most studies stimulated the posterior deltoid and the supraspinatus to reduce glenohumeral subluxation. Participants were treated for 4–6 h daily for 4–6 weeks. Outcomes included extent of glenohumeral subluxation, pain-free lateral range of motion (ROM), and motor impairment. In general, stimulation parameters were adjusted iteratively by skilled personnel to help participants accommodate to the discomfort of surface stimulation and minimize the risk for muscle fatigue. Skilled personnel also placed the electrodes on motor points to maximize reliability of stimulation. The Cochrane Review concluded that NMES improves pain-free passive external rotation ROM and reduces subluxation, but does not improve shoulder pain or motor impairment [24]. A meta-analysis by Ada and Foongchomcheay concluded that surface NMES reduces or prevents subluxation and improves motor impairment in the subacute phase but not in the chronic phase [25]. Recent evidence-based reviews and practice guidelines now all recommend surface NMES for the prevention and treatment of post-stroke shoulder pain [26–28].

Intramuscular systems

Despite the evidence for therapeutic benefit, the clinical implementation of surface NMES for shoulder pain in hemiplegia has been difficult. The primary reason for this is the difficulty of use, which requires skilled personnel to ensure reliable and tolerable stimulation. This was predicted by Baker and Parker, the authors of the first RCT of surface NMES, when they concluded, "until implanted electrode systems become

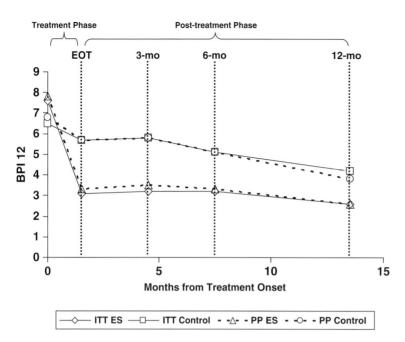

Figure 22.2 Results of a multicenter randomized clinical trial of percutaneous intramuscular electrical stimulation (ES) for the treatment of hemiplegic shoulder pain. Per-protocol (PP; dashed lines) and intent-to-treat (ITT; solid lines) approaches showed that percutaneous intramuscular ES significantly reduces hemiplegic shoulder pain (Brief Pain Inventory Question 12) for up to 12 months after completion of treatment compared to controls who were treated with a cuffed hemisling. (Reproduced with permission, from [32] Copyright © 2005 by Lippincott Williams and Wilkins.)

available ... long-term use of surface electrical stimulation can be managed by only a few patients with hemiparesis and their families" [29].

Two implanted NMES systems are under investigation: an injectable system with an external antenna, and a percutaneous system with an external stimulator. The injectable microstimulator is presently under investigation for various applications, including post-stroke shoulder dysfunction. Uncontrolled observational studies suggested feasibility and effectiveness in reducing glenohumeral subluxation and associated pain [30,31]. Preliminary controlled trials in support of commercialization are in their early stages. The stimulators are permanently implanted and, if shoulder pain recurs, additional treatments can be provided without an additional invasive procedure.

The percutaneous system includes helical intramuscular electrodes, a "pager" size stimulator, and a connector. Electrodes are placed in a minimally invasive procedure under local anesthesia. Electrodes traverse the skin and remain across the skin for the duration of treatment. After completion of treatment, the electrodes are removed by gentle traction. A multicenter RCT demonstrated clinically important pain reduction that is maintained for up to 12 months after completion of treatment (Figure 22.2) [32]. Post-hoc analysis revealed that stroke survivors treated within 18 months of stroke are most likely to experience treatment success [33]. This approach is undergoing

additional clinical studies in support of commercialization opportunities.

Post-stroke shoulder pain: summary and future directions

The preponderance of evidence suggests that surface NMES is effective in reducing post-stroke shoulder subluxation, increasing pain-free lateral rotation ROM, and facilitating motor recovery, especially for those in the acute phase of stroke. At present, it is unclear whether NMES renders any therapeutic benefit for those with shoulder pain in the absence of glenohumeral subluxation. Most surface NMES studies were conducted with the daily assistance of skilled personnel who ensured reliable and tolerable stimulation. While numerous evidence-based reviews and practice guidelines recommend surface NMES for post-stroke shoulder pain [26–28], clinical implementation has been limited, as the present healthcare environment cannot accommodate the necessary daily assistance of skilled personnel.

Additional studies are needed to address the various methodological limitations in order to more definitively address the question of clinical effectiveness. A large, multicenter, single-blinded RCT is needed that clearly defines the optimal subject population, identifies potential confounders, and evaluates long-term outcomes. The trial should be clinically relevant and focus on pain as the primary outcome, with activity limitations, societal participation, and quality of life as secondary outcomes. Motor impairment and biomechanical and physiological measures may be included for elucidation of mechanisms. Although surface NMES systems may ultimately prove effective, issues of pain during stimulation, compliance, reliability of stimulation, and need for skilled personnel may only be addressed by the intramuscular systems presently under investigation.

Neuroprostheses

The objective of a neuroprosthesis is the safe and efficient completion of functional tasks for those with more severe paralysis where motor relearning strategies are not amenable. Historically, neuroprostheses development focused on application to the spinal cord injury (SCI) population, including grasp and release function for persons with tetraplegia [34], and transfer and limited ambulation function for persons with paraplegia [35]. Given the success of neuroprostheses in the SCI population, it is reasonable to explore the feasibility of neuroprostheses in the stroke population.

Upper limb applications

Figure 22.3 shows the component of a typical implanted upper limb neuroprosthesis utilized by a person with C5 tetraplegia. The system provides functional lateral or palmar hand grasp by stimulating multiple forearm and hand muscles. The system is typically controlled by a position transducer mounted on the part of the body where control is retained.

However, other control sources, such as EMG activity and switches, may also be used. Systems may use surface or implanted components.

In 1973, Rebersek and Vodovnik published the first paper on the use of a hand neuroprosthesis in hemiplegia [36]. Surface NMES opened the hand, while closing was mediated by termination of the stimulation and subject's own volitional ability. Some participants demonstrated progressive improvements in the number of plugs and baskets they could manipulate with the device. In 1975, Merletti and associates evaluated a similar surface NMES device and demonstrated that participants were able to move small baskets or bottles from one defined area to another with the device [37]. However, the authors noted that performance of functional tasks required considerable amounts of mental concentration and in several cases increased voluntary effort was associated with tremors, spasticity, and erratic shoulder movement. Alon and associates tested the previously described hybrid NMES–orthosis neuroprosthesis and reported significant improvements in the completion of specific ADL tasks [38].

Due to the limitations of surface NMES, Merletti and associates suggested that an implanted system might be more efficacious [37]. Accordingly, Chae and Hart evaluated a percutaneous intramuscular system [39]. The system was able to open a spastic hemiparetic hand as long as the limb was in a resting position and participants did not try to assist the stimulation. However, when they tried to assist the stimulation, especially during functional tasks, hand opening was significantly reduced due to increased finger flexor hypertonia.

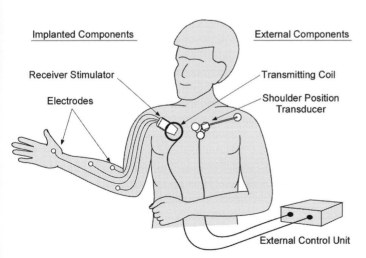

Implanted Components   External Components

Receiver Stimulator

Electrodes

Transmitting Coil

Shoulder Position Transducer

External Control Unit

Figure 22.3 An implanted 8-channel hand neuroprosthesis system for persons with C5 tetraplegia. (Courtesy, Cleveland Functional Electrical Stimulation Center.)

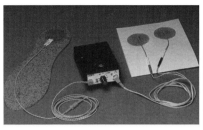
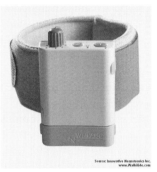
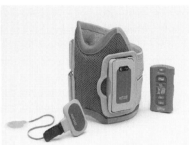

Figure 22.4 Three FDA-approved transcutaneous peroneal nerve stimulators. The Odstock Dropped Foot Stimulator (left-top; courtesy of the Department of Medical Physics and Biomedical Engineering, Salisbury District Hospital, Salisbury, UK) and the wireless L300 (left-bottom; courtesy of Bioness Inc., Valencia, CA) uses a heel switch to trigger ankle dorsiflexion. The WalkAide (right; courtesy of Innovative Neurotronics, Austin, TX) uses a tilt sensor to trigger ankle dorsiflexion.

Lower limb applications

In 1961, Lieberson and associates described a surface peroneal nerve stimulator that dorsiflexed the ankle during the swing phase of gait [15]. A systematic review of seven case series and one RCT since this initial study reported a 38% pooled improvement in walking speed with the device, relative to no device [40]. The authors concluded, "... review suggests a positive orthotic effect of functional electrical stimulation on walking speed" [40].

Despite demonstrated effectiveness, surface peroneal nerve stimulation is not routinely prescribed in the United States. Likely reasons include difficulty with electrode placement and the availability of custom-molded ankle–foot-orthoses (AFO). The United States Food and Drug Administration recently approved three surface peroneal nerve stimulators (Figure 22.4); two of these use electrodes embedded in a cuff, which may facilitate electrode placement. A recent study also demonstrated the comparability of the peroneal nerve stimulator to an AFO in improving hemiplegic gait [41]. These changes may facilitate broader clinical prescription and usage of these devices.

Some of the inherent limitations of surface peroneal nerve stimulation might be addressed by implantable systems. At present, two implantable peroneal nerve stimulators are available. A dual-channel device developed in the UK stimulates the deep and superficial peroneal nerves. A four-channel device, developed in Denmark, utilizes a nerve cuff with four tri-polar electrodes, oriented to activate different nerve fibers within the common peroneal nerve. Both devices have the CE mark in Europe but are not yet available in the US. Both systems demonstrated improvements in walking speed in two recent studies [42,43].

Neuroprostheses: summary and future directions

At present, a hand neuroprosthesis may allow stroke survivors to complete a limited number of selected functional tasks. However, a clinically viable system that provides broad functional benefit is not yet available. A viable system will allow stroke survivors to perform bilateral tasks or provide significant assistance to facilitate completion of tasks that are difficult to perform with only the unaffected limb. The system will be controlled with minimal effort to avoid triggering generalized hypertonia or "associated reactions." Finally, the system will "turn off" overactive muscles to address the problems of spasticity, associated reactions, co-activations, co-contractions, and delay in termination of muscle contractions.

In contrast to upper limb neuroprostheses, lower limb neuroprostheses are closer to clinical viability. Surface peroneal nerve stimulators are superior to no device in improving overall mobility, may be equivalent to an ankle–foot-orthosis, and are ready for clinical implementation. Implanted peroneal nerve stimulation devices are available in Europe and are likely to be equivalent to the surface devices with respect to function. They may be appropriate for those who experience significant improvement in mobility with the surface system but have difficulty with electrode placement, skin irritation, painful sensation of stimulation, or donning and doffing of the device.

Although the development of lower limb neuroprostheses for hemiplegia is further along than upper limb systems, several issues remain to be further elucidated. Studies must document clinical effectiveness with respect to mobility and quality of life and not just walking speed. Large RCTs that compare stimulation of peroneal nerves with standard of care, such as ankle–foot-orthosis, are needed to further demonstrate clinical relevance. For implanted systems, potential benefits over surface systems must be demonstrated given the added risks and costs associated with an invasive procedure. Finally, ambulation is a multijointed task. Future devices should explore multichannel devices that also control the knee and hip and not just the ankle.

Emerging techniques

As noted above, future development of neuroprostheses will need to incorporate control strategies that are near effortless and more intuitive. In addition, while neuroprostheses are effective in activating weak muscles, they do little in reducing unwanted motor activity such as spasticity, co-contractions, and associated reactions. Emergence of advanced techniques such as brain-controlled interfaces and high-frequency block may usher in a new era of promising opportunities for neuroprostheses.

Brain-controlled interfaces for neuroprostheses

The emerging field of brain–computer interfaces (BCI) is focused on developing technologies that will allow people with paralysis (from brainstem stroke, spinal cord injury, and neuromuscular disease) to use "brain signals" for control of external devices. There are a number of methods for recording cortical activity, including scalp-recorded electroencephalography, brain-surface recorded electrocorticography, and intracortically recorded neuronal ensemble activity

including local field potentials and the action potentials from single neurons [44]. Voluntary upper extremity movement is largely governed by the output from primary motor cortex and premotor cortex (see also Chapters 10 and 11), which are important generators of the movement signals that have been disconnected from their targets due to paralyzing disease or illness. Toward the development of a cortically controlled neuroprosthesis, there have been extensive studies in animals documenting the ability to not only "decode" the activity of ensembles of individual neurons in these and other cortical areas, but to allow monkeys to direct the movement of a computer cursor [45] or a robot arm [46] simply from the real-time decoded output of its motor cortex.

Following the demonstration of a unidirectional movement of a computer cursor controlled by the motor cortical activity of a gentleman with brainstem stroke [47], and the proofs-of-concept monkey studies, early clinical trials of an intracortically based neuroprosthesis, "BrainGate"*, were launched. These studies (see www.braingate2.org) have thus far demonstrated that a person with tetraplegia from SCI can control a computer cursor, open and close a prosthetic hand, and move a robotic arm, all from the neural activity recorded by a tiny microelectrode array implanted chronically into the motor cortex [48]. More recently, a person with brainstem stroke has used the same technology to gain point-and-click control over a cursor [49], and to use that neurally recorded activity for functionally useful tasks. The control of these external devices was achieved while the trial participants simply imagined the movement of their paralyzed limb.

As described above, it is hoped that the cortical activity generated during the intent or attempt to move a paralyzed limb can be converted into a powerful controller for implanted limb neuroprostheses. Recently there has been an initial preclinical demonstration of a motor cortex-controlled FES device. After monkeys were trained to play a video game with their hand (requiring only isometric flexion and extension), recording electrodes were placed in the motor cortex and stimulating electrodes were placed in the wrist muscles. Wrist movements were then temporarily paralyzed with a peripheral nerve block. A brain-to-FES system was then turned on, and the animals quickly learned to modulate motor cortical neurons for the direct activation of the wrist muscles, and they again successfully performed the video game [50].

Anticipated next steps in this research include the intracortical control of a "virtual arm" based on a realistic model of FES-enabled arm dynamics [51]. Work toward a fully implanted brain-to-FES system also progresses; such a system may serve both therapeutic and functional purposes in the future.

High-frequency block

Many stroke survivors exhibit significant spasticity, co-activation of synergistic muscles, co-contraction of antagonists, and delay in termination of motor activation after volitional activation. These manifestations limit the clinical utility of available neuroprostheses. While standard clinical approaches such as oral medications and chemoneurolysis may provide some symptom relief, side effects are common, the effect may be too global, or the nerve may be damaged; more importantly, these approaches do not provide rapid initiation and termination of tone reduction.

One innovative approach is high-frequency alternating current (HFAC) block of the peripheral nerve [52]. The mechanism of HFAC block remains uncertain, but there are several postulated mechanisms. Using a model of the unmyelinated axon based on the Hodgkin–Huxley equations, Zhang and associates [53] concluded that HFAC block was due to activation of potassium channels. Bhadra and associates [54] used a mammalian myelinated axon model and reported that during HFAC block, the axons showed a dynamic steady-state depolarization of multiple nodes, strongly suggesting a depolarization mechanism with opening of Na^+ channels. However, placing the nerve in a stronger depolarizing field actually resulted in conduction failure, because it forces the inactivation Na^+ gate to remain closed.

The block typically has three phases: an onset response; a period of asynchronous firing; and a steady state of complete or partial block [52]. Using frequencies between 10 and 30 kHz at amplitudes between 2 and 10 V, complete and reversible blocks can be obtained. The block is gradable and can be quickly reversed. Thus the approach can provide both a partial block, similar to that produced by botulinum toxin and phenol neurolysis, or the block can be complete. HFAC block may be combined with an intelligent control system that varies the block based on sensed activity. For example, overpowering flexor spasticity often prevents NMES-mediated hand opening among stroke survivors, especially after volitional closure or during functional use of the limb [39]. By monitoring the myoelectric signal of the flexor and extensor muscles, it may be possible to identify the intention of the patient and partially block the finger flexors while activating the finger extensors with electrical stimulation when hand opening is desired. A similar approach may be implemented in the lower limb, where equinovarus tone and extensor synergy patterns can lead to significant gait deviations and limit the clinical implementation of neuroprostheses. HFAC block is still in the animal trials phase, but human feasibility trials are anticipated in the next several years.

Electrical stimulation approaches to stroke recovery: conclusions

Recent advances in clinical medicine and biomedical engineering are making the clinical implementation of NMES systems to enhance the ADL and mobility of persons with hemiparesis more feasible. NMES for motor relearning in hemiplegia is a promising application of goal-oriented repetitive movement therapy. Multicenter clinical trials to confirm effectiveness and fundamental studies to elucidate mechanisms are still needed. Surface NMES for the treatment of shoulder subluxation and pain in hemiplegia has yielded encouraging results. While future large-scale multicenter clinical trials will likely confirm effectiveness, the more invasive approaches may prove to be most appropriate for clinical implementation. The development of the hand neuroprosthesis for stroke survivors is in its infancy and must await further technical and scientific developments. Similarly, multichannel, multijoint lower-limb neuroprostheses need further development. However, surface peroneal stimulators appear to be effective in improving hemiplegic gait and should be included in the clinical armamentarium. Still, if NMES is to have a major impact on the quality of life of stroke survivors, additional technological advances in the form of cortical control and real-time control of hypertonia will need to be integrated into emerging systems.

Acknowledgments

This work was supported in part by grants R01HD49777, R01HD044816, and K24HD054600 from the National Institute for Child Health and Human Development (JC) and the Office of Research and Development, Rehabilitation R&D Service, Department of Veterans Affairs; National Institute for Child Health and Human Development, National Center for Medical Rehabilitation Research; and the Doris Duke Charitable Foundation (LRH).

Conflict of interest

Dr. Chae serves as a consultant to NDI Medical, a medical device company with commercial interest in a device presented in this chapter.

Dr. Hochberg received clinical trial support from Cyberkinetics Neurotechnology Systems, Inc. Cyberkinetics has ceased operations.

*CAUTION: Investigational Device is limited by US Federal law to investigational use.

References

1. Lee RG, van Donkelaar P. Mechanisms underlying functional recovery following stroke. *Can J Neurol Sci.* 1995;**22**:257–63.

2. Nudo RJ, Plautz EJ, Frost SB. Role of adaptive plasticity in recovery of function after damage to motor cortex. *Muscle Nerve.* 2001;**24**:1000–19.

3. Rushton D. Functional Electrical Stimulation and rehabilitation – An hypothesis. *Med Engng Phys.* 2003;**25**:75–8.

4. de Kroon JR, van der Lee JH, IJzerman MJ, *et al.* Therapeutic electrical stimulation to improve motor control and functional abilities of the upper extremity after stroke: A systematic review. *Clin Rehabil.* 2002;**16**:350–60.

5. de Kroon JR, Ijzerman MJ, Chae J, *et al.* Relation between stimulation characteristics and clinical outcome in studies using electrical stimulation to improve motor control of the upper extremity in stroke. *J Rehabil Med.* 2005;**37**:65–74.

6. Meilink A, Hemmen B, Seelen H, *et al.* Impact of EMG-triggered neuromuscular stimulation of the wrist and finger extensors of the paretic hand after stroke: A systematic review of the literature. *Clin Rehabil.* 2008;**22**:291–305.

7. de Kroon JR, Izjerman MJ. Electrical stimulation of the upper extremity in stroke: cyclic versus EMG-triggered stimulation. *Clin Rehabil.* 2008;**22**:690–7.

8. Chae J, Harley MY, Hisel TZ, *et al.* Intramuscular electrical stimulation for upper limb recovery in chronic hemiparesis: An exploratory randomized clinical trial. *Neurorehabil Neural Repair.* 2009;**23**:569–78.

9. Alon G, Levitt AF, McCarthy PA. Functional electrical stimulation enhancement of upper extremity functional recovery during stroke rehabilitation: A pilot study. *Neurorehabil Neural Repair.* 2007;**21**:207–15.

10. Alon G, Levitt AF, McCarthy PA. Functional electrical stimulation (FES) may modify the poor prognosis of stroke survivors with severe motor loss of the upper extremity: A preliminary study. *Am J Phys Med Rehabil.* 2008;**87**:627–36.

11. Thrasher TA, Zivanovic V, McIlroy W, *et al.* Rehabilitation of reaching and grasping function in severe hemiplegic patients using functional electrical stimulation therapy. *Neurorehabil Neural Repair.* 2008;**22**:706–14.

12. Turk R, Burridge JH, Davis R, *et al.* Therapeutic effectiveness of electric stimulation of the upper-limb poststroke using implanted microstimulators. *Arch Phys Med Rehabil.* 2008;**89**:1913–22.

13. Knutson JS, Harley MY, Hisel TZ, *et al.* Improving hand function in stroke survivors: A pilot study of contralaterally controlled functional electric stimulation in chronic hemiplegia. *Arch Phys Med Rehabil.* 2007;**88**:513–20.

14. Kowalczewski J, Gritsenko V, Ashworth N, *et al.* Upper-extremity functional electric stimulation-assisted exercises on a workstation in the subacute phase of stroke recovery. *Arch Phys Med Rehabil.* 2007;**88**:833–9.

15. Lieberson W, Holmquest H, Scot D, *et al.* Functional electrotherapy: Stimulation of the peroneal nerve synchronized with the swing phase of the gait of hemiplegia patients. *Arch Phys Med Rehabil.* 1961;**42**:101–05.

16. Robbins SM, Houghton PE, Woodbury MG, *et al.* The therapeutic effect of functional and transcutaneous electric stimulation on improving gait speed in stroke patients: A meta-analysis. *Arch Phys Med Rehabil.* 2006;**87**:853–9.

17. Yan T, Hui-Chan CW, Li LS. Functional electrical stimulation improves motor recovery of the lower extremity and walking ability of subjects with first acute stroke: A randomized placebo-controlled trial. *Stroke.* 2005;**36**:80–5.

18. Stein RB, Chong S, Everaert DG, *et al.* A multicenter trial of a footdrop stimulator controlled by a tilt sensor. *Neurorehabil Neural Repair.* 2006;**20**:371–9.

19. Bogataj U, Gros N, Kljajic M, *et al.* The rehabilitation of gait in patients with hemiplegia: A comparison between conventional therapy and multichannel functional electrical stimulation therapy. *Phys Ther.* 1995;**75**:490–502.

20. Daly JJ, Roenigk K, Holcomb J, *et al.* A randomized controlled trial of functional neuromuscular stimulation in chronic stroke subjects. *Stroke.* 2006;**37**:172–8. Epub 2005 Dec 1.

21. Van Ouwenaller C, Laplace PM, Chantraine A. Painful shoulder in hemiplegia. *Arch Phys Med Rehabil.* 1986;**67**:23–6.

22. Sheffler LR, Chae J. Neuromuscular electrical stimulation in neurorehabilitation. *Muscle Nerve.* 2007;**35**:562–90.

23. Snels IA, Dekker JH, van der Lee JH, *et al.* Treating patients with hemiplegic shoulder pain. *Am J Phys Med Rehabil.* 2002;**81**:150–60.

24. Price CI, Pandyan AD. Electrical stimulation for preventing and treating post-stroke shoulder pain: A systematic Cochrane review. *Clin Rehabil.* 2001;**15**:5–19.

25. Ada L, Foongchomcheay A. Efficacy of electrical stimulation in preventing or reducing subluxation of the shoulder after stroke: A meta-analysis. *Aust J Physiother.* 2002;**48**:257–67.

26. Bates B, Choi JY, Duncan PW, *et al.* Veterans Affairs/Department of Defense Clinical Practice Guideline for the Management of Adult Stroke Rehabilitation Care: Executive summary. *Stroke.* 2005;**36**:2049–56.

27. Khadilkar A, Phillips K, Jean N, *et al.* Ottawa panel evidence-based clinical practice guidelines for post-stroke rehabilitation. *Top Stroke Rehabil.* 2006;**13**:1–269.

28. Teasell RW, Foley NC, Bhogal SK, *et al.* An evidence-based review of stroke rehabilitation. *Top Stroke Rehabil.* 2003;**10**:29–58.

29. Baker LL, Parker K. Neuromuscular electrical stimulation of the muscles surrounding the shoulder. *Phys Ther.* 1986;**66**:1930–7.

30. Dupont Salter AC, Bagg SD, Creasey JL, *et al.* First clinical experience with BION implants for therapeutic electrical stimulation. *Neuromodulation.* 2004;**7**:38–47.

31. Shimada Y, Davis R, Matsunaga T, *et al.* Electrical stimulation using implantable radiofrequency microstimulators to relieve pain associated with shoulder subluxation in chronic hemiplegic stroke. *Neuromodulation.* 2006;**9**:234–8.

32. Chae J, Yu DT, Walker ME, *et al.* Intramuscular electrical stimulation for hemiplegic shoulder pain: A 12-month follow-up of a multiple-center, randomized clinical trial. *Am J Phys Med Rehabil.* 2005;**84**:832–42.

33. Chae J, Ng A, Yu DT, *et al.* Intramuscular electrical stimulation for shoulder pain in hemiplegia: Does time from stroke onset predict treatment success? *Neurorehabil Neural Repair.* 2007;**16**:16.

34. Peckham PH, Keith MW, *et al.* Efficacy of an implanted neuroprosthesis for restoring hand grasp in tetraplegia: A multicenter study. *Arch Phys Med Rehabil.* 2001;**82**:1380–8.

35. Dutta A, Kobetic R, Triolo RJ. Ambulation after incomplete spinal cord injury with EMG-triggered functional electrical stimulation. *IEEE Trans Biomed Engng.* 2008;**55**:791–4.

36. Rebersek S, Vodovnik L. Proportionally controlled functional electrical stimulation of hand. *Arch Phys Med Rehabil.* 1973;**54**:378–82.

37. Merletti R, Acimovic R, Grobelnik S, *et al.* Electrophysiological orthosis for the upper extremity in hemiplegia: Feasibility study. *Arch Phys Med Rehabil.* 1975;**56**:507–13.

38. Alon G, McBride K, Ring H. Improving selected hand functions using a noninvasive neuroprosthesis in persons with chronic stroke. *J Stroke Cerebrovasc Dis.* 2002;**11**:99–106.

39. Chae J, Hart R. Intramuscular hand neuroprosthesis for chronic stroke survivors. *Neurorehabil Neural Repair.* 2003;**17**:109–17.

40. Kottink AI, Oostendorp LJ, Buurke JH, *et al.* The orthotic effect of functional electrical stimulation on the improvement of walking in stroke patients with a dropped foot: A systematic review. *Artif Organs.* 2004;**28**:577–86.

41. Sheffler LR, Hennessey MT, Naples GG, *et al.* Peroneal nerve stimulation versus an ankle foot orthosis for correction of footdrop in stroke: Impact on functional ambulation. *Neurorehabil Neural Repair.* 2006;**20**:355–60.

42. Burridge JH, Haugland M, Larsen B, *et al.* Phase II trial to evaluate the ActiGait implanted drop-foot stimulator in established hemiplegia. *J Rehabil Med.* 2007;**39**:212–8.

43. Kottink AI, Hermens HJ, Nene AV, *et al.* A randomized controlled trial of an implantable 2-channel peroneal nerve stimulator on walking speed and activity in poststroke hemiplegia. *Arch Phys Med Rehabil.* 2007;**88**:971–8.

44. Hochberg LR, Donoghue JP. Sensors for brain–computer interfaces. *IEEE Engng Med Biol Mag.* 2006;**25**:32–8.

45. Serruya MD, Hatsopoulos NG, Paninski L, *et al.* Instant neural control of a movement signal. *Nature.* 2002;**416**:141–2.

46. Velliste M, Perel S, Spalding MC, *et al.* Cortical control of a prosthetic arm for self-feeding. *Nature.* 2008;**453**:1098–101.

47. Kennedy PR, Bakay RA, Moore MM, *et al.* Direct control of a computer from the human central nervous system. *IEEE Trans Rehabil Engng.* 2000;**8**:198–202.

48. Hochberg LR, Serruya MD, Friehs GM, *et al.* Neuronal ensemble control of prosthetic devices by a human with tetraplegia. *Nature.* 2006;**442**:164–71.

49. Kim S, Simeral J, Hochberg L, *et al.* Multi-state decoding of point-and-click control signals from motor cortical activity in a human with tetraplegia. 2007 CNE '07 3rd International IEEE/EMBS Conference on Neural Engineering; 2007: 486–9.

50. Moritz CT, Perlmutter SI, Fetz EE. Direct control of paralysed muscles by cortical neurons. *Nature.* 2008;**456**:639–42.

51. Blana D, Hincapie JG, Chadwick EK, *et al.* A musculoskeletal model of the upper extremity for use in the development of neuroprosthetic systems. *J Biomech.* 2008;**41**:1714–21.

52. Bhadra N, Kilgore KL. High-frequency electrical conduction block of mammalian peripheral motor nerve. *Muscle Nerve.* 2005;**32**:782–90.

53. Zhang X, Roppolo JR, de Groat WC, *et al.* Mechanism of nerve conduction block induced by high-frequency biphasic electrical currents. *IEEE Trans Biomed Engng.* 2006;**53**:2445–54.

54. Bhadra N, Lahowetz EA, Foldes ST, *et al.* Simulation of high-frequency sinusoidal electrical block of mammalian myelinated axons. *J Comput Neurosci.* 2007;**22**:313–26.

23 Growth factors as treatments for stroke

Seth P. Finklestein & JingMei Ren

Broadly speaking, growth factors are defined as endogenous proteins that, working through high-affinity receptors, promote cell survival, proliferation, and differentiation. Growth factors can be grouped into superfamilies. Factors found in the CNS with effects on brain cells include members of the neurotrophin, fibroblast growth factor (FGF), transforming growth factor-β (TGF-β), epidermal growth factor (EGF), and hematopoietic growth factor families, among others.

The endogenous expression of many growth factors is upregulated in the mammalian brain following stroke. Moreover, because of the availability of recombinant growth factors and their effects on CNS cells, a literature has arisen on the potential usefulness of the exogenous administration of growth factors in stroke. This consists of a well-developed preclinical literature in animal models of cerebral ischemia, as well as a nascent literature on clinical trials of growth factor administration in human stroke. Note too that growth factors are a major mechanism by which stem cell therapies exert their effects (see Chapter 24).

In considering this literature overall, it is important for the reader to be aware of several fundamental distinctions, including differences between focal vs. global cerebral ischemia, and between permanent vs. temporary ischemia [1]. Perhaps the most important distinction is between acute stroke vs. stroke recovery. In the early stages of focal stroke, there exists tissue in which cells are frankly dead (infarct "core"), surrounded by tissue in which cells are injured but not yet necrotic (the "ischemic penumbra"). Acute stroke therapies are targeted at increasing blood flow to the ischemic brain or otherwise antagonizing the death of injured but still salvageable cells in the ischemic penumbra. Generally, such treatments are effective in preclinical studies for only a few hours after the onset of ischemia and are recognized by their effect in decreasing infarct size and thereby reducing

neurological deficits after ischemia. Despite decades of effort and dozens of clinical trials of putative acute stroke treatments, including numerous "neuroprotective" agents, only thrombolytic (clot-busting) therapies have shown value in human clinical trials of acute stroke therapies.

After focal ischemia has occurred and infarcts are fixed in size, animals and humans can recover to some degree in terms of neurological deficits following stroke. This recovery occurs during days to weeks, and depends on intact regions of brain that "take over" or compensate for loss of function incurred by focal brain infarction. The cellular underpinnings of recovery may include new neuronal sprouting and synapse formation in uninjured regions of brain, as well as progenitor cell proliferation, migration and differentiation [2,3]. Although regions of focal brain damage are not regenerated by these phenomena, functional recovery does occur. Treatments that enhance stroke recovery are likely to include those that promote neuronal outgrowth and synapse formation, as well as progenitor cell proliferation and differentiation. In animal models, recovery-promoting treatments are recognized by their ability to enhance neurological recovery without necessarily reducing infarct volume. Because of the time course of stroke recovery, such treatments are likely to be effective when given within days to weeks after stroke. To date, few clinical trials of stroke recovery-promoting agents have been undertaken.

This review will cover preclinical and clinical literature on the exogenous administration of selective growth factors in stroke, including basic fibroblast growth factor (bFGF, FGF-2), osteogenic protein-1 (OP-1, BMP-7), erythropoietin (EPO), and granulocyte colony-stimulating factor (G-CSF). This review will focus on preclinical studies in acute stroke and stroke recovery following focal ischemia in mature

Brain Repair After Stroke, ed. S. C. Cramer and R. J. Nudo. Published by Cambridge University Press.
© Cambridge University Press 2010.

animals, and on the few clinical trials that have been undertaken using these growth factors. This chapter represents an update of a previous review on this subject [1].

Basic fibroblast growth factor (FGF-2, bFGF)

Basic fibroblast growth factor (FGF-2, bFGF), a member of the fibroblast growth factor superfamily, is sometimes referred to as a "promiscuous" factor because of its mitogenic, survival-promoting, and differentiating effects on a host of cell types throughout the body. In particular, FGF-2 and its high-affinity receptors are widely distributed throughout the mammalian brain, including in neurons, glia, endothelia, and progenitor cells. The expression of FGF-2 and its receptors is upregulated after brain injury or stroke [4]. In vitro, FGF-2 protects neurons against a number of toxins and insults, including anoxia, hypoglycemia, excitatory amino acid toxicity, and free radical damage, among others, and promotes neurite outgrowth (especially axonal) from cultured neurons [5,6].

There is a robust literature of the effects of exogenously administered FGF-2 in animal models of acute stroke and stroke recovery. In an early study of acute stroke, Koketsu et al. [7] found that the intracerebroventricular infusion of FGF-2 for 3 days before ischemia reduced infarct volume in a model of focal ischemia/reperfusion in rats. In later studies, Fisher et al. [8] found that intravenous infusion of FGF-2, starting 30 min after permanent middle cerebral artery occlusion (MCAo), reduced infarct volume, and Jiang et al. [9] found that intravenous administration of FGF-2 at the time of reperfusion reduced infarct volume in a model of temporary MCAo in rats. In the case of permanent MCAo, infarct size is reduced if FGF-2 is administered up to 3 h after the onset of ischemia [10]. The mechanism of infarct reduction in these studies may be twofold: First, FGF-2 is a potent arteriolar vasodilator, and increases regional cerebral blood flow (rCBF) at the borders of focal infarcts [11,12]. Second, independent of these rCBF effects, FGF-2 reduces apoptotic cell death and increases expression of the anti-apoptotic protein bcl-2 at the borders of focal infarcts [13].

These initial findings in rodent models of acute stroke have been expanded subsequently. Watanabe et al. [14] found that intracerebroventricular administration of a viral vector containing the FGF-2 gene reduced infarct volume in a model of temporary MCAo in rats. Liu et al. [15] found that labeled FGF-2 administered at 2 h after permanent MCAo entered ischemic brain tissue and remained there for up to 14 days after stroke. Ma et al. [16] found that intranasally administered FGF-2 decreased infarct volume following temporary MCAo in rats.

In addition to these preclinical studies showing the effects of FGF-2 in reducing infarct size in acute stroke, other studies demonstrate the recovery-promoting effects of FGF-2. In these studies, FGF-2, administered at 1 or more days after ischemia, did not reduce infarct volume, but did promote neurological recovery. In early studies, Kawamata et al. [17,18] administered FGF-2 by intracisternal injection beginning at one day after permanent MCAo in rats and found no reduction in infarct volume, but enhancement of sensorimotor recovery of the affected (contralateral) limbs during the first month after stroke. Similar results were attained with a dimerized FGF-2, which may be more potent and stable than the monomer [19]. Further studies established that the mechanisms of enhanced recovery following FGF-2 treatment may be twofold: (1) stimulation of new neuronal sprouting and synapse formation in undamaged regions of brain, and (2) stimulation of progenitor cell proliferation, migration, and differentiation in brain [18,20,21].

Other groups have expanded on these findings. Leker et al. [22] injected a viral vector containing the FGF-2 gene into peri-infarct cortex following permanent MCAo in rats and found enhanced sensorimotor recovery and increased neurogenesis in treated animals. Wang et al. [23] administered FGF-2 intranasally at 1–6 days after temporary MCAo in rats and found improved sensorimotor recovery as well as increased progenitor cell proliferation and neurogenesis in treated animals.

A paper by Won et al. [24] emphasizes possible age differences in response to FGF-2 treatment following stroke in rats. Aged (14-month-old) male rats received FGF-2 intraventricularly for 3 days, beginning at either 48 h before, or 24 or 96 h after temporary MCAo. A comparison group of young mature (3-month-old) rats received a similar dosage regimen of FGF-2, beginning at 24 h after temporary MCAo. Both aged and young mature animals showed enhanced behavioral recovery when FGF-2 treatment was begun up to 24 h after stroke. Interestingly, young adult rats also showed reduction in infarct volume when FGF-2 treatment was begun 24 h after stroke, whereas aged animals did not. These results in aged rats are consistent with previous reports showing enhancement of recovery without infarct reduction when FGF-2 treatment is begun at one day after stroke [17,18,20]. The results in young rats differ, however, from other data showing that the effective time window for infarct reduction by FGF-2 lasts for only a few hours after stroke [10].

Two studies have examined the expression of FGF-2 following human stroke. In a study of postmortem human brain, Issa et al. [25] found increased FGF-2 levels within infarcts as well as increased FGF-2 and FGF-2 mRNA levels in tissue surrounding focal infarcts. Increased FGF-2 immunoreactivity was localized in neurons, astrocytes, macrophages, and endothelia in these regions. Guo et al. [26] found elevations in serum FGF-2 levels in human stroke patients, lasting up to 14 days after stroke. Interestingly, higher FGF-2 serum levels were correlated to improved clinical outcome.

Because of the above reports of the neuroprotective (infarct-reducing) effects of FGF-2 in preclinical studies, two human clinical trials of FGF-2 treatment in acute stroke were initiated. In a North American trial [27], FGF-2 (5 or 10 mg) was administered intravenously for 8 h, beginning within 6 h of onset of ischemic stroke. This study was prematurely terminated due to an apparent excess of adverse outcomes in FGF-2-treated patients. In a European/Australian trial [28], the same dose (5 or 10 mg) of FGF-2 was given intravenously, also within 6 h of stroke onset, but over a longer time period (24 h), resulting in lower FGF-2 serum concentrations. No excess adverse outcomes were seen among FGF-2-treated patients in this study. The trial was terminated prematurely due to projected futility on primary efficacy outcome measures. Post-hoc analysis, however, revealed a subgroup with apparent improved clinical outcome – specifically, those patients in whom FGF-2 treatment was begun at 5 h or later after stroke onset. These results suggest that FGF-2 may have greater utility when give later than sooner after stroke, i.e. as a recovery-promoting rather than as an acute stroke drug. To date, no clinical trials of the stroke recovery-promoting effects of FGF-2 have been initiated.

Osteogenic protein-1 (OP-1, BMP-7)

Osteogenic protein-1 (OP-1, BMP-7) is a member of the bone morphogenetic protein subfamily of the transforming growth factor-β superfamily. OP-1 was originally described by its ability to promote osteoblast proliferation and bone formation in mesenchymal tissue [29]. OP-1 is also expressed elsewhere, including kidneys, bladder, and brain. OP-1 stimulates dendritic outgrowth from cultured neurons [30].

In a preclinical study of acute stroke, OP-1 was administered intracortically or intracerebroventricularly at 30 min, 24 h, or 72 h before temporary MCAo. At 24 h after ischemia, infarct volume (and consequent neurological impairment) was reduced only in animals receiving OP-1 pretreatment at 24 h before ischemia [31].

Most preclinical studies of OP-1 in stroke have been done in models of stroke recovery. In an early study, Kawamata et al. [32] administered OP-1 by intracisternal injection at 1 and 4 days after permanent MCAo in rats. Sensorimotor recovery of the affected limbs (contralateral to infarcts) was enhanced by OP-1 treatment in a dose-dependent manner. In a follow up study, Ren et al. [33] explored the effective time window of OP-1 administration. OP-1 administered intracisternally at 1 and 3, and 3 and 5, but not 7 and 9 days after permanent MCAo enhanced sensorimotor recovery of the affected limbs in rats. As in the previous study, no reduction in infarct volume was observed.

Liu et al. [34] administered OP-1 intracisternally at 24 h after temporary MCAo in rats. At 48 h, they found improved total neurological scores in OP-1 treated animals that were associated with increased cerebral blood flow and glucose utilization in some regions of the ipsilateral (but not contralateral) hemisphere. Chang et al. [35] administered OP-1 intravenously at 24 h after temporary MCAo in rats. These investigators found enhanced recovery of body asymmetry and total locomotor activity in OP-1 treated animals. Overall, these preclinical data suggest that OP-1 exerts cytoprotective as well as recovery-promoting effects after stroke. Clinical trials of OP-1 in stroke have yet to be undertaken.

Erythropoeitin (EPO)

Erythropoietin (EPO) is a glycoprotein named for its ability to stimulate proliferation of red cell precursors in the bone marrow. EPO and its high-affinity receptor (EPO-R) are expressed in the mammalian brain – in neurons, glia, and endothelial cells. Following focal stroke, EPO expression is upregulated in peri-infarct tissue, and the EPO/EPO-R system participates in the proliferation, migration, and differentiation of neuronal precursor cells from the SVZ and in the process of angiogenesis in peri-infarct tissue [36,37].

Several preclinical studies have documented the effects of exogenously administered EPO in rodent models of focal stroke. In studies using neuroprotective paradigms, several authors have shown neuron sparing and infarct-reducing effects of EPO when given systemically or intranasally just before and/or up to 6 h after focal temporary, permanent, or embolic occlusion of the MCA [38–42].

In a study using a stroke recovery-promoting paradigm, Wang et al. [43] found that systemic administration of EPO at 24 h after embolic MCA occlusion did not reduce infarct volume, but did improve recovery of sensorimotor function. Behavioral recovery was accompanied by enhanced angiogenesis at infarct borders, and neurogenesis within the SVZ. In a remarkable study, Kolb et al. [44] found that the intracerebroventricular co-administration of the combination of EPO + epidermal growth factor (EGF) (but neither one alone), up to 7 days after focal infarction, resulted in the regeneration of cortical tissue and recovery of sensorimotor function. This stimulated a second study evaluating effects of two sequential growth factors. Belayev et al. [45] found that administration of 3 daily doses of i.v. EPO to rats beginning 6 days after stroke onset, and following 3 doses of i.m. beta-hCG initiated 24 h after stroke onset, was associated with improved behavioral outcome and an 82% reduction in infarct volume.

Preliminary clinical trials of EPO in acute stroke were undertaken by Ehrenreich and colleagues [46]. A small safety trial (N=18) established that EPO at the dose administered (3.3×10^4 IU/50 ml/30 min i.v. daily for 3 days) was safe in stroke patients. In a larger efficacy trial (N=40), patients with MCA stroke (< 80 years) were randomized to receive EPO (at this same dose) or placebo, starting within 8 h of acute stroke. All preselected endpoints (NIH Stroke Scale (NIHSS), Scandinavian Stroke Scale, Barthel Index (BI), modified Rankin Scale, and evolution of infarct size by MR) showed a trend or significant results in favor of EPO treatment. In EPO-treated patients, there were expected increases in CSF EPO levels and in peripheral reticulocyte counts. These promising preliminary findings are currently being expanded in a larger clinical trial.

Granulocyte colony-stimulating factor (G-CSF)

Granulocyte colony-stimulating factor (G-CSF) is a glycoprotein that stimulates the proliferation and mobilization of granulocytes from bone marrow. G-CSF and its high-affinity receptor are also found in the brain, including in neurons, glia, endothelia, and neural progenitor cells. G-CSF appears to have several effects in the intact and post-stroke brain, including enhancing neuronal survival and proliferation and stimulating blood vessel growth. The effects of G-CSF on the post-stroke brain may include stimulation of granulocyte infiltration into infarcted tissue as well as direct effects on G-CSF receptors.

Several studies have examined the infarct-reducing (neuroprotective) effects of G-CSF in rodent models of acute stroke. In models of temporary MCAo in rats and mice, several studies have shown reduction in infarct volume and corresponding reduction in neurological deficits when G-CSF was administered between 0.5 and 6 h after the onset of ischemia [47–54]. Other studies have shown reduction in infarct volume when G-CSF was administered between 0 and 3 h after permanent MCAo [55,56].

Relatively fewer studies have been done to look at later effects of G-CSF administration. Six et al. [57] and Shyu et al. [58] showed reduction in infarct volume when G-CSF was administered at 24 h after temporary MCAo in mice or rats, respectively. Lee et al. [49] reported diminution in infarct volume and improved sensorimotor outcome when G-CSF was administered starting up to 4 days after temporary MCAo in rats. Schneider et al. [59] found improved sensorimotor outcome when G-CSF was administered starting at 24 or 72 h after focal photothrombotic infarction in rats.

Minnerup et al. [60] undertook a meta-analysis of 13 published studies of G-CSF treatment in rodent models of stroke, and found a strong relationship between the total dose of G-CSF administered and the degree of reduction in infarct size, regardless of the time of initiation of G-CSF treatment. These results, as well as the results of the individual studies cited above, are surprising, in that apparent infarct size-reducing effects were seen when G-CSF was administered after 24 h (indeed up to 4 days) after the onset of focal stroke. In this regard, the literature on G-CSF differs from that on some of the other growth factors discussed above.

In a small clinical study, Shyu et al. randomized seven patients to receive G-CSF within 1 week of the onset of acute ischemic stroke and compared clinical outcome at 6 months to results in three patients receiving standard treatment [61]. There were no major adverse events in patients receiving G-CSF. Change scores of outcome on several neurological rating scales (including the NIHSS, the European Stroke Scale (ESS), and the BI) tended to be higher in patients receiving G-CSF vs. standard care. As expected, the circulating white blood cell count transiently increased after G-CSF treatment. In a double-blind placebo-controlled dose-escalation trial of patients receiving G-CSF (N=24) vs. placebo (N=12), beginning at 7–30 days after stroke, no adverse outcomes were seen in G-CSF treated patients [62]. A dose-dependent leukocytosis was seen after G-CSF treatment. There were no differences in clinical outcome (by BI, modified Rankin Scale (mRS), or Scandinavian Neurological Stroke Score (SNSS)) between G-CSF and placebo treated patients at 10 or 90 days after stroke.

Conclusions

The foregoing summarizes current work on the pre-clinical and clinical development of four specific growth factors as treatments for acute stroke and stroke recovery. Future directions in this field include refinements in preclinical models, clinical trial design, and the use of growth factors along with stem cells, especially in the development of stroke recovery-promoting treatments.

As noted above, virtually all preclinical studies have been done using rodent models of stroke. Among many important differences between human and rodent stroke are differences in brain anatomy, and differences in the degree and time course of stroke recovery. The rodent brain is smooth (lissencephalic) in surface. Rodents with large unilateral strokes show clumsiness in the contralateral extremities, which recovers toward a plateau within 1 month after stroke. By contrast, humans have a convoluted (gyrencephalic) and considerably more complex brain. Patients with moderate to large unilateral strokes are often markedly weak (paralyzed) in the opposite extremities, and recovery reaches a plateau at 3 months after stroke. Gyrencephalic monkeys show neurological deficits and a recovery course similar to humans. In a preliminary study, Moore *et al.* [63] trained rhesus monkeys to retrieve food pellets from wells of various sizes, and then made focal ischemic lesions in motor cortex controlling arm and hand movement. Following stroke, there was initial paralysis of contralateral arm and hand movement that recovered toward a plateau by 3 months. At that time, monkeys were again able to retrieve pellets from the largest wells, but were still considerably impaired in retrieving pellets from the smallest ones. Moreover, this recovery appeared compensatory, in that, rather than using a thumb–forefinger "pincer" grasp, monkeys now used a palm-grasping strategy to retrieve pellets. This strategy was entirely efficient for large (but not small) wells. The close similarity of phenomenology of motor stroke recovery in gyrencephalic primates compared to humans suggests that primate models may be useful as a penultimate step in advancing promising stroke recovery-promoting treatments to human clinical trials.

In addition to improved preclinical modeling, clinical trial design (see also Chapter 16) can be optimized for growth factors and other putative stroke recovery-promoting agents. Clinical trials of acute stroke (thrombolytic and neuroprotective) agents generally have a short time window to enrollment after stroke (within 3–6 h), and rely on composite clinical rating scales that combine outcome in several neurological modalities (motor, sensory, cognition, coordination, etc.). However, since neurological modalities may recover to different extents with different time courses after stroke, "modality-specific" outcome measures may represent a more sensitive and specific way with which to assess effects of putative stroke recovery-promoting treatments [64]. Examples of modality-specific outcomes include specific tests of arm/hand function, gait, or language. Moreover, since the effective time window for administration of recovery-promoting agents is likely to encompass days or even weeks after stroke, both baseline and post-treatment scores can be obtained, and informative "change scores" calculated, for each patient. The use of modality-specific endpoints may extend, and does not obviate, the concurrent use of standard composite outcome measures.

Finally, with specific regard to polypeptide growth factors, one of the mechanisms by which these agents may promote recovery is through stimulation of endogenous progenitor cell proliferation, differentiation and migration after stroke. As the isolation and availability of exogenous progenitor and stem cell populations advances, there may be advantages to the co-administration of cells and stimulating growth factors as treatments for stroke. Going forward, the field of growth factor treatment of stroke is likely to benefit greatly from advances in preclinical modeling, clinical trial design, and cell therapy.

References

1. Ren JM, Finklestein SP. Growth factor treatment of stroke. *Current Drug Targets – CNS Neurol Disord*. 2005;**39**:121–5.

2. Cramer SC. Repairing the human brain after stroke: I. Mechanisms of spontaneous recovery. *Ann Neurol*. 2008;**63**:272–87.

3. Cramer SC. Repairing the human brain after stroke. II. Restorative therapies. *Ann Neurol*. 2008;**63**:549–60.

4. Speliotes EK, Caday CG, Do T, *et al*. Increased expression of basic fibroblast growth factor (bFGF) following focal cerebral infarction in the rat. *Mol Brain Res*. 1996;**39**:31–42.

5. Finklestein SP, Kemmou A, Caday CG, *et al*. Basic fibroblast growth factor protects cerebrocortical neurons against excitatory amino acid toxicity in vitro. *Stroke*. 1993;**24**(suppl I): I-141–3.

6. Walicke P, Cowan WM, Ueno N, *et al*. Fibroblast growth factor promotes survival of dissociated hippocampal neurons and enhances neurite extension. *Proc Natl Acad Sci USA*. 1986;**83**:3012–6.

7. Koketsu N, Berlove DJ, Moskowitz MA, *et al*. Pretreatment with intraventricular basic fibroblast growth factor (bFGF) decreases infarct size following focal cerebral ischemia in rats. *Ann Neurol*. 1994;**35**:451–7.

8. Fisher M, Meadows ME, Do T, *et al*. Delayed treatment with intravenous basic fibroblast growth factor reduces infarct size following permanent focal cerebral ischemia in rats. *J Cereb Blood Flow Metab*. 1995;**15**:953–9.

9. Jiang N, Finklestein SP, Do T, *et al*. Delayed intravenous administration of basic fibroblast growth factor (bFGF) reduces infarct volume in a model of focal cerebral ischemia/reperfusion in the rat. *J Neurol Sci*. 1996;**139**:173–9.

10. Ren J, Finklestein SP. Time dependence of infarct reduction by intravenous basic fibroblast growth factor (bFGF) following focal cerebral ischemia in rats. *Eur J Pharmacol*. 1997;**327**:11–6.

11. Rosenblatt S, Irikura K, Caday CG, *et al*. Basic fibroblast growth factor (bFGF) dilates rat pial arterioles. *J Cereb Blood Flow Metab*. 1994;**14**: 70–4.

12. Huang Z, Chen K, Huang PL, *et al*. bFGF ameliorates focal ischemic injury by blood flow-independent mechanisms in eNOS mutant mice. *Am J Physiol*. 1996;**272**:H1401–05.

13. Ay I, Sugimori H, Finklestein SP. Intravenous basic fibroblast growth factor (bFGF) decreases DNA fragmentation and prevents downregulation of Bcl-2 expression in the ischemic brain following middle cerebral artery occlusion in rats. *Mol Brain Res*. 2001;**87**:71–80.

14. Watanabe T, Okuda Y, Nonoguchi N, *et al*. Postichemic intraventricular administration of FGF-2 expressing adenoviral vectors improves neurologic outcome and reduces infarct volume after transient focal cerebral ischemia in rats. *J Cereb Blood Flow Metab*. 2004;**24**:1205–13.

15. Liu Y, Lu JB, Ye ZR. Permeability of injured blood brain barrier for exogenous bFGF and protection mechanism of bFGF in rat brain ischemia. *Neuropathology*. 2006;**26**:257–66.

16. Ma YP, Ma MM, Cheng SM, *et al*. Intranasal bFGF-induced progenitor cell proliferation and neuroprotection after transient focal cerebral ischemia. *Neurosci Lett*. 2008;**30**:93–7.

17. Kawamata T, Alexis NE, Dietrich WD, *et al*. Intracisternal basic fibroblast growth factor (bFGF) enhances behavioral recovery following focal cerebral infarction in the rat. *J Cereb Blood Flow Metab*. 1996;**16**:542–7.

18. Kawamata T, Dietrich WD, Schallert T, *et al*. Intracisternal basic fibroblast growth factor (bFGF) enhances functional recovery and upregulates the expression of a molecular marker of neuronal sprouting following focal cerebral infarction. *Proc Natl Acad Sci USA*. 1997;**94**:8179–84.

19. Berry D, Ren JM, Kwan C-P, *et al*. Dimeric fibroblast growth factor-2 enhances functional recovery after focal cerebral ischemia. *Rest Neurol Neurosci*. 2005;**23**:.1–6.

20. Kawamata T, Ren JM, Cha CH, *et al*. Intracisternal antisense oligonucleotide to growth associated protein-43 (GAP-43) blocks the recovery-promoting effects of basic fibroblast growth factor (bFGF) after focal stroke. *Exp Neurol*. 1999;**158**:89–96.

21. Wada K, Sugimori H, Bhide PB, *et al*. Effect of basic fibroblast growth factor treatment on brain progenitor cells after permanent focal ischemia in rats. *Stroke*. 2003;**34**:2722–8.

22. Leker RR, Soldner F, Velasco I, *et al*. Long-lasting regeneration after ischemia in the cerebral cortex. *Stroke*. 2007;**38**:153–61.

23. Wang ZL, Cheng SM, Ma MM, *et al*. Intranasally delivered bFGF enhances neurogenesis in adult rats following cerebral ischemia. *Neurosci Lett*. 2008;**28**:30–5.

24. Won SJ, Xie L, Kim SH, *et al*. Influence of age on the response to fibroblast growth factor-2 treatment in a rat model of stroke. *Brain Res*. 2006;**1123**:237–44.

25. Issa R, Alqteishat A, Mitsios N, *et al*. Expression of basic fibroblast growth factor mRNA and protein in the human brain following ischemic stroke. *Angiogenesis*. 2005;**8**:53–62.

26. Guo H, Huang L, Cheng M, *et al.* Serial measurement of serum basic fibroblast growth factor in patients with acute cerebral infarction. *Neurosci Lett.* 2006;**393**:56–9.

27. Clark WM, Schim JD, Kasner SE, *et al.* Trafermin in acute ischemic stroke: Results of a phase II/III randomized efficacy study. *Neurology.* 2000;**54**:A88.

28. Bogousslavsky J, Victor SJ, Salins EO, *et al.* Fiblast (Trafermin) in acute stroke: Results of the European–Australian Phase II/III safety and efficacy trial. *Cerebrovasc Dis.* 2002;**14**:239–51.

29. Sampath TK, Maliakal JC, Hauschka PV, *et al.* Recombinant human osteogenic protein-1 (hOP-1) induces new bone formation in vivo with a specific activity comparable with mature bovine osteogenic protein and stimulates osteoblast proliferation and differentiation in vitro. *J Biol Chem.* 1992;**267**:20 352–62.

30. LeRoux P, Behar S, Higgins D, *et al.* OP-1 enhances dendritic growth from cerebral cortical neurons in vitro. *Exp Neurol.* 1999;**160**:151–63.

31. Lin SZ, Hoffer BJ, Kaplan P, *et al.* Osteogenic protein-1 protects against cerebral infarction induced by MCA ligation in adult rats. *Stroke.* 1999;**30**:126–33.

32. Kawamata T, Ren J, Chan TCK, *et al.* Intracisternal osteogenic protein-1 enhances functional recovery following focal stroke. *NeuroReport.* 1998;**9**:1441–5.

33. Ren J, Kaplan PL, Charette MF, *et al.* Time window of intracisternal osteogenic protein-1 in enhancing functional recovery after stroke. *Neuropharmacology.* 2000;**39**:860–5.

34. Liu Y, Belayev L, Zhao W, *et al.* The effect of bone morphogenetic protein-7 (BMP-7) on functional recovery, local cerebral glucose utilization and blood flow after transient focal cerebral ischemia in rats. *Brain Res.* 2001;**905**:81–90.

35. Chang CF, Lin SZ, Chiang YH, *et al.* Intravenous administration of bone morphogenetic protein-7 after ischemia improves motor function in stroke rats. *Stroke.* 2003;**34**:558–64.

36. Tsai PT, Ohab JJ, Kertesz N, *et al.* A critical role of erythropoietin receptor in neurogenesis and post-stroke recovery. *J Neurosci.* 2006;**26**:1269–74.

37. Carmichael ST. Cellular and molecular mechanisms of neural repair after stroke: Making waves. *Ann Neurol.* 2006;**59**:735–42.

38. Brines ML, Ghezzi P, Keenan S, *et al.* Erythropoietin crosses the blood–brain barrier to protect against experimental brain injury. *Proc Natl Acad Sci USA.* 2000;**97**:10 526–31.

39. Siren AL, Fratelli M, Brines M, *et al.* Erythropoietin prevents neuronal apoptosis after cerebral ischemia and metabolic stress. *Proc Natl Acad Sci USA.* 2001;**98**:4044–9.

40. Yu YP, Xu QQ, Zhang Q, *et al.* Intranasal recombinant human erythropoietin protects rats against focal cerebral ischemia. *Neurosci Lett.* 2005; **387**: 5–10.

41. Li Y, Lu Z, Keogh CL, *et al.* Erythropoietin-induced neurovascular protection, angiogenesis, and cerebral blood flow restoration after focal ischemia in mice. *J Cereb Blood Flow Metab.* 2007;**27**:1043–54.

42. Wang Y, Zhang ZG, Rhodes K, *et al.* Post-ischemic treatment with erythropoietin or carbamylated erythropoietin reduces infarction and improves neurological outcome in a rat model of focal cerebral ischemia. *Br J Pharmacol.* 2007;**151**:1141–2.

43. Wang L, Zhang Z, Wang Y, *et al.* Treatment of stroke with erythropoietin enhances neurogenesis and angiogenesis and improves neurological function in rats. *Stroke.* 2004;**35**:1732–7.

44. Kolb B, Morshead C, Gonzalez C, *et al.* Growth factor-stimulated generation of new cortical tissue and functional recovery after stroke damage to the motor cortex of rats. *J Cereb Blood Flow Metab.* 2007;**27**:983–97.

45. Belayev L, Khoutorova L, Zhao KL, *et al.* A novel neurotrophic therapeutic strategy for experimental stroke. *Brain Res.* 2009;**1280**:117–23.

46. Ehrenreich H, Hasselblatt M, Dembowski C, *et al.* Erythropoietin therapy for acute stroke is both safe and beneficial. *Mol Med.* 2002;**8**:495–505.

47. Schabitz WR, Kollmar R, Schwaninger M, *et al.* Neuroprotective effect of granulocyte colony-stimulating factor after focal cerebral ischemia. *Stroke.* 2003;**34**:745–51.

48. Gibson CL, Bath PM, Murphy SP. G-CSF reduces infarct volume and improves functional outcome after transient focal cerebral ischemia in mice. *J Cereb Blood Flow Metab.* 2005;**25**:431–9.

49. Lee ST, Chu K, Jung KH, *et al.* Granulocyte colony-stimulating factor enhances angiogenesis after focal cerebral ischemia. *Brain Res.* 2005;**1058**:120–8.

50. Schneider A, Kruger C, Steigleder T, *et al.* The hematopoietic growth factor G-CSF is a neuronal ligand that counteracts programmed cell death and drives neurogenesis. *J Clin Invest.* 2005;**115**:2083–98.

51. Komine-Kobayashi M, Zhang N, Liu M, *et al.* Neuroprotective effect of recombinant human granulocyte colony-stimulating factor in transient focal ischemia of mice. *J Cereb Blood Flow Metab.* 2006;**26**:402–13.

52. Solaroglu I, Tsubokawa T, Cahill J, *et al.* Anti-apoptotic effect of granulocyte colony-stimulating factor after focal cerebral ischemia in the rat. *Neuroscience.* 2006;**143**:965–74.

53. Yanqing Z, Yu-Min L, Jian Q, *et al.* Fibronectin and neuroprotective effect of granulocyte colony-

stimulating factor in focal cerebral ischemia. *Brain Res.* 2006;**1098**:161–9.

54. Sehara Y, Hayashi T, Degushi K, *et al.* Decreased focal inflammatory response by G-CSF may improve stroke outcome following transient middle cerebral artery occlusion in rats. *J Neurosci Res.* 2007;**85**:2167–74.

55. Gibson CL, Jones NC, Prior MJ, *et al.* G-CSF suppresses edema formation and reduces interleukin-1beta expression after cerebral ischemia in mice. *J Neuropathol Exp Neurol.* 2005;**64**:763–9.

56. Zhao LR, Singhal S, Duan WM, *et al.* Brain repair by hematopoietic growth factors in a rat model of stroke. *Stroke.* 2007;**38**:2584–91.

57. Six I, Gassan G, Mura E, *et al.* Beneficial effect of pharmacological mobilization of bone marrow in experimental cerebral ischemia. *Eur J Pharmacol.* 2003;**458**:327–8.

58. Shyu WC, Lin SZ, Yang HI, *et al.* Functional recovery of stroke rats induced by granulocyte colony-stimulating factor-stimulated stem cells. *Circulation.* 2004;**110**:1847–54.

59. Schneider A, Wysocki R, Pitzer C, *et al.* An extended window of oppoortunity for G-CSF treatment in cerebral ischemia. *BMC Biol.* 2006;**4**:36.

60. Minnerup J, Heidrich J, Wellmann J, *et al.* Meta-analysis of the efficacy of granulocyte-colony stimulating factor in animal models of focal cerebral ischemia. *Stroke.* 2008;**39**:1855–61.

61. Shyu WC, Lin SZ, Lee CC, *et al.* Granulocyte colony-stimulationg factor for acute ischemic stroke: A randomized controlled trial. *CMAJ.* 2006;**174**:927–33.

62. Sprigg N, Bath PM, Zhao L, *et al.* Granulocyte-colony-stimulating factor mobilizes bone marrow stem cells in patients with subacute ischemic stroke. The Stem Cell Trial of Recovery EnhanceMent After Stroke (STEMS) pilot randomized, controlled trial (ISRCTN 16784092). *Stroke.* 2006;**37**:2979–83.

63. Moore TI, Killiany RJ, Finklestein S, *et al.* Non-human primate model of motor recovery after cortical stroke. *Soc Neurosci Abstr.* 2003:**414**.1.

64. Cramer SC, Koroshetz WJ, Finklestein SP. The case for modality-specific outcome measures in clinical trials of stroke recovery-promoting agents. *Stroke.* 2007;**38**:1393–5.

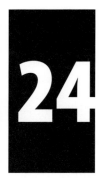

24 Cellular approaches to stroke recovery

Yi Li & Michael Chopp

Stroke is a leading cause of long-term disability. Recovery from stroke is a challenging journey that can last a lifetime. Therapeutic options have until now been limited to the first hours after disease onset. However, once the damage from a stroke event has maximized, little can be done to recover premorbid function. Experimental animal data suggest that restorative cell approaches may be an effective alternative to conventional disease management strategies of ischemic stroke. Therefore, this chapter focuses on the use of cellular approaches in the restorative treatment of stroke.

Endogenous stem cells and progenitor cells in the adult brain after stroke

Stem cells are undifferentiated cells capable of self-renewal, production of a large number of differentiated progeny, and regeneration of tissues. Generally, it has been thought that damage to the brain could not be repaired, as adult neurons could not be replaced. However, convincing evidence has emerged showing that neurogenesis in the adult central nervous system (CNS) is an ongoing physiological process [1]. Neural stem cells (NSCs) and neural progenitor cells (NPCs), the source of the new neurons, are present mainly at two sites in the adult brain. One is the subventricular zone (SVZ) in the lateral ventricles. The SVZ feeds new neurons into the olfactory bulb to continuously maintain the sense of smell [2]. The other site is the subgranular zone (SGZ) of the dentate gyrus in the hippocampus, a brain region involved in learning and memory [3]. Although NSCs/NPCs are a continuous source for new neurons in the brain, the turnover of these cells is vanishingly low under physiological conditions. Moreover, the turnover rate of NSCs is influenced by pathological

conditions in the brain. After ischemic brain injury, significantly more neurons are generated in the neurogenic zones and these new neurons tend to migrate toward the site of damage [4]. It seems that the brain tries to repair itself, possibly but not exclusively by replacing the damaged cells with an amplified endogenous pool of stem and progenitor cells. The replacement, though, is not extensive. After a few weeks, only 0.2% of the cells destroyed by ischemic attack are replaced and as many as 80% of the new neurons produced die [5].

It is necessary to amplify the endogenous neurorestorative response of the brain to stroke, to stimulate intrinsic neurorestorative pathways so that we can further improve neurological function after stroke. Preclinical data demonstrate that after stroke, the brain expresses an array of developmental genes and proteins, particularly in the boundary of the ischemic lesion, reminiscent of the developing brain [6]. We can capitalize on this attempted return to youth and amplify these restorative processes to rewire and restructure the CNS so as to minimize loss of function.

Stem and progenitor cells respond to key growth, differentiation and migration factors [7]. These factors are likely to differ depending on the tissue, degree of injury, and the stem cells involved [7]. Various molecules can enhance the intrinsic neurogenic capacity. Pharmacological intervention targeting enhancement of endogenous neurogenesis has become an important strategy in stroke research. For example, biological molecules capable of increasing endogenous neurogenesis after stroke in animal models include brain-derived neurotrophic factor (BDNF), epidermal growth factor (EGF), fibroblast growth factor 2 (bFGF), stem cell factor (SCF), vascular endothelial growth factor (VEGF), and others [8]. Moreover, similar effects on endogenous neurogenesis have been reported using clinically available drugs such as

Brain Repair After Stroke, ed. S. C. Cramer and R. J. Nudo. Published by Cambridge University Press.
© Cambridge University Press 2010.

statins, sildenafil, and erythropoietin (EPO) and carbamylated erythropoietin (CEPO) after middle cerebral artery occlusion (MCAo) in adult rodents [9]. Recently, the benefits of high density lipoproteins (HDL) as restorative factors have been investigated, with evidence demonstrating that Niaspan, a slow-release form of niacin which increases HDL, improves neurogenesis and functional outcome when administered well after stroke onset [9]. These data support the hypothesis that increasing neurogenesis is related to recovery of function.

Interestingly, many of the aforementioned agents, if not all, increase neurogenesis, synaptogenesis, and angiogenesis. Acute ischemic stroke causes a disturbance of neuronal circuitry and disruption of the blood–brain barrier that lead to functional disabilities. Angiogenic events are highly coupled to neurogenesis and synaptic activity [9]. Newly formed vasculature expresses BDNF, which acts to recruit neuroblasts from the SVZ to the site of vascular alteration [10]. Angiopoietin 1 and its receptor Tie2 are also upregulated in the ischemic brain in response to BMSC therapy and contribute to the maturation and stabilization of this newly formed vasculature [11]. Indeed, the relationship between angiogenesis and neurogenesis is under intense investigation. Goldman and his colleagues found that new neurons localize to angiogenic vessels within the parenchyma [12]. Palmer and others suggested that migrating neuroblasts and newly formed vessels are closely coupled, and the latter might provide a "vascular niche" for the survival of stem cells and their descendants [13]. Taken together, these experimental data suggest that endothelial cells foster conditions leading to the local proliferation and survival of neural stem cells. Therefore, promoting angiogenesis may prompt endogenous neurogenesis after stroke. Future drug development may consider that neurogenesis, synaptogenesis, and angiogenesis act in concert to stimulate repair and enhance recovery from stroke.

Exogenous stem cells and progenitor cells in the adult brain after stroke

Tissue-specific neural stem cells

Stem cells from the CNS provide a source of well-characterized tissue-specific cells. They can be categorized into embryonic, fetal, and adult stem cells according to their source. Embryonic neural progenitor cells transplanted in a rat model of MCAo demonstrated potent therapeutic effects examined behaviorally along with neuroradiological assessment using magnetic resonance imaging (MRI) [14]. Fetal cortical cells survive after stroke in adult rats, and the adult hosts have a regenerative capacity sufficient to innervate the grafted tissue [15]. Because of ethical dilemmas and practical concerns regarding teratoma formation with embryonic and fetal stem cells, increased attention has been directed to adult-derived cells for therapeutic application to neural injury. This has been fueled by primary observations that adult brain stem cells can be harvested, expanded, and then reimplanted and may have the capacity to integrate into the injured brain microenvironment and transdifferentiate into neural cells or, possibly and more importantly, serve as a source for beneficial growth and restorative factors [16].

Following the discovery of the ability to generate neurons and astrocytes from isolated cells of the adult mammalian brain in 1992 [17], NSCs/NPCs were found to be continuously generated in the adult rodent brain. Endogenous NPCs are activated in response to ischemia, both in rodents [5] and humans [18]. We delivered ferromagnetic labeled adult SVZ cells intracisternally into rats 48 h after MCAo [19]. MRI analysis showed that SVZ cells targeted the ischemic boundary zone, and that these cells also selectively migrated within the cerebrospinal fluid into parenchyma at a mean speed of 65±14.6 microns/h. Neurological function evaluation showed that the deficit ameliorating effect of SVZ cell treatment was apparent at 28 days after stroke. Other studies also demonstrate that transplanted NSC-generated cells migrated to the lesion, differentiated into neurons with axons that projected to appropriate targets, and expressed appropriate neurotransmitters and receptors [20]. Tissue-specific neural stem cells under investigation for reduction of neurological deficits after stroke in rat, mouse, gerbil, and monkey include immortalized cell lines (for review see [21]), including C17.2-mouse neural precursors, MHP36-mouse hippocampal stem cells, NT2N-human postmitotic neurons, porcine fetal cells–striatal progenitors, and various stem or progenitor cells. As a source of new neurons throughout the life span of mammals, NSCs/NPCs are good candidates for the treatment of stroke. The first cell-based therapy for the treatment of stroke employed cells (the Ntera 2/ce.D1 human embryonic carcinoma-derived cell line) injected into the brain of patients 6 months after stroke [22]. Twelve patients were treated and no cell-related adverse effects were reported and outcome measurements were consistent with a trend of improved neurological scores.

Restorative treatment of stroke with bone marrow stromal cells (BMSCs)

A growing number of studies indicates that a classification of stem and progenitor cells based solely on tissue compartment of origin may greatly underestimate the potential of cell-based therapies. Non-tissue-specific adult cells provide a feasible and a clinically realistic approach to the restoration of lost brain function after stroke. These cells, derived from bone marrow, peripheral blood, adipose tissue, and olfactory mucosa, act as central repositories for multipotent stem cells that can repopulate neural tissues [16]. There is optimism concerning the clinical applications of autologous adult cells in stroke, based on promising results obtained in experimental studies and initial clinical trials [23–25]. Success in future clinical trials will depend on careful investigation at the experimental level, to test safety, optimize treatment protocols, and to elucidate the underlying biological principles involved in improving neurological function. Among the cell candidates for restorative treatment, a leading source is BMSCs. As a prototype of cell-based therapy, we focus discussion on BMSCs as a source of cells for inducing functional recovery after stroke.

BMSCs have great potential as therapeutic agents, since they are easy to isolate and can be expanded from patients without serious ethical and technical problems, and may provide an unlimited cell source for cell therapy. BMSCs are a heterogeneous population of plastic-adherent cells, which arise from the supporting structure in bone marrow, and are distinguished from hematopoietic cells by adherence to plastic in culture. According to the International Society for Cellular Therapy, the biological characteristic of a multipotent mesenchymal stromal cell (MSC) is defined by the following criteria [26]: (a) its property of adherence to plastic; (b) its phenotype: CD14− or CD11b−, CD19− or CD79−, CD34−, CD45−, HLA-DR−, CD73+, CD90+, CD105+; and (c) its capacity to be differentiated into three lineages, chondrocyte, osteoblast, and adipocyte. The last decade has witnessed extensive studies of BMSCs as a candidate for stroke therapy [23,24]. We have demonstrated that treatment of experimental

stroke with BMSCs significantly improves functional outcome [23,27,28]. In these studies, various effective doses of BMSCs derived from donor rats, mice, or humans were transplanted into post-stroke animals intracerebrally, intracisternally, intra-arterially, or intravenously from 1 day [23] to 1 month [28] after MCAo. BMSCs have been found to selectively target injured tissue and significantly promote functional recovery for at least 1 year post-stroke [27]. Males and females [28,29] and young and older animals with stroke have robust functional improvement with cell-based therapies [24].

Homing of BMSCs to sites of injury, including the ischemic brain, is believed to occur through a complex multistep process. Although the mechanisms underlying this targeted movement are not fully understood, some studies suggest that chemotactic factors are responsible. Our preference has been to administer cells by an intravenous route [23]. These BMSCs target the injured or compromised microvasculature, localize to the ischemic border tissue, and encompass the lesion, where the cells stimulate recovery. Homing signals may result from local damage and influence the migration of BMSCs to specific sites, in a manner reminiscent of white blood cell homing. Inflammatory factors, such as monocyte chemoattractant protein-1, macrophage inflammatory protein-1alpha, and interleukin-8 appear to promote selective BMSC migration [30]. Several recently published studies demonstrate that expression of stromal-cell-derived factor 1 (SDF-1) on endothelial cells and the SDF-1 receptor, CXCR4, on the BMSCs mediate selective targeting of intravenously injected BMSCs to activated endothelial cells within compromised cerebral tissue [28,31].

After BMSCs enter the injured brain, the next question is how these cells exert their beneficial effects. Tissue replacement, as the mechanism by which BMSCs promote their beneficial effects, is highly unlikely for the following reasons: (1) only a very small fraction of BMSCs express neural markers [23], and even if all the cells were to differentiate into neurons and other parenchymal cells, only a minute volume of the infarcted tissue would be replaced; and (2) the functional benefit of cells is detected in many cases a few days after treatment, inconsistent with the time required for newly formed cells to integrate and function properly in the complex neural circuitry of the brain. The overwhelming body of data indicates that bioactive factors secreted by BMSCs in response to the local environment underlie the tissue restorative effects to support the adjacent cells and tissues [24]. Our studies demonstrate that ischemic brain extracts induce production of trophic growth factors by BMSCs [32], and BMSC transplantation facilitates and amplifies endogenous neuroprotective and neuro-restorative mechanisms [33]. The well-characterized BMSCs that are employed in this therapy are not necessarily stem cells, but progenitor and differentiated cells that escape immune system surveillance and survive in the CNS. Possible mechanisms by which BMSCs improve neurological outcome after stroke are presented in Figure 24.1. With various routes of administration, most BMSCs target and localize to the ischemic boundary zone (IBZ) [27,28]. The IBZ tissue is potentially salvageable and multiple processes of cell repair are present. BMSCs survive in the adult ischemic brain and secrete neurotrophic and growth factors that create a favorable environment to promote brain repair [24]. BMSCs induce cerebral tissue to activate endogenous restorative responses in injured brain, which include neurogenesis, synaptogenesis, and angiogenesis [24]. These restorative events are highly coupled.

How do scattered BMSCs in the ischemic brain promote neurological functional recovery? We propose that BMSCs, as a small biomaterial "factory," stimulate the neurorestorative processes, especially

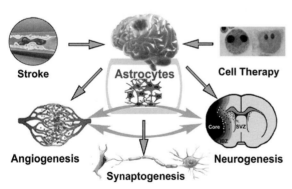

Figure 24.1 Mechanisms of action supporting the treatment of stroke with bone marrow stromal cells (MSCs). The majority of MSCs (white dots) are present in the ischemic boundary zone (IBZ) and secrete an array of neurotrophins and growth factors to coax brain cells to form functional tissue. Restorative events may be mediated by MSCs directly, and/or indirectly by "reactive" astrocytes via an astrocyte–vessel–neuron network to increase angiogenesis, neurite outgrowth, synaptogenesis in the IBZ, as well as cell proliferation, migration and differentiation from neurogenesis (black dots) in the subventricular zone (SVZ, the largest source of neural stem and progenitor cells in the adult CNS) into the damaged brain to improve functional recovery.

by activating the major endogenous repair mediator in the CNS, the astrocyte. The parenchymal cells that most prominently respond to the exogenous MSCs are astrocytes [33], and neuronal plasticity in the adult animal may utilize mechanisms that are active during development. Astrocytes in the developing brain direct neurites through their synthesis of cell surface and extracellular matrix molecules. Astrocytes have traditionally been viewed as supporters of neuronal function. Only recently, a very active role for astrocytes has been emerging in physiology and pathophysiology. Astrocytes are the most abundant cells in the adult CNS and greatly outnumber neurons. Astrocytes are coupled to one another in a cellular network (homocellular and heterocellular junctions) via gap junction intercellular communication (GJIC) by channels composed primarily of connexin43 (Cx43), which is an astrocyte-specific functional protein in brain [34]. GJIC allows direct intercellular diffusion of ions and signaling molecules. Brain capillary endothelial cells form a functional barrier between blood and brain (BBB). Morphological arrangement separates the vessels from the neuronal perikaryon and their processes, and astrocytic end-feet cover almost the entire surface of capillaries of adult brain. With their finely branching processes enveloping all cellular components throughout the CNS, astrocytes contact all parts of neurons, i.e. soma, dendrites, axons, and synapse terminals. Astrocytes, thus, function as a syncytium of interconnected cells identifying the astrocyte–vessel–neuron network in brain, rather than as individual cells. These characteristics of astrocytes allow oxygen and glucose, ions and molecules to cross from the blood to neurons. Astrocytes provide many supportive activities essential for neuronal function under physiological circumstances, which include homeostatic maintenance of extracellular ionic environment and pH, clearance and release of extracellular glutamate, provision of metabolic substrates for neurons, and the sculpting and maintenance of synapses [35].

In addition, astrocytes become reactive in response to all CNS insults [36]. Distal astrocytic processes can undergo morphological changes in a matter of minutes, a remodeling that modifies the geometry and diffusion properties of the extracellular space and relationships with adjacent neuronal elements, especially synapses [35]. Where astrocytic processes are mobile then, astrocytic–neuronal interactions become highly dynamic, a plasticity that has important functional consequences since it modifies extracellular ionic homeostasis, neurotransmission, gliotransmission, and ultimately neuronal function at the cellular and system levels. Astrocytes influence long-term recovery after brain injury, through neurite outgrowth, synaptic plasticity, or neuron regeneration, which are mediated by astrocyte surface molecule expression and trophic factor release. The roles reactive gliosis take after brain injury are varied. Rapidly expanding astrocytic processes create both physical and functional walls surrounding the ischemic core, which extend the time available for marshalling endogenous repair mechanisms, e.g. redirection of blood flow to still salvageable parts of the brain and redirection of neurite sprouting and synapse formation to build a new circuitry. However, astrocytes can also form scars that inhibit axonal regeneration [36]. Our data suggest that astrocytes promote brain plasticity and recovery from stroke [33], and that the beneficial effects of reactive astrocytes are enhanced in the ischemic brain after BMSC transplantation, and thereby promote appropriate neurite outgrowth and extension and myelination of axons to the injured hemisphere. The glial scar adjacent to the infarct is significantly reduced and more permeable than in control non-treated rats subjected to ischemic stroke [37]. Cells reduce scar tissue formation and very importantly reduce inhibitory glycoproteins. When inhibited, these proteins are permissive of neurite outgrowth and axonal remodeling in both the brain and spinal cord. In the adult animal after stroke, axons may also acquire their potential for outgrowth from neighboring astrocytes and establish contacts with existing circuits in the CNS.

Our studies demonstrate that white matter areas, in the striatum and the corpus callosum, are more intact and enlarged after BMSC treatment than in control non-treated rats subjected to MCAo [37]. A somewhat neglected but obviously important area of interest is the response of the spinal cord to stroke and restorative cell therapy. Motor and somatosensory response requires communication with the spinal cord, via the corticospinal tract (CST). Thus, recovery of function may be associated with plasticity in the CST and the spinal cord. Anterograde and retrograde labeling of the CST demonstrates a remarkable pattern of neurite outgrowth from the intact to the denervated spinal cord which significantly correlates with somatosensory functional recovery [38]. Retrograde labeling of bilateral forelimbs also demonstrates crossed connections in the contralateral and ipsilateral brain

hemispheres amplified by BMSCs. Downregulation of inhibitory glycoproteins may contribute to this robust rewiring in the brain and spinal cord. To sum up, constitutive reparative responses are facilitated by a series of interactions between BMSCs and host cells after stroke, fostering the remodeling of brain tissue, reducing scar tissue, and facilitating synaptic and vascular reconstitution.

Changes in white matter in response to either a cellular or a pharmacological restorative therapy can be readily monitored using magnetic resonance imaging–diffusion tensor imaging techniques (MRI–DTI) [39]. Tissue, in which the diffusion tensor for water is isotropic, is cavitated. The more anisotropic the diffusion constant for water, the more structure is present in the tissue [40]. Water moves easily along white matter fibers, and these structural changes in white matter and axonal growth may become evident using DTI [40]. Preclinical data demonstrate that cell therapy evokes white matter changes in the corpus callosum, the striatum, and in the boundary region of the ischemic lesion which is sensitive to the DTI, and significant correlations between functional recovery and a DTI-based parameter, Fractional Anisotropy (FA), may find clinical application [39].

Other cell sources for restorative treatment of stroke: view within article

Other sources of non-tissue-specific adult stem cells for use in stroke therapy include cells derived from hematological stem cells, peripheral blood, umbilical cord blood, adipose cells, and olfactory mucosa.

Bone marrow-derived pluripotent hematopoietic stem cells (HSCs) have the ability to reconstitute all cells of the blood. It has been suggested, based on statistical arguments, that individual stem cells can give rise to clones with full hematopoietic capacity. The hematopoietic stem cell can be highly enriched up to 10 000-fold and delivered to marrow-ablated recipients to fully reconstitute the blood [41]. Systemically applied HSCs reduce cerebral postischemic inflammation, attenuate peripheral immune activation, and mediate neuroprotection after ischemic stroke [42].

Filgratism (granulocyte colony stimulating factor, G-CSF)-mobilized peripheral blood progenitor cells (PBPCs) have been employed as a preferred source of autologous stem cells, in light of the faster hematological recovery and lesser supportive care requirement exhibited by PBPC transplants [43]. Transplanted G-CSF-mobilized PBPCs in rats after MCAo significantly reduced the stroke-induced hyperactivity compared with nontransplanted stroked animals [43]. Preclinical data suggest that peripheral blood-derived HSCs are as efficient in promoting functional improvement following MCAo as intravenous transplantation in rats [43].

The identification of endothelial progenitor cells (EPCs) in peripheral blood with the ability to differentiate into endothelial cells broke the paradigm that vasculogenesis was only an embryogenic process. Use of EPCs in experimental models [44] and patients [45] of cerebral ischemia suggest EPCs can form new vessels in ischemic areas and thus promote recovery after ischemic events. The increase of circulating EPC after acute ischemic stroke was associated with good functional outcome and reduced infarct growth in 25 patients compared with 23 patients with poor outcome [45]. These findings suggest that EPCs participate in neurorepair after ischemic stroke. These studies suggest that EPC can be used as a potential cell-based therapeutic agent in stroke, since EPCs may play an important role in tissue vascularization and endothelium homeostasis.

Umbilical cord blood cells (UCBCs) are a promising source of HSCs because of their availability, weak immunogenicity, and low risk of mediating viral transmission. Infusion of human UCBCs into rats after MCAo improved behavioral recovery [46]. UCBCs secrete neuroprotective molecules, enhance neovascularization and endogenous neurogenesis, and reduce inflammation in the ischemic brain [47]. These aforementioned effects, not cell replacement, may underlie the therapeutic benefits of UCBCs in ischemic brain.

Adipose tissue-derived stem cells (ADSCs) share many of the characteristics of the BMSCs, including extensive proliferative potential and the ability to undergo multilineage differentiation. To test the effects of ADSCs on experimental stroke, these cells were directly implanted into the brain of rats after MCAo [48]. ADSCs migrated toward the ischemic area, and they also traveled far distances to the contralateral cortex. Transplanted rats had significantly better recovery in motor and somatosensory behavior compared with animals that only received saline. The benefits strongly support current hypotheses that transplanted stem cells after stroke provide and induce trophic support of injured brain.

Murine olfactory ensheathing cells (OECs) promote central nervous system axonal regeneration in a murine model of stroke [49]. OECs also induce a neuroplastic effect which reduces neurological dysfunction caused by hypoxic/ischemic stress. Rats with intracerebral implantation of human OECs/olfactory nerve fibroblasts (hOECs/ONFs) showed more improvement on behavioral measures of neurological deficit following stroke than control rats. [18F]fluoro-2-deoxyglucose PET (FDG-PET) showed increased glucose metabolic activity in the hOEC/ONF-treated group compared with controls. Both hOECs/ONFs and endogenous homing stem cells enhanced neuroplasticity in the rat and mouse ischemic brain.

Conclusion

The non-tissue-specific adult stem cells, whether they be MSC, HSCs, PBPCs, EPCs, UCBCs, ADSCs, or OECs, when injected into the adult do not repopulate the adult brain tissue; they produce an array of factors including angiogenic and neurotrophic factors which initiate a restorative cascade of recovery. The targets of cellular therapy are distinct from neuroprotective effects of acute intervention to reduce the volume of cerebral infarction and the sequelae of secondary cell death, whether by necrosis or apoptosis. After many years of failed clinical trials of neuroprotective drugs and in light of the compelling scientific evidence supporting neurorestoration, cell-based therapy is poised to be tested further in a translational setting for stroke patients. Among various cell sources, adult-derived cells stand out because: (1) cells can be obtained readily and expanded in culture; (2) autologous transplantation circumvents the risk of rejection and graft-versus-host reaction; some cells, e.g. BMSCs, are not rejected and can be administered allogeneically; (3) intravenous transplantation is an essentially non-invasive way to administer cells; and (4) safety of cell administration has been demonstrated in experimental animals. Indeed, Bang and others have reported data from a clinical trial [25], in which 1×10^8 culture expanded autologous BMSCs were administered intravenously into 5 patients with ischemic stroke. Neurological outcome was significantly improved in treated patients and no adverse effects were detected. Additional trials for stroke are under way, and these early studies will hopefully spur application of this promising restorative therapy.

We now know that the injured brain is highly malleable and the entire intact brain responds to injury and stroke, by producing new brain cells (neurogenesis), new vasculature (angiogenesis and arteriogenesis), and new wiring (synaptogenesis and axonal growth), and these events collectively improve neurological function after stroke [50]. Although a complete picture of the cellular approach acting as a catalyst endogenous mechanism is still lacking, some aspects have been identified, notably, stimulating bioactive factors to enhance neurite outgrowth, angiogenesis, neurogenesis, and synaptogenesis [24]. Cell-based therapy induces recovery of function post-stroke by stimulating endogenous restorative mechanisms and not by replacing infarcted tissue. Adult cerebral tissues are highly plastic and amenable to change given the appropriate microenvironment. The field of restorative neurology for the treatment of stroke is rapidly progressing and cell approaches can be used to amplify recovery of function in the injured brain. Cell-based restorative therapies initiated days or weeks after stroke hold tremendous promise for millions of disabled stroke survivors.

Acknowledgments

This work was supported by NINDS grants PO1 NS42345 and PO1 NS23393.

References

1. Gage FH. Mammalian neural stem cells. *Science.* 2000;**287**:1433–8.

2. Alvarez-Buylla A, Seri B, Doetsch F. Identification of neural stem cells in the adult vertebrate brain. *Brain Res Bull.* 2002;**57**:751–8.

3. Eriksson PS, Perfilieva E, Bjork-Eriksson T, *et al.* Neurogenesis in the adult human hippocampus. *Nature Med.* 1998;**4**:1313–7.

4. Zhang R, Zhang Z, Wang L, *et al.* Activated neural stem cells contribute to stroke-induced neurogenesis and neuroblast migration toward the infarct boundary in adult rats. *J Cereb Blood Flow Metab.* 2004;**24**:441–8.

5. Arvidsson A, Collin T, Kirik D, *et al.* Neuronal replacement from endogenous precursors in the adult brain after stroke. *Nature Med.* 2002;**8**:963–70.

6. Cramer SC, Chopp M. Recovery recapitulates ontogeny. *Trends Neurosci.* 2000;**23**:265–71.

7. Blau HM, Brazelton TR, Weimann JM. The evolving concept of a stem cell: Entity or function? *Cell.* 2001;**105**:829–41.

8. Wiltrout C, Lang B, Yan Y, *et al.* Repairing brain after stroke: A review on post-ischemic neurogenesis. *Neurochem Int.* 2007;**50**:1028–41.

9. Chopp M, Li Y, Chen J, *et al.* Brain repair and recovery from stroke. *Eur Neurol.* 2008;**3**:2–5.

10. Wang L, Zhang Z, Wang Y, *et al.* Treatment of stroke with erythropoietin enhances neurogenesis and angiogenesis and improves neurological function in rats. *Stroke.* 2004;**35**:1732–7.

11. Zacharek A, Chen J, Cui X, *et al.* Angiopoietin1/Tie2 and VEGF/Flk1 induced by MSC treatment amplifies angiogenesis and vascular stabilization after stroke. *J Cereb Blood Flow Metab.* 2007;**27**:1684–91.

12. Leventhal C, Rafii S, Rafii D, *et al.* Endothelial trophic support of neuronal production and recruitment from the adult mammalian subependyma. *Mol Cell Neurosci.* 1999;**13**:450–64.

13. Palmer TD, Willhoite AR, Gage FH. Vascular niche for adult hippocampal neurogenesis. *J Comp Neurol.* 2000;**425**:479–94.

14. Takahashi K, Yasuhara T, Shingo T, *et al.* Embryonic neural stem cells transplanted in middle cerebral artery occlusion model of rats demonstrated potent therapeutic effects, compared to adult neural stem cells. *Brain Res.* 2008;**1234**:172–82.

15. Grabowski M, Brundin P, Johansson BB. Fetal neocortical grafts implanted in adult hypertensive rats with cortical infarcts following a middle cerebral artery occlusion: Ingrowth of afferent fibers from the host brain. *Exp Neurol.* 1992;**116**:105–21.

16. Roh JK, Jung KH, Chu K. Adult stem cell transplantation in stroke: Its limitations and prospects. *Curr Stem Cell Res Ther.* 2008;**3**:185–96.

17. Reynolds BA, Weiss S. Generation of neurons and astrocytes from isolated cells of the adult mammalian central nervous system. *Science.* 1992;**255**:1707–10.

18. Jin K, Wang X, Xie L, *et al.* Evidence for stroke-induced neurogenesis in the human brain. *Proc Natl Acad Sci USA.* 2006;**103**:13 198–202.

19. Zhang ZG, Jiang Q, Zhang R, *et al.* Magnetic resonance imaging and neurosphere therapy of stroke in rat. *Ann Neurol.* 2003;**53**:259–63.

20. Magavi SS, Macklis JD. Induction of neuronal type-specific neurogenesis in the cerebral cortex of adult mice: Manipulation of neural precursors in situ. *Brain Res Dev Brain Res.* 2002;**134**:57–76.

21. Bacigaluppi M, Pluchino S, Martino G, *et al.* Neural stem/precursor cells for the treatment of ischemic stroke. *J Neurol Sci.* 2008;**265**:73–7.

22. Kondziolka D, Wechsler L, Goldstein S, *et al.* Transplantation of cultured human neuronal cells for patients with stroke. *Neurology.* 2000;**55**:565–9.

23. Chen J, Li Y, Wang L, *et al.* Therapeutic benefit of intravenous administration of bone marrow stromal cells after cerebral ischemia in rats. *Stroke.* 2001;**32**:1005–11.

24. Chopp M, Li Y. Treatment of neural injury with marrow stromal cells. *Lancet Neurol.* 2002;**1**:92–100.

25. Bang OY, Lee JS, Lee PH, *et al.* Autologous mesenchymal stem cell transplantation in stroke patients. *Ann Neurol.* 2005;**57**:874–82.

26. Dominici M, Le Blanc K, Mueller I, *et al.* Minimal criteria for defining multipotent mesenchymal stromal cells. The International Society for Cellular Therapy position statement. *Cytotherapy.* 2006;**8**:315–7.

27. Shen LH, Li Y, Chen J, *et al.* One-year follow-up after bone marrow stromal cell treatment in middle-aged female rats with stroke. *Stroke.* 2007;**38**:2150–6.

28. Shen LH, Li Y, Chen J, *et al.* Therapeutic benefit of bone marrow stromal cells administered 1 month after stroke. *J Cereb Blood Flow Metab.* 2007;**27**:6–13.

29. Li Y, McIntosh K, Chen J, *et al.* Allogeneic bone marrow stromal cells promote glial–axonal remodeling without immunologic sensitization after stroke in rats. *Exp Neurol.* 2006;**198**:313–25.

30. Wang L, Li Y, Chen J, *et al.* Ischemic cerebral tissue and MCP-1 enhance rat bone marrow stromal cell migration in interface culture. *Exp Hematol.* 2002;**30**:831–6.

31. Cui X, Chen J, Zacharek A, *et al.* Nitric oxide donor upregulation of stromal cell-derived factor-1/chemokine (CXC motif) receptor 4 enhances bone marrow stromal cell migration into ischemic brain after stroke. *Stem Cells (Dayton, Ohio).* 2007;**25**:2777–85.

32. Qu R, Li Y, Gao Q, *et al.* Neurotrophic and growth factor gene expression profiling of mouse bone marrow stromal cells induced by ischemic brain extracts. *Neuropathology.* 2007;**27**:355–63.

33. Gao Q, Li Y, Chopp M. Bone marrow stromal cells increase astrocyte survival via upregulation of phosphoinositide 3-kinase/threonine protein kinase and mitogen-activated protein kinase kinase/extracellular signal-regulated kinase pathways and stimulate astrocyte trophic factor gene expression after anaerobic insult. *Neuroscience.* 2005;**136**:123–34.

34. Rouach N, Glowinski J, Giaume C. Activity-dependent neuronal control of gap-junctional communication in astrocytes. *J Cell Biol.* 2000;**149**:1513–26.

35. Theodosis DT, Poulain DA, Oliet SH. Activity-dependent structural and functional plasticity of astrocyte–neuron interactions. *Physiol Rev.* 2008;**88**:983–1008.

36. Sofroniew MV. Reactive astrocytes in neural repair and protection. *Neuroscientist.* 2005;**11**:400–07.

37. Shen LH, Li Y, Chen J, *et al.* Intracarotid transplantation of bone marrow stromal cells increases axon–myelin remodeling after stroke. *Neuroscience.* 2006;**137**:393–9.

38. Liu Z, Li Y, Qu R, *et al.* Axonal sprouting into the denervated spinal cord and synaptic and postsynaptic protein expression in the spinal cord after transplantation of bone marrow stromal cell in stroke rats. *Brain Res.* 2007;**1149**:172–80.

39. Jiang Q, Zhang ZG, Ding GL, *et al.* MRI detects white matter reorganization after neural progenitor cell treatment of stroke. *NeuroImage.* 2006;**32**:1080–9.

40. Beaulieu C. The basis of anisotropic water diffusion in the nervous system – A technical review. *NMR Biomed.* 2002;**15**:435–55.

41. Morrison SJ, Weissman IL. The long-term repopulating subset of hematopoietic stem cells is deterministic and isolatable by phenotype. *Immunity.* 1994;**1**:661–73.

42. Schwarting S, Litwak S, Hao W, *et al.* Hematopoietic stem cells reduce postischemic inflammation and ameliorate ischemic brain injury. *Stroke.* 2008;**39**:2867–75.

43. Willing AE, Vendrame M, Mallery J, *et al.* Mobilized peripheral blood cells administered intravenously produce functional recovery in stroke. *Cell Transplant.* 2003;**12**:449–54.

44. Rouhl RP, van Oostenbrugge RJ, Damoiseaux J, *et al.* Endothelial progenitor cell research in stroke: A potential shift in pathophysiological and therapeutical concepts. *Stroke.* 2008;**39**:2158–65.

45. Sobrino T, Hurtado O, Moro MA, *et al.* The increase of circulating endothelial progenitor cells after acute ischemic stroke is associated with good outcome. *Stroke.* 2007;**38**:2759–64.

46. Newcomb JD, Ajmo CT, Jr, Sanberg CD, *et al.* Timing of cord blood treatment after experimental stroke determines therapeutic efficacy. *Cell Transplant.* 2006;**15**:213–23.

47. Vendrame M, Gemma C, de Mesquita D, *et al.* Anti-inflammatory effects of human cord blood cells in a rat model of stroke. *Stem Cells Dev.* 2005;**14**:595–604.

48. Kang S, Lee D, Bae Y, *et al.* Improvement of neurological deficits by intracerebral transplantation of human adipose tissue-derived stromal cells after cerebral ischemia in rats. *Exp Neurol.* 2003;**183**:355–66.

49. Shyu WC, Liu DD, Lin SZ, *et al.* Implantation of olfactory ensheathing cells promotes neuroplasticity in murine models of stroke. *J Clin Invest.* 2008;**118**:355–66.

50. Lindvall O, Kokaia Z, Martinez-Serrano A. Stem cell therapy for human neurodegenerative disorders – How to make it work. *Nature Med.* 2004;**10**:S42–50.

Index

Aachener Aphasie Test, 187
ABI *see* acquired brain injury (ABI)
ACA (anterior cerebral artery), 71
Accelerated Skill Acquisition Program
    (ASAP), 227–9
  components, 227–8
  definition, 228–9
  models, 227
  outcomes, 228
  principles, 228
{*N*-}acetylaspartate–creatine ratios, 151
acetylcholine, 188
acquired brain injury (ABI)
  impacts, 233
  incidence, 233
  rehabilitation treatments, 233–4
  survivors, 233
  acrobatic tasks, rats, 28–9
acrobatic training
  efficacy, 28–9
action observation
  in post-stroke motor learning, 237–8
Action Research Arm Test (ARAT),
    186, 239
Activate-Initiate-Monitor intervention,
    156
activation patterns
  and stroke recovery, 95
active motor thresholds (AMTs), 104
activin, 12–13
activities of daily living (ADL), 233
  basic, 151
  effects on post-stroke depression
      treatment, 153–4
  instrumental, 151
  post-stroke depression effects on,
      151–2, 154–5
acute stroke
  brain events
      and subsequent repair, 87–96
acute stroke survivors
  robotic therapy, 197
acute stroke therapies
  goals, 259
  and nature of stroke, 167
  recanalization strategies, 89
  selection issues, 82
  thrombolysis, 88
  timing issues, 87
acute stroke trials

and repair-based stroke trials,
    173–4
and repair-based stroke trials
    compared, 174
vs. placebo, 173
ADAMTS 1
  expression, 16
ADAMTS 4
  expression, 16
ADC (apparent diffusion coefficient),
    60–1
adipose tissue-derived stem cells
    (ADSCs)
  in stroke recovery, 272
adjunct light therapy, 156
adjuvant therapies
  motor map plasticity promotion,
      7–8
ADL, *See* activities of daily
      living (ADL)
ADRS. *See* Aphasic Depression Rating
      Scale (ADRS), 146
ADSCs (adipose tissue-derived stem
      cells)
  in stroke recovery, 272
affected hemisphere
  stroke recovery, 105–7
affective depression, 150
AFOs (ankle–foot-orthoses), 252
African-Americans
  stroke recovery, 166
Afrotheria (Superorder), 67–8
age
  and cerebrovascular hemodynamics,
      114–15
  and post-stroke recovery therapies,
      36–7
  and stroke recovery, 166
aggrecan
  induction, 15
  mechanisms, 14
aggression, 155
aging
  and environmental factors, 52–3
AIXTENT program, 140
alertness training
  computerized, 140
alexithymia, 150
alternating currents, 213
Alzheimer's disease

mouse models, 52
and vascular dementia, 52
American Association of Neural
    Transplantation and Repair,
    190
American Heart Association, 233
American Stroke Association, 164
AMES (Assisted Movement with
    Enhanced Sensation), 198
AMPA receptors, 24–5
amphetamines, 184
  and aphasia recovery, 185
  applications, 40
  and motor function recovery,
      185
  and stroke recovery, 167–8, 185
amplitude/stimulus function (ASF),
    150–1
AMTs (active motor thresholds), 104
anatomical substrates
  of recovered motor function, 115–16
anesthesia protocols, 59
anger
  proneness, 155
  and stroke, 146–7
angiogenesis, 73
  and neurogenesis, 12, 268
  post-stroke, 17
angiopoietin 1, 268
animal–human translation issues
  drug use, 81–2
  stroke heterogeneity, 80–1
  stroke recovery research, 77–82
animal models
  advantages, 1, 80–1, 103
  behavioral experience, 27–8
  ischemic injuries, 80
  limitations, 1
  motor function improvement, 105
  motor maps, 1
  neuropharmacology, 183–5
      experimental studies, 184–5
  primates as, 69
      issues, 69
  skilled reaching, 29
animal stroke studies
  functional brain activation, 58
  functional magnetic resonance
      imaging, 58–60
  magnetic resonance imaging, 57

animal studies
 focused training, 29
 growth factors in stroke
  therapies, 263
 neuroplasticity mechanisms, 67
 and repair-based stroke trials, 174
 synaptic plasticity, 94
animals
 old
  mortality issues, 81
  pre-clinical stroke research, 81
  post-stroke recovery therapies,
   35–44
 young
  pre-clinical stroke research, 81
ankle–foot-orthoses (AFOs), 252
anosognosia, 154
anterior cerebral artery (ACA), 71
anthropoid primates, 68–9
anticholesterol drugs
 and stroke therapies, 82
anticholinergic drugs
 and stroke therapies, 81–2
anticoagulation, 87
antidepressants, 37
 post-stroke depression
  recovery, 153
 post-stroke depression treatment,
  154–5
 post-stroke emotional disorder
  treatment, 155
 prophylactic
  in post-stroke depression
   prevention, 157
 response rates, 155
 and stroke recovery, 184
 and stroke therapies, 82
 treatment
  and post-stroke mortality, 153–4
antihypertension drugs
 and stroke therapies, 82
anti-platelet therapy, 87
anxiety
 and depression, 148
 and post-stroke depression
  lesion locational issues, 149–50
 and stroke, 146
anxious depression, 155
apathetic depression, 150
aphasia
 brain reorganization
  therapy impacts, 129
 conduction, 129–30
 constraint-induced therapy, 129
 future research, 130
 longitudinal studies, 127–8
 measures, 146
 and network approach, 129–30
 neuroimaging trials, 187–8
 recovery

acute phase imaging, 125–6
 and amphetamines, 185
 chronic phase imaging, 128–9
 imaging studies, 125–30
 reorganization
  imaging dynamics, 126–8
 subcortical, 125–6
Aphasia Quotient, 187
Aphasia Test Battery, 187
Aphasic Depression Rating Scale
 (ADRS), 146
apomorphine
 and neglect recovery, 184
apparent diffusion coefficient (ADC),
 60–1
ARAS (ascending reticular activating
 system), 137,
ARAT (Action Research Arm Test),
 186, 239
Archonta (Superorder), 67–8
area
 and dexterity, 2–3
arm exercise
 robotic therapy, 197
 robotic vs. other therapies, 198–200,
  201
ARM Guide, 197, 199
ARMOR robot, 199, 200
arterial emboli
 composition, 92
 origin, 92
arterial spin labeling (ASL), 57–8
arthritis
 and stroke, 37, 81
ASAP. See Accelerated Skill Acquisition
 Program (ASAP)
ascending reticular activating system
 (ARAS), 137
ASF (amplitude/stimulus function),
 150–1
ASL (arterial spin labeling), 57–8
aspiration lesions
 effects, 80
 primates, 70–1
Assisted Movement with Enhanced
 Sensation (AMES), 198
astrocytes, 50, 270
 generation, 268–9
 in post-stroke recovery
  therapies, 42
 roles, 35, 50, 270–1
ATF3, 14
atherosclerosis
 and stroke, 37
attention,
 brain mapping
  after stroke, 133–41
 and brain reorganization, 141
 functional mapping studies,
  136–9

psychology of, 133
 see also selective attention, spatial
  attention
attention deficits
 after brain injury, 133–4
 lateralized, 133
 non-lateralized, 134
auditory stimuli
 in post-stroke motor learning, 237
Australia
 post-stroke depression studies,
  146
Auto-Cite, 201
axonal growth inhibitory molecules
 occurrence, 13
axonal regeneration
 and developmental axonal
  outgrowth, 15
axonal sprouting, 7, 11
 contralateral cortex, 12
 induction, 11–12
 inhibition, 14–15
 occurrence, 11, 13
 peri-infarct cortex, 12
 rodent models, 11
 timing factors, 13

baboons
 evolution, 68–9
 grasp recovery, 70
 spasticity, 70
bADL (basic activities of daily living),
 151, 152
Barthel Index, 153, 167, 178,
 189–90
basic activities of daily living (bADL),
 151, 152
basic fibroblast growth factor (bFGF),
 40–1, 259–60, 267–8
 expression, 78–9
 functions, 260
 infusion, 41
 occurrence, 260
 in stroke therapies, 260–1
  human studies, 261
  rodent models, 260–1
BATRAC device, 201
BCIs. See brain–computer interfaces
 (BCIs)
BDI (Beck Depression Inventory),
 145, 155
BDNF. See brain derived neurotrophic
 factor (BDNF)
BDNF gene, 8, 49–50
Beck Depression Inventory (BDI),
 145, 155
behavior
 and environment, 47
behavioral deficits
 and hemispatial neglect, 135

behavioral experience
  animal models, 27–8
  and brain injuries, 25
  and environmental complexity,
    27–8
behavioral experience manipulations
  and degenerative responses,
    23–4
  and degenerative–regenerative
    cascade, 26
  and regenerative responses,
    23–4
behavioral impairments
  and stroke, 1
behavioral influences
  on post-stroke neuronal events,
    23–31
behavioral manipulations
  and other interventions combined,
    29–30
behavioral repertoires
  mammals, 39–40
behavioral training
  and post-injury pharmacological
    manipulations, 29–30
benzodiazepine, 52
  and motor recovery, 184
  neuroprotectant activity, 184
Betz cells, 72, *See also* corticospinal
  (CS) neurons
bFGF. *See* basic fibroblast growth factor
  (bFGF)
bicuculline, 60
bilateral training, 202
BiManuTrac, 198, 200
biomarkers
  and repair-based stroke trials,
    176–8
block myelin-associated growth
    inhibitors, 12
blood glucose levels
  and stroke recovery, 167
blood oxygenation level-dependent
    (BOLD) fMRI, 57–8, 88
  activity, 138
  age factors, 114–15
  applications, 58, 177
  in cerebrovascular disease,
    113–15
  correlation approaches, 114
  limitations, 114
  low frequency signals, 60
  principles, 113
  signal fluctuations, 139
  signal reduction, 114
  signal shape, 113–14
BMP-7. *See* osteogenic protein-1
  (OP-1)
BMSCs. *See* bone marrow stromal cells
  (BMSCs)

Bobath approach, 220, 221, 223
  and stroke outcomes, 222
  treatment–outcome relationships,
    221–2
BOLD fMRI. *See* blood oxygenation
    level-dependent (BOLD)
    fMRI
bone marrow stromal cells (BMSCs),
    270
  advantages, 269
  homing, 269
  in stroke recovery, 269–71
    mechanisms, 269–71
  trials, 272
brain
  degenerative processes, 24, 43–4
  regenerative processes, 24
  reparative processes, 43–4
brain activity
  hyperactivity, 128
  lateralization, 119
brain adaptation
  future research, 130
brain centers
  functional independence issues,
    129–30
brain–computer interfaces (BCIs)
  development, 253–4
  field of study, 253
brain damage. *See* brain injuries
brain derived neurotrophic factor
    (BDNF), 37, 40, 148,
    267–8
  and environmental enrichment,
    49–50
  expression, 268
  polymorphisms, 166
  Val66Met polymorphism,
    49–50
brain disorders
  and environmental enrichment, 52
brain events
  in acute stroke period
    and subsequent repair, 87–96
brain functions
  loss, 130
  organization, 129
brain infarcts
  determinants, 88
  magnetic resonance imaging,
    88–9
  pathogenesis, 89
  recovery, 87–8, 94–5
brain injuries. *See also* acquired brain
    injury (ABI), *See also* traumatic
    brain injury (TBI)
  and attention deficits, 133–4
  and behavioral experience, 25
  functional recovery
    lesion-dependent, 80

  locational issues, 80
  and motor system reconfiguration,
    120
  responses
    gender differences, 38
  tissue loss
    compensation strategies, 37
  unilateral, 27
brain ischemia
  etiology, 87
  and stroke, 87
brain lesions
  and post-stroke depression
    locational issues,
    149–50
brain mapping
  of attention
    after stroke, 133–41
  of neglect
    after stroke, 133–41
  post-stroke
    motor system, 113–20
  rats, 63
brain plasticity
  and environmental enrichment,
    52
  occurrence, 23
brain reorganization, *See also* post-
    stroke brain reorganization
  aphasia
    imaging dynamics, 126–8
    therapy impacts, 129
  and attention, 141
  environmental enrichment, 23
  optimization, 23
  and post-stroke recovery,
    116–17
  and rehabilitative training, 23
  and self-taught behavioral change,
    26–7
brain repair
  and perfusion–diffusion mismatch,
    88–9
brain repair after stroke
  clinical applications, 173
  clinical trial methodologies
    issues, 173–8
  definition, 173
  mammals, 77
  and potential clinical applications,
    173
  therapies
    classes, 178
  tissue targeting issues, 173
brain tissue
  preservation
    and stroke recovery, 168
brain-controlled interfaces
  neuroprostheses, 253–4
BrainGate, 253

BrdU, 50
brevican
   induction, 15
Broca's area, 126–7, 129–30,
bromocriptine
   and stroke recovery, 167–8
Brunnstrom approach, 220,
   and stroke outcomes, 221
butyrophenones
   and neglect recovery, 184

cAMP/CREB pathway, 7
Canadian Stroke Network, 225
Canadian Stroke Registry, 166
CAP23, 13
   PI3 kinase mediation, 13–14
capacity, 227–8
   evidence for, 228
carbamazepine, 109
   and motor recovery, 184
carbamylated erythropoietin (CEPO),
   267–8
case control studies, 163
Caucasians
   stroke recovery, 166
CCL2, 17
cell adhesion molecules
   induction, 13–14
cell behavior
   mouse cortex, 48
cell death, 36
cell transplantation therapy, 190
cells
   genesis
      after motor cortex lesions, 42
   sources
      in stroke recovery, 271–2
cellular approaches
   future trends, 272–3
   targets, 272
   to stroke recovery, 267–73
cellular concepts
   of neural repair after stroke,
      11–12
Centers for Disease Control and
      Prevention, 233
central motor conduction time, 109
central nervous system (CNS)
   astrocytes, 270
   connectivity changes, 234
   drug effects, 184
   injury, 7, 13, 14–15, 178
   neurogenesis, 267
   neuroplastic mechanisms, 1
   norepinephrine effects, 183
   repair, 42, 51
   stem cells, 268
   tissue morphology, 15
CEPO (carbamylated erythropoietin),
   267–8

Cercopithecoidea (baboons,
      macaques), 68–9
cerebral arterial circle, 75
cerebral artery occlusion, 87
   effects, 88
cerebral blood flow
   neglect studies, 139
cerebral ischemia. See also focal
      cerebral ischemia, See also
      global cerebral ischemia
   unilateral, 58–9
cerebral metabolic rate of oxygen
      (CMRO$_2$), 57
cerebral perfusion
   depression, 88
cerebrovascular disease
   and stroke, 91
   blood oxygenation level-dependent
      fMRI in, 113–15
cerebrovascular hemodynamics
   and age, 114–15
cerebrovascular reactivity
   impairment, 114
CES (cranial electrical stimulation), 207
Chedoke–McMaster Stroke
      Assessment Scale, 223–5
chimpanzees
   evolution, 68–9
   grasp recovery, 70
   spasticity, 70
choline–creatinine ratios, 151
chondroitin sulfate proteoglycan
      neurocans
   induction, 13
chondroitin sulfate proteoglycans
      (CSPGs), 14–15
   mechanisms, 14
   post-stroke responses, 15
chromatin, 52
chronic stroke
   motor imagery studies, 239
CIMT. See constraint-induced
      movement therapy (CIMT)
cingulate motor areas, 72,
      115–16
Cirstea, M. C., 234–5, 241
citalopram, 153, 155, 186
c-jun, 12, 13
clinical depression
   stroke survivors, 37
clinical trial methodologies
   for brain repair after stroke
      issues, 173–8
clinical trials
   neuropharmacology, 185–7
clonidine
   and motor recovery, 184
CMRO$_2$ (cerebral metabolic rate of
      oxygen), 57
CNS. See central nervous system (CNS)

Cochrane Collaboration, 240–1
Cochrane Collection, 220
Cochrane Review, 187
cognitive approaches
   future trends, 241–2
   in post-stroke motor learning, 236–41
   to stroke recovery, 233–42
   techniques and evidence, 234–41
cohort studies, 164
Communicative Ability Log, 187
computed tomography (CT), 57
   dense artery sign, 92
   perfusion imaging, 88
computer games
   applications, 195
conduction aphasia, 129–30
Consensus Panel on Hemiplegic Arm
      and Hand, 223–5
Consolidated Standards of Reporting
      Trials (CONSORT), 190
constant current stimulators, 209–10
constraint-induced movement therapy
      (CIMT), 164, 234
   advantages, 77–8, 80
   applications, 77
   disadvantages, 80
   efficacy, 234
   and upper extremity motor
      performance, 3
contralateral cortex
   axonal sprouting, 11–12,
contralesional dorsal premotor cortex
   disruption, 118
   signal changes, 118
contralesional hemisphere
   activity, 116–17
   physiological changes, 107
   stroke recovery, 107
   studies, 107
contralesional motor cortex activity,
      94–5, 117–18
   disruption, 118
   enhanced, 58
   and limb movement, 5
contralesional motor regions
   disinhibition, 207
Copenhagen Stroke Study, 164, 165–6
   age factors, 166
Corbetta–Shulman model, 137
cortical excitability
   after stroke
      changes, 103–10
   measures, 103
cortical injury
   neuroanatomical plasticity after, 74
   spasticity after, 70
cortical lesions, 104
   and neglect, 135
cortical motor system
   regions, 115–16

cortical neurons
  sprouting, 13
cortical reorganization
  of emotional processing, 158
cortical stimulation (CS)
  effects, 213–14
  human studies, 30
  low-intensity, 29–30
  motor map plasticity enhancement,
    7–8
cortical stimulation and rehabilitative
    training (CS-RT)
  efficacy, 7–8
cortical stimulation experiments, 6
cortical transplants
  rats, 51
corticospinal (CS) neurons
  primate brains, 70, 72
  terminations, 70
corticospinal excitability
  transcranial magnetic stimulation
    measures, 109–10
corticospinal function
  measurement, 2–3, 103–4
corticospinal system
  integrity, 119–20
    and post-stroke motor recovery, 3
  and motor evoked potentials, 3
corticospinal tract (CST), 117, 271
  functional integrity, 103
  primate brains, 69–70
CPG21, 12
cranial electrical stimulation (CES),
    207
Cretaceous, 68–9
critical lesions
  concept of, 130
critical period. See ischemic critical
    period
cross sectional studies, 164
CS. See cortical stimulation (CS)
CS neurons. See corticospinal (CS)
    neurons
CSPGs. See chondroitin sulfate
    proteoglycans (CSPGs)
CS-RT (cortical stimulation and
    rehabilitative training)
  efficacy, 7–8
CST. See corticospinal tract (CST)
CT. See computed tomography (CT)
cyclic neuromuscular electrical
    stimulation, 247–8
  efficacy, 249
  upper limb motor learning, 248
cytoskeletal molecules
  induction, 13–14

degenerative processes
  brain, 24, 43–4
degenerative responses, 23

and behavioral experience
    manipulations, 23–4
degenerative–regenerative cascade,
    25–6
  and behavioral experience
    manipulations, 26
dementia
  and stroke, 149
  and stroke recovery, 168
dendrites
  and environmental enrichment,
    47–8
  growth, 27
  overproduction, 26–7
dendritic spines
  and environmental enrichment,
    47–8
dendritic sprouting, 11
  occurrence, 11
dendritic tree, 47
Denmark
  neuroprostheses, 252
dense artery sign, 92
dentate gyrus (DG), 50
depression. See also post-stroke
    depression
  and anxiety, 148
  prevalence, 157
  rating scales, 145–6
  risk factors, 147–8, 152
  and self-esteem, 148
  and stroke recovery, 167
  as stroke risk factor, 147
depression-dysexecutive syndrome,
    150
deprived housing
  use of term, 47
desipramine
  and motor recovery, 184
DESTRO study, 146, 147
developmental axonal outgrowth
  axonal regeneration, 15
dexterity
  and area, 2–3
  recovery, 5
dextroamphetamine
  and stroke recovery, 185
dextromethorphan, 210–11
DG (dentate gyrus), 50
diabetes
  and stroke, 37, 81
Diagnostic and Statistical Manual
    of Mental Disorders (DSM-IV),
    145
  depression, 145
diaschisis, 128
  concept of, 125
  use of term, 3–4, 125
diazepam
  and motor recovery, 184

diffusion tensor imaging (DTI),
    60–1
  advantages, 61–2
  applications, 177, 271
  limitations, 61–2
  neuroplasticity studies, 62
  principles, 61
  procedures, 61–2
diffusion weighted imaging (DWI), 93
  abnormalities, 88–9
  applications, 88
disinhibition
  of contralesional motor regions, 207
distal axonal branch formation, 12
DNA microarrays, 50
donepezil
  and stroke recovery, 187
dopamine
  mechanisms, 189
  and stroke recovery, 184
dopaminergic drugs
  and neglect recovery, 184
  and stroke recovery, 184
dorsal attention networks, 135
dorsal network abnormalities
  and neglect, 137–9
dorsal premotor cortex (PMd), 72,
    115–16, See also contralesional
    dorsal premotor cortex, See also
    ipsilesional dorsal premotor
    cortex
dorsal root ganglion (DRG), 14
dose–response relationships
  and brain repair after stroke, 174
DRG (dorsal root ganglion), 14
droperidol
  and neglect recovery, 184
drug use
  and animal–human translation
    issues, 81–2
drugs
  and repair-based stroke trials, 175
DSM-IV. See Diagnostic and Statistical
    Manual of Mental Disorders
    (DSM-IV)
DTI. See diffusion tensor imaging
    (DTI)
dual responses, 6
Duncan, P. W., 233
Dunsky, A., 239
DWI. See diffusion weighted imaging
    (DWI)

EC. See environmental complexity (EC)
edemas
  development, 35
EEG. See electroencephalography (EEG)
EGF. See epidermal growth factor (EGF)
egocentric frames of reference, 133–4
elbow representations, 6

electrical stimulation (ES). *See also*
  neuromuscular electrical
  stimulation (NMES)
  effects, 247
  mechanisms, 43
  percutaneous intramuscular, 250
  post-stroke recovery therapies, 43
  stroke recovery, 247–54
  future trends, 254
electroencephalography (EEG), 118
  directed coherence, 118
electromagnetic approaches
  to stroke recovery, 207–14
electromagnetic stimulation
  evaluation, 207–8
electromyographic (EMG) activity, 2, 239
  biofeedback, 240–1
  measurements, 197
  onset, 107
electromyographically (EMG) mediated
  neuromuscular electrical
  stimulation (NMES), 247–8
  efficacy, 249
  upper limb motor relearning, 248
electromyographic-triggered
  functional electrical stimulation
  (EMG-FES), 199, 200
emboli
  injection into internal carotid artery,
  71
EMG activity. *See* electromyographic
  (EMG) activity
EMG mediated NMES. *See*
  electromyographically (EMG)
  mediated neuromuscular
  electrical stimulation (NMES)
EMG-FES (electromyographic-
  triggered functional electrical
  stimulation), 199, 200
emotional disorders
  and stroke, 145
emotional incontinence, 155
emotional processing
  cortical reorganization of, 158
emotional symptoms
  stroke patients, 145
encephalization of function
  primates, 70
endogenous stem cells
  activation, 41
  in adult brain after stroke, 267–8
endothelial cells, 12
endothelial progenitor cells (EPCs)
  roles, 272
  in stroke recovery, 272
endovascular occlusion, 71
environment
  and behavior, 47
  and neurogenesis, 50–1
  and repair-based therapies, 174–5

environmental complexity (EC)
  advantages, 28
  and behavioral experience, 27–8
  and functional improvements, 28
  and functional recovery, 40
  manipulating, 27–8
environmental effects
  on functional outcomes after stroke,
  47–53
environmental enrichment
  advantages, 52–3
  and brain disorders, 52
  and brain plasticity, 52
  and brain reorganization, 23
  and dendrites, 47–8
  and dendritic spines, 47–8
  and fetal transplantation, 51
  and forepaw training, 51
  and hippocampus changes, 50
  and interventions, 51–2
  rats, 47
  and somatosensory maps, 48
environmental factors
  and aging, 52–3
Eocene, 68–9
EPCs. *See* endothelial progenitor cells
  (EPCs)
EphB1
  induction, 15
EphB2, 15
ephrin A5
  induction, 13, 15
epidemiological research
  in stroke recovery, 168–9
epidemiological studies
  experimental, 164
  types of, 163–4
epidemiology
  definition, 163
  of stroke recovery, 163–9
epidermal growth factor (EGF), 259,
  267–8
  applications, 41–2
epidural cortical stimulation, 207–8
  in stroke recovery, 208–9
epidural motor cortex stimulation, 7
epileptic patients
  movement control studies, 2
EPO. *See* erythropoietin (EPO)
EPSPs (excitatory postsynaptic
  potentials), 6
error-amplification strategies, 195
erythropoietin (EPO), 259–60, 267–8
  applications, 41–2
  functions, 261
  roles, 17
  in stroke therapies, 261–2
ES. *See* electrical stimulation (ES)
escitalopram, 157
ethnicity

and stroke recovery, 166
Euarchontoglires (Superorder), 67–8
EVEREST Study, 168
evidence-based treatment, 227
evolution
  humans, 68–9
  primates, 67–9
excitatory postsynaptic potentials
  (EPSPs), 6
EXCITE Trial. *See* Extremity
  Constraint Induced Therapy
  Evaluation (EXCITE) Trial
exercise
  and post-stroke depression, 156–7
  in rehabilitation treatments, 79
  wheel-running, 79
exogenous stem cells
  in adult brain after stroke, 268–72
experience
  and post-stroke brain, 23, 30–1
  and repair-based therapies, 174–5
  time-dependent post-stroke
  processes sensitive to, 23–6
extracranial artery
  dissection, 91–2
Extremity Constraint Induced Therapy
  Evaluation (EXCITE) Trial,
  164, 222–3, 227
  age factors, 166
  dosage issues, 165
  and plateau effect, 165–6

FA. *See* fractional anisotropy (FA)
family life
  and post-stroke depression, 154
feedback
  extrinsic, 240, 241
  intrinsic, 240–1,
  and post-stroke motor learning, 240–1
FES. *See* functional electrical
  stimulation (FES)
fetal neocortical cells, 51
fetal transplantation
  and environmental enrichment, 51
fever
  and stroke recovery, 167
FGF (fibroblast growth factor), 259
FGF-2. *See* basic fibroblast growth
  factor (bFGF)
FGF22, 12–13
fibroblast growth factor (FGF), 259
filgratism, 271–2
FIM (Functional Independence
  Measure), 153, 185–6, 197
FLAME trials, 186–7
FL-SMC. *See* forelimb region of rat
  sensorimotor cortex (FL-SMC)
fluanisone
  and neglect recovery, 184
fluoxetine, 153–4, 155, 186

applications, 37, 60, 155
and hemiparesis, 188
FM score. *See* Fugl-Meyer (FM) score
fMRI. *See* functional magnetic
    resonance imaging (fMRI)
focal cerebral ischemia, 259
    and global cerebral ischemia
        compared, 259
focal electrocoagulation
    primates, 71–2
focal ischemic infarcts, 43
    consequences, 126
focused training
    animal studies, 29
    efficacy, 29
forelimb impairment
    functional recovery, 51
    neural outcomes, 78
forelimb movement studies
    animals, 26
    rats, 4, 27, 61, 79
forelimb region of rat sensorimotor
    cortex (FL-SMC)
    electrolytic lesions, 77–8
    injury, 77, 78–9, 80
forelimbs
    disuse, 78–9
    overuse, 78
    stimulation, 59
forepaw training
    and environmental enrichment, 51
fractional anisotropy (FA), 61
    increase, 62
    reduced, 61–2
    stroke recovery studies, 168
fractured somatotopy, 2
Framingham Heart Study, 147
Fugl-Meyer (FM) score
    upper extremity, 196–7, 198
Fugl-Meyer Assessment Scale, 220,
        238, 239
Fugl-Meyer Motor Scale, 185–6
Fugl-Meyer scale, 152
functional brain activation
    animal stroke studies, 58
functional brain imaging
    contributions, 113, 125
functional brain responses
    changes, 60
functional electrical stimulation
    (FES)
    motor cortex-controlled, 253–4
    use of term, 247
functional goals
    vs. treatment, 226
functional imaging, 135
    early studies, 115
functional imaging studies, 94–5
Functional Independence Measure
    (FIM), 153, 185–6, 197

functional magnetic resonance imaging
    (fMRI)
    alternative approaches, 60
    with anesthesia protocols, 59
    animal stroke studies, 58–60
    aphasia studies, 125, 126–7, 128
    applications, 57–8
    hand grip studies, 116, 117
    hemiparesis, 188
    language-specific activation, 127
    limitations, 59
    longitudinal studies, 116–17
    motor system studies, 115
    of post-stroke brain reorganization,
        57–64
    post-stroke studies, 119–20
    principles, 57–8
    procedures, 57–60
    resting-state, 60
    stroke rehabilitation studies, 96
    transcranial direct current
        stimulation studies, 213
    treatment strategy effects, 60
functional mapping studies
    of attention, 136–9
    of spatial neglect, 136–9
functional motor recovery
    mechanistic bases, 67
functional outcomes after stroke
    environmental effects, 47–53
functional recovery
    and environmental complexity, 40
    factors affecting, 26
    following motor cortex injury, 67
    lesion-dependent, 80
    and neurophysiological map
        plasticity, 72–4
functional representations
    changes, 94–5

GABA. *See* gamma-aminobutyric acid
    (GABA)
GABA-benzodiazepine-receptor
    expression, 94
GABAergic agonists, 106
    and stroke therapies, 81–2
GABAergic inhibition
    studies, 107
GABAergic neurotransmission, 95
GADD45
    activation, 14
galanin
    activation, 14
gamma-aminobutyric acid (GABA)
    expression, 94
    and stroke recovery, 184
gap junction intercellular
    communication (GJIC), 270
GAP43, 13
    expression

decrease, 80
    PI3 kinase mediation, 13–14
G-CSF. *See* granulocyte colony-
    stimulating factor (G-CSF)
gender
    and stroke recovery, 166–7
gender differences
    brain injury responses, 38
    post-stroke recovery
        therapies, 38
gene expression, 48–50
    changes, 12–13
gene expression profiling
    and biological meaning, 12–13
    development, 12
gene–environment interactions, 47
genetic factors
    motor map plasticity enhancement, 8
genetics
    and stroke recovery, 166
Genetics and Environmental Risk
        Factors for Hemorrhagic
        Stroke, 163
Gentle-S robot, 200
GJIC (gap junction intercellular
        communication), 270
glia
    injury-induced proliferation, 26
glial cells, 41
global cerebral ischemia
    and focal cerebral ischemia
        compared, 259
gloves
    pneumatic, 199
glutamate
    expression, 94
glutamate/glutamine–creatinine ratios,
        151
glutaminergic synapses, 47
granulocyte colony-stimulating factor
        (G-CSF), 259–60
    functions, 262
    in stroke therapies, 262–3
grasp recovery
    primates, 70
gray matter
    damage, 87–8
Greater Cincinnati/Northern Kentucky
        Stroke Study, 166, 167
    infection studies, 167
growth factors
    applications, 40–1
    classification, 259
    clinical trial designs, 263
    definition, 259
    expression, 259
    in stroke therapies, 259–63
        animal studies, 263
        future trends, 263
        mechanisms, 263

growth inhibitory molecular programs
  post-stroke neuronal sprouting,
    14–15
growth promoting molecular programs
  post-stroke neuronal sprouting,
    13–14

HADS. *See* Hospital Anxiety and
    Depression Scale (HADS)
haloperidol
  and neglect recovery, 184
Hamilton Rating Scale for Depression
    (HRSD), 145, 155, 156
hand grip
  functional magnetic resonance
    imaging studies, 116, 117
hand movements
  and interhemispheric inhibition,
    107–8
  maps, 4
hand neuroprostheses, 251
hand representations, 73
  site changes, 115
  in supplementary motor area, 73–4
Hand Wrist Assistive Rehabilitation
    Device (HWARD), 196,
    197, 200
hand/wrist/forearm exercise
  robotic therapy, 197–8
  robotic vs. non-robotic technologies,
    201
  robotic vs. other therapies,
    199, 200
HDLs (high density lipoproteins), 268
health care management
  post-stroke depression, 156
health care utilization
  and post-stroke depression, 154
Heart and Stroke Foundation of
    Ontario, 223–5
heart disease
  and stroke, 81
Heilman–Mesulam model, 137
hematopoietic growth factor, 259
hematopoietic stem cells (HSCs)
  peripheral blood-derived, 272
  sources, 272
  in stroke recovery, 271
hemidecortication, 70
hemiparesis
  functional magnetic resonance
    imaging, 188
  neuroimaging trials, 188–9
  pharmacology mechanisms, 189
  transcranial magnetic stimulation,
    188–9
hemiplegia
  gait deviation, 248–9
  neuroprostheses, 251
hemiplegic shoulder pain, 250

hemispatial neglect, 133
  and behavioral deficits, 135
  left, 139
  right, 139
hemispheres
  targeting, 211
hemispheric balance
  changing, 117–19
hemodynamic insufficiency, 114
heparin sulfate proteoglycans,
    14–15
HFAC block. *See* high frequency
    alternating current (HFAC)
    block
Hif1, 13–14
high density lipoproteins (HDLs), 268
high frequency alternating current
    (HFAC) block
  mechanisms, 254
  phases, 254
high frequency block
  neuroprostheses, 254
hippocampus
  astrocytes, 50
  changes
    and environmental enrichment, 50
histone
  acetylation, 52
hNT cells
  implantation, 190
Hodgkin–Huxley equations, 254
Hominoidea (apes, humans), 68–9
homotopic contralateral
    somatosensory cortex, 47
Hospital Anxiety and Depression Scale
    (HADS), 146
  emotional status, 152
HRSD (Hamilton Rating Scale for
    Depression), 145, 155
HSCs. *See* hematopoietic stem cells
    (HSCs)
[5-]HT. *See* serotonin
5-HTTLPR, 150, *See* inability to control
    anger or aggression (ICAA)
humans
  cerebral arterial circle, 75
  corticospinal neuron terminations,
    70
  evolution, 68–9
  motor cortex lesions, 67
  and primates compared, 70, 74–5
HWARD (Hand Wrist Assistive
    Rehabilitation Device), 196,
    197, 200
hypercapnia, 114
hypertension
  and stroke, 37, 81
hypokinesia
  directional, 133
hypometabolism, 139

hypothermia
  in stroke therapies, 92

iADL (instrumental activities of daily
    living), 151
IBZ (ischemic boundary zone), 269–70
ICA (internal carotid artery)
  emboli injection, 71
ICAA (inability to control anger or
    aggression), 146–7, 150
ICD-10 (International Classification of
    Diseases), 145
ICF (intracortical facilitation), 110
ICMS. *See* intracortical
    microstimulation (ICMS)
IDAPs (intensity dependence of the
    auditory-evoked potentials),
    150–1
idazoxan
  and motor recovery, 183–4
IFG (inferior frontal gyrus), 125
IGF1, 12–13
IGF2, 12–13
IHI. *See* interhemispheric inhibition
    (IHI)
imaging
  aphasia recovery studies, 125–30
immunosuppression
  and lesion growth, 93–4
impairments
  training focused on, 28–9
IN-1, 7
inability to control anger or aggression
    (ICAA), 146–7, 150
infections
  and stroke recovery, 167
inferior frontal gyrus (IFG), 125
inflammation
  postischemic, 93
  and post-stroke neurogenesis, 17
inflammatory cytokine/chemokine
    signaling
  and post-stroke neurogenesis, 17
information provision
  and post-stroke depression,
    156–7
injuries
  and synaptic changes, 24–5
InMotion2, 197
inosine, 12
instrumental activities of daily living
    (iADL), 151
insula
  infarcts, 89–91
intensity
  concept of, 219, 229
  contemporary approaches, 222–3,
    224
  definitions, 219
  issues, 223–5

literature searches, 220
perspectives, 225–9
and stroke rehabilitation, 219–20
treatment–outcome relationships, 229
Bobath approach, 221–2
Brunnstrom approach, 220
proprioceptive neuromuscular facilitation, 221
intensity dependence of the auditory-evoked potentials (IDAPs), 150–1
intensity of practice, 225
intensive physical therapeutic approaches
to stroke recovery, 219–29
interconnectivity, 2
interhemispheric inhibition (IHI), 110
brain models, 212
characteristics, 107
and hand movements, 107–8
interhemispheric inhibitory interactions, 211
interhemispheric interactions
after stroke
changes, 103–10
and stroke recovery, 107–8
internal carotid artery (ICA)
emboli injection, 71
International Classification of Diseases (ICD-10), 145
International Society for Cellular Therapy, 269
inter-regional interactions
measures, 110
interventions
and behavioral manipulations combined, 29–30
and environmental enrichment, 51–2
intracortical excitability
measures, 110
intracortical facilitation (ICF), 110
intracortical microstimulation (ICMS), 2, 3, 73
applications, 72
hand movement studies, 4
primary motor cortex studies, 6
intrinsic motivation, 228
ipsilateral corticospinal projections
sprouting, 26
ipsilateral motor cortex
active, 125
ipsilesional activity, 116–17
ipsilesional dorsal premotor cortex
activity, 5
disruption, 118
ipsilesional forelimb
impairments, 27
training, 27

ipsilesional hemisphere, 208
activity, 117
ipsilesional motor cortex
increased excitability, 208
ipsilesional motor regions
increased inhibition, 207
ipsilesional sensorimotor cortex
diminished activation, 58
tissue injury, 58–9
irritability, 155
ischemia. *See also* cerebral ischemia
and language function, 125
permanent vs. temporary, 259
ischemic boundary zone (IBZ), 269–70,
ischemic brain damage
diffusion-weighted MRI studies, 60–1
ischemic cortex
reactivation, 90
ischemic critical period. *See also*
juvenile critical period
characterization, 16
future research, 16
importance of, 17–18
post-stroke neuronal sprouting, 16
ischemic injuries
animal models, 80
Italy
post-stroke depression studies, 146, 147

juvenile critical period, 16

knowledge of performance, 240, 241
modalities, 241
knowledge of results, 241
feedback, 241

L300, 252
lacunar infarcts, 91
language function
and ischemia, 125
neural reorganization, 126–7
language network
dysfunction, 125
function, 125
language pathways, 129
language recovery
models, 128
language-specific activation
functional magnetic resonance imaging, 127
laughing
antidepressant treatment, 155
Laurasiatheria (Superorder), 67–8
layer 2/3 pyramidal neurons
abundance, 48
L-dopa, 213
left temporal infarction
longitudinal studies, 127–8

lentiform nucleus
infarcts, 89–91
lesion growth
and immunosuppression, 93–4
lesion–behavior interactions, 27
leukoaraiosis
and stroke recovery, 168
levodopa
and hemiparesis, 189
and stroke recovery, 186
chronic dosage, 186
single dosage, 186
LHS. *See* London Handicap Scale (LHS)
LICI (long interval intracortical inhibition), 106–7, 110
Lokomat robot, 196, 200
London Handicap Scale (LHS), 152
applications, 152
long interval intracortical inhibition (LICI), 106–7, 110
long term depression (LTD), 6, 210–11
long term potentiation (LTP), 6, 210–11
blocking, 212–13
lower limb motor relearning, 248–9
lower limbs
neuroprostheses, 252
LTD (long term depression), 6, 210–11
LTP. *See* long term potentiation (LTP)
lymphocytes
accumulation, 93–4

M1. *See* primary motor cortex
macaques
cerebral arterial circle, 75
corticospinal neuron terminations, 70
endovascular occlusion, 71
evolution, 68–9
grasp recovery, 70
spasticity, 70
macrophages
accumulation, 93–4
MADRS. *See* Montgomery–Asberg Depression Rating Scale (MADRS)
MAG. *See* myelin-associated glycoprotein (MAG)
magnetic resonance imaging (MRI), 57,
See also functional magnetic resonance imaging (fMRI),
See also structural magnetic resonance imaging
activity-induced manganese-dependent, 60
advantages, 64
animal stroke studies, 57
brain infarcts, 88–9
future trends, 64
magnetic-source, 60
measures, 177
perfusion imaging, 88

magnetic resonance imaging (MRI), (cont.)
  post-stroke depression studies, 149
  repair-based stroke trial endpoints, 176
maladaptive behavioral experience, 30
mammals. *See also* rodents
  behavioral repertoires, 39–40
  brain repair after stroke, 77
  cladograms, 68
  phyletic relationships, 67
  Superorders, 67–8
manganese-enhanced magnetic resonance imaging (MEMRI), 60–1
  applications, 63–4
  limitations, 64
  principles, 62
  procedures, 62–4
  variations, 63
maprotiline, 186
MARCKS
  induction, 13–14
marmosets
  corticospinal neuron terminations, 70
  evolution, 69
  NXY-059 studies, 74
matrix metalloproteinases
  expression, 16
  secretion, 17
MCA. *See* middle cerebral artery (MCA)
MCAo. *See* middle cerebral artery occlusion (MCAo)
MCP-1, 17
medial prefrontal cortex regeneration
  rats, 41
MEMOS, 197
MEMRI. *See* manganese-enhanced magnetic resonance imaging (MEMRI)
MEPs. *See* motor evoked potentials (MEPs)
mesenchymal stromal cells (MSCs), 269
Mesulam model, 137
Mesulam target cancellation task, 134
metabolic changes
  in post-stroke depression, 151
methylphenidate
  and hemiparesis, 188
  and motor recovery, 183–4
  and stroke recovery, 185–6
MI. *See also* motor imagery (MI)
Michigan Stroke Registry, 166
microaneurysm clips, 71
microarray analysis, 12
microglia, 50–1
  roles, 35
middle cerebral artery (MCA)
  ligation, 47

occlusion, 38, 53, 89, 93
  embolic, 89–91
  permanent, 92–3
  perfusion–diffusion mismatch, 88
  unilateral occlusion, 58, 63–4
middle cerebral artery occlusion (MCAo)
  advantages, 71
  approaches, 71
  endovascular, 71
  growth factor studies, 260–1, 262
  NXY-059 studies, 74
  primates, 71
  rodents, 49, 267–8
  timing factors, 80
MIME device, 198–9
Mini-Mental State Examination (MMSE), 146
Miocene, 68–9
miotic cells, 50
mirtazapine, 157
MIT-MANUS, 196, 197, 199, 200
MMSE (Mini-Mental State Examination), 146
moclobemide
  and stroke recovery, 187
modified Rankin Scale, 153, 178
moesin
  activation, 14
molecular mechanisms
  of neuronal repair after stroke, 11–18
monkeys, *See also* squirrel monkeys; macaques; marmosets
  evolution, 68–9
  hand movement studies, 4
  New World, 68–9
  Old World, 68–9
  stroke studies, 263
monoaminergic drugs
  and hemiparesis, 188
monoamines
  roles, 189
Montgomery–Asberg Depression Rating Scale (MADRS), 145
  reliability, 146
motivation, 227–8
  enhancement, 228
  intrinsic, 228
  psychological theories of, 228
motor areas
  retraining, 5–6
  roles, 4–5
motor behavior
  animal models, 1
motor compensation
  use of term, 3
motor cortex
  focal lesions, 6
  and motor relearning, 247
motor cortex injury

functional recovery, 67
motor cortex lesions
  cellular genesis, 42
  humans, 67
motor cortex organization
  primates, 72
motor cortex reorganization
  neural bases of
    synaptic plasticity, 6
motor evoked potentials (MEPs), 2, 94, 95, 177, 207
  amplitude, 103–4, 109
    reduction, 104
  and corticospinal system, 3
  interpretation issues, 103
  latency, 109
  maximal, 109
  in post-stroke recovery studies, 119
  production, 103
  recording, 109
motor function
  recovered
    anatomical substrates of, 115–16
  recovery
    and amphetamines, 185
  rehabilitation, 234–5
motor function improvement
  animal models, 105
  neural substrates for, 1–8
motor imagery (MI), 238–40
  affected arm impairment reduction, 238
  affected leg retraining after stroke, 239
  chronic stroke studies, 239
  definition, 238
  efficacy
    for affected arm in stroke, 238–9
  mechanisms, 239–40
  neural mechanisms, 238
  reaching kinematics improvement, 238–9
motor improvement
  and motor map reorganization, 6
  neural strategies, 4
motor learning. *See also* post-stroke motor learning
  ability
    studies, 235–6
  implicit, 235
  in stroke rehabilitation, 236
    implications, 236
motor map organization
  principles, 2–3
motor map plasticity, 1–8
  importance of, 8,
  as model
    for post-stroke functional improvement studies, 1

promotion
    adjuvant therapies, 7–8
    and synaptogenesis, 6
motor map plasticity enhancement
    cortical stimulation, 7–8
    pharmacological stimulation, 7
motor map reorganization
    determinants, 6
    and motor improvement, 6
motor maps
    animal models, 1
    post-stoke, 113–20
    recruitment, 6
    restoration, 4, 6
    retraining, 6
motor practice, 119, 233
motor recovery
    and norepinephrine, 183
    stroke rehabilitation
        active participation, 234–5
    use of term, 3
motor rehabilitation, 4, 5, 7
    roles, 4
motor relearning, 247–9
    definition, 247
    future trends, 249
    lower limb, 248–9
    and motor cortex, 247
    principles, 247–8
    theoretical issues, 247–8
    upper limb, 248
motor representations
    changes, 106
motor skill learning
    and synaptic potentiation, 6
motor skill training
    efficacy, 29
motor system. See also cortical motor
        system
    functional imaging
        early studies, 115
    physiology, 108
    post-stroke brain reorganization,
        115
    post-stroke human brain mapping,
        113–20
    reconfiguration
        and brain injuries, 120
motor threshold (MT), 103–4, 109
    changes
        factors affecting, 104
motor training
    effects on primary motor cortex
        functional topography, 72–3
    squirrel monkeys, 72–3
mouse cortex
    cell behavior, 48
mouse models
    Alzheimer's disease, 52
movement

post-stroke rehabilitation, 195
movement control
    early studies, 2
movement representations
    reorganization, 7
    restoration, 7
    and retraining, 6
    topography, 1
movement tracking games, 201
movement training
    robotic vs. non-robotic, 196
movements
    assisting patients to complete, 202
    coding, 133
moyamoya disease, 92
MRI. See magnetic resonance imaging
        (MRI)
MSCs (mesenchymal stromal cells), 269
MT. See motor threshold (MT)
music
    and post-stroke depression, 156–7
myelin-associated glycoprotein
        (MAG), 14–15
    induction, 15
myelin-associated inhibitory factors, 7

NARIs. See noradrenaline reuptake
        inhibitors (NARIs)
NARP, 12
National Institute of Neurological
        Disorders and Stroke (NINDS)
        tPA Study Group, 167
NDT (neurodevelopmental treatment),
        219–20
neglect. See also spatial neglect
    anatomical bases, 135–9
    anatomical studies, 135
    brain mapping
        after stroke, 133–41
    cerebral blood flow studies, 139
    and dorsal network abnormalities,
        137–9
    future research, 140–1
    occurrence, 133–4
    post-stroke recovery, 140
        neural correlates, 139
    subtypes, 133, 135, 140
    treatment
        and neuroimaging, 141,
        and ventral network damage, 137–9
neglect recovery
    and dopaminergic drugs, 184
neocortex
    neuroblasts in, 50–1
Neogene, 68–9
NeReBot, 197
nerve growth factor (NGF)
    applications, 40–1
nerve growth factor-induced gene A
        (NGFI-A)

down regulation, 49–50
    expression, 48–9
nerve growth factor-induced gene B
        (NGFI-B)
    expression, 48–9
network approach
    and aphasia, 129–30
neural mechanisms
    and electrical stimulation, 43
neural plasticity
    animal studies, 26–7
neural progenitor cells (NPCs)
    generation, 268–9
    localization, 267
neural reorganization
    of language function, 126–7
neural repair
    after stroke
        cellular concepts, 11–12
    mechanisms, 17–18
neural stem cells (NSCs)
    applications, 41
    generation, 268–9
    localization, 267
    tissue-specific
        in stroke recovery, 268–9
    trials, 189–90
neural strategies
    for post-stroke motor improvement,
        3–6
neural substrates
    for motor function improvement,
        1–8
neural tissue
    loss of, 1
neuroanatomical plasticity
    after cortical injury, 74
neuroblasts
    in neocortex, 50–1
neurocan
    induction, 15
neurochemicals
    and synaptic plasticity, 7
neurodegenerative cascade,
        35–6,
neurodevelopmental treatment (NDT),
        219–20
neurogenesis, 11, 48–50
    and angiogenesis, 268
    effects on, 267–8
    and environment, 50–1
    induction, 12
    inhibition, 17
    mechanisms, 267
neurogenesis and angiogenesis, 12
neuroglia
    classification, 50–1
neuroimaging
    and neglect treatment, 141,
    and pharmacology, 187–9

neuroimaging (cont.)
  in post-stroke depression,
      149–50
  technologies, 57
  trials
      in aphasia, 187–8
      in hemiparesis, 188–9
neurological traits
  humans and primates compared, 74–5
neuromodulatory agents
  and non-invasive brain stimulation,
      212–13
  and transcranial direct current
      stimulation, 213
neuromuscular electrical stimulation
      (NMES), 247, See also
      electromyographically (EMG)
      mediated neuromuscular
      electrical stimulation (NMES),
      See also cyclic neuromuscular
      electrical stimulation, See also
      neuroprostheses
  implanted, 250
  in motor relearning, 247–8
  types of, 247–8
neuromuscular treatment techniques, 220
  issues, 226–7
neuronal growth cone function, 12
neuronal network remodeling, 37
neuronal networks
  mapping, 63–4
neuronal plasticity
  factors affecting, 26
neuronal repair
  molecular mechanisms
      after stroke, 11–18
neuronal stem cells
  roles, 41–2
neuronal tracing, 64
neurons
  generation, 268–9
  migration, 12
  regeneration, 14, 87–8
neuropharmacology
  animal models, 183–5
      experimental studies, 184–5
  clinical trials, 185–7
  in stroke recovery, 183–90
neurophysiological maps
  derivation, 72
  plasticity
      and functional recovery, 72–4
neurophysiological studies
  stroke patients, 207
neuropilin 1
  induction, 13, 15
neuroplastic mechanisms
  in central nervous system, 1
neuroplasticity
  diffusion tensor imaging studies, 62

mechanisms
  animal studies, 67
  and robot-assisted movement
      therapy, 195–6
neuroprostheses, 247–8, 251–3
  applications
      lower limbs, 252
      upper limbs, 251
  brace-transcutaneous, 248
  brain-controlled interfaces, 253–4
  cost effectiveness, 249
  developments, 253–4
  future trends, 252–3
  goals, 251
  hand, 251
  high frequency block, 254
  implanted, 251
  upper limb motor leaning, 248
  use of term, 247
neuroprotectants. See neuroprotective
      agents
neuroprotection, 73
  failure, 92
  field of study, 36
neuroprotective agents, 92, 184
  applications, 35–6
neurotrophic factors, 48–50
  production, 40–1
neurotrophins, 259
  applications, 26
neurovascular coupling, 59
  mechanisms, 113
New World monkeys, 68–9
NG2, 14–15
NGF. See nerve growth factor (NGF)
NGFb, 12–13
NGFI-A. See nerve growth factor-
      induced gene A (NGFI-A)
NGFI-B. See nerve growth factor-
      induced gene B (NGFI-B)
nicotine
  applications, 40
NIH Stroke Scale, 167, 178
NINDS. See National Institute of
      Neurological Disorders and
      Stroke (NINDS)
NMES. See neuromuscular electrical
      stimulation (NMES)
Nogo
  applications, 26
  expression, 16
Nogo-A, 7, 12, 14–15
  induction, 13
noise
  random, 213
nondysphoric depression, 150
non-human primates. See primates
non-invasive brain stimulation
  efficacy, 213–14
  and neuromodulatory agents, 212–13

and sensorimotor activities, 212–13
noninvasive testing, 103
non-lateralized deficits
  and neglect, 137
non-pharmacological treatment
  post-stroke depression, 156
non-robotic technology
  and robotic technology compared,
      201
noradrenaline reuptake inhibitors
      (NARIs), 154
  post-stroke depression treatment,
      155
norepinephrine
  and motor recovery, 183
norepinephrine agonists
  experimental studies, 184
  and stroke recovery, 183–4
norepinephrine antagonists
  experimental studies, 184
  and stroke recovery, 183–4
Northstar Neuroscience, Inc., 234
nortriptyline, 153–4
  applications, 155
Notch pathway, 13
NPCs. See neural progenitor cells
      (NPCs)
NSCs. See neural stem cells (NSCs)
NT2N cells
  implantation, 190
nucleus basalis of Meynert
  lesioning, 6
NudelHolz device, 201
NXY-059, 74

Odstock Dropped Foot Stimulator, 252
OECs (olfactory ensheathing cells)
  in stroke recovery, 272
OKS (optokinetic stimulation), 140
Old World monkeys, 68–9
olfactory ensheathing cells (OECs)
  in stroke recovery, 272
olfactory nerve fibroblasts (ONFs), 272
Oligocene, 68–9
oligodendrocyte myelin glycoprotein
      (OMgp), 14–15
oligodendrocytes, 50–1
OMgp (oligodendrocyte myelin
      glycoprotein), 14–15
ONFs (olfactory nerve fibroblasts), 272
OP-1. See osteogenic protein-1 (OP-1)
optokinetic stimulation (OKS), 140
osteogenic protein-1 (OP-1), 259–60
  functions, 261
  in stroke therapies, 261

p21/waf1
  induction, 13–14
Paleogene, 68–9
paraplegia, 251

paresis, 113
Parkinson's degeneration
  rat models, 30
paroxetine, 184
participation. *See also* restricted
      participation
  and post-stroke depression,
      152–3
  and stroke rehabilitation for motor
      recovery, 234–5
pathological crying
  antidepressant treatment, 155
Paul Coverdell National Acute Stroke
      Registry, 163
PBPCs. *See* peripheral blood progenitor
      cells (PBPCs)
PEDro, 220
perfusion imaging, 88
  applications, 88–9
perfusion–diffusion mismatch
  relevance to prognosis and repair,
      88–9
peri-infarct cortex
  axonal sprouting, 12
  tissue survival, 115
perilesion cortex
  degeneration, 30
perilesional motor cortex
  tissue repair, 58
perilesional motor cortex activity
  reinstatement, 58
perilesional somatosensory cortex
  enhanced activity, 60
perineuronal nets, 16
  reduction, 16
peripheral blood progenitor cells
      (PBPCs)
  in stroke recovery, 271–2
  transplantation, 271–2
PET. *See* positron emission
      tomography (PET)
pharmacological magnetic resonance
      imaging (phMRI), 60
pharmacological stimulation
  motor map plasticity
      enhancement, 7
pharmacology. *See also*
      neuropharmacology
  mechanisms
    hemiparesis, 189
  and neuroimaging, 187–9
  and stem cells, 189–90
phenobarbital
  and motor recovery, 184
phenoxybenzamine
  and motor recovery, 184
phentermine
  and motor recovery, 183–4
phenylpropanolamine
  and motor recovery, 183–4

phenytoin
  and motor recovery, 184
  and stroke recovery, 167
phMRI (pharmacological magnetic
      resonance imaging), 60
phosphocan
  induction, 15
photocoagulation, 71
phyletic relationships
  mammals, 67
physiological measures
  and treatment strategies, 108–9
physiotherapy
  and acute stroke trials, 174
  outside, 174–5
PI3 kinase
  mediation, 13–14
piracetam
  and aphasia, 187–8
  and stroke recovery, 187
plasticity, 3
  stimulation
    and robotic therapy, 202
  in treatments
    initiation, 36
plateau effect
  in stroke recovery, 165–6
PMd. *See* dorsal premotor cortex
      (PMd)
PMv. *See* ventral premotor cortex
      (PMv)
pneumatic gloves, 199
Pneu-WREX, 196, 200
PNF. *See* proprioceptive
      neuromuscular facilitation
      (PNF)
polydendrocytes
  NG2-positive, 50–1
Porch Index of Communicative Ability,
      185
positron emission tomography (PET), 57
  aphasia studies, 128
  applications, 177
  motor system studies, 115
  serial, 187–8
Posner spatial orienting task, 134,
      138, 140
post-injury pharmacological
      manipulations
  and behavioral training, 29–30
post-ischemic inflammatory
      infiltration, 93–4
post-stroke axonal sprouting, 15
post-stroke brain
  and endogenous stem cells, 267–8
  and exogenous stem cells,
      268–72
  and experience, 23, 30–1
  and progenitor cells, 267–72,
post-stroke brain reorganization, 174

functional magnetic resonance
      imaging, 57–64
  motor system, 115
  structural magnetic resonance
      imaging, 57–64
post-stroke brain repair. *See* brain
      repair after stroke
post-stroke deficits
  and stroke recovery patterns, 165
post-stroke depression
  and anxiety
    lesion locational issues, 149–50
  cause and effect, 147–51
  comorbidities, 148
  consequences, 158
  diagnosis, 145–6
  effects, 145–59
    studies, 149
  on activities of daily living, 151–2
  epidemiological reasoning, 147–9
  etiology, 147–8
  evolution, 146–7
    causes, 148–9
  and exercise, 156–7
  and family life, 154
  frequency, 146–7
  future research, 158
  health care management, 156
  and health care utilization, 154
  incidence, 146
  and information provision, 156–7
  issues, 154
  metabolic changes, 151
  and music, 156–7
  neuroimaging evidence, 149–50
  neuroscience reasoning, 149–51
  and participation, 152–3
  prevalence, 146
  prevention
    prophylactic antidepressant
        treatment, 157
    strategies, 156–7
  and quality of life, 152–3
  recovery implications, 151–4
  risk factors, 158
  and serotonergic system, 150–1
  treatment
    antidepressants, 154–5
    effects on activities of daily living,
        153–4
    non-pharmacological, 156
    options, 154–7, 158
post-stroke effects
  degenerative responses, 23
  regenerative responses, 23
post-stroke emotional disorders
  treatment
    antidepressant, 155
post-stroke emotional symptoms
  frequency, 146–7

post-stroke fatigue
  etiology, 147–8
  frequency, 147
  risk factors, 148
  studies, 155
post-stroke functional improvements
  studies
    motor map plasticity as model
      for, 1
post-stroke interventions
  primate studies, 74
post-stroke mortality
  and antidepressant treatment, 153–4
post-stroke motor improvement
  motor map plasticity, 1–8
  neural strategies for, 3–6
post-stroke motor learning, 235–6
  action observation, 237–8
  auditory stimuli, 237
  cognitive approaches, 236–41
  and feedback, 240–1
  information/instruction provision,
    236–40
  verbal information, 236–7
post-stroke neurogenesis, 16–17
  induction, 12
  and inflammation, 17
  and inflammatory cytokine/
    chemokine signaling, 17
  occurrence, 17
post-stroke neuronal events
  behavioral influences, 23–31
post-stroke neuronal sprouting
  growth inhibitory molecular
    programs, 14–15
  growth promoting molecular
    programs, 13–14
  ischemic critical period, 16
post-stroke personality changes, 147
post-stroke recovery
  availability, 38
  and brain reorganization, 116–17
  cause and effects, 158
  mechanisms, 116
  from neglect, 140
  predicting, 119–20
  treatment, 158
  upper limb function, 113, 117
post-stroke recovery research
  rodents, 35
post-stroke recovery therapies,
  end point measures, 38–9
  age factors, 36–7
  in animals, 35–44
  astrocytes, 42
  cell-based, 41–3
  electrical stimulation, 43
  enrichment issues, 40
  experience issues, 40
  gender differences, 38

hormonal status, 38
intensity issues, 35–6
issues, 35–40
measurement issues, 38–40
organismal factors, 36–8
pharmacotherapy, 40–1
plasticity, 36
sex status, 38
timing issues, 35–6
and vascular system, 42–3
post-stroke rehabilitation
  of movement, 195
post-stroke shoulder pain, 249–51
  electrical stimulation
    future trends, 250–1
    intramuscular systems,
      249–50
    surface systems, 249
    theoretical issues, 249
prazosin
  and motor recovery, 184
pre-clinical stroke research
  old animals, 81
  young animals, 81,
premotor cortex, 115–16
prenatal infarct, 115
pre-stroke fatigue
  risk factors, 148
primary motor cortex, 115–16
  BOLD responses, 113–14
  functional organization, 6
  functional topography
    and motor training, 72–3
  functions, 1
  infarctions, 5
  lesions, 5
  movement representations, 1
  premotor areas, 72
  primates, 72
primary sensorimotor cortex
  damage, 120
  ischemic damage prevention, 60
primate brains
  corticospinal neurons, 70, 72
  corticospinal tract, 69–70
  injury, 69
  size, 69
  stroke recovery research, 69–70
  white matter–gray matter ratios, 69
primates. See also monkeys
  as animal models, 69
    issues, 69
  anthropoid, 68–9
  aspiration lesions, 70–1
  cladograms, 68
  encephalization of function, 70
  evolution, 67–9
  focal electrocoagulation, 71–2
  grasp recovery, 70
  and humans compared, 70, 74–5

middle cerebral artery occlusion, 71
motor cortex organization, 72
post-stroke intervention studies, 74
primary motor cortex, 72
secondary motor areas, 115–16
spasticity, 70
strepsirrhine, 68–9
stroke models, 70–2
stroke recovery
  comparative perspectives, 67–75
stroke recovery studies, 67–70
  practical and ethical issues, 69
progenitor cells. See also endothelial
  progenitor cells (EPCs), See also
  peripheral blood progenitor
  cells (PBPCs)
  in adult brain after stroke, 267–72,
  factors affecting, 267–8
prognosis
  and perfusion–diffusion mismatch,
    88–9
proprioceptive neuromuscular
  facilitation (PNF)
  and stroke outcomes, 221
  treatment–outcome relationships, 221
propriospinal projections, 116
protease activity
  roles, 17
  upregulation, 16
proton magnetic resonance
  spectroscopy, 151
psychoactive drugs
  and stroke therapies, 81–2
psychomotor stimulants
  applications, 40
pyramidal neurons
  dendritic morphology, 48
pyrexia, 167

quality of life (QoL)
  factors affecting, 53
  and post-stroke depression, 152–3

race
  and stroke recovery, 166
random effects analysis, 115
random noise, 213
range of motion (ROM)
  lateral, 249
rat models
  Parkinson's degeneration, 30
rats
  acrobatic tasks, 28–9, 49
  brain imaging, 62
  brain maps, 63
  cortical stimulation studies, 29–30
  cortical transplants, 51
  and environmental enrichment, 47
  exercise
    forced vs. voluntary, 79

fMRI stroke studies, 58–60
forelimb movement studies, 4, 27,
    61, 79
forelimb stimulation, 59
medial prefrontal cortex
    regeneration, 41
neural plasticity studies, 26–7
skilled reaching, 29
stroke studies
    age factors, 36–7
transcranial direct current
    stimulation, 209
rCBF. See regional cerebral blood flow
    (rCBF)
RCs. See recruitment curves (RCs)
reaching kinematics
    improvement, 238–9
reach-to-grasp. See skilled reaching
Reasons for Geographic And Racial
    Differences in Stroke
    (REGARDS) Study, 164
reboxetine, 155
    and hemiparesis, 188–9
    and stroke recovery, 187
recanalization
    in acute stroke therapies, 89
    early, 93
    rapid, 93
recombinant tissue plasminogen
    activator (rtPA), 92
recovery
    and social complexity, 30
recruitment, 4–6,
    motor maps, 6
    use of term, 4–5
recruitment curves (RCs), 109
    gradient, 109
reference electrodes
    locational issues, 210
REGARDS (Reasons for Geographic
    And Racial Differences in
    Stroke) Study, 164
regenerative processes
    brain, 24
regenerative responses, 23
    and behavioral experience
        manipulations, 23–4
regional cerebral blood flow (rCBF), 87
    increase, 260
rehabilitation. See also motor
        rehabilitation
    use of term, 113
rehabilitation training, 4
rehabilitation treatments
    acquired brain injury, 233–4
    exercise, 79
    factors affecting, 77
    gains, 119
    intensity issues, 77–80
    limitations, 77

optimal timing issues, 77–80
    and stroke recovery, 164
    and transcranial direct current
        stimulation, 212–13
rehabilitative training
    and brain reorganization, 23
religious beliefs
    and stroke, 148
repair-based stroke trials
    and acute stroke trials, 173–4
    and acute stroke trials compared, 174
    and animal studies, 174
    baseline measures, 175
    and biomarkers, 176–8
    blinding issues, 175
    covariates, 175
    and drugs, 175
    endpoints, 175, 176
        domain-specific, 176,
    study design issues, 175
    surrogate markers, 176–7
repair-based therapies
    and environment, 174–5
    and experience, 174–5
    and training, 174–5
reparative processes
    brain, 43–4
reperfusion injury, 92–3
repetitive transcranial magnetic
        stimulation (rTMS), 207–8
    applications, 128–9
    in stroke recovery, 208
    studies, 156
    thrombolysis, 183
repetitive-task practice (RTP), 234,
    approaches, 234
restoration, 3–4, 5–6
    motor maps, 4, 6
    movement representations, 7
    use of term, 3
restricted participation
    determinants, 152
retarded depression, 155,
retinal ganglion cell (RGC), 14
retraining, 5–6
    motor maps, 6
    and movement representations, 6
RGC (retinal ganglion cell), 14
rhesus monkeys
    stroke studies, 263
Rho kinase
    inhibition, 13–14
right hemisphere injury
    and spatial neglect, 136
rightward spatial bias
    and neglect, 137
Riks-Stroke Registry, 166
Rivermead Motor Assessment, 186
Robo, 15
robot-assisted movement therapy

efficacy, 195–6
    research, 195
robotic approaches
    to stroke recovery, 195–203
robotic arm trainers, 197
robotic movements
    naturalistic, 202
robotic technology
    and non-robotic technology
        compared, 201
robotic therapy
    acute stroke survivors, 197
    arm exercise, 197
    benefits, 201–2
    definition, 195
    future research, 202–3
    hand/wrist/forearm exercise,
        197–8
    intense, 202
    optimization, 202–3
    and plasticity stimulation, 202
robotic therapy devices
    advantages, 195
    applications, 195
    clinical studies, 196–8
    design goals
        evaluation, 202
    and non-robot therapies
        compared
        no differences, 198–9
        robotic benefits, 199–200
    publications, 196
robots
    definition, 195
rocking chairs, 201
rodent models
    axonal sprouting, 11
    basic fibroblast growth factor in
        stroke therapies, 260–1
    disadvantages, 70
    granulocyte colony-stimulating
        factor in stroke therapies,
        262
    osteogenic protein-1 in stroke
        therapies, 261
    stroke, 263
rodents. See also rats
    middle cerebral artery occlusion, 49,
        267–8
    post-stroke recovery research, 35
ROM (range of motion)
    lateral, 249
rTMS. See repetitive transcranial
    magnetic stimulation
    (rTMS)
RTP. See repetitive-task practice
    (RTP)
rtPA (recombinant tissue plasminogen
    activator), 92
Rutgers Glove, 197

SADQ (Stroke Aphasic Depression Questionnaire), 146
saliency maps, 133
Scandinavian Stroke Scale, 153
SCF (stem cell factor), 267–8
SCG10, 13–14, 15
SCILT (Spinal Cord Injury Locomotor Trial), 222–3
SCLIP, 13–14
SDF-1 (stromal-cell-derived factor 1), 17, 269
secondary motor areas
    primates, 115–16
    projections, 116
seizures
    and stroke, 37–8
selection, 133
selective attention
    use of term, 133
selective serotonin reuptake inhibitors (SSRIs), 151, 154
    applications, 37
    post-stroke depression treatment, 155
    and stroke recovery, 186–7
        chronic dosage, 186
        pending studies, 186–7
        single dosage, 186
self-efficacy, 228
self-esteem
    and depression, 148
self-taught behavioral change
    and brain reorganization, 26–7
semaphorin 3a
    induction, 15,
Sensorimotor Active Rehabilitation Training (SMART) Arm, 201
sensorimotor activities
    and non-invasive brain stimulation, 212–13
serotonergic pathway
    studies, 188
serotonergic system
    and post-stroke depression, 150–1
serotonin
    roles, 189
sertraline, 157
SGZ (subgranular zone), 267
short interval intracortical inhibition (SICI), 106, 110
    contralesional hemisphere studies, 107
    spatial distribution, 106–7
shoulder pain. *See also* post-stroke shoulder pain
    hemiplegic, 250
SICI. *See* short interval intracortical inhibition (SICI)
signal-to-noise ratio (SNR)
    reduced, 114–15

sildenafil, 62, 267–8
silent period
    use of term, 95
skilled reaching
    animal models, 29
    improvements, 29
skills, 227–8
SLF (superior longitudinal fasciculus)
    lesions, 135
Slit, 15
SMA. *See* supplementary motor area (SMA)
SMART (Sensorimotor Active Rehabilitation Training) Arm, 201
SNR (signal-to-noise ratio)
    reduced, 114–15
social complexity
    and recovery, 30
socio-economic factors
    and stroke recovery, 168
somatosensory evoked potentials, 95
somatosensory maps
    and environmental enrichment, 48
spasticity
    after cortical injury, 70
    primates, 70
spatial attention
    definition, 133
spatial neglect, 133–4, *See also* hemispatial neglect
    functional mapping studies, 136–9
    models, 137
    and right hemisphere injury, 136
    tests, 134
spatial orienting
    biases, 139
Spaulding, S. J., 234
speech
    spontaneous, 129–30
Spinal Cord Injury Locomotor Trial (SCILT), 222–3
SPIO (superparamagnetic iron oxide) particles, 190
spiroperidol
    and neglect recovery, 184
SPRR1, 12, 13
SPRR1a
    activation, 14
squirrel monkeys
    corticospinal neuron terminations, 70
    evolution, 69
    forelimb movement studies, 26
    motor training, 72–3
    primary motor cortex infarctions, 5, 74
    skilled reaching, 29
SSRIs. *See* selective serotonin reuptake inhibitors (SSRIs)

STAIR consensus conference, 74
Stat3, 14
statins, 267–8
stem cell factor (SCF), 267–8
stem cells. *See also* neural stem cells (NSCs), *See also* hematopoietic stem cells (HSCs)
    adipose tissue-derived, 272
    characterization, 268
    definition, 267
    factors affecting, 267–8
    and pharmacology, 189–90
    tagging, 190
    trials, 189–90
stimulation targets
    defining, 208
stimulus–response mapping, 133
strepsirrhine primates, 68–9
stroke
    acute period, 87
    age factors, 36–7
    and anger, 146–7
    and anxiety, 146
    and behavioral impairments, 1
    and brain ischemia, 87
    classification, 89
    comorbidities, 37–8, 81
        and stroke recovery, 167–8
    damage quantification, 103–5
    and dementia, 149
    and emotional disorders, 145
    epidemiological studies
        types of, 163–4
    incidence, 77, 173
    mechanisms, 35
    modeling, 38
    molecular mechanisms of neuronal repair, 11–18
    nature of
        and acute treatment, 167
    prevalence, 173
    and religious beliefs, 148
    risk factors
        depression, 147
    rodent models, 263
    and seizures, 37–8
    types of, 89–92
        pathogenesis, 90
    and vascular dementia, 52
Stroke Aphasic Depression Questionnaire (SADQ), 146
stroke evolution
    determinants, 88–9
stroke heterogeneity
    animal–human translation issues, 80–1
stroke models
    primates, 70–2
stroke outcomes
    and Bobath approach, 222

and Brunnstrom approach, 221
models, 169
and proprioceptive neuromuscular
facilitation, 221
stroke pathophysiology
imaging technologies, 57
stroke patients
contralesional motor cortex activity, 5
emotional symptoms, 145
neurophysiological studies, 207
survival issues, 81
stroke recovery
and activation patterns, 95
affected hemisphere, 105–7
bone marrow stromal cells in, 269–71
cellular approaches, 267–73
cognitive approaches, 233–42
contralesional hemisphere, 107
electrical stimulation, 247–54
future trends, 254
electromagnetic approaches, 207–14
epidemiological research
importance of, 168–9
epidemiology, 163–9
definition, 163
epidural cortical stimulation, 208–9
intensive physical therapeutic
approaches, 219–29
interhemispheric interactions, 107–8
neuropharmacology in, 183–90
outcomes, 169
patterns, 164–6
and post-stroke deficits, 165
plateau effect, 165–6
predictors, 168–9,
primate brain studies, 69–70
primate studies, 67–70
practical and ethical issues, 69
primates
comparative perspectives, 67–75
and rehabilitation treatments, 164
repetitive transcranial magnetic
stimulation, 208
robotic approaches, 195–203
specific factors, 166–8
integration, 168
statistics, 164
therapeutic options, 267
time factors, 164–5
tissue-specific neural stem cells in,
268–9
transcranial direct current
stimulation, 209–11
transcranial magnetic stimulation
studies, 105–8
stroke recovery research
animal–human translation issues,
77–82
stroke recovery-promoting agents, 259
stroke registries

epidemiological studies, 163
stroke rehabilitation
approaches, 108
early commencement, 95–6
and intensity, 219–20
motor learning strategies, 236
implications, 236
for motor recovery
active participation, 234–5
requirements, 52
stroke survivors
impairment variations, 38
medications, 37
stroke therapies. See also acute stroke
therapies
approved, 173
dosage issues, 165
drug issues, 81–2
growth factors, 259–63
selection issues, 82
timing issues, 87
stroke units
advantages, 53
stromal-cell-derived factor 1 (SDF-1),
17, 269
structural magnetic resonance imaging
of post-stroke brain reorganization,
57–64
procedures, 60–4
structural plasticity, 11
subcortical aphasia, 125–6
subgranular zone (SGZ), 267
subventricular zone (SVZ), 12, 267, 270
astrocytes, 50
cell proliferation, 16–17, 268–9
proliferating cells, 50
Sunnybrook Stroke Study, 167
superior longitudinal fasciculus (SLF)
lesions, 135
superparamagnetic iron oxide (SPIO)
particles, 190
supplementary motor area (SMA), 72,
115–16
hand representations, 73–4
surface peroneal nerve stimulation, 252
SVZ. See subventricular zone (SVZ)
Sweden
post-stroke depression studies,
146, 148
Riks-Stroke Registry, 166
synapses
growth, 27
synaptic changes
and injuries, 24–5
synaptic efficacy
changes, 6
synaptic plasticity, 7, 103
animal studies, 94
and motor cortex reorganization, 6
signaling pathways, 7

synaptic potentiation
and motor skill learning, 6
synaptic strength
changes, 6
synaptogenesis, 268
and motor map plasticity, 6

task parameter modulation
and task-related activities, 118
task-related activities
and task parameter modulation, 118
task-specific training, 229
TBI (traumatic brain injury), 233
tDCS. See transcranial direct cortical
stimulation (tDCS)
temporo-parietal junction (TPJ) cortex,
136, 140
damage, 135
tenascin, 14–15
tetraplegia, 251
neuroprostheses, 251,
brain-controlled interfaces, 253
TGFb pathway, 13
TGFb1, 12–13
TGF-β (transforming growth factor-β),
259
therapeutic electricity
concept of, 207
historical background, 207
thrombolysis, 87, 91, 92
in acute stroke therapies, 88
Tie2, 268
time-dependent post-stroke processes
experience sensitive, 23–6
tissue loss
compensation strategies, 37
TMS. See transcranial magnetic
stimulation (TMS)
TOAST Study, 167
total map area, 109–10
total map volume, 109–10
tPA
mechanisms, 16
TPJ cortex. See temporo-parietal
junction (TPJ) cortex
training
bilateral, 202
focused on impairments, 28–9
and repair-based therapies,
174–5
task-specific, 229
timing factors, 29
transcallosal disinhibition, 107
transcallosal projections
degeneration, 27
transcranial direct current stimulation
(tDCS)
functional magnetic resonance
imaging studies, 213
setup, 210

transcranial direct current stimulation (tDCS), 7
advantages, 209
applications, 207
effects on brain tissue, 210–11
and neuromodulatory agents, 213
and rehabilitation treatments, 212–13
in stroke recovery, 209–11
safety issues, 210
transcranial magnetic stimulation (TMS), 2, 94, 95, 118, 207–8
advantages, 108
applications, 2, 141, 207
corticospinal excitability measures, 109–10
disruption induction, 5
hemiparesis, 188–9
inter-regional interactions measures, 110
intracortical excitability measures, 110
limitations, 104
map center of gravity, 105–6, 109–10
measures, 106
improvements over time, 105
issues, 105
motor map restoration, 4
paired-pulse, 95
principles, 109
recovery mechanism studies, 105–8
stroke damage quantification, 103–5
stroke rehabilitation studies, 96
techniques, 106
virtual lesion studies, 108
transcutaneous peroneal nerve stimulators, 252
transforming growth factor-β (TGF-β), 259
transient receptor potential (trp) channels, 35–6
transplantation
of lost cells, 41
traumatic brain injury (TBI), 233
trazodone
and motor recovery, 184
treatment
evidence-based, 227
vs. functional goals, 226
treatment strategies
and physiological measures, 108–9
trp (transient receptor potential) channels, 35–6

T-WREX, 196, 201
type I stroke, 89
type II stroke, 89–91, 94
type III stroke, 91
type IV stroke, 91–2
type IV-specific phosphodiesterase (PDE 4) inhibitors, 7
Tα1 tubulin
activation, 13–14

UCBCs (umbilical cord blood cells)
in stroke recovery, 272
umbilical cord blood cells (UCBCs)
in stroke recovery, 272
United Kingdom (UK)
neuroprostheses, 252
United States (US)
electrical stimulation, 252
epidemiological studies, 169
post-stroke depression studies, 151–2
United States Food and Drug Administration, 252
upper extremity motor performance
and constraint induced movement therapy, 3
upper extremity rehabilitation, 220
gains, 198
problem solving issues, 226
professional attitudes, 225–6
upper limb function
post-stroke recovery, 113, 117
upper limb motor relearning, 248
upper limbs
neuroprostheses, 251

Val66Met polymorphism, 49–50, 148
vascular dementia
and stroke, 52
vascular endothelial growth factor (VEGF), 267–8
vascular system
and post-stroke recovery therapies, 42–3
VECTORS (Very Early Constraint-Induced Movement during Stroke Rehabilitation) Trial, 165, 174
VEGF (vascular endothelial growth factor), 267–8
VEGF1, 13
VEGF2, 13

ventral frontal cortex (VFC), 136
ventral network
damage
and neglect, 137–9
ventral premotor cortex (PMv), 26, 69–70, 72, 73, 115–16
hand representations, 73
verbal information
in post-stroke motor learning, 236–7
versican
induction, 15
Very Early Constraint-Induced Movement during Stroke Rehabilitation (VECTORS) Trial, 165, 174
VFC (ventral frontal cortex), 136
vigabatrin
and motor recovery, 184
virtual arms, 253–4
virtual lesions, 209
transcranial magnetic stimulation studies, 108
visual cortex
histone acetylation, 52
visual stimuli
coding, 133
Vividness of Movement Imagery Questionnaire, 239–40
voxels
suprathreshold, 114–15

WalkAide, 252
Wallerian degeneration, 12
Wernicke's area, 129–30
wheel-running exercise, 79
white matter
abundance, 53
changes, 271
damage, 87–8, 135
periventricular, 89–91
tracts
preservation, 168
white matter disease
and stroke recovery, 168
white matter–gray matter ratios
primate brains, 69

Xenarthra (Superorder), 67–8

yohimbine
and motor recovery, 183–4